COLOR ATLAS OF AIDS

COLOR ATLAS OF AIDS

second edition

Alvin E. Friedman-Kien, MD
Professor, Department of Dermatology
and Microbiology
New York University Medical Center
New York, New York

Clay J. Cockerell, MD
Associate Professor, Departments of Dermatology and Pathology
University of Texas Southwestern Medical Center at Dallas
Dallas, Texas

W.B. SAUNDERS COMPANY
A Division of Harcourt Brace & Company
Philadelphia London Toronto Montreal Sydney Tokyo

W.B. SAUNDERS COMPANY
A Division of Harcourt Brace & Company

The Curtis Center
Independence Square West
Philadelphia, Pennsylvania 19106

Library of Congress Cataloging-in-Publication Data

Color atlas of AIDS / [edited by] Alvin E. Friedman-Kien, Clay J. Cockerell—2nd ed.

p. cm.

Includes bibliographical references and index.
ISBN 0-7216-4949-1

1. AIDS (Disease)—Atlases. I. Friedman-Kien, Alvin E. II. Cockerell, Clay J.
[DNLM: 1. Acquired Immunodeficiency Syndrome—atlases. 2. Skin Manifestations—atlases.
WC 17 C719 1996]

RC607.A26C654 1996
616.97'92075—dc20

DNLM/DLC 95-20377

The author wishes to thank Janssen Pharmaceutica for its support for color illustration separations and color printing.

COLOR ATLAS OF AIDS, second edition ISBN 0-7216-4949-1

Printed in the United States of America

Last digit is the print number: 9 8 7 6 5 4 3 2 1

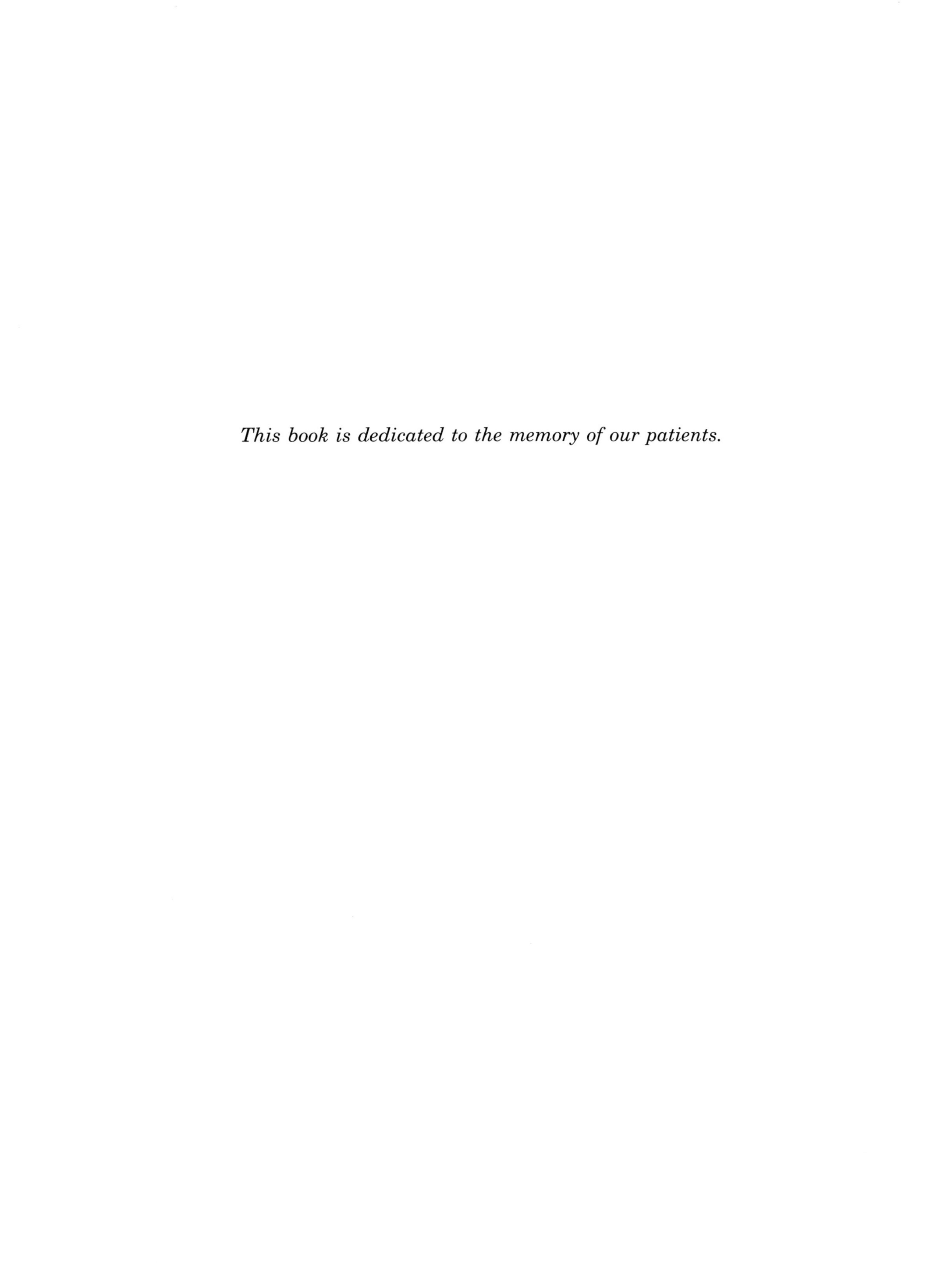

This book is dedicated to the memory of our patients.

CONTRIBUTORS

Aby Buchbinder, MD, CM
Assistant Professor, Cornell University Medical College, New York; Attending Physician, North Shore University Hospital, Manhasset, New York
Clinical Manifestations and Histopathologic Features of Classic, Endemic African, and Epidemic AIDS-Associated Kaposi's Sarcoma

Clay J. Cockerell, MD
Associate Professor, Departments of Dermatology and Pathology, University of Texas Southwestern Medical Center at Dallas, Dallas, Texas
Clinical Manifestations and Histopathologic Features of Classic, Endemic African, and Epidemic AIDS-Associated Kaposi's Sarcoma; Cutaneous Manifestations of HIV Infection

Robert Colebunders, MD, PhD
Professor of Tropical and Infectious Diseases, Institute of Tropical Medicine and the University of Antwerp; Head, HIV/STD Clinic and Hospitalization Unit, Institute of Tropical Medicine, Antwerp, Belgium
HIV Infection in Africa

Charles Farthing, MD
Clinical Assistant Professor of Medicine, University of California, Los Angeles, UCLA School of Medicine; Medical Director, AIDS Health Care Foundation, Los Angeles, California
AIDS—A Historical Overview

Dorothy Nahm Friedberg, MD, PhD
Clinical Associate Professor of Ophthalmology, New York University School of Medicine; Attending Physician, New York Eye and Ear Infirmary, New York, New York
Ocular Complications of HIV Infection

Alvin E. Friedman-Kien, MD
Professor, Department of Dermatology and Microbiology, New York University Medical Center, New York, New York
Clinical Manifestations and Histopathologic Features of Classic, Endemic African, and Epidemic AIDS-Associated Kaposi's Sarcoma; Cutaneous Manifestations of HIV Infection

Deborah Greenspan, BDS, DSc, ScD(hc)
Clinical Professor, Department of Stomatology, University of California, San Francisco, School of Medicine, San Francisco, California
Oral Manifestations of HIV Infection

John S. Greenspan, BDS, PhD, FRCPath, ScD(hc)
Professor, Oral Pathology; Chair, Department of Stomatology; Director, Oral AIDS Center; Director, AIDS Clinical Research Center, University of California, San Francisco, School of Medicine, San Francisco, California
Oral Manifestations of HIV Infection

Yao-Qi Huang, MD
Assistant Professor of Microbiology and Dermatology, New York University Medical Center, New York, New York
Clinical Manifestations and Histopathologic Features of Classic, Endemic African, and Epidemic AIDS-Associated Kaposi's Sarcoma

Elly T. Katabira, MRCP
Lecturer in Medicine, Makerere University Medical School; Lecturer, Department of Medicine, Mulago Hospital, Kampala, Uganda
HIV Infection in Africa

Kenneth H. Mayer, MD
Professor of Medicine and Community Health and Director, Brown University AIDS Program, Brown University School of Medicine, Providence; Chief, Infectious Disease Division, Memorial Hospital of Rhode Island, Pawtucket, Rhode Island
Opportunistic Infections in Patients with HIV Infection

Ross E. McKinney, Jr., MD
Associate Professor of Pediatrics, Assistant Professor of Microbiology, and Acting Chief of Pediatric Infectious Diseases, Duke University School of Medicine, Durham, North Carolina
Mucocutaneous Manifestations of Pediatric HIV Infection

Steven M. Opal, MD
Associate Professor of Medicine and Director, Infectious Disease Fellowship Program, Brown University School of Medicine, Providence; Head, Infection Control, and Staff Physician, Infectious Disease Division, Memorial Hospital of Rhode Island, Pawtucket, Rhode Island
Opportunistic Infections in Patients with HIV Infection

Neil S. Prose, MD
Associate Professor of Medicine (Dermatology) and Pediatrics, Duke University School of Medicine, Durham, North Carolina
Mucocutaneous Manifestations of Pediatric HIV Infection

PREFACE

Since the pandemic now known as the acquired immunodeficiency syndrome (AIDS) was first recognized in the United States in 1981, our knowledge of the spectrum of the disease caused by the human immunodeficiency virus (HIV) and of the varied clinical manifestations has expanded considerably.

The second edition of the *Color Atlas of AIDS* is designed to serve as a convenient visual aid and reference for health care providers, including physicians, nurses, physician assistants, medical students, and paramedical personnel. We have included superb clinical photographs of the many mucocutaneous manifestations of the various HIV-related diseases and photomicrographs of the typical histopathology of the different skin and mucosal conditions frequently seen in the HIV-infected host.

This second edition incorporates a vast amount of new information about HIV-related disease that has been elucidated since the first edition of the *Color Atlas of AIDS* was published. Each chapter includes a list of carefully selected references to enable the reader to acquire additional in-depth information about specific aspects of HIV-related diseases and AIDS.

Also included in this edition of the *Atlas* are new chapters written by leading physicians on the ophthalmologic, oral, and pediatric aspects of diseases associated with HIV infection and AIDS. Furthermore, the clinical manifestations of HIV infection and AIDS noted in Africa are presented in a new chapter. This section is illustrated with photographs that emphasize many of the opportunistic infections seen in these patients, especially infections that are different from those seen in Europe and the United States.

Our aim was to create a work that will help those who care for patients with HIV infection to become better acquainted with the broad manifestations of HIV-related diseases in order to enable the caregivers to lessen the suffering that patients face from the multiple opportunistic disorders that commonly afflict them—from the early acute HIV exanthem to the advanced symptomatic, life-threatening diseases that often complicate AIDS. We hope that the second edition of the *Color Atlas of AIDS* will serve this purpose and these goals.

Alvin E. Friedman-Kien, MD
Clay J. Cockerell, MD

INTRODUCTION

Color Atlas of AIDS is an important addition to any physician's library. The acquired immunodeficiency syndrome (AIDS), caused by the retrovirus known as human immunodeficiency virus (HIV), was recognized as a distinctive clinical entity more than a decade ago. Since that time, the acquisition of knowledge about the molecular foundations and clinical expression of this devastating disease has proceeded at an unprecedented pace. The development of effective (albeit not curative) antiretroviral therapies, coupled with the recognition and suppression of opportunistic infections, is translating into attenuation of disease progression and prolongation of survival for the HIV-infected individual. Ironically, it is this prolongation of survival in the profoundly immunocompromised state that, in turn, is leading to an increasing incidence and broadening spectrum of aggressive HIV-associated malignancies. Drug-resistant infectious pathogens such as multidrug-resistant tuberculosis, *Mycobacterium avium* complex, fungi such as *Aspergillus* species plus imidazole-resistant *Candida albicans* and *Cryptococcus neoformans,* and viruses (e.g., herpesviruses and papillomaviruses) capable of inducing systemic infection or malignant transformation are emerging in this clinical setting as well.

The skin and mucosal surfaces are common sites of clinical pathology in the HIV-infected individual. Not surprisingly, the etiologies of these pathologic lesions are diverse, and the clinical expressions are protean, which most likely reflects a combination of humoral and cellular immune imbalances of varying proportion. Superimposed in some cases are skin or mucosal infections with bacterial or fungal pathogens, or various viruses—for example, Epstein-Barr virus, cytomegalovirus, herpes zoster and herpes simplex, and human papillomavirus (HPV)—that can cause mucocutaneous exanthems, mucosal lesions, or both, even in the absence of HIV or profound immunosuppression.

Perhaps the prototypical cutaneous and mucosal manifestations of HIV infection are found in Kaposi's sarcoma (KS). This complex malignancy is characterized by a transformed spindle cell whose origins are still not clear and may reside in endothelial cells (vascular, lymphatic, or both) or pluripotent mesenchymal (Schwann) cells. In the setting of AIDS, this cell arises in multiple foci in diverse tissues. With the AIDS epidemic, KS has risen from an intriguing but unusual neoplasm to a prominent challenge, occurring in approximately 20% of all AIDS patients, and, until recently, serving as the index marker of AIDS in 30 to 40% (now the "AIDS-defining" illness in roughly 10%). In fact, Dr. Friedman-Kien and his colleagues defined the onset of the AIDS epidemic 15 years ago by recognizing the clinical intersection of two uncommon diseases whose occurrence implied profound immunodeficiency—namely, fulminant KS and *Pneumocystis carinii* infection—in a cluster of young gay men.

In the 7 years that have passed since the first edition of Dr. Friedman-Kien's *Color Atlas of AIDS,* a great deal has been learned about the pathogenesis of AIDS-KS, in particular the exuberant production of growth-promoting, inflammatory, and angiogenic cytokines by both AIDS-KS cells and multiple surrounding interactive cell types such as HIV-infected T cells and monocytes, fibroblasts, and vascular endothelium. Most prominent among the host factors are basic-fibroblast growth factor (b-FGF), interleukin (IL)-1 beta, and IL-6. In addition, two factors are perhaps unique to AIDS-KS, namely, a specific *k*-FGF encoded by the constitutively expressed "KS" oncogene (identical to the *hst* oncogene on chromosome 11q12–13 found in stomach cancers) and the newly-detected oncostatin M, a structurally distinct glycoprotein produced by activated T cells that binds to the active subunit of the IL-6 receptor, enhances IL-6 production by vascular endothelium, and induces AIDS-KS cells to assume the spindle configuration. In addition to the panoply of host-derived growth factors, AIDS-KS and normal mesenchymal cells proliferate in response to the HIV Tat protein, which is encoded by the HIV transactivating gene *tat,* secreted extracellularly by HIV-infected T cells and monocytes, and then taken up by proximate AIDS-KS cells.

Thus, AIDS-KS is under autocrine and paracine stimulation by host and viral factors that induce tumor and vascular proliferation, vascular permeability, and HIV replication. Such stimulation seems pivotal to the transformation process on the molecular level. It also seems critical to the histopathologic evolution and the net clinical expression of AIDS-KS, both in its mucocutaneous manifestations and in its visceral organ involvement (pulmonary and gastrointestinal, most especially)—inflammation, vascular permeability, and neoangiogenesis. Indeed, AIDS-KS may provide an extreme clinical representation of intense and unmitigated cytokine pathophysiology. The continued unraveling of cell-cytokine interactions provides some innovative therapeutic leads that are just now coming to clinical testing, for instance, growth factor blockage and antiangiogenesis approaches.

Recent molecular studies combined with epidemiologic observations raise the possibility that something other than growth factors may drive the emergence and perpetuation of KS. To this end, the detection of DNA sequences from the highly conserved E6 gene of HPV-16 (an oncogenic strain of HPV) in KS cells from up to 30% of both HIV-positive and HIV-negative homosexual and nonhomosexual men and women raises the issue of HPV acting in the capacity of at least an "agent provocateur" in the pathogenesis of KS in a substantial number of patients. The E6 gene encodes a transforming oncoprotein that exerts its oncogenic activity by binding and degrading the p53 tumor suppressor protein. The potential role of HPV in the emergence or perpetuation of KS, although still speculative, is theoretically substantiated by the presence of the E6 gene. As this intriguing possibility is further dissected, it too may offer a novel target for both therapy and prevention of KS arising in HIV-infected and non–HIV-infected individuals. In a sense, this book helps us visualize the final common pathway of these diverse factors.

Although AIDS-KS may be the classic AIDS-related malignancy, the spectrum of HIV-related cancers and their clinical mucocutaneous presentations continues to evolve. For instance, the anogenital (anal and cervical) cancers associated with HPV are gaining importance as major opportunistic complications of HIV infection. This is especially true for cervical cancer, which has risen to prominence as HIV affects increasing numbers of women. Indeed, both HIV-infected men and women have strikingly high incidences of HPV-associated anal and cervical epithelial dysplasia (as high as 40–60% in some series) and intraepithelial neoplasia.

The manifestations of HIV infection continue to diversify over time, in concert with changes in the epidemiology, biology, and natural history of the disease. Some changes reflect the impact of antiretroviral and other anti-infective or antitumor therapies on the overall pace of disease progression. The salutary changes brought about by clinical awareness and implementation of therapeutic and preventive strategies, however, may in part be counterbalanced by the emergence of new opportunistic complications that demand clinical recognition, molecular dissection, and development of targeted therapies. This elegant second edition of the *Color Atlas of AIDS,* like its predecessor, chronicles these changes and provides a comprehensive view of the clinical expressions of HIV infection. Let us pray that a third edition be rendered unnecessary owing to medical progress.

Samuel Broder, MD
Former Director
National Cancer Institute
Bethesda, Maryland

CONTENTS

AIDS—A HISTORICAL OVERVIEW

Charles Farthing

1

THE FIRST REPORTS

Acquired immunodeficiency syndrome (AIDS) was first recognized and described as a clinical entity in mid-1981, when Friedman-Kien in New York described a cohort of gay men with the previously very rare Kaposi's sarcoma and Gottlieb in Los Angeles described another cohort of gay men with the also previously rare disease *Pneumocystis carinii* pneumonia; both of these diseases were known to be linked to immunosuppression.[1,2] Many additional reports followed rapidly of the same two illnesses and of other illnesses linked to immunosuppression that were occurring in gay men across the United States. These cases were well documented at the Centers for Disease Control and Prevention (CDC) in Atlanta and were collectively reported in the journal *Morbidity and Mortality Weekly Review* (MMWR) as cases of the so-called gay-related immunodeficiency syndrome. By the time of reporting, 40% of the patients had already died. To those watching the figures, it became apparent that a disastrous epidemic was unfolding that would lead to the deaths of many thousands of young people. Even more worrying were reports that many gay men without gay-related immunodeficiency syndrome had persistent lymphadenopathy, fatigue, and depressed $CD4^+$ lymphocyte counts on immune function testing—something index cases also had. Experts speculated that these individuals might have prodromal gay-related immunodeficiency syndrome.

NOT ONLY GAY MEN

By the end of 1981, several cases of *P. carinii* pneumonia had been reported in nonhomosexual intravenous drug users.[3] This resulted in a change of name, from gay-related immunodeficiency syndrome to acquired immunodeficiency syndrome. Further opportunistic infections were described, and in 1982 AIDS was defined by the CDC as the occurrence of not only *P. carinii* pneumonia and Kaposi's sarcoma but also cerebral toxoplasmosis, cryptococcal meningitis, esophageal candidiasis, cytomegalovirus retinitis, progressive mucocutaneous herpes simplex, and progressive multifocal leukoencephalopathy in an individual with no other known cause of immunosuppression.[3] The occurrence of AIDS in both gay men and intravenous drug users provided a vital epidemiologic clue as to the cause of the epidemic, for occurrence in these two groups mimics exactly the epidemiology of hepatitis B. The logical assumption was that a new virus, spreading in a manner that was almost identical to that of the hepatitis B virus (HBV), was the causative agent. Despite the logic of this hypothesis that was favored by the CDC, speculation as to the cause was rife and varied from the plausible—amyl or butyl nitrites being inhaled as a sexual stimulant, especially by gay men (although this practice had been in use for 20 years or more, and victims of coronary artery disease had used amyl nitrite for years without immunosuppression being noted—to the absurd—the frequent application of 1% hydrocortisone to the perianal skin of gay men being absorbed and resulting in severe immunosuppression.

In 1982, AIDS was reported in hemophiliacs who had been recipients of the blood clotting product factor VIII[4] and in recipients of blood transfusions.[5] The case for a virus that was transmitted in a manner similar to that of HBV was strengthened considerably. Virtual proof that an infectious agent was the cause came later the same year when it was reported that 40 of the first 248 gay men diagnosed with AIDS in the United States had had sex with one of the index patients or with someone who had.[6]

THE DISCOVERY OF HIV

In June 1983, Barre-Sinoussi and Montagnier reported from the Pasteur Institute in Paris the discovery of a new retrovirus isolated from a lymph node of a gay man with persistent lymphadenopathy.[7] They called this new virus the lymphadenopathy-associated virus (LAV). They postulated that LAV was the cause of AIDS. Doubt remained, however, as initial reports of testing for antibodies to LAV showed that only 20% of AIDS patients were definitely infected; at the same time, Gallo of the National Institutes of Health in Bethesda, Maryland, was favoring the known retrovirus human T-cell lymphotropic virus type I (HTLV-I) as the cause. Uncertainty remained until 1984, when Gallo reported the isolation of a new retrovirus he called human T-cell lymphotropic virus type III (HTLV-III).[8] The results of serum antibody testing for the virus were positive in almost 100% of AIDS patients. Subsequent work revealed that LAV and HTLV-III were the same virus and that the reason the initial antibody testing for LAV had shown a low incidence in AIDS patients earlier was the insufficient sensitivity of the LAV antibody test. In 1987, an international nomenclature committee decided that the new virus should be termed the *human immunodeficiency virus,* or HIV, rather than either LAV or HTLV-III.

HIV-2

In 1987, Clavel and colleagues isolated a second retrovirus from

AIDS patients in West Africa, which he termed *HIV-2*.[9] Related to but genetically quite distinct from HIV-1, HIV-2 is more closely related to simian immunodeficiency virus (formally called STLV-III). Simian immunodeficiency virus is a virus isolated from African monkeys that apparently is nonpathogenic to them but causes an AIDS-like illness when Asian monkeys are infected. HIV-2 causes AIDS in a manner that is identical to that of HIV-1 but allows a longer disease-free period. It seems that HIV-2 is derived from simian immunodeficiency virus.

THE CHARACTERIZATION OF HIV INFECTION

With the development of a reliable antibody test to detect the presence of HIV in an infected individual, a more accurate picture of the full clinical spectrum, time course, and geographic distribution of HIV infection could be determined.

The vast majority of gay men and intravenous drug users with persistent lymphadenopathy who were being followed, as well as many others, were found to be positive for HIV antibodies, confirming the worst fears of physicians and proving that the number of individuals infected with the virus that causes AIDS is many times greater than the number of those reported with AIDS itself. The HIV antibody test also revealed that HIV infection was widespread in Haiti and in central Africa, where almost as many women as men were found to be infected. This made it clear that HIV could be spread by heterosexual as well as homosexual intercourse, and many individual case reports confirmed this. The reason HIV was occurring mainly in gay men in the United States and in other Western countries was presumably because it was introduced first into the homosexual community, where it spread rapidly with relatively little opportunity to reach heterosexual men and women, because gay men seldom practice heterosexual intercourse.

With the use of the HIV antibody test, it also became clear that individuals were dying of illnesses that they had acquired secondary to immunosuppression caused by HIV, yet their deaths were not classified as being caused by AIDS. Their fatal illnesses were not the previously very rare opportunistic infections or tumors such as *P. carinii* pneumonia or Kaposi's sarcoma but more familiar illnesses such as tuberculosis (TB) and lymphoma. Other persons were noted to be dying from a progressively disabling neurologic syndrome involving dementia (AIDS dementia complex) and from a progressive wasting syndrome without apparent development of any secondary infections or tumors. Both the AIDS dementia complex and the wasting syndrome seemed to be a direct effect of HIV itself. Because of these observations, in 1987 the CDC revised the definition of AIDS yet again and added an additional fourteen illnesses (including extrapulmonary TB, lymphoma, dementia, and wasting syndrome) that would define an individual as having AIDS if he or she were also HIV positive. In addition, a clause was added to include the few individuals with HIV infection who developed opportunistic illnesses but who remained HIV antibody negative.[10]

In January 1993, the definition of AIDS was expanded once more to include all those who are HIV antibody positive and suffering from pulmonary TB, recurrent bacterial pneumonias, or invasive cervical carcinoma or who have a $CD4^+$ lymphocyte count below $200/mm^3$ (normal range: $500-1200/mm^3$).[11]

Aside from the list of major opportunistic illnesses that define AIDS, many lesser non–life-threatening clinical manifestations of HIV infection have been described.[12] A number of mucocutaneous manifestations were reported. Shingles, dermatophyte infections, folliculitis, and seborrheic dermatitis frequently occur 1 to 3 years before an AIDS diagnosis. In the mouth, oral thrush, ulcerative gingivitis, and the new phenomenon of hairy leukoplakia are important clinical clues to the presence of underlying immunosuppression and HIV infection. Patients suffering only these more minor manifestations are often referred to as suffering from the AIDS-related complex, or ARC.

In 1985, a syndrome of acute HIV infection was described as a 1- to 3-week self-limiting illness with a viral exanthem variably associated with sore throat, arthralgia, oral aphthous ulcers, diarrhea, meningoencephalitis, and a short period of marked immunosuppression with low $CD4^+$ lymphocyte levels that may lead to the development of oral or even esophageal candidiasis and *P. carinii* pneumonia.[13] The HIV antigen is generally positive during this acute HIV illness, but seroconversion to HIV antibody positive does not occur until 4 to 6 weeks after the patient presents. Occurrence of an opportunistic infection at this stage of the illness when the immunosuppression is transitory probably should not define a case as AIDS.

Individuals have now been followed clinically from the onset of the acute illness until the development of AIDS, which has provided a view of the general shape of HIV in disease. After the acute illness, CD4 cell levels may remain depressed or return to normal, but in either case most patients remain clinically well for several years. This has been referred to as a period of latent disease; however, if immune function tests are performed regularly, a fall in $CD4^+$ lymphocytes with time is usually seen, indicating continuous viral activity rather than latency, even though the patient may be totally asymptomatic. Studies with quantitative polymerase chain reaction confirm that a high rate of HIV replication is ongoing during the period of apparent clinical latency—even in those whose $CD4^+$ lymphocyte counts appear stable.[14] Other work shows that early in disease HIV is largely contained in the lymph nodes, where it remains active during the latency period, depleting the CD4 cell population and slowly destroying the lymph node architecture.[15] After a variable period of 1 to 10 years or more, manifestations of ARC develop, and then a few years later, the patient's disease status changes to AIDS with the development of one of the index illnesses. However, AIDS may occur without preceding ARC symptoms or signs.

At this time, the percentage of HIV-infected individuals who will ultimately progress to AIDS is still uncertain. Experience to date indicates that after 10 years of infection, 50% have developed AIDS, another 25% have developed ARC, and only approximately 5% have a CD4 lymphocyte count still within the normal range.[16] As cohorts of HIV-infected individuals are followed longer, the percentage that develops AIDS may rise even higher.

THE CHARACTERIZATION OF HIV

Considerable progress has been made in retrovirology and in understanding HIV since its discovery in 1983. The HIV is a lentivirus related to the animal retroviruses visna (which causes a slow, degenerative brain disease in sheep and goats) and equine infectious anemia virus. The HIV infects human $CD4^+$ lymphocytes (the CD4 protein-antigen on the surface of the lymphocyte acting as the receptor of the virus), macrophages, and neuroglial cells. It buds from cells, taking a small part of the cell's membrane as its own. Its membrane is studded with viral proteins of molecular weight 41,000 (gp41), attached to which are larger viral protein molecules (gp120) that interact with the CD4 receptor. The cone-shaped core of the virus is composed principally of a protein of 24,000 molecular weight (p24), a single strand of RNA, and the enzyme reverse transcriptase (RT), the last being essential in the replication of a retrovirus for conversion of its genetic code from RNA to DNA before integration of viral genetic material with that of the host cell. The HIV viral genome has been sequenced, and even which mutations result in resistance to different antiviral drugs (e.g., zidovudine, didanosine) has been documented. Recent work has confirmed that an infected individual usually becomes infected with just one strain of HIV, but soon after infection the virus mutates progressively into many different quasispecies. Once an individual has become infected, superinfection with a strain from another individual does not seem to occur. At some point in the course of infection, a syncytium-inducing mutant may arise. This means that a viral isolate from a patient induces lymphocytes in tissue culture to fuse into syncytia. Development of a syncytium-inducing mutant correlates with the development of a more aggressive disease and a more rapid decline in CD4 cell numbers.[17]

There has been debate in the scientific literature regarding why CD4 cells decline in HIV infection—direct viral killing by HIV being thought to be unlikely by some because the quantity of virus in the blood stream was thought to be too low. It now seems likely that direct viral killing is the likely mechanism—the previous estimates of viral burden in the blood being too low and the large viral load in the lymph glands (up to 25% of $CD4^+$ cells being infected) having not been taken into account previously. The very considerable rebound in CD4 count that can occur when powerful antiretroviral drugs are used (such as the protease inhibitor ABT538, which can produce a 300% rise in CD4 count within 1 week) also suggests that it is viral replication that is destroying CD4 cells and that control of viral replication is the key to controlling or curing AIDS. It is now estimated that 10 billion (10×10^{10}) virus copies are produced every day in the average infected individual.

INFECTION CONTROL

Early in the AIDS epidemic, the disease engendered great fear, as people worried that it might be highly contagious. Epidemiologists showed early on that its spread was limited to that of a sexually transmitted disease that was also spread by blood and blood product transfusion and by intravenous drug use (as is HBV). Subsequent epidemiologic study has shown HIV to be somewhat less contagious than HBV: 0.5% of needle stick injuries to health care workers from HIV antigen carriers resulted in seroconversion compared with 17% of such injuries from HBV "e" antigen carriers. No seroconversion in health care workers injured by solid needles (suture needles) has been reported, and of the 30 confirmed seroconversions in health care workers in the United States none has occurred in a surgeon.[18]

Considerable concern that infected health care workers may be a risk to patients arose in 1992 when it was reported that a dentist in Florida had infected five of his patients.[19] DNA sequence analysis subsequently confirmed that the patients were infected by the same strain of HIV as the dentist.[20] This case remains an isolated unexplained instance. The possibility of homicidal activity on the part of the dentist has been suggested, but no evidence has been found to support this conjecture. Extensive investigations of patients operated on by other HIV-infected dentists and surgeons have not unearthed a single additional case of health care worker–to–patient transmission.

Extensive studies have shown HIV to be easily destroyed by hot soapy water, bleach, and heat sterilization. Universal precautions are recommended for the care of AIDS patients, meaning that gloves should be worn when exposure to any bodily secretions is likely. Gloves are little protection against a needle stick injury, however, and the most important single protective measure is the careful and immediate disposal of hypodermic needles to protect against the definite though statistically small risk of seroconversion should injury occur. Masks are only necessary if the patient is coinfected with a highly contagious respiratory pathogen, such as TB, and gowns are required only when significant splash injury might occur, such as during surgical procedures. Any spills of bodily fluids should be sterilized quickly using sodium hypochlorite (bleach).[21]

SURROGATE MARKERS

Even before HIV was isolated, it was realized that the $CD4^+$ lymphocyte count was a useful prognostic marker for HIV infection. Two patients may both look well, but if one has a normal CD4 cell level and another a very low one, then almost certainly the two are at very different stages in their HIV infection and have very different prognoses. The individual with the very low count may be expected to develop AIDS much sooner. Although statistically this assumption holds up well, the CD4 count does not predict well for every patient.

In 1987, the HIV p24 antigen assay became available and has proved to be a useful additional surrogate marker. Although usually present with the initial acute illness, p24 antigen disappears from the blood with the development of HIV antibody but often reappears later in the disease as antibody concentration falls—either before or after the development of clinical disease. For any individual, the p24 antigen assay may not predict well, and many patients develop AIDS without the reappearance of p24 antigen. The p24 antigen assay improved our ability to assess anti-HIV therapy. When an antiviral drug such as zidovudine (often called AZT) is given to a patient, p24 antigen usually falls faster and more impressively than the CD4 cell count rises. Direct measurement of plasma viremia by quantitative polymerase chain reaction and branch chain DNA assay has further improved the physician's ability to determine rapidly if an antiviral drug is effective in vivo. It has become standard in HIV antiviral trials to monitor patients with frequent viremia measurements. These tests may also prove useful in monitoring anti-HIV therapy in the HIV clinic.[22]

DEVELOPMENT OF A VACCINE

Enormous efforts have been made, and continue to be made, to create a vaccine that is effective against HIV. From the outset this has been a daunting task, because until recently no natural state of immunity against HIV appeared to exist; the virus seemingly established chronic infection (with or without disease progression) in every infected individual. A report of an infant who was infected with HIV at birth and seems to have cleared the infection spontaneously is perhaps one exception.

Most HIV vaccine research has focused on the development of protein subunit vaccines that utilize either gp120 or gp160. These vaccines raise antibodies in vaccinated individuals but do not appear to be protective in animal models to strains other than the strain of HIV from which they were developed. These vaccines have also been used in therapeutic trials in HIV-infected individuals in an attempt to boost the host's immune response and to improve the prognosis. Pilot studies of this approach looked hopeful initially, with augmentation of T-cell proliferative responses to HIV antigens and modest rises in CD4 lymphocyte counts in treated individuals. Subsequent studies have not confirmed these initial results.

Perhaps the most exciting vaccine research has been that with a *nef* gene–deficient simian immunodeficiency virus in an attempt to produce a live attenuated virus vaccine. Such a vaccine has proved protective in macaque monkeys, who develop AIDS from wild-type simian immunodeficiency virus but not from the vaccine strain. Vaccinated monkeys remain infected but stay well and cannot be superinfected with a pathogenic strain.[23] Unfortunately, infant macaques born to vaccinated and apparently protected adult female macaques have subsequently developed AIDS. A live attenuated strain may also prove to be protective in humans, but testing such a vaccine poses huge ethical problems.

TREATMENT

Initially, the only treatments available for AIDS patients were those for the major opportunistic illnesses.

Trimethoprim-sulfamethoxazole (Bactrim) and pentamidine are still the main drugs for treatment of *P. carinii* pneumonia, but several alternative regimens have been developed, that is, atovaquone (Mepron), dapsone-pyrimethamine, primaquine-clindamycin, and trimetrexate. Major improvements in patient survival occurred when physicians realized what others treating the immunocompromised had known for years, namely, that treatment for opportunistic infections must be commenced early and empirically. Now in nearly all centers, treatment is begun as soon as *P. carinii* pneumonia is suspected, and efforts to prove the diagnosis follow subsequently. The addition of steroids to treatment regimens for moderate to severe *P. carinii* pneumonia has resulted in improved patient survival. A further major development in AIDS therapy has been secondary, and now more recently primary, prophylaxis against *P. carinii* pneumonia with the use of oral trimethoprim-sulfamethoxazole (the best prophylaxis if tolerated), aerosolized pentamidine, or dapsone. Primary prophylaxis is recommended for patients with CD4 counts below 200/mm^3, as in these patients, the risk of *P. carinii* pneumonia is high.[21]

New treatments for other opportunistic infections are being developed continuously. Foscarnet, as well as ganciclovir (DHPG), is now available as a treatment for cytomegalovirus retinitis, and recent data show that oral ganciclovir has a useful role to play in primary prophylaxis against cytomegalovirus disease. Fluconazole and itraconazole are now available to treat candidiasis and cryptococcal and other fungal infections, and new combination antituberculous regimens containing the azolides clarithromycin or azithromycin are showing good effect against disseminated atypical mycobacterial complex infection.[22] Rifabutin (Mycobutin) and clarithromycin (Biaxin) have proved to be useful as prophylactic agents against mycobacterial complex infection. Pyrimethamine in combination with sulfadiazine or clindamycin is an effective therapy against cerebral toxoplasmosis, and trimethoprimsulfamethoxazole has been found to be a useful primary prophylaxis against toxoplasmosis in AIDS patients. Paromomycin (Humatin) is now thought to be a useful agent for the treatment of cryptosporidial diarrhea, and albendazole is being assessed as a therapy against the recently described opportunistic gastrointestinal infection due to Microsporida protozoa. Experience with chemotherapy against Kaposi's sarcoma and lymphoma has resulted in improved regimens, and techniques of local destruction of Kaposi's sarcoma lesions such as cryotherapy and intralesional chemotherapy have been developed.[13] Lipid encapsulation of daunorubicin (DaunoXome) and doxorubicin (Adriamycin, Doxil) has produced two new powerfully effective and less toxic chemotherapeutic agents for the treatment of Kaposi's sarcoma. Unfortunately, no successful treatment has yet been developed for progressive multifocal leukoencephalopathy, although trials with cytosine arabinoside (cytarabine, ara-C) have shown some efficacy.

In 1984, it was reported that the thymidine analogue zidovudine (AZT or Retrovir), an RT inhibitor, was an effective antiviral in vitro against HIV infection and had resulted in improvement in well-being, improvement in CD4 cell counts, and resolution of fungal nail infections in patients with AIDS. Subsequently, a large-scale, placebo-controlled, double-blind study in AIDS patients showed improvement in survival in the AZT-treated group. Ever since the completion of this study, AZT has been in widespread clinical use. In 1989 research documented that AZT-resistant strains of HIV could be detected in AZT-treated patients, and codons coding for AZT resistance were identified in the HIV genome. This was something that by then many clinicians thought was occurring, because patients could be seen to improve clinically and p24 antigen levels fell with introduction of the drug; however, 6 to 12 months later the patient would begin to deteriorate again clinically and the p24 antigen would again become detectable in the blood.

Since 1990, first in clinical trials and then owing to U.S. Food and Drug Administration approval, other nucleoside analogue RT inhibitor antiretrovirals have become available for clinical use: didanosine or ddI (Videx), zalcitabine or ddC (Hivid), stavudine or d4T (Zerit), and lamivudine or 3TC. Clinical trials have indicated that ddI has a potency similar to that of AZT, but probably because of the resistance phenomenon switching to ddI after 16 weeks of AZT therapy is advantageous. Other studies have shown that ddC is a less powerful agent than AZT. Both ddI and ddC share the side effects of peripheral neuropathy and pancreatitis and do not share the principal side effect of AZT, which is anemia. Some data have shown that d4T is also an effective RT inhibitor, well tolerated but for a significant incidence of peripheral neuropathy. 3TC monotherapy has been found to be of limited value, because early (average 1 month) high-level drug resistance occurs.

In the 1980s and early 1990s a diverse group of drugs called the nonnucleoside RT inhibitors, nevirapine being the best known, caused excitement, as they proved to be powerful nontoxic antiretrovirals. Unfortunately, as a group they have not proved very useful clinically because HIV develops very early (3–6 weeks) high-level resistance to all these compounds.

In 1992 and 1993 clinical trials began with antiretrovirals of an entirely different class—the protease inhibitors. These drugs inhibit not RT but the viral protease enzyme that is responsible for cleaving the precursor protein of the virus's core proteins after the virus buds from the cell. Many such compounds are in development, and startling CD4 count rises of 100 cells and higher have been noted with indinavir (Crixivan) from Merck and ritonavir (Norvir) from Abbott. The early clinical trials with these compounds have changed thinking on the pathogenesis of HIV and have brought about a realization that the immune system can recover if HIV can be brought under control. Unfortunately, these trials have also proved that early viral resistance can occur with these compounds as well.

The hope for the future now appears to lie firmly with the use of combination therapy. Combinations are more powerful, and they delay or prevent the onset of drug resistance. Very encouraging results were reported in 1994 with the use of AZT and 3TC in combination: CD4 rises were recorded that are fourfold greater and sustained four times longer than those seen with AZT monotherapy. Similar results have been seen with a d4T-ddI regimen. Even more impressive results have been seen when RT inhibitors have been combined with protease inhibitors in either double or triple combinations. With an AZT-3TC-indinavir regimen, viral load has been suppressed to undetectable limits (<200 copies/ml) in 90% of patients, and this level has been sustained for 6 months. We can now think of putting patients with HIV infection in remission, which may last a long time if therapy is started early enough with full doses of a multiple drug regimen and is continued without interruption.

SOCIAL CHANGE

The AIDS epidemic is the first major epidemic that the world has faced in many decades, and it is having a profound effect on society. It is an epidemic of a sexually transmitted disease, and like that of syphilis that preceded it, it was initially treated by society with a degree of fear and loathing. People with AIDS were shunned, and prejudice flourished—especially against the minority groups most at risk. With the passage of time and with more accurate information about the risks and the risk groups, attitudes (at least in the cities most affected) have noticeably changed for the better. The need to talk frankly about how to make sex safer and to educate about sex and safer sex at a young age is now apparent to many, if not most, people.

The attitudes not only of persons in society at large but also of persons most at risk have also changed. Initially, many, if not the majority of, gay men and intravenous drug users practiced denial and continued risky practices as before. As more of their number fell ill, however, their attitude changed, and many began taking necessary precautions. Of late there are worrisome signs that many gay men are reverting to previously used unsafe practices. Early in the epidemic, gay spokespersons were advising gay men not to take the HIV antibody test because to be found to be HIV positive would lead to depression and to prejudice. Now with a change in the level of prejudice in society and with more options for treatment and prophylaxis, their advice has largely changed to an encouragement to be tested early so that early intervention can take place.

The AIDS epidemic has forced change in the medical world. Politically active infected individuals have forcibly stated that they wish to be involved in a major way with the way their disease is treated and investigated. They point out that placebo-controlled studies of potentially life-saving drugs are not acceptable and that before major studies are drawn up, there should be consultations with representatives of those who will be involved. This is exactly what is happening now in many clinical trials organizations throughout the United States, including the AIDS Clinical Trials Group, which coordinates large multicenter AIDS trials. All anti-HIV treatment trials will be RT inhibitor controlled and not placebo controlled in the foreseeable future. Representatives of several risk group organizations attend every major scientific AIDS research meeting. This represents a major change from the way clinical studies were organized 10 years ago.

SUMMARY

Acquired immunodeficiency syndrome has been a recognized clinical entity now for just 15 years. During that time in the United States alone, it is estimated that 1 to 2 million persons may have been infected with HIV. Estimates of numbers infected worldwide are as high as 10 million. Over these 15 years, considerable progress has been made: the disease and all its protean manifestations have been described accurately, the way it spreads and where it is spreading have been recorded accurately, and the cause has been discovered and is well understood (more detailed information is available about HIV than about any other virus). Drugs have been discovered that slow down the replication of HIV and are in widespread use. A cure or a vaccine, however, seems unlikely in the near future. The major hopes for the present appear to be continued education to prevent the spread of AIDS and to promote the development of better antiviral agents to keep HIV suppressed and, ideally, to allow infected individuals to live a close-to-normal life span (if treatment is commenced at an early enough stage in the course of the infection and continued indefinitely).

References

1. Friedman-Kien AE. Disseminated Kaposi's sarcoma syndrome in young homosexual men. J Am Acad Dermatol 1981;5:468–471.
2. Gottlieb MS, Schroff R, Schanker HM, et al. *Pneumocystis carinii* pneumonia and mucosal candidiasis in previously healthy homosexual men. Evidence of a new acquired cellular immunodeficiency. N Engl J Med 1981;305:1425.
3. Centers for Disease Control. Update on acquired immunodeficiency syndrome (AIDS), United States. MMWR 1982;31:507–514.
4. Centers for Disease Control. *Pneumocystis carinii* pneumonia among persons with hemophilia A. MMWR 1982; 31:365–367.
5. Centers for Disease Control. Possible transfusion-associated acquired immune deficiency (AIDS). MMWR 1982; 31:652–654.
6. Centers for Disease Control. A cluster of Kaposi's sarcoma and *Pneumocystis carinii* pneumonia among homosexual male residents of Los Angeles and Orange County, California. MMWR 1982; 31:305–307.
7. Barre-Sinoussi F, Chwemann JC, Rey F, et al. Isolation of a T-lymphocyte retrovirus from a patient at risk for acquired immune deficiency syndrome (AIDS). Science 1983;220:868–871.
8. Gallo RC, Salahuddin SZ, Popovic M, et al. Frequent detection and isolation of cytopathic retrovirus (HTLV-III) from patients with AIDS and at risk for AIDS. Science 1984;224:500–504.
9. Calvel F, Guetard F, Bravi-Vezinet F, et al. Isolation of a new human retrovirus from West African patients with AIDS. Science 1986;233:343.
10. Centers for Disease Control. Revision of the CDC surveillance case definition for the acquired immunodeficiency syndrome. MMWR 1987;36(1S):1–13.
11. Centers for Disease Control and Prevention. 1993 Revised classification system for HIV infection and expanded surveillance of definition for AIDS among adolescents and adults. MMWR 1992;41(RR-17).
12. Friedman-Kien AE, Farthing C. Human immunodeficiency virus infection: A survey with special emphasis on mucocutaneous modifications. Sem Dermatol 1990;9:167–177.
13. Cooper DA, Gold J, Maclean P. Acute AIDS retrovirus infection. Lancet 1985;1:537–540.
14. Piatak M, Saag MS, Yang LC, et al. High levels of HIV-1 plasma during all stages of infection determined by competitive PCR. Science 1993;259:1719–1754.
15. Pantaleo G, Graziosi C, Demarest JF, et al. HIV infection is active and progressive in lymphoid tissue during the clinically latent stage of disease. Nature (Lond.) 1993;362:355–358.
16. Moss AR, Bacchetti P. Natural history of HIV infection. AIDS 1989;3:55–61.
17. Koot M, Keet IPM, Voss AHV, et al. Prognostic value of HIV-1 syncytium-inducing phenotype for rate of $CD4^+$ cell depletion and progression to AIDS. Ann Intern Med 1993;118:681–688.
18. Rogers DE, Gellin BG. The bright spot about AIDS: It is very tough to catch. AIDS 1990;4:695–696.
19. Ciesielski C, Marians D, Ou C-Y, et al. Transmission of human immunodeficiency virus in a dental practice. Ann Intern Med 1992;116:798–805.
20. Ou C-Y, Ciesielski CA, Myers G, et al. Molecular epidemiology of HIV transmission in a dental practice. Science 1992;256:1165–1171.
21. National Commission on AIDS. America living with AIDS. Washington, DC: US Government Printing Office, 1991.
22. Lagakos SW. Surrogate markers in AIDS clinical trials: Conceptual basis, validation, and uncertainties. Clin Infect Dis 1993;(suppl 1):S22–S25.
23. Desrosiers RC, Wyand MS, Kodama T, et al. Vaccine protection against simian immunodeficiency virus infection. Proc Natl Acad Sci USA 1989;86: 6353–6357.

OPPORTUNISTIC INFECTIONS IN PATIENTS WITH HIV INFECTION

Kenneth H. Mayer
Steven M. Opal

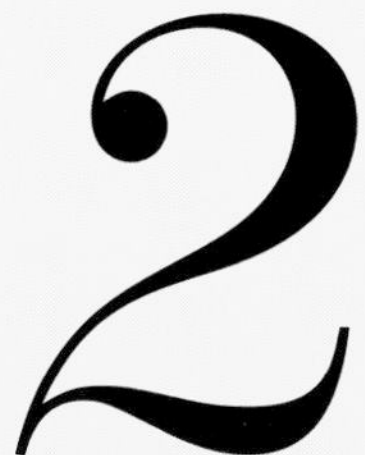

Infection with the human immunodeficiency virus (HIV) may result in clinically inapparent immunologic abnormalities or may culminate in life-threatening illnesses due to a multiplicity of viral, bacterial, fungal, or protozoal pathogens, as well as opportunistic malignancies.[1,2] A unifying feature of these disparate processes, which may affect many organ systems and thus may result in varied clinical presentations, is the underlying immunologic derangement that occurs after retroviral infection.[3] The primary insult has been thought to be due to a diminution of both the absolute number and the functioning of T-helper or T-inducer, lymphocytes; however, HIV affects other circulating cells of the immune system including monocyte-macrophages and tissue-associated antigen processing cells, such as microglia and enteric M cells.[4]

The relation between the immune dysfunction and the development of opportunistic infections in acquired immunodeficiency syndrome (AIDS) is further complicated by the fact that some of the infections result from the exposure of immunoincompetent individuals to ubiquitous agents, such as *Pneumocystis carinii* or *Candida albicans,* whereas other illnesses usually represent the reactivation of latent infections, such as those from *Toxoplasma gondii* or herpes simplex. The prevalence of different AIDS-associated illnesses may vary among risk groups. Persons from Africa and the Caribbean tend to have more toxoplasmosis and *Mycobacterium tuberculosis* infections and relatively less *P. carinii* infection than persons from the United States and western Europe.[5] Putative cofactors, such as recreational drug use, exposure to other immunosuppressive viruses (e.g., cytomegalovirus [CMV] and Epstein-Barr virus), age at the time of HIV infection, and genetically determined immune response loci, have been thought to modify the expression of disease among individuals, and their roles are being evaluated in ongoing studies.

ETIOLOGY

The ultimate origin of the HIV epidemic is still uncertain, but to date the earliest clinical isolates were found in central Africa. A genetically similar retrovirus has been isolated from wild African green monkeys.[6] Another retrovirus, found in western Africa, has been identified that is remarkably similar to this simian immunodeficiency virus (SIV) and has been called HIV-2.[7] The evolutionary relationships between SIV and HIV-1 and HIV-2 are undergoing further clarification. It is possible that mutations in simian retroviruses in close contact between primates and humans in Africa may explain the fairly recent appearance of HIV in human populations. Although SIV does not result in clinical disease in infected African green monkeys, macaques develop lethal immunodeficiency after receiving SIV via an intravenous injection.[8]

Human immunodeficiency virus has biologic and structural similarities to other human T-lymphotropic viruses (HTLV-I and HTLV-II) but is more closely related to visna (a slow virus that causes neurologic destruction in sheep) and other lentiviruses.[9] It encodes several unique regulatory gene products, which makes it structurally more complex than most of the other known animal retroviruses.[10] All of the primate retroviruses possess at least three common genes—*env, pol,* and *gag*—coding for envelope proteins, the reverse transcriptase enzyme, and core proteins, respectively. Figure 2–1 depicts HIV budding off the cell membrane of an infected lymphocyte.

The HIV genome is 9000 base pairs in size, with a divergence of up to 10% in its genetic material between isolates found in San Francisco and in central Africa.[11–14] The *env* gene contains the most divergent regions; some areas are hypervariable and appear to be unique for each isolate, whereas other regions are constant between multiple strains.[15] The *gag* gene codes for several structural proteins, of which the p24 protein appears to be the most highly antigenic and may be one of the first antibodies to be detected after infection with HIV.[16] The regulatory genes are distinctive and include *tat,*[17] *vif, nef,* and *rev* genes that modulate replication efficiency and virulence.[18] These gene products trigger the activation of other HIV genes, resulting in rapid transcription and translation, which may lead to an acceleration of viral replication up to 1000 times the basal rate. The *tat* and other regulatory gene products appear to exert their greatest effect at the posttranscriptional level.[19–21] Complex interactions among proteins encoded by these regulatory genes also affect HIV latency, reactivation, and cytotropism.

PATHOGENESIS

Although the transmission of HIV infection has been associated with intimate sexual contact as well as parenteral exposure to infected blood and blood products, the initial events in the pathogenesis of HIV infection are not certain. Human immunodeficiency virus has been shown to be able to infect T-helper lymphocytes,[22] monocytes-macrophages,[23] and neuroglial cells of macrophage lineage,[24] as well as many other cell lines in tissue culture. It is able to enter target T-helper lymphocytes via binding of the envelope glycoprotein (gp120) to the CD4 antigenic determinant of the lymphocyte[25] (Fig. 2–2). Following attachment and entry into the lymphocyte, the viral RNA is transcribed, as a result of the action of reverse transcriptase, into single-stranded DNA. Some of this DNA remains free in the cytoplasm and may partially account for a cytopathic effect on target cells.[26] However, most of the DNA is integrated into the host chromosome as proviral DNA, which may remain latent as part of the host genome indefinitely. This observation indicates that after the initial infection with HIV, the host remains infected indefinitely.

Although the virus may remain dormant for months to years, proviral DNA may become activated in response to antigenic signals. Under in vitro conditions, effective antigenic stimuli have included mitogens, exposure to other viruses, and certain immunosuppressive agents.[27,28] Activated proviral DNA can produce gene products at extraordinarily rapid rates under the influence of several regulatory genes, with the production of multiple copies of free virus and the associated destruction of the host cell[17,18] (see Fig. 2–1). The precise mechanisms of cellular destruction are not certain at present. Giant cell formation, including the recruitment of uninfected lymphocytes, has been demonstrated in vitro.[29] Lymphocytes that are infected with HIV appear to undergo accelerated maturation and are functionally impaired, responding inadequately to new stimuli. Likewise, the function of monocytes-macrophages that are directly infected by HIV is severely impaired.[23]

Mononuclear cells that are infected with HIV do not respond appropriately to new antigenic stimuli, resulting in impaired production of lymphokines and monokines.[30] It is not known whether soluble mediators are produced that have a deleterious effect on the immune system. The immune dysregulation due to the T lymphocyte and monocyte infection results in alterations of humoral immunity as well. Many individuals with HIV infection have polyclonal hypergammaglobulinemia but are unable to respond appropriately to new antigenic stimuli by producing new antibodies.[31] Infants and children with congenitally acquired HIV infection are often hypogammaglobulinemic because their B cells have not become sensitized to ubiquitous antigens in the environment. This hypogammaglobulinemia is associated with recurrent infections with pyogenic bacteria in patients with pediatric AIDS as well as in severely compromised adults who have survived for long periods of time.[32]

The loss of cell-mediated immunity results in patients becoming susceptible to a wide range of opportunistic infections and malignancies. It is not known whether the extreme cachexia seen in individuals with progressive HIV infection is due to multiple infections that recur in impaired hosts or to the elaboration of humoral factors such as tumor necrosis factor (cachectin), which independently augment their constitutional symptoms. The extreme debilitation of individuals after recurrent opportunistic infections plus the inability to eradicate many of these pathogens (e.g., CMV, *Mycobacterium avium-intracellulare, Cryptosporidium*) results in the high lethality of HIV infection.

Human immunodeficiency virus itself may have direct effects on specific organs in addition to its effects on the immune system. The direct effects of HIV on the

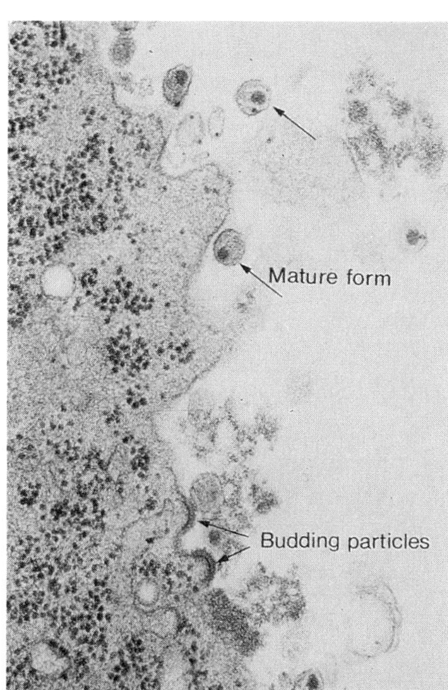

FIGURE 2–1. Human immunodeficiency virus (HIV)

Electron micrograph of HIV budding off a T lymphocyte.

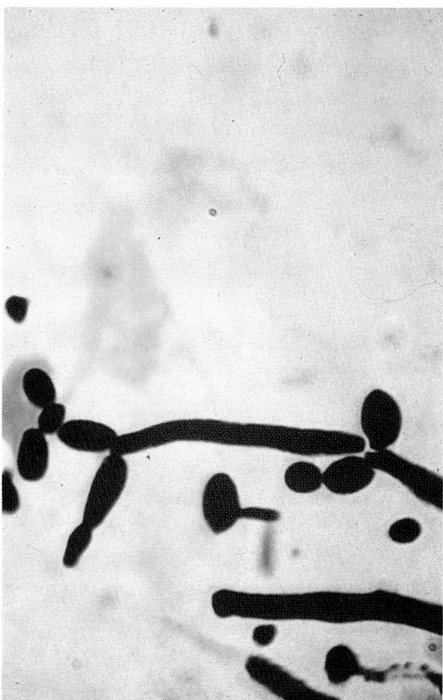

FIGURE 2–2. *Candida albicans*

Potassium hydroxide stain of tongue scraping reveals budding yeast forms of *C. albicans* causing thrush. (Courtesy of Jonathan W. M. Gold, MD, Associate Director, Special Microbiology Laboratory, Memorial Sloan-Kettering Cancer Center, New York.)

central nervous system appear to be second only to its effects on the immune system as a cause of morbidity and mortality. The virus can multiply in central nervous system cells of macrophage lineage.[24] A number of cell lines derived from the central nervous system have been productively infected in vitro with HIV. At least a third of patients with advanced HIV infection may show progressive neurologic deterioration, and neurodevelopmental delays may be common among infants and children who are infected with HIV.[33]

THE DIAGNOSIS OF AIDS AND HIV INFECTION

Since the initial case definition of AIDS was developed before the elucidation of HIV as the etiologic agent, the diagnosis of AIDS then required that an individual with no other reason for cellular immunodeficiency have one of a specific list of opportunistic infections or malignancies. Subsequently, the Centers for Disease Control and Prevention (CDC) developed a classification schema that incorporated new insights that had been made in recent years about the natural history of HIV infection as the epidemic has increasingly affected more diverse populations.[34] The revision of the CDC case definition of AIDS to include invasive cervical neoplasia reflects the increasing number of women infected with HIV, and the inclusion of pulmonary tuberculosis (TB) reflects the burgeoning interactive epidemics abetted by inner city poverty. The specific diagnosis of HIV infection requires the use of corroborative serologic screening tests (see subsequent discussion), but the diagnosis of AIDS may be made by diagnosing a clinical illness associated with severe cell-mediated immunodeficiency or by determining that an HIV-infected person has a CD4 count below 200 cells/mm^3.[35]

The most commonly employed screening test is the enzyme-linked immunosorbent assay (ELISA) in which disrupted virus proteins are applied to the surfaces of wells and microtiter plates or on beads. Many companies have utilized these technologies to develop HIV screening tests that can be done rapidly with a high degree of reproducibility. Serum is added to these plates, and if antibodies to HIV are present, they are sandwiched between the surfaces of the plate and an anti-antibody, which is conjugated to a chemical that can produce a color change when an additional specific reagent is added. Thus, a positive response is usually detected through a colorimetric reaction in a spectrophotometer, with cutoffs being set on the basis of panels of known standards. The choice of the cutoff point has been set toward the more sensitive side so that the predictive value of the test is least accurate in low-prevalence populations; this approach is clearly desirable for ensuring the safety of the blood supply but necessitates secondary corroborative tests in seropositive individuals, particularly in those from low-risk groups.[36]

Other tests for antibody detection include the Western blot assay,[37] the radioimmunoprecipitation assay, and the cytoplasmic or membrane immunofluorescence test.[38] Second-generation tests are being developed that include assays of antibodies to purified recombinant antigens,[39] as well as tests to detect directly the presence of free serum antigen.[40,41] Polymerase chain reaction (PCR) detection of HIV proviral DNA and free virus RNA have also been developed that can assist in the determination of viral load.[42] The clinical utility of these and other newer tests are being evaluated through follow-up with larger cohorts over longer periods of time to better assess the natural history of HIV infection.

False-positive ELISA results are more commonly found in multiparous women, drug users who are exposed to multiple human antigens, and individuals who have collagen vascular diseases.[43,44] Therefore, the Western blot or another more specific test is necessary to corroborate the presence of HIV infection, particularly in low-risk individuals. Even the Western blot test may occasionally yield a false-positive result,[45] especially in intravenous drug users.

In high-risk populations, the correlation of positive ELISA test results with positive Western blot studies has been excellent; frequently, more than 93% of individuals who have positive ELISA findings have corroborative Western blot studies.[36] Although in theory, the gold standard for the diagnosis of HIV infection should be the ability to grow HIV from the patient's blood, growth of the virus in tissue culture has not been consistent, even in patients with clear-cut HIV infection.[46] A number of factors probably contribute to this, of which an important one is the very low titers of virus (usually no more than 1 in 1000 peripheral blood lymphocytes are infected) in the blood of infected patients. Other problems in confirming the antibody test results with viral culture include technical difficulties of the culture techniques and the possibility that humoral factors such as neutralizing antibodies may limit the ability to grow the virus from infected hosts at different stages of illness. Newer diagnostic techniques such as the use of the

PCR technique to detect proviral DNA (integrated virus) and infectious HIV RNA have advanced the understanding of the level of HIV replication throughout the course of HIV infection.[47] Rare individuals have had blood cultures that were positive for HIV without initially generating detectable antibodies[48,49]; the vast majority of these individuals, presumably recently infected at the time their blood was tested, have subsequently seroconverted.

In addition to their use in the detection of infected patients who may benefit from antiretroviral therapy and treatments to forestall common opportunistic complications of HIV disease, such as *P. carinii* pneumonia, screening tests for HIV are now used in the United States to screen the nation's blood supply, to assist clinicians in interpreting new patterns of infection among members of high- and low-risk groups, and as an adjunct in counseling for specific patients to maximize risk reduction education. Over the past year, HIV diagnostic tests have been utilized more than 20 million times.

CLINICAL MANIFESTATIONS OF AIDS

ACUTE RETROVIRAL SYNDROME

After an initial intimate exposure in which HIV is transmitted, the newly infected person may remain asymptomatic for long periods of time or may develop an acute mononucleosis-like febrile illness within 3 to 6 weeks.[50] The symptoms include fever, malaise, and generalized lymphadenopathy, which frequently lasts for about a week and then subsides completely. Other manifestations may include arthralgias, aseptic meningitis, and maculopapular or urticarial rashes.[51] However, in one prospective study of a high-risk group in Amsterdam, the majority of newly infected individuals did not record any focal symptoms other than fever around the time of seroconversion.[40,41] Thus, it is not known what proportion of patients develop an "acute retroviral syndrome," but such a reaction may portend a higher viral burden after seroconversion and has been associated with more rapid progression of HIV. From the small number of individuals who have been studied intensively, antibodies to HIV are generally detectable within 4 to 12 weeks after a transmitting exposure.[52] The time between infection by HIV and seroconversion appears to be similar whether the exposure is via contaminated blood or sexual contact. Newer studies indicate that HIV is active at all stages of the chronic disease[49] and ultimately results in AIDS-associated infections or neoplasia in the majority of those infected. Although HIV may not be cultured readily from the blood during the often long clinically asymptomatic period, the virus can be detected readily in lymphoid tissues, including the bone marrow, spleen, and peripheral nodes. In these sequestered sites, ongoing HIV replication results in a silent increase in the viral burden and progressive subclinical immunosuppression.[53]

ASYMPTOMATIC INFECTION

Worldwide, the majority of individuals currently infected with HIV are asymptomatic. The rates of development of AIDS and other clinical sequelae are uncertain at the present time because not enough large cohorts have been followed for sufficiently long periods of time. Cofactors such as strain variations in HIV virulence, coinfection with other immunosuppressive viruses (e.g., CMV), malnutrition, immunogenetic differences, or a combination of these may play a role in the ultimate expression of illness after exposure to the retrovirus. After more than 13 years follow-up of a group of initially asymptomatic homosexually active males in a San Francisco hepatitis B cohort study, more than half had developed CDC-defined AIDS, and less than 10% were asymptomatic with normal laboratory test results.[54] The rest of the men could be described using an intermediate group of heterogeneous categories, including being asymptomatic with laboratory evidence of immunocompromise (i.e., CD4 lymphocyte counts lower than 500 cells/mm^3) or having clinical symptoms that were not AIDS-defining, including mild constitutinal manifestations, thrush, or other chronic mucocutaneous conditions; or both. These data suggest a tendency to progress from clinical conditions of less severity to those of more severity without any evidence of improvement in immunologic function or clinical symptoms over time.

PROGRESSIVE GENERALIZED LYMPHADENOPATHY

Individuals at increased risk for HIV infection may have lymphadenopathy for many reasons other than the presence of HIV infection, including chronic infections with Epstein-Barr virus, CMV, toxoplasmosis, or secondary syphilis. However, early in the AIDS epidemic, it was recognized that a large number of high-risk individuals had developed generalized lymphadenopathy.[55] In a male homosexual San Francisco cohort followed for about 3 years in the early years of the epidemic, 9% of the men with generalized lymphadenopathy developed AIDS.[56] Subsequent studies have found higher rates of progression of illness in individuals with generalized lymphadenopathy[57]; however, rates of development of clinical illness over time have been difficult to assess because the time of development of lymphadenopathy or of HIV seroconversion is frequently not known. A subgroup of individuals with generalized lymphadenopathy seem to do well for long periods of time, as long as they are without systemic manifestations. The onset of constitutional symptoms, minor opportunistic infections such as thrush or zoster, persistent hematologic abnormalities including leukopenia, lymphopenia, hypergammaglobulinemia, and an increase in the erythrocyte sedimentation rate, or a combination of these developments may be a harbinger of the subsequent development of more serious opportunistic processes.

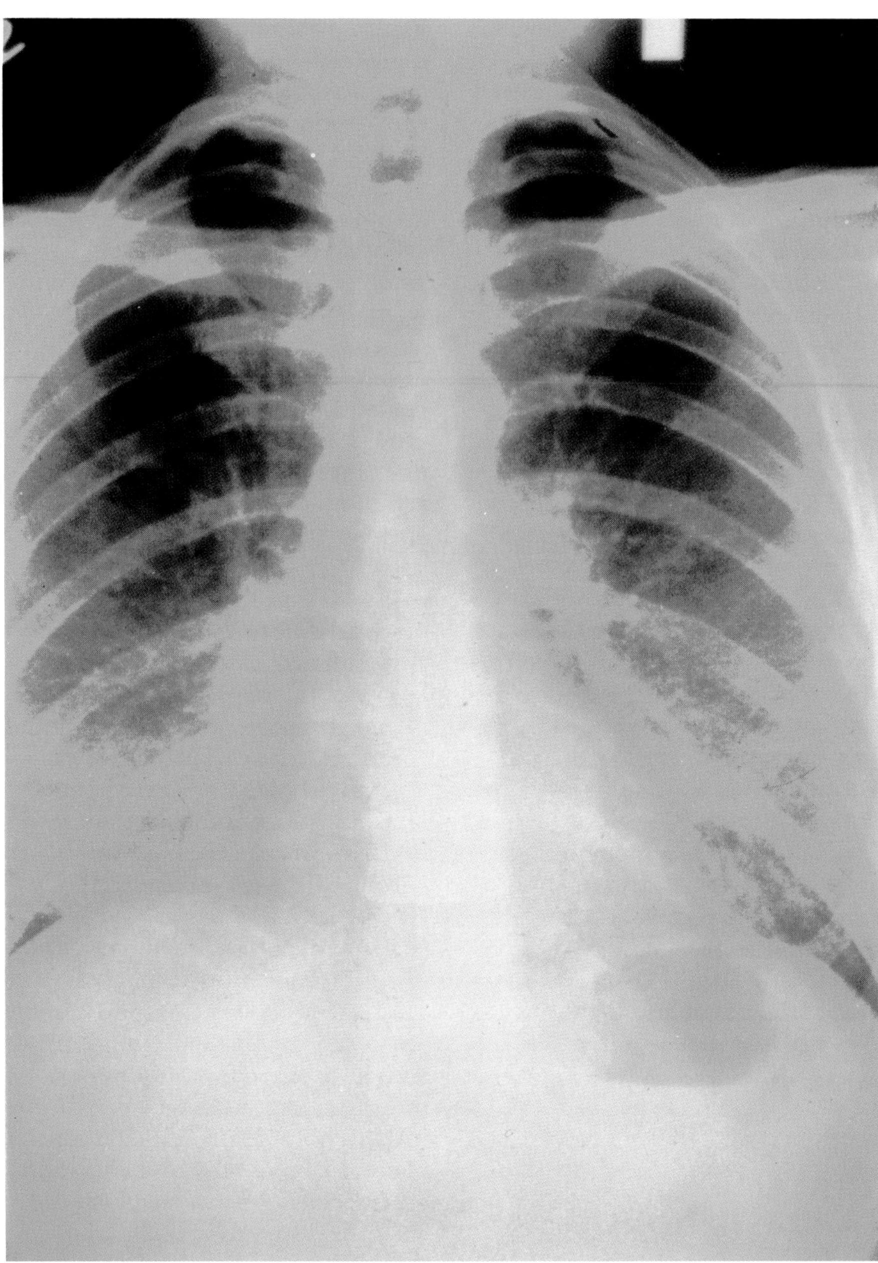

FIGURE 2–3. *Pneumocystis carinii*
Chest radiograph showing bilateral lower lobar interstitial infiltrates.

SYMPTOMATIC HIV INFECTION

Various investigators have described signs and symptoms that did not fit in the CDC's classification for AIDS initially but suggested that individuals had infections associated with HIV and might be at increased risk of developing full-blown AIDS.[56,57] This led to the description of an AIDS-related complex (ARC) that eluded a precise and uniformly accepted case definition; hence, most reports about symptomatic HIV disease describe the clinical manifestations and associated immune status (e.g., CD4 count). In addition to generalized lymphadenopathy, symptoms that suggested the presence of progressive HIV infection included persistent fevers, diarrhea, anorexia, weight loss, and malaise that were not due to other underlying illnesses. The high prevalence of other infections that can produce these symptoms independently (e.g., CMV, Epstein-Barr virus, and other viral infections) has decreased the utility of particular symptom complexes for the diagnosis and staging of progressive HIV infection. The presence of oropharyngeal candidiasis has been suggested to be a particularly serious negative prognostic feature of individuals in this group[58] (see Fig. 2–2). Individuals who develop thrush, have constitutional symptoms, or have CD4 cell counts of 200 cells/mm^3 or lower may develop opportunistic infections at rates exceeding 10% per year.[57–59] Severe depression of the T-lymphocyte subpopulation has been associated with the rapid onset of more severe manifestations of immunodeficiency.[60]

PROTOZOAN INFECTIONS

Pneumocystis carinii

P. carinii is common in the environment so that the majority of immunocompetent children in the United States have detectable antibodies to this organism.[61] In addition to wide geographic dispersion, *P. carinii* has been found in multiple mammalian genera. Human cases of *P. carinii* pneumonitis have been noted in most countries. The initial epidemics were described among malnourished and premature infants in refugee camps after World War II. Before the AIDS epidemic, the most frequent descriptions of *P. carinii* pneumonitis were of patients, particularly children, with hematologic malignancies.

The clinical disease usually affects only the lungs (Figs. 2–3 and 2–4), although parasitemia and liver, spleen, and lymph gland involvement have been noted. One report suggested that ocular involvement was present in a patient with AIDS.[62] The organism may be found in either a cystic or a trophozoite form. Cysts are spheric or cup-shaped, and the wall stains brownish-black with Gomori's methenamine silver nitrate stain (see Fig. 2–4) and purple-violet with toluidine blue staining.[63] Neither method will stain the trophozoite. Up to eight sporozoites may be found within a cyst, which may be demonstrated by Giemsa (Fig. 2–5), Wright's, Gram-Weigert, polychrome methylene blue, or hematoxylin and eosin stains (Fig. 2–6), which also stain trophozoites but not the cyst wall.

Infection occurs after cyst forms are aerosolized and then multiply in pulmonary alveolar macrophages, which may be associated with septal inflammation. If the organism proliferates extensively, a diffuse desquamative alveolitis may ensue. The alveolar lumen may fill with large numbers of organisms and macrophages, and the alveolar walls may thicken

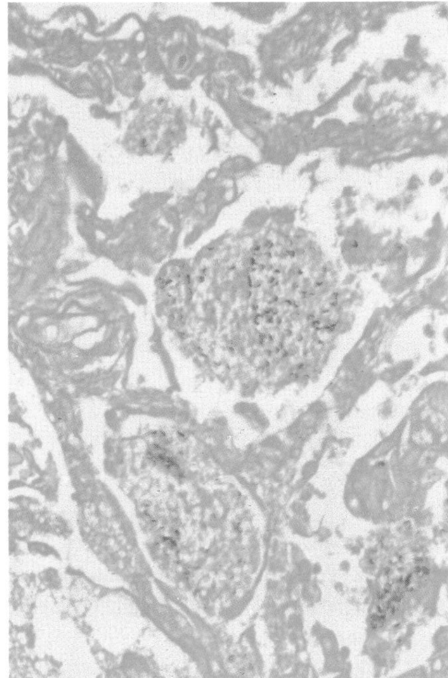

FIGURE 2–4. *Pneumocystis carinii* cysts These cysts are in alveolar spaces, stained black by Gomori's methenamine silver stain. (From Still Picture Archives, Centers for Disease Control and Prevention, Atlanta, Georgia.)

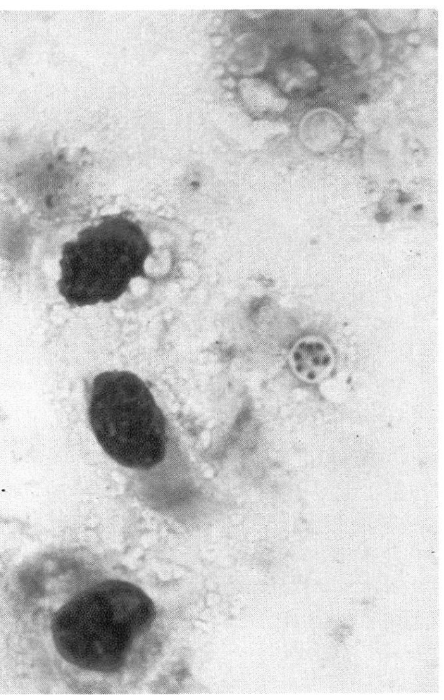

FIGURE 2–5. *Pneumocystis carinii* *P. carinii,* lung impression smear; Giemsa stain (×1125). (From Still Picture Archives, Centers for Disease Control and Prevention, Atlanta, Georgia.)

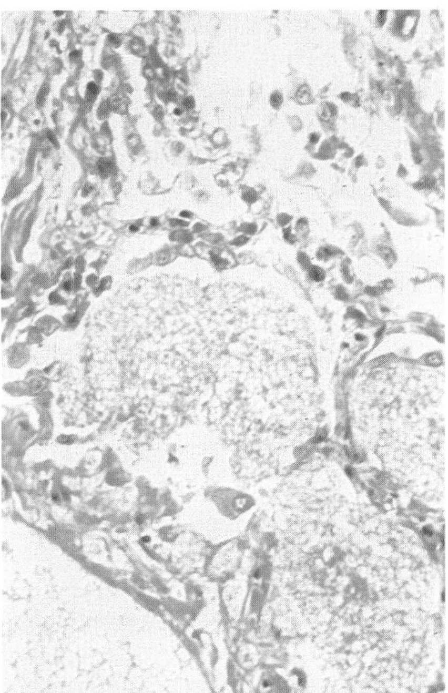

FIGURE 2–6. Pneumocystis carinii *P. carinii* in alveolar spaces in human lung; hematoxylin and eosin stain. (From Still Picture Archives, Centers for Disease Control and Prevention, Atlanta, Georgia.)

because of interstitial plasma cell infiltration, which results in a diffuse interstitial pneumonitis that tends to be more prominent in the lower lobes (see Fig. 2–3). The chest radiograph, however, cannot be diagnostic by itself, as other types of interstitial pneumonitis may be seen with AIDS.[64,65]

The clinical findings may appear subacutely or abruptly, most often including tachypnea and fever. A dry, nonproductive cough may be present, but more nonspecific symptoms such as anxiety, dyspnea on exertion, and malaise are more common. Evidence of pneumonitis on chest radiograph is generally only apparent after symptoms have been present for more than a week. Pallor and cyanosis may be associated with more advanced illness. Rales are often absent, and the arterial oxygen tension may be in the normal range.

The diagnosis can be made with bronchoalveolar lavage without a transbronchial biopsy.[66–68] The use of induced sputum examination has been advocated and may be a useful first step in establishing a diagnosis.[69] The majority of the patients respond to their first course of therapy with trimethoprim-sulfamethoxazole, dapsone, or pentamidine. However, more than a third of patients manifest allergic reactions to these drugs (e.g., rash, granulocytopenia, hypoglycemia) and thus require a change in therapy.[70] Since relapses are frequent, it is suggested that individuals be treated for at least 3 weeks with systemic therapy.[71] Atovaquone, pyrimethamine (Fansidar), trimethoprim alone, and trimetrexate with folinic acid have been used with some success.[72,73] In severe cases, the adjunctive use of systemic corticosteroids may be necessary.[74,75] *P. carinii* prophylaxis using oral trimethoprim-sulfamethoxazole, dapsone, or pentamidine and other second-line agents is indicated for all HIV-infected individuals with CD4 counts lower than 200 cells/mm^3 and for all persons who have had an initial episode of *P. carinii* pneumonia.[76]

Toxoplasma gondii

T. gondii is an obligate intracellular protozoan that is ubiquitous in nature, resulting in varying degrees of infection and disease in animals and humans. Infection may be transmitted to many species of carnivores through the ingestion of cysts that release viable trophozoites after the cyst wall is disrupted by gastric enzymes. Humans may also become infected congenitally and through environmental contact. The typical scenario for the latter is by handling cat litter, with fecal contamination and subsequent oocyst ingestion. These invade the mucosa of the gastrointestinal tract and from there disseminate widely through the body, most commonly encysting in the brain (Figs. 2–7 and 2–8), heart, or skeletal muscle. Infection persists for the life of the host, with reactivation occurring most frequently if the host becomes immunodeficient.

The majority of AIDS patients with toxoplasmosis have findings referable to the central nervous system,[77,78] which may manifest subacutely as personality changes (e.g., apathy, depression), as acute meningoencephalitis, or commonly as a space-occupying lesion. Myocarditis, pneumonitis, and adult chorioretinitis have also been noted. Rarely, *T. gondii* may be found in the lymph nodes of persons with chronic generalized lymphadenopathy. The most common presenting symptoms include seizures, focal neurologic deficits, and encephalopathy.[79] Computed tomography scans frequently demonstrate the presence of one or multiple space-occupying lesions whose ring is enhanced by the use of contrast dye (Fig. 2–9). The diagnosis of *T. gondii* encephalitis often is based on the clinical presentation, serodiagnosis, and response to empiric therapy with sulfonamides and pyrimethamine. The use of brain biopsy may be necessary to establish a definitive diagnosis in atypical cases, particularly because individuals in some of the high-risk groups, such as intravenous drug users, may present in the same fashion with pyogenic brain abscesses.

Positive serologic findings, such as on the Sabin-Feldman dye test or the IgM indirect fluorescent antibody test, have been unreliable in the diagnosis of toxoplasmosis in patients with AIDS; however, negative results on serologic testing are strong evidence against this diagnosis. The demonstration of trophozoites in body fluids or tissue by Wright's or Giemsa stains is diagnostic. Tissue cysts may be seen with the periodic acid–Schiff stain, which stains the tachyzoites within the cyst. They may reflect chronic infection, so the clinical history is important in deciding the significance of finding only cysts without invasive tachyzoites. Increased numbers of tissue cysts in a specific location may be helpful in establishing a diagnosis of reactivated central nervous system toxoplasmosis, which can only be diagnosed definitively by brain biopsy.[79] Patients tend to respond to therapy with pyrimethamine and sulfadiazine but may relapse because the cyst forms are resistant to these agents.[80] Immunocompromised patients with cerebral toxoplasmosis must be treated for life. Patients who are infected with HIV often may manifest sulfa allergies in the course of therapy, limiting the effectiveness of the most commonly used regimen. Other drugs that are under investigation for the treatment of HIV-associated invasive toxoplasmosis include dapsone, clindamycin, as well as the newer macrolides such as azithromycin and clarithromycin.

Cryptosporidiosis

Cryptosporidium parvum and other enteric coccidial parasites, such as Microsporida and *Isospora belli,* have been recognized as human pathogens only over the last 15 years[81] but have been increasingly associated as causes of HIV-associated enteropathy as the AIDS epidemic has matured.[82] Human immunodeficiency virus itself can infect gut mucosal M cells, which are of macrophage origin, and result in immune dysfunction, leading to symptoms and increased gastrointestinal susceptibility to colonization and disease caused by enteric parasites.[83] The spectrum of illness caused by these organisms is now appreciated to range from subclinical manifestations such as transient diarrhea in immunocompetent individuals to fulminant profuse cholera-like diarrhea in individuals whose immune systems are not intact[84] (Fig. 2–10). Many patients with AIDS have severe watery diarrhea, but in only a fraction of them can this be documented to be caused by *Cryptosporidium* infection. Because *Cryptosporidium* may grow profusely on the surface of the small bowel, needed nutrients may not be readily absorbed, resulting in malnutrition and diarrhea (see Fig. 2–10).[84] Occasionally, the organism may be

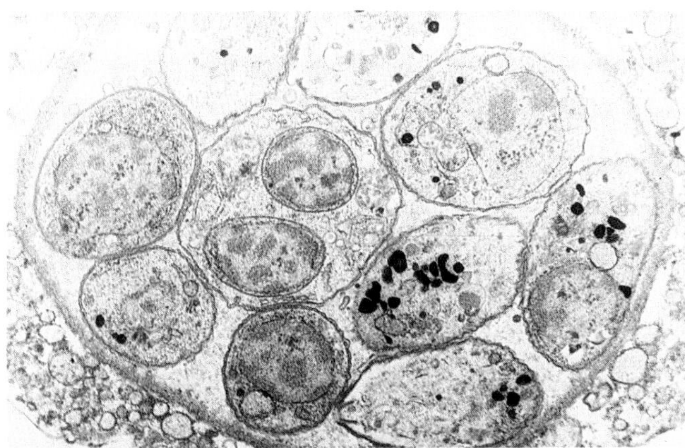

FIGURE 2–7. *Toxoplasma*
Toxoplasma cyst, electron micrograft. (From Still Picture Archives, Centers for Disease Control and Prevention, Atlanta, Georgia.)

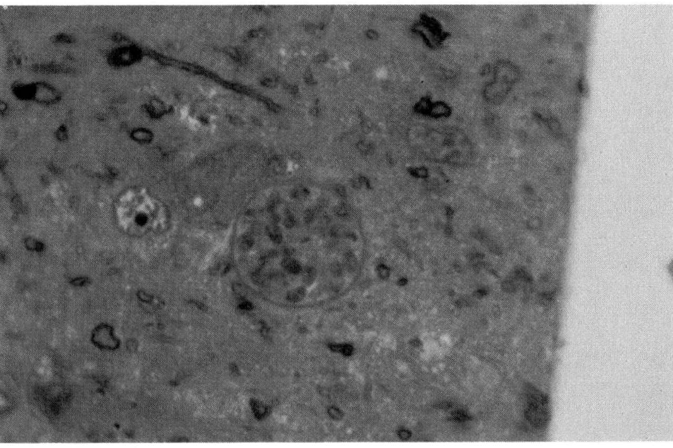

FIGURE 2–8. Toxoplasmosis
Toxoplasmosis, section of brain (×1200). (From Still Picture Archives, Centers for Disease Control and Prevention, Atlanta, Georgia.)

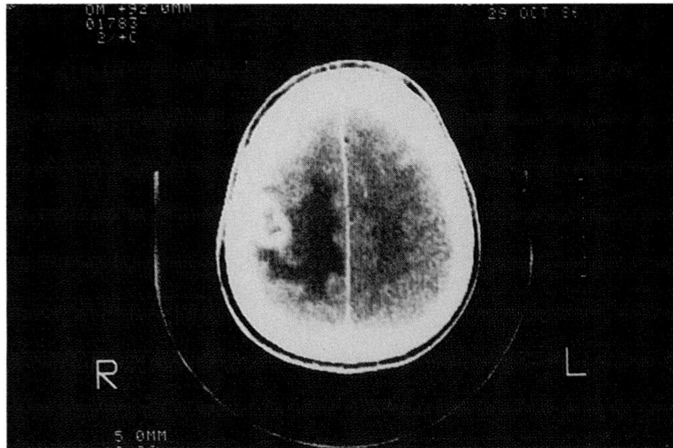

FIGURE 2–9. Toxoplasmosis
Toxoplasmosis, space-occupying lesion on computed tomography scan.

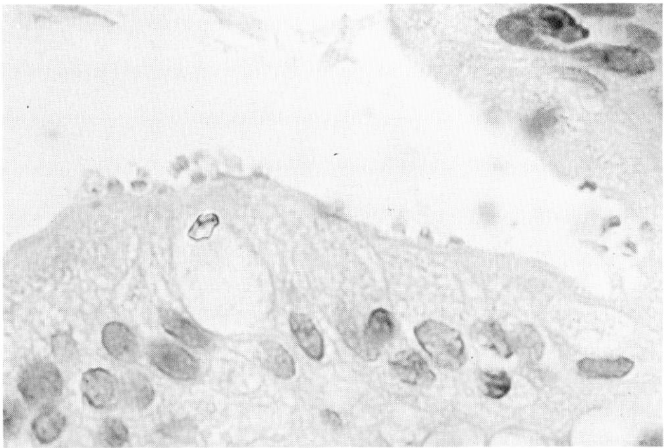

FIGURE 2–10. Cryptosporidiosis
Cryptosporidiosis, small bowel biopsy; high-power magnification. (Courtesy of Jonathan W. M. Gold, MD, Associate Director, Special Microbiology Laboratory, Memorial Sloan-Kettering Cancer Center, New York.)

isolated from other organs such as the gallbladder (associated with a sclerosing cholangitis-like syndrome)[85] as well as the lungs, but the primary morbidity is from the profuse, watery diarrhea that has been resistant to most antibiotic regimens in patients with AIDS. Symptoms may wax and wane, ranging from a few soft stools per day to a constant watery stream of diarrhea, with associated inanition.

The organism cannot be identified by conventional stool staining techniques; however, it can be seen on iodine-stained wet mounts or in acid-fast stains of stool smears. However, the yield on identifying the organism is best if a sucrose flotation gradient technique is utilized (Fig. 2–11).[86] The organism can be visualized on biopsy specimens of gastrointestinal mucosa by light or electron microscopy.

The therapy of cryptosporidiosis has been generally unsuccessful. Clinical studies have utilized a wide range of antiprotozoal drugs such as furazolidone, dimethylfluoro-ornithine (DMFO) and tetracycline, spiramycin, and antimalarials; however, the best success to date has been with newer macrolide antibiotics, such as azithromycin and clarithromycin.[87–90] Nonetheless, an adequate response has not been uniform, and relapses have occurred when the drug was discontinued. A nonabsorbable aminoglycoside, paromomycin, has been shown to be helpful in milder cases.[91] Studies are under way to evaluate combining macrolides and paromomycin to increase therapeutic efficacy and to prevent relapse. Infection with *I. belli* can cause symptoms that mimic cryptosporidiosis, but it responds to treatment with trimethoprim-sulfamethoxazole therapy.[92] Another coccidial cause of malabsorption is microsporidiosis, which may be hard to diagnose but which may respond to albendazole therapy.[93] The medical management of cryptosporidiosis and other enteric parasites in HIV-infected patients also includes nutritional repletion, either through enteral or parenteral supplementation, and the use of antimotility drugs and may include the addition of drugs that reverse the profound catabolism that patients may experience (e.g., somatostatin, medroxyprogesterone, dronabinol [Marinol]), several of which are still being assessed in clinical trials.[94]

Other Protozoa

Giardia lamblia *and* Entamoeba histolytica

Although infection with *Giardia lamblia* (Fig. 2–12) or *Entamoeba histolytica* (Figs. 2–13 and 2–14) is not itself suggestive of immunodeficiency or of HIV infection, these organisms are found in sexually active adults more frequently than in the general population. Infected individuals may be asymptomatic carriers or may have persistent diarrhea, cramps, and constitutional symptoms. Chronic infection may result in malabsorption and malnutrition, and may possibly exacerbate HIV progression by stimulating the immune system of HIV-infected individuals. Thus, prompt diagnosis by checking stools for cysts and trophozoites, and offering subsequent antiparasitic therapy, if necessary, is desirable.

Visceral Leishmaniasis

Another protozoan parasite that may infect HIV-infected patients is *Leishmania donovani,* the etiologic agent of visceral leishmaniasis.[95,96] Visceral leishmaniasis (kala-azar) is increasingly recognized as an opportunistic infection in AIDS patients from the Mediterranean region and from Africa. The organism is an intracellular pathogen (Fig. 2–15) that requires a coordinated, cell-mediated immune response by the host to control the infection. The organism is transmitted by sand flies as flagellated promastigotes (Fig. 2–16). The organisms disseminate throughout the body following cutaneous inoculation. They are taken up by macrophages, where they lose their flagella and reside as intracellular amastigotes for years.

Leishmaniasis may cause fever, weight loss, hepatosplenomegaly, pancytopenia, and death in immunocompromised patients. Diagnosis may be difficult and frequently requires specialized culture techniques from the bone marrow or skin lesions. The organism may occasionally be seen on Giemsa stains of the peripheral blood smear.[97] Treatment generally consists of pentavalent antimony compounds; immunotherapy with interferon-γ may also be useful.[98]

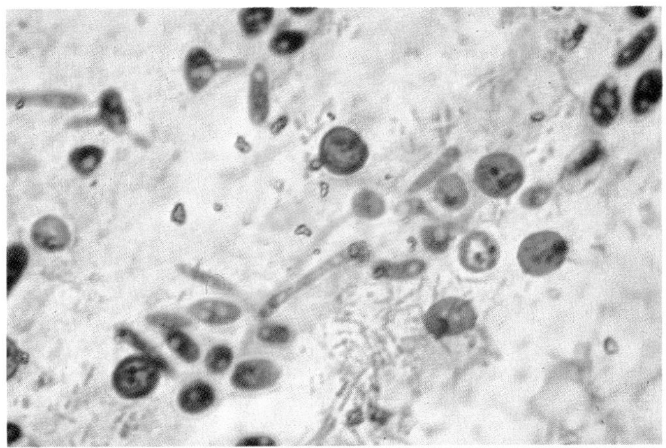

FIGURE 2–11. Cryptosporidiosis

Cryptosporidiosis, modified cold Kinyoun acid-fast stain under oil immersion lens; oocysts (acid-fast) stain red; yeast cells (not acid-fast) stain green; direct fecal smear. (Courtesy of Pearl Ma, MD, Director, Microbiology, St. Vincent's Hospital, New York.)

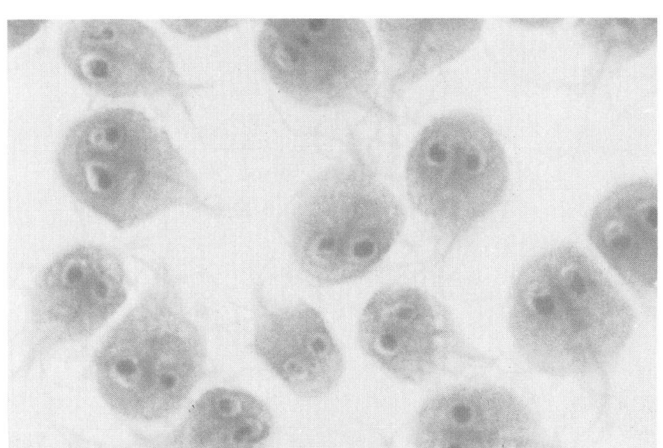

FIGURE 2–12. *Giardia lamblia*

G. lamblia trophozoite from duodenal aspirate.

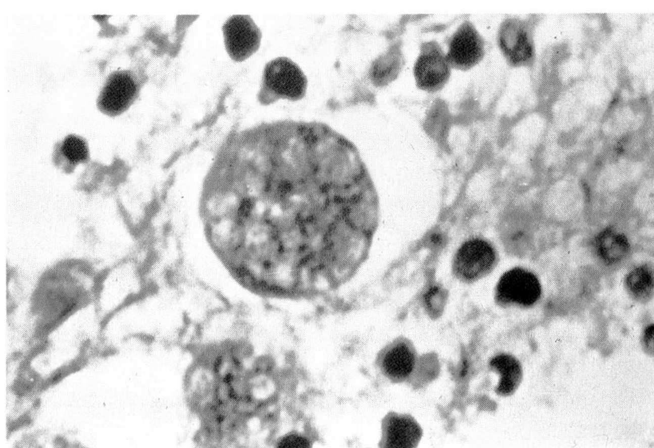

FIGURE 2–13. *Entamoeba histolytica*

E. histolytica cyst in bowel preparation, surrounded by red blood cells.

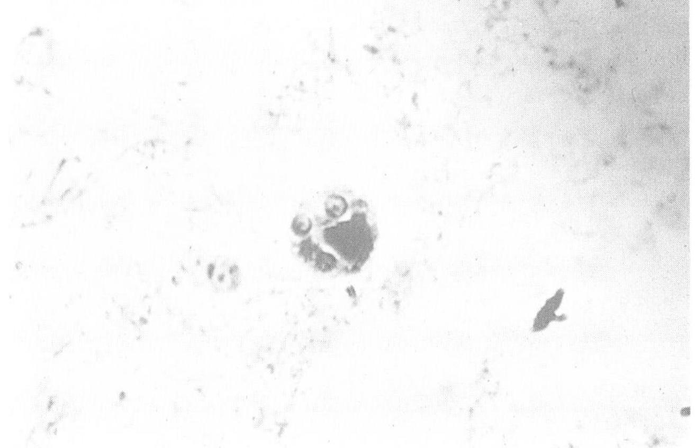

FIGURE 2–14. *Entamoeba histolytica*

E. histolytica cyst with four nuclei and prominent chromatoidal body.

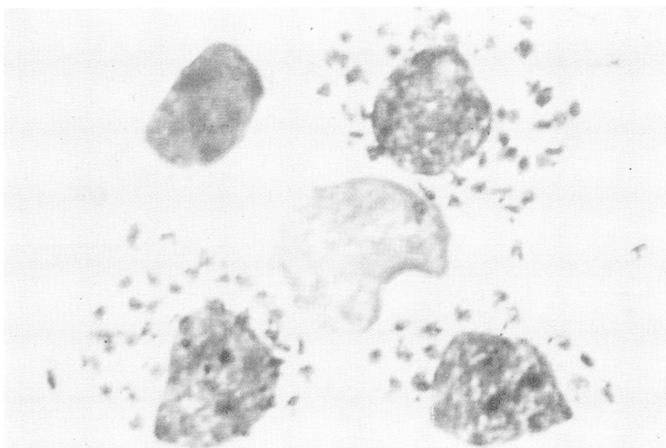

FIGURE 2–15. Visceral leishmaniasis

Intracellular forms (×1200). Amastigote forms within the cytoplasm of histiocytes.

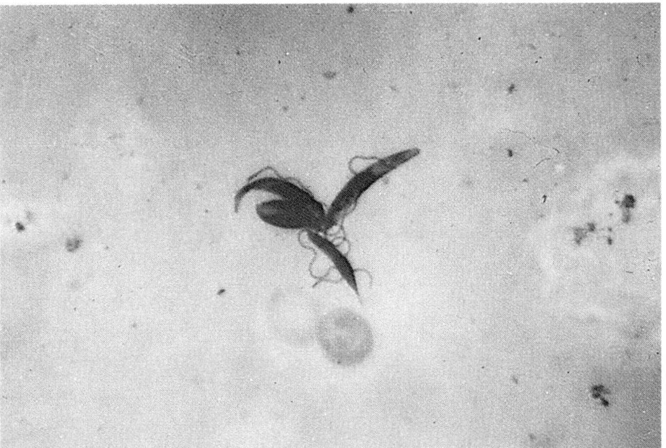

FIGURE 2–16. Visceral leishmaniasis

Flagellated promastigotes (×1200). Infectious form found in the gut of sand flies.

FUNGAL INFECTIONS

Candida albicans

Candidal infections of the mucous membranes and the skin are common occurrences in patients with AIDS and related disorders. It is rare to see invasive or disseminated disease, except in patients who have long-standing intravenous lines or are extremely debilitated and cachetic. Case reports of candidal endocarditis or other systemic involvement have been noted (Figs. 2–17 and 2–18).

Oropharyngeal candidiasis, or thrush, has been noted to be a common feature of AIDS-related symptoms in several of the risk groups.[58] Thrush is an uncommon finding in individuals who have not received broad spectrum antibiotics or corticosteroids or who do not have other underlying immunologic or metabolic diseases. In the increasing number of recently HIV-infected women, new or recurrent episodes of candidal vaginitis may be the first clinical manifestation of altered mucosal immunity.[99] Whereas thrush tends to occur only after the CD4 count falls below levels seen in persons without HIV infections, recurrent candidal vaginitis may occur in women with CD4 counts higher than 500 cells/mm^3.

Candidal esophagitis is distinctly uncommon except among persons with AIDS, so that individuals who are at risk for the syndrome who complain of dysphagia should undergo prompt endoscopy so that early treatment can be instituted (Fig. 2–19). The differential diagnosis of dysphagia in these individuals also includes herpes simplex and CMV esophagitis as well. Mucosal candidal infections frequently respond rapidly to therapy with nystatin or clotrimazole troches or mouthwash. However, some individuals, particularly those with esophagitis, need treatment with one of the newer imidazoles, such as fluconazole, and rarely, refractory cases should be treated with systemic amphotericin B.

Cryptococcus neoformans

Cryptococcal infection in individuals with AIDS, as in those who have other immunologic disorders, may manifest subacutely as a mild headache with a low-grade fever.[100,101] More severe manifestations such as nausea, vomiting, and meningeal signs may subsequently develop. The cerebrospinal fluid usually reveals pleocytosis, low glucose, and high protein. Definitive studies include the India ink test (Fig. 2–20), the latex agglutination test for the cryptococcal antigen, and fungal cultures. In addition to causing cryptococcal meningitis, this organism may develop into mass lesions of the central nervous system (cryptococcomas) (Fig. 2–21). Patients with AIDS may also present with extrameningeal disease, including hepatic (Fig. 2–22), pulmonary (Fig. 2–23), dermatologic (Fig. 2–24), lymphadenopathic, and peritoneal involvement. The demonstration of this organism from any site in a patient with AIDS is a sufficient indication for the institution of prompt therapy.

Therapeutic regimens include amphotericin B with or without flucytosine or high-dose imidazole therapy (e.g., fluconazole).[102] Unfortunately, because the immunologic deficit in patients with AIDS does not remit during the course of therapy, relapses have been noted, and therefore individuals with AIDS who have cryptococcal disease need lifetime courses of therapy to prevent relapse.

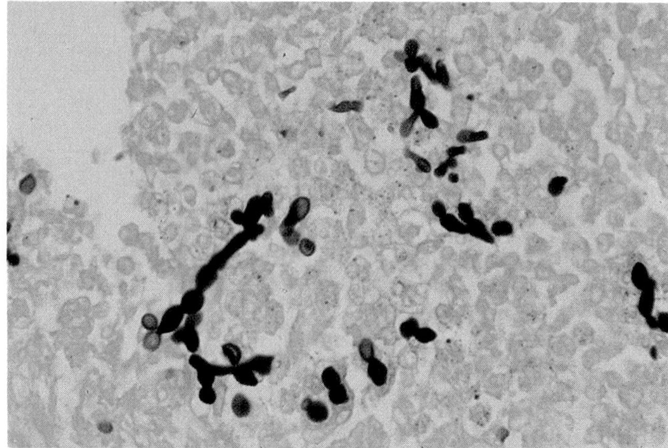

FIGURE 2–17. *Candida albicans*

C. albicans in human heart tissue; Gomori's stain (×500). (From Still Picture Archives, Centers for Disease Control and Prevention, Atlanta, Georgia.)

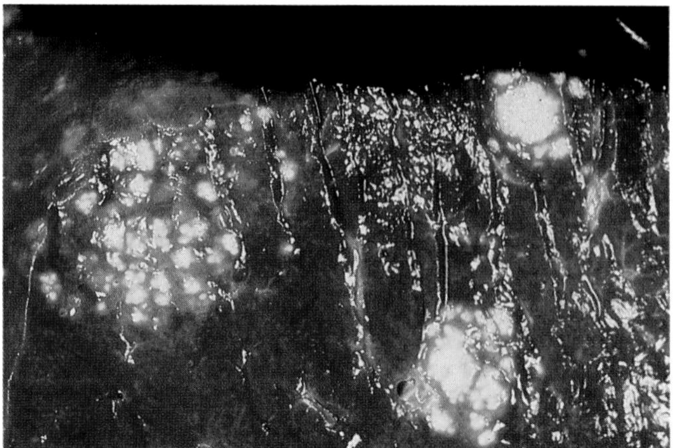

FIGURE 2–18. *Candida albicans*

Human liver showing multiple granulomas caused by *C. albicans.* (From Still Picture Archives, Centers for Disease Control and Prevention, Atlanta, Georgia.)

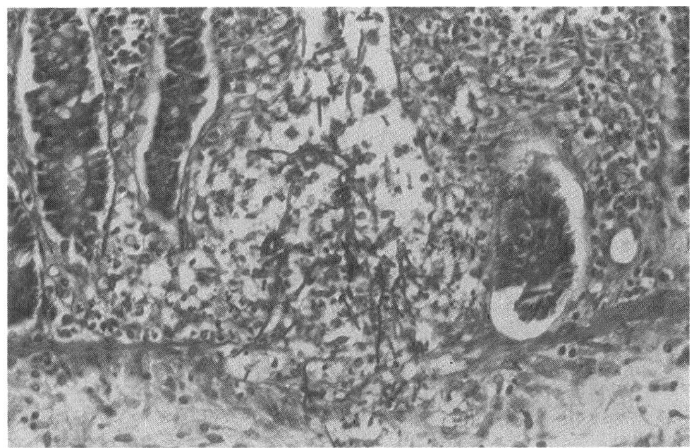

FIGURE 2–19. Candidal abscesses

Esophageal biopsy reveals candidal abscesses, pseudohyphae extending through submucosa; periodic acid–Schiff stain. (From Still Picture Archives, Centers for Disease Control and Prevention, Atlanta, Georgia.)

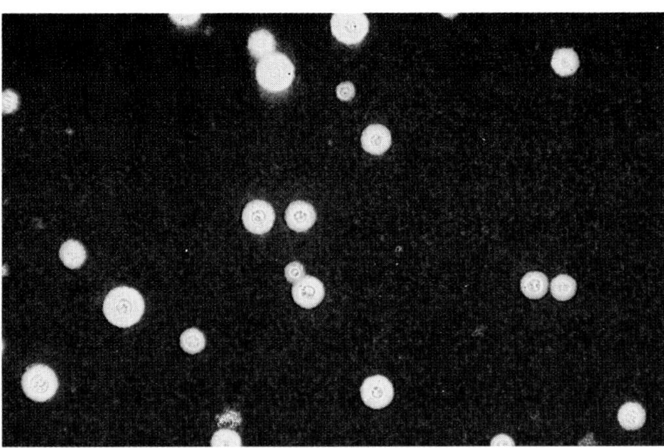

FIGURE 2–20. *Cryptococcus neoformans*

Photomicrograph showing *C. neoformans;* India ink mount (×475). (From Still Picture Archives, Centers for Disease Control and Prevention, Atlanta, Georgia.)

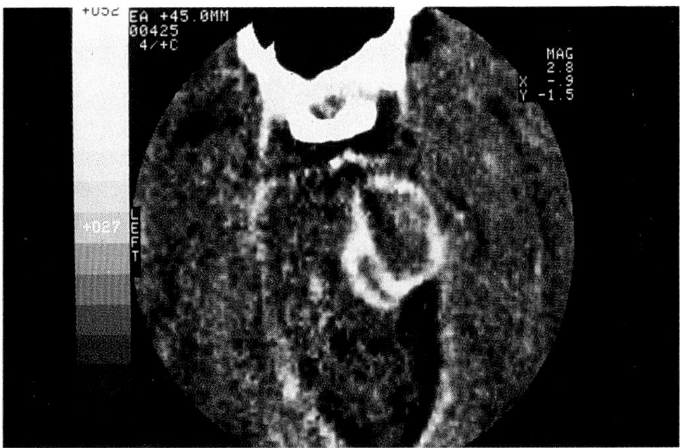

FIGURE 2–21. Cryptococcal abscess

Cryptococcal abscess of the brain stem on computed tomography scan. (From Still Picture Archives, Centers for Disease Control and Prevention, Atlanta, Georgia.)

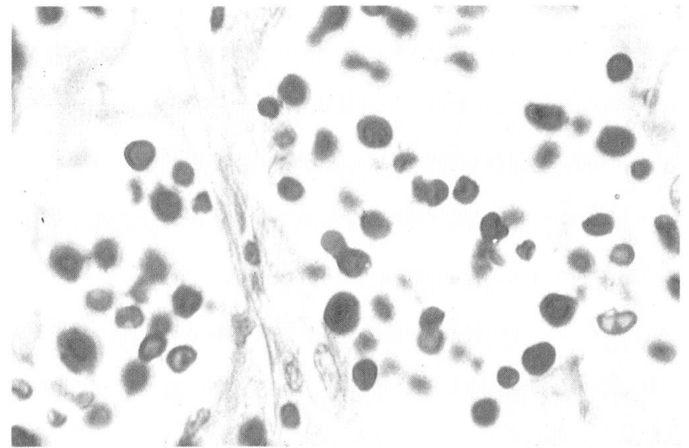

FIGURE 2–22. Cryptococcosis

Cryptococcosis—tissue section of liver; periodic acid–Schiff stain (×980). (From Still Picture Archives, Centers for Disease Control and Prevention, Atlanta, Georgia.)

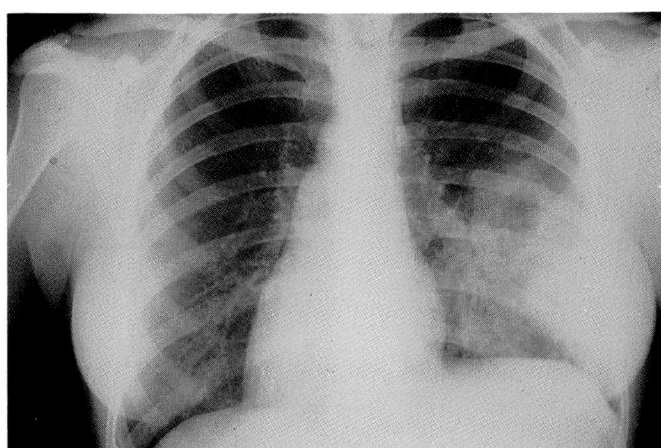

FIGURE 2–23. Cryptococcosis

Radiograph of patient showing nonencapsulated cryptococcosis. (From Still Picture Archives, Centers for Disease Control and Prevention, Atlanta, Georgia.)

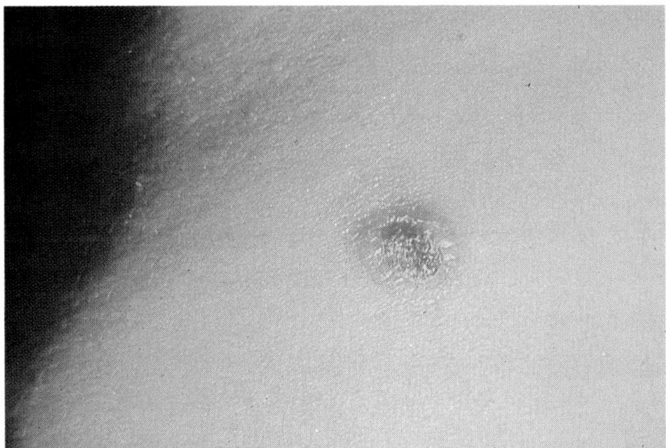

FIGURE 2–24. Cryptococcosis

Cryptococcosis—skin lesion (close-up); disseminated case. (From Still Picture Archives, Centers for Disease Control and Prevention, Atlanta, Georgia.)

Other Fungi

Immunocompromised patients, including those with AIDS, may develop disseminated fungal infections with a large number of other pathogens. *Aspergillus* infection is uncommon in AIDS patients but may result in a necrotizing pneumonitis (Fig. 2–25) or may spread widely and invade virtually any organ (Fig. 2–26). Where histoplasmosis and coccidioidomycosis are endemic diseases (the Midwest and South and the desert southwestern United States, respectively), retroviral-induced immunodeficiency may result in disseminated infection (Figs. 2–27 and 2–28).

BACTERIAL INFECTIONS

Mycobacterium avium-intracellulare

Before the advent of the AIDS epidemic, *M. avium-intracellulare* was known to be a ubiquitous environmental contaminant that rarely caused disseminated disease in adults. In patients with AIDS, however, it has been found in up to one fifth of the number of cases that have been followed prospectively, manifesting with fever, weight loss, and debilitation.[103,104] The organism may be cultured from blood, lymph nodes, liver, spleen, lung, and bone marrow.[105] Granulomas may not be present, so the actual contribution of this organism to the morbidity of patients with AIDS is not always clear.[106] Several patients with *M. avium-intracellulare* infection have had chronic diarrhea, and the organism has been found on small bowel biopsy specimens (Fig. 2–29).[107]

The organisms are acid-fast but are somewhat longer and thicker than *M. tuberculosis* on staining. Cultures tend to grow more rapidly than those of *M. tuberculosis* and may often be recognized in 2 to 3 weeks (Fig. 2–30). In addition to the acid-fast bacteria stain of blood cultures and other tissues, the organism may be demonstrated in macrophages utilizing the periodic acid–Schiff stain.

The treatment of this organism usually requires multiple antimycobacterial drugs because of high levels of resistance.[108] In addition to its sensitivity to some of the usual tuberculostatic medications such as isoniazid, ethambutol, and aminoglycosides, the organism is often sensitive to clofazimine and rifabutin, a rifampin derivative.[109] Treatment often utilizes four of these drugs.[110] However, progressive cachexia, anemia, and fevers may be seen in individuals despite treatment with an optimal regimen, as the organism may manifest resistance rapidly. Rifabutin has been shown to be effective in the prophylaxis of *M. avium-intracellulare* infection in patients with CD4 counts of fewer than 100 cells/mm^3.

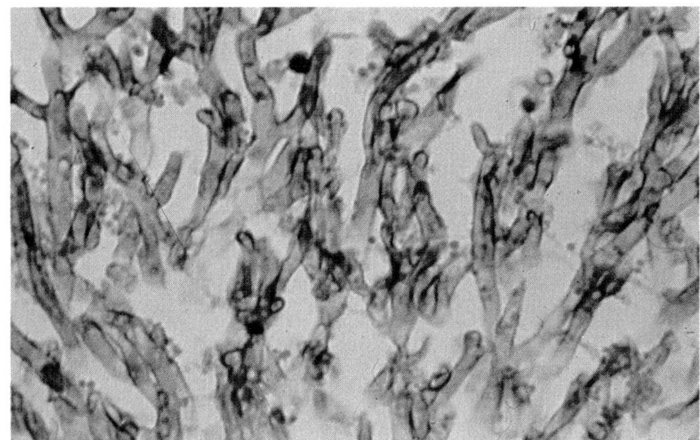

FIGURE 2–25. *Aspergillus fumigatus*

A. fumigatus; hematoxylin and eosin stain of lung tissue with "forked stick" branching hyphae.

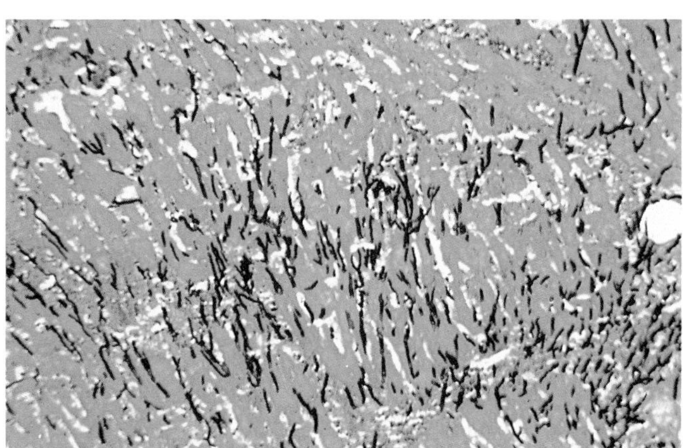

FIGURE 2–26. *Aspergillus fumigatus*

A. fumigatus; Gomori's methenamine silver stain of fungal invasion of myocardium.

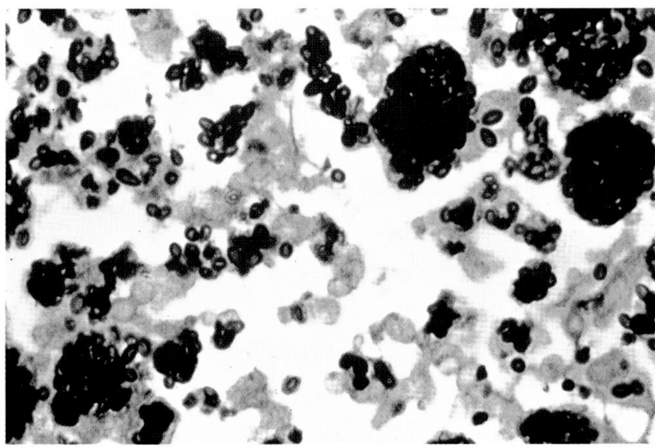

FIGURE 2–27. Histoplasmosis

Histoplasmosis; Gomori's methenamine silver stain of lung, revealing narrow-based budding.

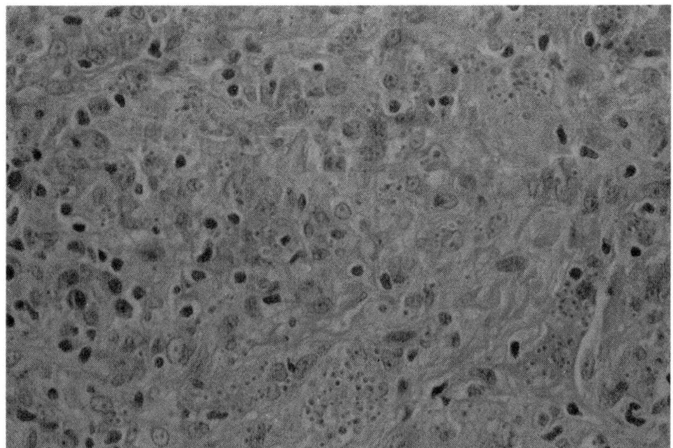

FIGURE 2–28. Histoplasmosis

Histoplasmosis; periodic acid–Schiff stain.

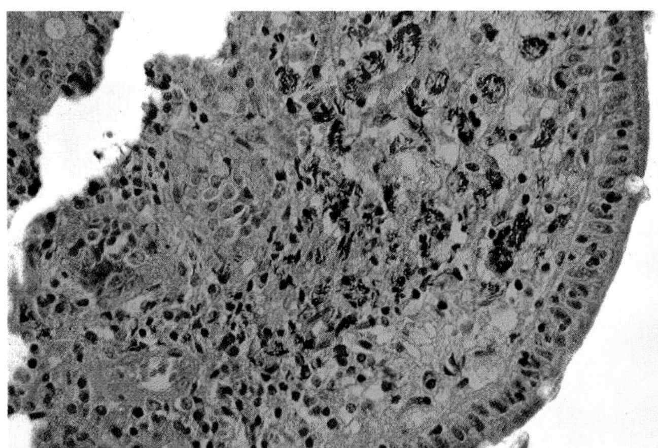

FIGURE 2–29. Mycobacterial infection

Mycobacterial infection of small bowel; acid-fast stain. Biopsy specimen. (Courtesy of Jonathan W. M. Gold, MD, Associate Director, Special Microbiology Laboratory, Memorial Sloan-Kettering Cancer Center, New York.)

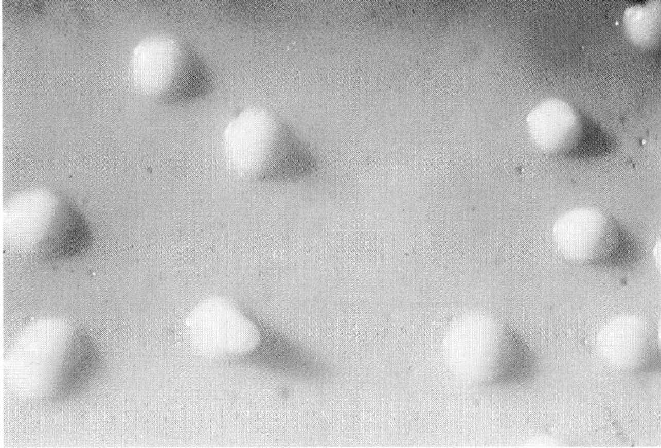

FIGURE 2–30. *Mycobacterium avium*

M. avium, colonial morphology. (From Still Picture Archives, Centers for Disease Control and Prevention, Atlanta, Georgia.)

Mycobacterium tuberculosis

Tuberculosis was initially recognized as a common comorbid condition in HIV-infected people from either the Caribbean, particularly Haiti, or central Africa[111] but is now increasingly found among all HIV-infected patients, regardless of national origin or HIV risk group. The specter of multidrug-resistant TB has heightened the clinical awareness of this manifestation of HIV-associated immunodeficiency, and, indeed, the AIDS epidemic has been associated with increased annual rates of TB in the United States in the last decade. Tuberculosis may manifest itself in a variety of ways in HIV-infected persons, ranging from a disseminated pulmonary pattern (Figs. 2–31 and 2–32) to extrapulmonary TB, including involvement of lymph nodes, liver (Fig. 2–33), spleen, bone marrow, and the gastrointestinal tract.

Therapy should begin with four active tuberculostatic drugs such as isoniazid, pyrazinamide ethambutol, and rifampin, given the increased prevalence of multidrug resistance and the high risk of occult metastatic TB foci in HIV-infected individuals.[112] The infection can usually be controlled with appropriate antituberculosis therapy and compliance with a 9-month course of therapy; however, because the immunodeficiency is generally not corrected in the course of treatment, patients are at an increased risk of relapse once medications are stopped. Multidrug resistance has led to the increased use of newer agents, such as the quinolones, or reliance on older, more toxic second-line drugs, such as aminoglycosides.

Bacillary Angiomatosis

Advances in molecular genetics have facilitated the search for the etiologic agent of bacillary angiomatosis, which may manifest as multiple, highly vascular cutaneous lesions in patients immunocompromised by HIV[113] (Fig. 2–34). The nodular lesions are usually distinctive, but biopsy may be necessary to differentiate them from those of Kaposi's sarcoma. Internal manifestations of bacillary angiomatosis may coexist with or without skin lesions. The lesions of hepatic peliosis are the most widespread manifestation of infection with this group of organisms. The most common agent of bacillary angiomatosis is a rickettsia-like organism, *Rochalimaea quintana,* but other related species may cause similar syndromes, for example, *Rochalimaea henslae.* In immunocompromised patients, these organisms may be associated with cat-scratch fever, and in AIDS patients, exposure to cats is associated with, but not necessary for, the development of bacillary angiomatosis and associated clinical sequelae.

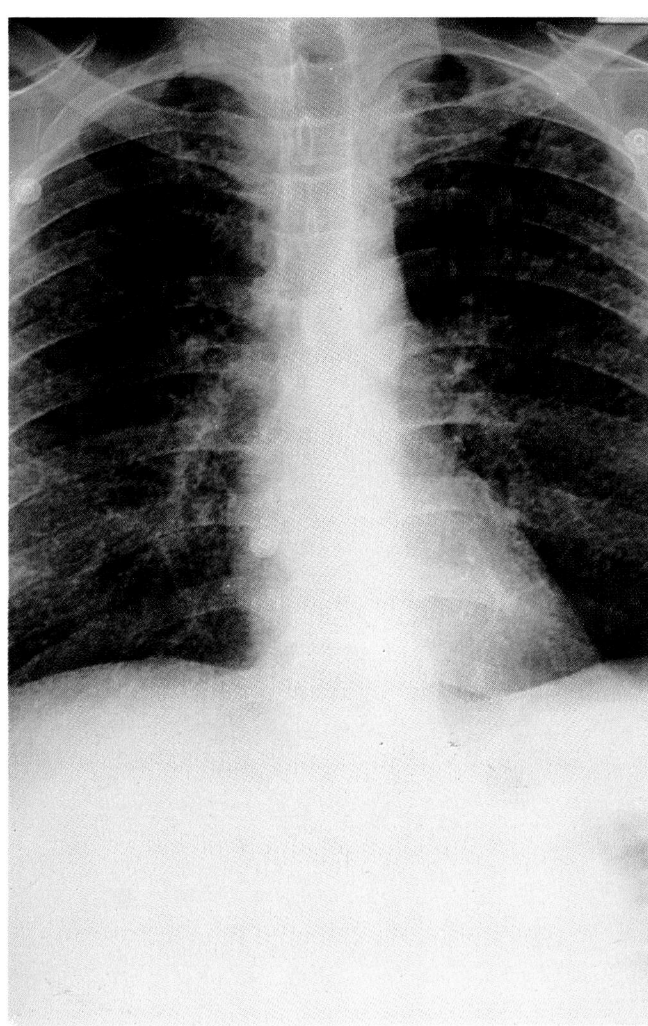

FIGURE 2–31. Miliary tuberculosis
Chest radiograph showing miliary tuberculosis.

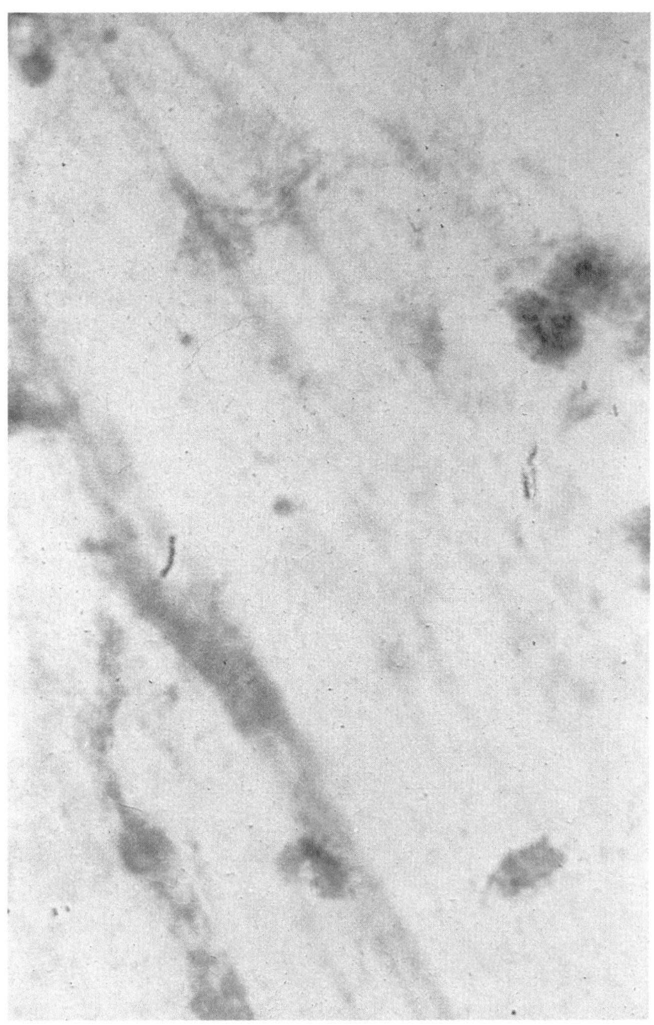

FIGURE 2–32. *Mycobacterium tuberculosis*
Ziehl-Neelsen stain of *M. tuberculosis.*

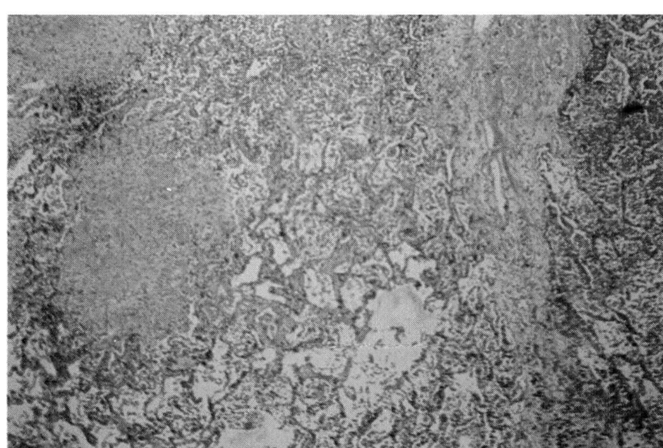

FIGURE 2–33. Hepatic granuloma
Liver—hematoxylin and eosin stain of hepatic granuloma.

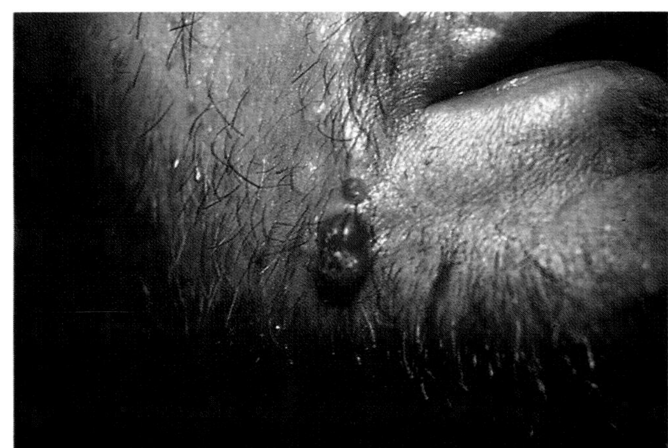

FIGURE 2–34. Bacillary angiomatosis
Cutaneous lesion of bacillary angiomatosis.

Salmonella Infection

Disseminated *Salmonella* infections have been associated with patients with other immunocompromised conditions, such as hematologic malignancies. Individuals from central Africa and Haiti and gay and bisexual men may have an increased prevalence of intestinal infections that are due to either environmental factors or specific behavioral practices. Individuals with AIDS who develop *Salmonella* infection of the gastrointestinal tract may have a higher incidence of persistent bacteremia.[113–115] These organisms may be routinely cultured using MacConkey, eosin-methylene blue, or *Salmonella-Shigella* (SS) media (Fig. 2–35) and are frequently controlled by conventional antibiotics, such as trimethoprim-sulfamethoxazole or newer quinolones. Severe *Campylobacter* intestinal infections with high-grade bacteremia have also been described in AIDS patients.[116] Given the ability for *Salmonella* to persist intracellularly in Peyer's patches in the gut, it is not surprising that the organism may be able to multiply and cause disseminated disease in immunocompromised patients with AIDS.

Other Bacteria

Immunocompromised patients with HIV infection may also be subject to disseminated infections with other bacteria that may be intracellular parasites. Thus, disseminated infection with *Nocardia* (Figs. 2–36 and 2–37) and *Legionella pneumophila* (Figs. 2–38 and 2–39) may be seen. Nocardiosis is generally treated with intravenous sulfonamides and legionellosis with systemic erythromycin.

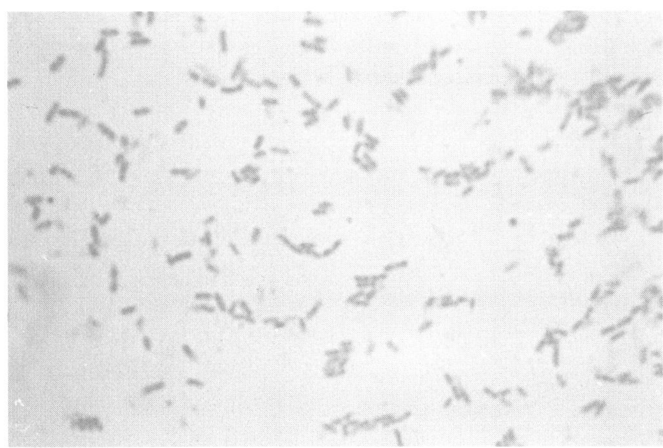

FIGURE 2–35. *Salmonella typhimurium*
Gram stain of blood subculture revealing *S. typhimurium*.

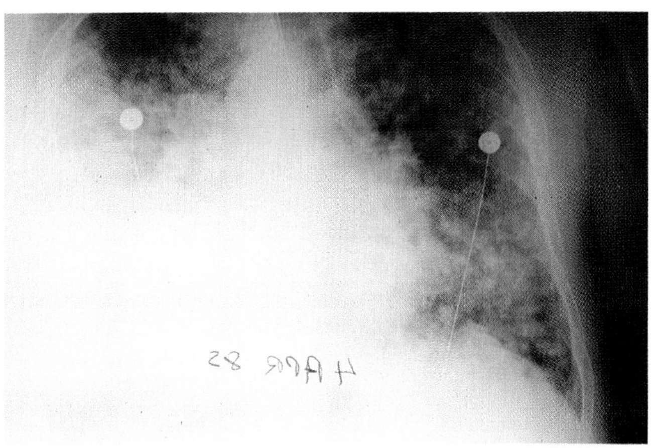

FIGURE 2–36. *Nocardia* pneumonia and pericarditis
Chest radiograph showing *Nocardia* pneumonia and pericarditis.

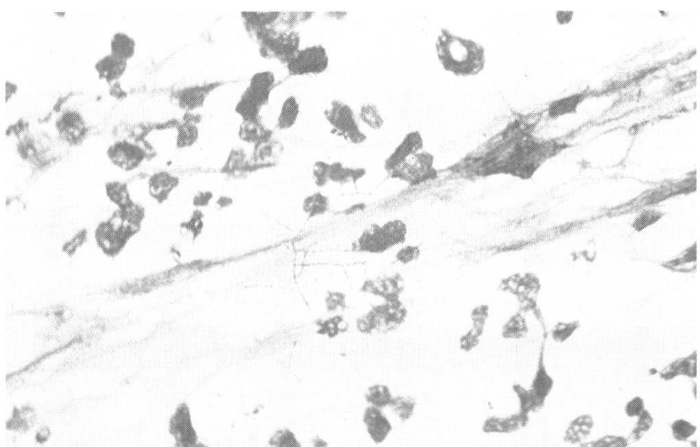

FIGURE 2–37. *Nocardia*
AVB stain of *Nocardia* from the lung, revealing branching acid-fast positive rods.

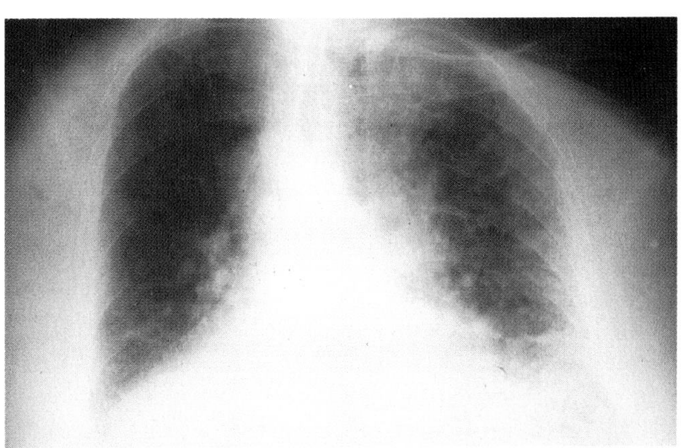

FIGURE 2–38. *Legionella pneumophila* pneumonia
Chest radiograph showing *L. pneumophila* pneumonia.

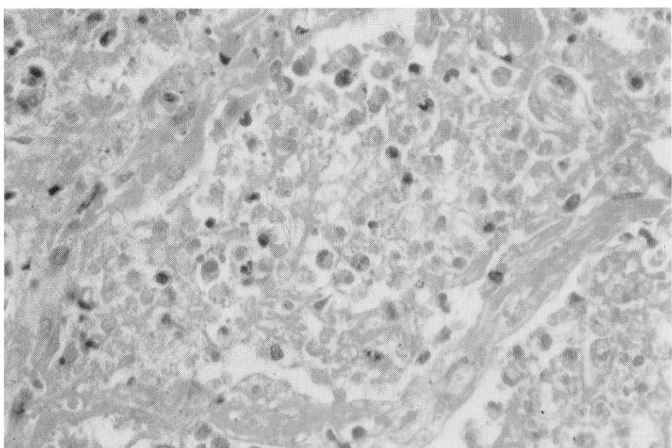

FIGURE 2–39. *Legionella* alveolitis
Hematoxylin and eosin stain—*Legionella* alveolitis.

VIRUSES

Herpes Simplex and Herpes Zoster

Exposure to herpes simplex earlier in life is a frequent finding in individuals who acquired AIDS because of sexual activity. Once individuals become immunodeficient because of HIV infection, herpes simplex may cause extensive mucosal and cutaneous ulcers in perioral or perirectal areas (Fig. 2–40).[117,118] Herpetic encephalitis or visceral involvement has not been commonly reported in individuals with AIDS. The major morbidity from these herpetic lesions is their failure to resolve, even with appropriate antiviral therapy using acyclovir. Clinical complaints may include rectal pain, bleeding, or discharge. The ulcers may be up to 10 cm in diameter. Newer treatment regimens that are under investigation include foscarnet as well as topical fluorothymidine, a fluorinated nucleoside.

Genital herpes may also occur in patients with AIDS; however, the progressive erosive disease noted with perioral and perianal involvement has not been reported. Part of the differential diagnosis of candidal esophagitis includes herpetic esophagitis and must be differentiated by endoscopy. Lesions that are suspected of being herpetic in origin may be swabbed, and Tzanck preparations using Wright's stain can be prepared for an immediate diagnosis (Fig. 2–41). The suspected herpetic ulcers can then be cultured. Patients with AIDS-related symptoms who have recurrent disease may be managed best with suppressive therapy using acyclovir, although the development of resistant strains may require the use of some of the newer investigational agents, such as topical fluorothymidine or systemic therapy with foscarnet.[119] The reactivation of herpes zoster that results in shingles may be seen frequently as an early manifestation of waning immunity in individuals with HIV infection (Fig. 2–42). Disseminated disease and encephalitis have been noted but are uncommon. Particularly severe cases may benefit from high-dose intravenous acyclovir.[120]

Cytomegalovirus

Cytomegalovirus is a ubiquitous cause of infection in individuals with AIDS that affects a wide variety of organ systems. Many individuals who are at increased risk for developing AIDS have previously been infected with CMV, and the deterioration of cellular immunity due to AIDS allows for latent CMV to reactivate and disseminate.[121] It is not known whether repeated exposure to the virus in gay and bisexual men results in hyperinfection with multiple strains and synergistic immunosuppression.

Most individuals with AIDS have persistent CMV viremia. It is therefore often difficult to determine the role that CMV is playing in the pathogenesis of specific clinical syndromes. Individuals who have not been exposed to HIV may have fever, malaise, and weight loss associated with primary CMV infection, and coinfection with HIV and other chronic herpesviruses, such as Epstein-Barr virus, makes it difficult to assess the independent contribution of CMV in the wasting syndromes of patients with AIDS.

Visceral involvement with CMV may be demonstrated by histologic staining with a demonstration of inclusion bodies such as the classic “owl's eye” pattern (Fig. 2–43). Culture alone is often insufficient evidence because contamination with peripheral blood leukocytes in patients who have CMV viremia makes it difficult to assess the morbidity due to CMV alone.

Cytomegalovirus may result in a pneumonitis that is most often diagnosed at autopsy.[122] In addition, hemorrhagic gastrointestinal disease,[123] hepatitis, and choreoretinitis[124] may be associated with CMV infection (Fig. 2–44). Hemorrhages and exudates found in the retina are more frequently due to CMV than to *T. gondii* in this population. Less common syndromes include CMV esophagitis, lymphadenitis, and adrenalitis.[125,126]

Ganciclovir, an acyclovir derivative, and foscarnet have been shown to be effective in the management of disseminated CMV infection, particularly retinitis.[127,128] In patients who are immunosuppressed because of renal transplants and who develop CMV infection, diminution of the immunosuppressive drugs has resulted in resolution of the CMV infection. It is unclear whether future, more efficacious immunostimulatory treatments for HIV will be effective in modifying the course of disseminated CMV disease.

Epstein-Barr Virus

Like CMV, Epstein-Barr virus can be isolated from many patients with AIDS and related disorders as well as from persons at increased risk for these syndromes.[119] The virus may result in fever, generalized lymphadenopathy, and malaise in individuals with or without exposure to HIV. It is, therefore, difficult to ascertain the independent role played by this virus in the pathogenesis of some of the disorders associated with AIDS. However, evidence of active Epstein-Barr virus that results in B-cell proliferation has been suggested as a

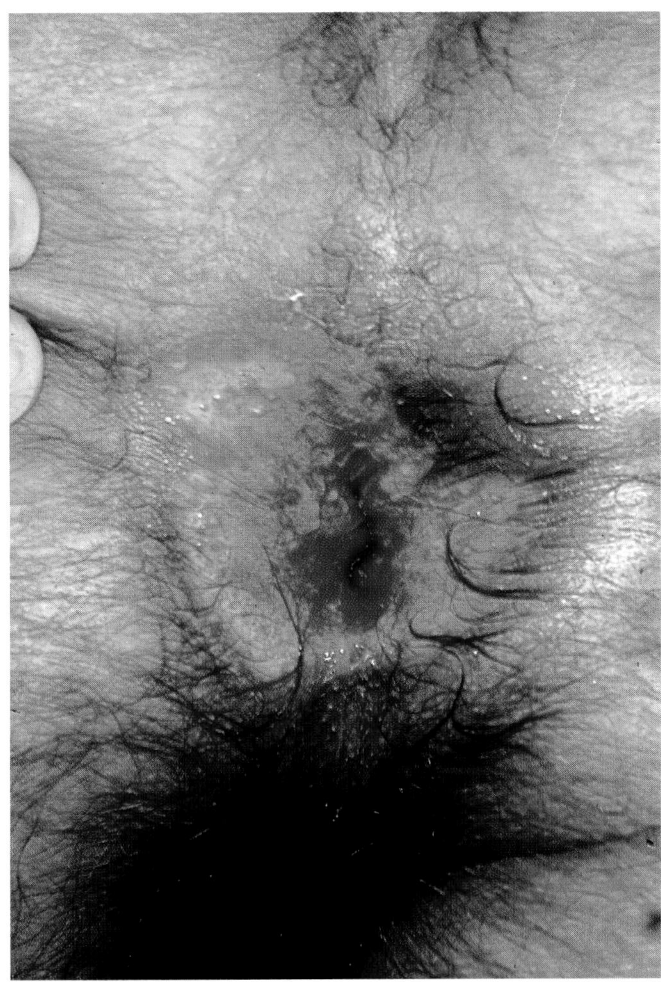

FIGURE 2–40. Herpes infection
Chronic mucocutaneous perianal herpes infection. (From Still Picture Archives, Centers for Disease Control and Prevention, Atlanta, Georgia.)

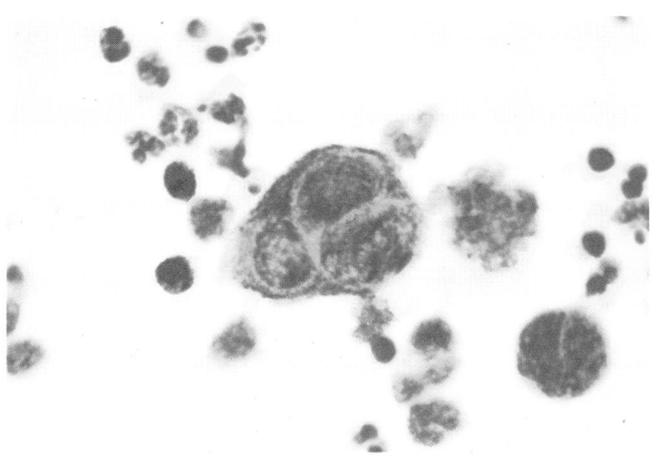

FIGURE 2–41. Herpes progenitalis
Herpes progenitalis, multinucleated giant cell, penile lesion; Tzanck preparation.

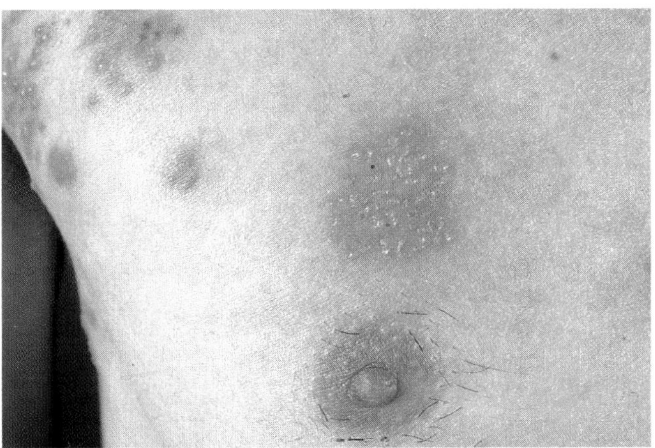

FIGURE 2–42. Varicella-zoster
Varicella-zoster—reactivation as shingles.

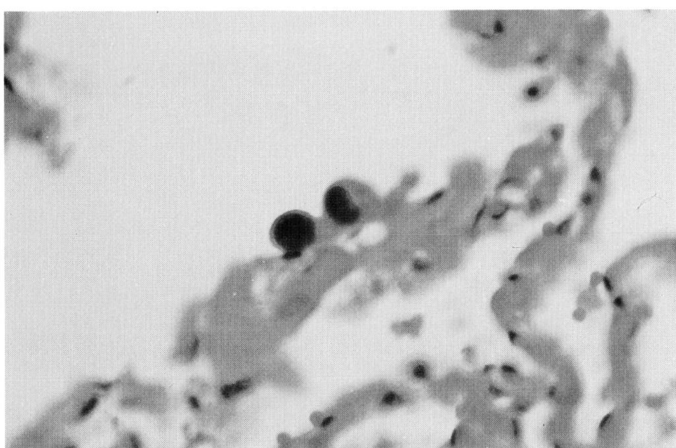

FIGURE 2–43. Cytomegalovirus
Cytomegalovirus—intranuclear inclusions in cells in lung biopsy. (Courtesy of Jonathan W. M. Gold, MD, Associate Director, Special Microbiology Laboratory, Memorial Sloan-Kettering Cancer Center, New York.)

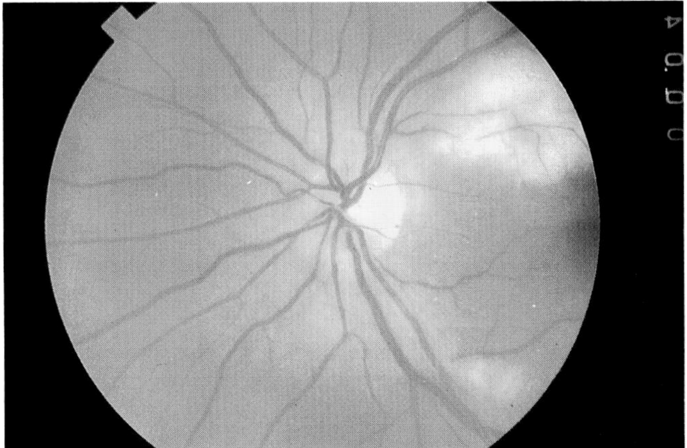

FIGURE 2–44. Cytomegalovirus retinitis
Cytomegalovirus retinitis—hemorrhage and exudate.

mechanism for the development of opportunistic lymphomas in individuals with AIDS. The diffuse lymphocytic interstitial pneumonitis described in the pediatric population with AIDS has been associated with active Epstein-Barr virus infection as well. Much more of the biology of the interaction of this virus with HIV remains to be clarified.

HELMINTHIC INFECTIONS

Strongyloides stercoralis may persist in human hosts for decades asymptomatically and reactivate when individuals become immunocompromised. Thus, persons with AIDS may develop disseminated disease without prior knowledge of infection, which may be manifested as diarrhea, abdominal pain, and intermittent pulmonary symptoms. Stool examination in the appropriate clinical context may be useful in establishing the diagnosis (Fig. 2–45). Patients can be treated with thiabendazole. *Trichuris* (whipworm) infection may be seen in homosexually active males (Fig. 2–46) and treated with mebendazole.

CONCLUSION

The many organisms that may cause significant illness in individuals with AIDS have certain features in common, particularly their ubiquitous presence in nature as well as the manner in which the immune system combats these organisms in immunocompetent hosts. Other organisms that require intact T-helper cell function have been described with increasing frequency in individuals with AIDS, such as strongyloidosis, histoplasmosis, and coccidioidomycosis. It is possible with increased observation of the epidemic that new pathogens will be identified that contribute to the significant morbidity and mortality of individuals with AIDS and related disorders.

Persons with AIDS and HIV infection are subject to multiple types of viral, bacterial, protozoal, and helminthic infections because of immune deficits, as well as lifestyle practices. The astute clinician must be aware that multisystem disease may be due to the spread of an unusual pathogen, that common organisms may manifest themselves in atypical ways, and that symptoms may be due to coinfection with multiple agents.

References

1. Barre-Sinoussi F, Chermann JC, Rety F, et al. Isolation of a T-lymphotropic retrovirus from a patient at risk for acquired immunodeficiency syndrome (AIDS). Science 1983; 220:868.
2. Gallo RC, Salahuddin SZ, Popovic M, et al. Frequent detection and isolation of cytopathic retroviruses (HTLV-III) from patients with AIDS and at risk for AIDS. Science 1984; 224:500.
3. Fauci AS, Macher AM, Longo DL, et al. Acquired immunodeficiency syndrome: Epidemiologic, clinical, immunologic, and therapeutic considerations. Ann Intern Med 1984;100:92–106.
4. Fauci AS. The human immunodeficiency virus: Infectivity and mechanisms of pathogenesis. Science 1988; 239:617–622.
5. Blaser MJ, Cohn DL. Opportunistic infections in patients with AIDS: Clues to the epidemiology of AIDS and the relative virulence of pathogens. Rev Infect Dis 1986;8:21.
6. Kanki PJ, Alroy J, Essex M. Isolation of a T-lymphotropic retrovirus related to HTLV-III/LAV from wild-caught African green monkeys. Science 1985; 230:951–954.
7. Kanki PJ, Barin F, M'Boup S, Allan JS, Romet-Lemonne JL, Marlink R, et al. New human T-cell retrovirus related to simian T-lymphotropic

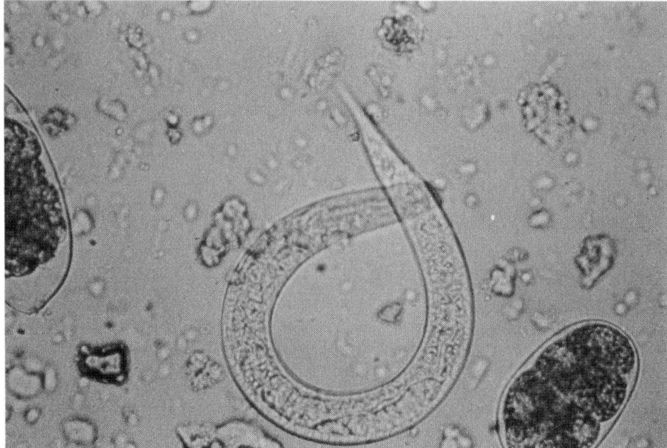

FIGURE 2–45. *Strongyloides stercoralis*
S. stercoralis—rhabditiform larvae on stool specimen.

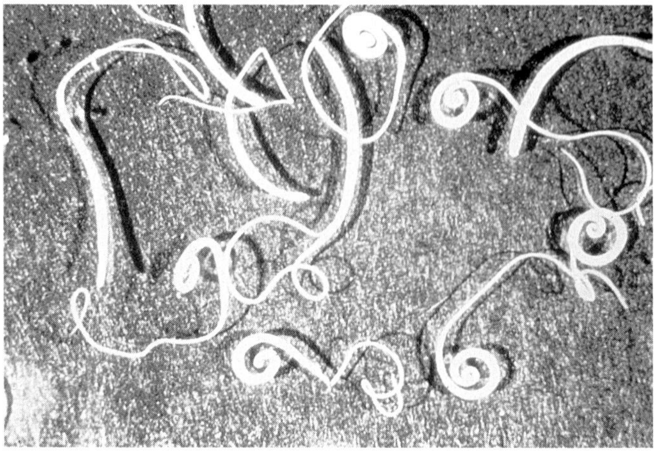

FIGURE 2–46. *Trichuris*
Trichuris (whipworm) from stool specimen.

virus type III ($STLV-III_{AGM}$). Science 1986;232:238–243.
8. Letvin NL, Daniel MD, Sehgal PK, Desrosiers RC, Hunt IM, Waldron JJ, et al. Induction of AIDS-like disease in macaque monkeys with T-cell tropic retrovirus STLV-III. Science 1985;230:71–73.
9. Sonigo P, Alizon M, Staskus K, Klatzman D, Cole S, Danos D, et al. Nucleotide sequence of the visna lentivirus: Relationship to the AIDS virus. Cell 1985;42:369–382.
10. Weiss R, Teich N, Varmus H, Coffin J, eds. The molecular biology of tumor viruses. 2d ed. RNA tumor viruses. Cold Spring Harbor, NY: Cold Spring Harbor Laboratory; 1987.
11. Ratner L, Haseltine W, Patarca R, Livak KJ, Starcich B, Josephs SF, et al. Complete nucleotide sequence of the AIDS virus, HTLV-III. Nature 1985;313:277–284.
12. Sanchez-Pescador R, Power MD, Barr PJ, Steiner KS, Stempien MM, et al. Nucleotide sequence and expression of an AIDS-associated retrovirus (ARV-2). Science 1985;227:484–492.
13. Wain-Hobson S, Sonigo P, Danos O, Cole S, Alizon M. Nucleotide sequence of the AIDS virus, LAV. Cell 1985;40:9–17.
14. Meusing MA, Smith DH, Cabradilla CD, Benton CV, Lasky LA, Capon DJ. Nucleic acid structure and expression of the human AIDS/lymphadenopathy retrovirus. Nature 1985;313:450–457.
15. Coffin JM. Genetic variation in AIDS viruses. Background paper. Washington, DC: Committee on a National Strategy for AIDS; 1986.
16. Dowbenko D, Bell J, Benton C, Groopman J, Nguyen H, Vetterlein D, et al. Bacterial expression of the AIDS retrovirus p24 GAG protein and its use as a diagnostic reagent. Proc Natl Acad Sci U S A 1985; 82:7748–7752.
17. Sodroski JG, Rosen C, Haseltine WA. Trans-activating transcriptional activation of the long terminal repeat of human T-lymphotropic virus in infected cells. Science 1984;225:381–385.
18. Sodroski JG, Goh WC, Rosen C, Tartar A, Portetella D, Burny A, et al. Replicative and cytopathic potential of HTLV-III/LAV with *sor* gene deletions. Science 1986;231:1549–1553.
19. Allan JS, Coligan JE, Lee TH, McCane MF, Kanki PJ, Groopman JE, et al. A new HTLV-III/LAV encoded antigen detected by antibodies from AIDS patients. Science 1985;230:810–813.
20. Lee TH, Coligan JE, Allan JS, McLane MF, Groopman JE, Essex M. A new HTLV-III/LAV protein encoded by a gene found in cytopathic retroviruses. Science 1985;236:1546–1549.
21. Fisher AG, Feinberg MB, Josephs SF, Harper ME, Marselle IM, Broder S, et al. Infectious mutants of HTLV-III with changes in the 3′ region and markedly reduced cytopathic effects. Science 1986;233:655–659.
22. Harper ME, Marsell LM, Gallo RC, et al. Detection of HTLV-III–infected lymphocytes in lymph nodes and peripheral blood from AIDS patients by in situ hybridization. Proc Natl Acad Sci U S A 1986;83:772–776.
23. Salahuddin Z, Rose RM, Groopman JE, et al. Human alveolar macrophages: One of the possible reservoirs of HTLV-III. Blood 1986;68:281–284.
24. Gartner S, Markovits P, Markovitz DM, Betts RF, Popovic M. Virus isolation from and identification of HTLV-III/LAV–producing cells in brain tissue from a patient with AIDS. JAMA 1986;256:2365–2371.
25. Dalgleish AG, Beverley PCL, Clapham PR, Crawford DH, Greaves MF, Weiss RA. The CD4 (T4) antigen is an essential component antigen of the receptor for the AIDS retrovirus. Nature 1984;312:763–767.
26. Klatzmann D, Barre-Sinoussi F, Nugeyre MT, et al. Selective tropism of lymphadenopathy associated virus (LAV) for helper-inducer T lymphocytes. Science 1984;225:59–63.
27. Folks T, Powell DM, Lightfoote MM, Benn S, Martin MA, Fauci AS. Induction of HTLV-III/LAV from a nonvirus-producing T-cell line: Implications for latency. Science 1986; 231:600–602.
28. Zagury D, Bernard J, Leonard R, Cheynier R, Feldman M, Sarin PS, et al. Immune induction of T cell death in long term culture of HTLV-III infected T cells: A cytopathogenic model for AIDS T-cell depletion. Science 1986;231:850–853.
29. Sodroski J, Goh WC, Rosen C, Campbell K, Haseltine WA. Role of HTLV-III/LAV envelope in syncytium formation and cytopathicity. Nature 1986;322:470–474.
30. Bowen DL, Lane HC, Fauci AS. Immunopathogenesis of the acquired immunodeficiency syndrome. Ann Intern Med 1985;103:704–709.
31. Lane HC, Depper JM, Greene WC, Whalen G, Waldmann TA, Fauci AS. Qualitative analysis of immune function in patients with the acquired immunodeficiency syndrome: Evidence for a selective defect in soluble antigen recognition. N Engl J Med 1985; 313:79–84.
32. Parks WP, Scott GB. An overview of pediatric AIDS: Approaches to diagnosis and outcome assessment. Background paper. Washington, DC: Committee on a National Strategy for AIDS; 1986.
33. Mintz M. Neurologic abnormalities. In: Yogev R, Connor EM, eds. Management of HIV Infection in Infants and Children. St. Louis: Mosby–Year Book; 1992:247–285.
34. Centers for Disease Control. 1993 revised classification system for HIV infection and expanded surveillance case definition for AIDS among adolescents and adults. MMWR 1992; 41(RR-17):1–19.
35. Centers for Disease Control. Guidelines for the performance of $CD4^+$ T-cell determinations in persons with human immunodeficiency virus infection. MMWR 1992;41(RR-8):1–17.
36. National Institutes of Health. The impact of routine HTLV-III antibody testing of blood and plasma on public health. Draft report of a consensus conference. Bethesda, Md, July 7–9, 1986.
37. Eyster ME, Goedert JJ, Sarngadharan MG, et al. Development and early natural history of HTLV-III antibodies in persons with hemophilia. JAMA 1985;253:2219–2223.
38. Sandstrom EG, Schooley RT, Ho DD, et al. Detection of human anti–HTLV-III antibodies by indirect immunofluorescense using fixed cells. Transfusion 1985;25:308–312.
39. Mortimer PP, Parry JV, Mortimer JY. Which anti–HTLV-III/LAV assays for screening and confirmatory testing? Lancet 1985;2:873–877.
40. Lange JMA, Coutinho RA, Krone WJA, Verdonck LF, Danner SA, van der Noordaa J, et al. Distinct IgG recognition patterns during progression of subclinical and clinical infection with LAV/HTLV-III. BMJ 1985; 292:228–230.
41. Goudsmit J, de Wolf F, Paul DA, et al. Expression of human immunodeficiency virus antigen (HIV-Ag) in serum and cerebro-spinal fluid during acute and chronic infection. Lancet 1986;11:177–180.
42. Ou CY, Kowk S, Mitchell S, Mack DH, Sninsky JJ, Krebs JW, Feorino P, Warfield D, Schochetman G. DNA amplification for direct detection of HIV-1 in DNA of peripheral blood mononuclear cells. Science 1988; 239:296–299.
43. Margan J, Tate R, Farr AD, Urbaniak SJ. Potential source of errors in HTLV-III antibody testing (letter). Lancet 1986;1:739–740.
44. Barr A, Dow BC, Arnott J, Crawford RS, Mitchell R. Anti–HTLV-III screening specificity and sensitivity (letter). Lancet 1986;1:1032.
45. Saag MS, Britz J. Asymptomatic blood donor with false positive HTLV-III Western blot (letter). N Engl J Med 1986;314:118.
46. Francis DP, Jaffe WH, Fultz PN, Getchell JP, McDougal JS, Feorino PM. The natural history of infection with the lymphadenopathy-associated virus human T-lymphotropic virus type III. Ann Intern Med 1985; 103:719–722.
47. Schnittman SM, Greenhouse JJ, Psallidopoulos MC, et al. Increasing viral burden in $CD4^+$ cells from patients with human immunodeficiency virus (HIV) infection reflects rapidly progressive immunosuppression and clinical disease. Ann Intern Med 1990;11:438–443.
48. Salahuddin SZ, Groopman JE, Markham PD, et al. HTLV-III in symptom-free seronegative persons. Lancet 1984;2:1418–1420.

49. Mayer KH, Stoddard AM, McCusker J, Ayotte D, Ferriani R, Groopman JE. Human T-lymphotropic virus type III in high-risk, antibody-negative homosexual men. Ann Intern Med 1986;104:194–196.
50. Cooper DA, Gold J, Maclean P, Donovan B, Finlayson R, Barnes TG, et al. Acute AIDS retrovirus infection: Definition of a clinical illness associated with seroconversion. Lancet 1985; 1:537–540.
51. Ho DD, Sarngadharan MG, Resnick L, et al. Primary human T-lymphotropic virus type III infection. Ann Intern Med 1985;103:880–883.
52. Curran JW, Meade Morgan W, Hardy AM, Jaffe HW, Darrow WW, Dowdle WR. The epidemiology of AIDS: Current status and future prospects. Science 1985;229:1352–1357.
53. Weiss RA. How does HIV cause AIDS? Science 1993;260:1273–1279.
54. Buchbinder S, Hessol N, O'Malley P, et al. HIV disease progression and the impact of prophylactic therapies in the San Francisco City Clinic Cohort: A 13-year follow-up. VII International Conference of AIDS. Vol. 2. Florence, Italy, June 16–21, 1991.
55. Mathur-Wagh U, Enlow RW, Spigland I, et al. Longitudinal study of persistent generalized lymphadenopathy in homosexual men: Relation to the acquired immunodeficiency syndrome. Lancet 1984;1:1033–1038.
56. Abrams DI, Mess TP, Volberding P. Lymphadenopathy: Update of a 40-month prospective study. Report presented at the International Conference on AIDS, Atlanta, Ga, April 15, 1985.
57. Goedert JJ, Biggar RJ, Weiss SH, et al. Three year incidence of AIDS among HTLV-III infected risk group members: A comparison of five cohorts. Science 1986;231:992–995.
58. Klein RS, Harris CA, Small CB, Moll B, Lesser M, Friedland GH. Oral candidiasis in high risk patients as the initial manifestation of the acquired immunodeficiency syndrome. N Engl J Med 1984;311:354–358.
59. Hughes WT: *Pneumocystis carinii* pneumonia. N Engl J Med 1977; 297:1381.
59. Phair J, Munoz A, Detels R, Kaslow R, Rinaldo C, Saah A. The risk of *Pneumocystis carinii* pneumonia among men infected with human immunodeficiency virus type 1. N Engl J Med 1990;322:161–165.
60. Hessol NA, Buchbinder SP. Predictors of HIV disease progression in the era of prophylactic therapies. In: Volberding P, Jacobson MA, eds. AIDS Clinical Review 1992. New York: Marcel Dekker; 1992:25–40.
61. Centers for Disease Control and Prevention. Guidelines for prophylaxis against *Pneumocystis carinii* pneumonia for persons infected with HIV. MMWR 1989;38:1–9.
62. Khadem M, Kalish SB, Goldsmith J, et al. Ophthalmologic findings in acquired immune deficiency syndrome (AIDS). Arch Ophthalmol 1984; 102:201.
63. Chalvardjian AM, Graw LA. A new procedure for the identification of *Pneumocystis carinii* cysts in tissue sections and smears. J Clin Pathol 1963;16:383.
64. Murray JF, Felton CP, Garay SM, et al. Pulmonary complications of the acquired immunodeficiency syndrome. Report of National Heart, Lung, and Blood Institute Workshop. N Engl J Med 1984;310:1682.
65. Kovacs JA, Hiemenz JW, Macher AM, et al. *Pneumocystis carinii* pneumonia: A comparison between patients with the acquired immunodeficiency syndrome and patients with other immunodeficiencies. Ann Intern Med 1984;100:663.
66. Blumenfeld W, Wager E, Hadley WK. Use of the transbronchial biopsy for diagnosis of opportunistic pulmonary infections in acquired immunodeficiency syndrome (AIDS). Am J Clin Pathol 1984;81:1.
67. Coleman DL, Dodek PM, Luce JM, et al. Diagnosis utility of fiberoptic bronchoscopy in patients with *Pneumocystis carinii* pneumonia and the acquired immunodeficiency syndrome. Am Rev Respir Dis 1983; 128:795.
68. Broaddus C, Dake MD, Stulbarg MS, Blumenfeld W, Hadley K, Golden JA, et al. Bronchoalveolar lavage and transbronchial biopsy for the diagnosis of pulmonary infections in the acquired immunodeficiency syndrome. Ann Intern Med 1985;102:747–752.
69. Bigby TD, Margolskee D, Curtis JL, Michael PF, Sheppard D, Hadley WK, et al. The usefulness of induced sputum in the diagnosis of *Pneumocystis carinii* pneumonia in patients with the acquired immunodeficiency syndrome. Am Rev Respir Dis 1986; 133:515–518.
70. Gordin FM, Simon GL, Wofsy CB, Mills J. Adverse reactions to trimethoprim-sulfamethoxazole in patients with AIDS. Ann Intern Med 1984; 100:495–499.
71. Haverkos HW. Assessment of therapy for *Pneumocystis carinii* pneumonia. Am J Med 1984;76:501–508.
72. Hughes WT, Smith BC. Efficiency of diaminodiphenylsulfone and other drugs in murine *Pneumocystis carinii* pneumonia. Antimicrob Agents Chemother 1984;26:436.
73. Safrin S. New developments in the management of *Pneumocystis carinii* disease. In: Volberding P, Jacobson MA, eds. AIDS Clinical Review 1992. New York: Marcel Dekker; 1992:95–112.
74. Bozzette SA, Sattler FR, Chiu J. A controlled trial of early adjunctive treatment with corticosteroids for *Pneumocystis carinii* pneumonia in the acquired immunodeficiency syndrome. N Engl J Med 1990; 323:1451–1457.
75. NIH–University of California Expert Panel for Corticosteroids as Adjunctive Therapy for PCP. Special report: Consensus statement on the use of corticosteroids as adjunctive therapy for *Pneumocystis* pneumonia in the acquired immunodeficiency syndrome. N Engl J Med 1990; 323:1500–1504.
77. Wong G, Gold JWM, Brown AE, et al. Central nervous system toxoplasmosis in homosexual men and parenteral drug abusers. Ann Intern Med 1984;100:36.
78. Luft BJ, Brooks RG, Conley FK, et al. Toxoplasmosis encephalitis in patients with acquired immune deficiency syndrome. JAMA 1984; 252:913.
79. Whelan MA, Kricheff II, Handler M, et al. Acquired immunodeficiency syndrome: Cerebral computed tomographic manifestations. Radiology 1983;149:477.
80. Mariuz PR, Benjamin JL. Toxoplasmic encephalitis. In: Volberding P, Jacobson MA, eds. AIDS Clinical Review 1992. New York: Marcel Dekker; 1992:105–130.
81. Current WL, Reese NC, Ernst JC, et al. Human cryptosporidiosis in immunocompetent and immunodeficient persons. N Engl J Med 1983; 308:1252.
82. Smith P, Lane H, Gill V, Manishewitz J, Quinnian G, Fauci A, Masur H. Intestinal infections in patients with the acquired immunodeficiency syndrome (AIDS). Ann Intern Med 1988;108:328–333.
83. Rodgers V, Fassett R, Kagnoff M. Abnormalities in intestinal mucosal T-cells in homosexual populations including those with the lymphadenopathy syndrome and acquired immunodeficiency syndrome. Gastroenterology 1986;90:552–558.
84. Soave R, Danner RL, Honig CL, Ma P, Hart CC, Nash T, et al. Cryptosporidiosis in homosexual men. Ann Intern Med 1984;100:504–511.
85. Margulis SJ, Honig CL, Soave R, Govoni AF, Mouradian JA, Jacobson IM. Biliary tract obstruction in the acquired immunodeficiency syndrome. Ann Intern Med 1986; 105:207–210.
86. Ma P, Soave R. Three-step stool examination with protracted watery diarrhea. J Infect Dis 1983;147:824.
87. Portnoy D, Whiteside ME, Bukley E, et al. Treatment of intestinal cryptosporidiosis with spiramycin. Ann Intern Med 1984;101:202.
88. Collier AC, Miller RA, Meyers JD. Cryptosporidiosis after marrow transplantation: Person-to-person transmission and treatment with spiramycin. Ann Intern Med 1984;101:205–206.
89. Rolston K, Fainstein V, Mansell P, Sjoerdsma A, Bodey GP. Alpha-di-

fluoromethylornithine (DFMO) in the treatment of cryptosporidiosis in AIDS patients: Preliminary evaluation. Abstracts of the International Conference on AIDS, Atlanta, Ga, April 14–17, 1985:77.
90. Blanshard C, et al. Azithromycin, paromomycin and letrazuril in the treatment of cryptosporidiosis. Abstract P28 of the Third European Conference on Clinical Aspects and Treatment of HIV Infection, Paris, 1992.
91. Marshall RJ, Flanigan TP. Paromomycin inhibits cryptosporidium infection of a human enterocyte cell line. J Infect Dis 1992;165:772–774.
92. Westerman EL, Christensen RP. Chronic *Isospora belli* infection treated with co-trimoxazole. Ann Intern Med 1979;91:413–414.
93. Dieterich D, et al. Treatment with albendazole for intestinal disease due to *Enterocytozoon bieneusi* in patients with AIDS. J Infect Dis 1994; 169:178–183.
94. Watson RR, ed. Nutrition and AIDS. Boca Raton, Fla: CRC Press; 1994.
95. Berenguer J, Moreno S, Carcenado E, Bernaldo de Quines JCL, Garcia de la Fuente A, Bouza E. Visceral leishmaniasis in patients infected with human immunodeficiency virus. Ann Intern Med 1989;111:129–132.
96. Sendino A, Barbado FJ, Mastaza JM, Fernandez-Martin J, Larrauri J, Vasquez-Rodriguez JJ. Visceral leishmaniasis with malabsorption syndrome in a patient with acquired immunodeficiency syndrome. Am J Med 1990;89:673–675.
97. Fillola G, Corberand JX, Laharraque PF, Lavenes H, Massip P, Recco P. Peripheral intramonocytic leishmaniasis in an AIDS patient. J Clin Microbiol 1992;30:3284–3285.
98. Badaro R, Falcoff E, Badaro FS, Carvalho EM, Pedral-Sampaio D, Barral A, et al. Treatment of visceral leishmaniasis with pentavalent antimony and interferon gamma. N Engl J Med 1990;322:16–21.
99. Imam N, Carpenter CCJ, Mayer KH, Fisher A, Stein M, Danforth SB. Hierarchical pattern of mucosal *Candida* infections in HIV seropositive women. Am J Med 1990;89:142–146.
100. Zuger A, Louie E, Holtzman RS, Simberkoff MS, Rahal JJ. Cryptococcal disease in patients with acquired immunodeficiency syndrome. Ann Intern Med 1986;104:234–240.
101. Kovacs JA, Polis M, Macher AM, et al. Cryptococcus infections in patients with acquired immunodeficiency syndrome (abstract 804). Abstracts of the 24th ICAAC. Washington, DC: American Society for Microbiology; 1984.
102. Powderly WG. New developments in the treatment of cryptococcal disease in AIDS. In: Volberding P, Jacobson MA, eds. AIDS Clinical Review 1992. New York: Marcel Dekker; 1992: 113–128.
103. Hawkins CC, Gold JWM, Whimbey E, Kiehn TE, Brannon P, Cammarata R, et al. *Mycobacterium avium* complex infections in patients with the acquired immunodeficiency syndrome. Ann Intern Med 1986; 105:184–188.
104. Greene JB, Sidhu GS, Lewin S, et al. *Mycobacterium avium-intracellulare:* A cause of disseminated life-threatening infection in homosexuals and drug abusers. Ann Intern Med 1982; 97:539.
105. Zakowski P, Fligiel S, Berlin GW, et al. Disseminated *Mycobacterium avium-intracellulare* in homosexual men dying of acquired immunodeficiency. JAMA 1982;248:2980.
106. Sohn CC, Schoroff RW, Kliewer KE, et al. Disseminated *Mycobacterium avium-intracellulare* infection in homosexual men with acquired cell-mediated immunodeficiency: A histologic and immunologic study of two cases. Am J Clin Pathol 1983;79:247.
107. Gillin JS, Urmacher C, West R, et al. Disseminated *Mycobacterium avium-intracellulare* infection in acquired immunodeficiency syndrome mimicking Whipple's disease. Gastroenterology 1983;85:1187.
108. Inderlied CB, Kemper CA. Disseminated *Mycobacterium avium* complex infection. In: Volberding P, Jacobson MA, eds. AIDS Clinical Review 1992. New York: Marcel Dekker; 1992: 131–172.
109. Woodley CL, Kilburn JO. In vitro susceptibility of *Mycobacterium avium* complex and *Mycobacterium tuberculosis* strains to a spiropiperidyl rifamycin. Am Rev Respir Dis 1982;126:586.
110. Wu M, Kolonoski PT, Yadegar S, Inderlied CB, Young LS. In vitro susceptibility of *Mycobacterium avium* complex (MAC) to novel antimycobacterial drugs. Program and Abstracts of the 26th Interscience Conference on Antimicrobial Agents and Chemotherapy, New Orleans, La, September 28–October 1, 1986:1102.
111. Pitchenik AE, Cole C, Russell BW, Fischl MA, Spira TJ, Snider DE. Tuberculosis, atypical mycobacteriosis and the acquired immunodeficiency syndrome among Haitian and non-Haitian patients in south Florida. Ann Intern Med 1984;101:641–654.
112. Johnson MP, Chaisson RE. Tuberculosis and HIV disease. In: Volberding P, Jacobson MA, eds. AIDS Clinical Review 1992. New York: Marcel Dekker; 1992:73–93.
113. Relman DA. Bacillary angiomatosis and *Rochalimaea* species. In: Remington JS, Swartz MN, eds. Current Clinical Topics in Infectious Diseases. Boston: Blackwell Scientific Publications; 1994.
114. Glaser JB, Morton-Kute L, Berger SR, Weber J, Siegel FP, Lopez C, et al. Recurrent *Salmonella typhimurium* bacteremia associated with the acquired immunodeficiency syndrome. Ann Intern Med 1985; 102:189–193.
115. Mayer KH, Hanson E. Recurrent salmonella infection with a single strain in the acquired immunodeficiency syndrome: Confirmation by plasmid fingerprinting. Diagn Microbiol Infect Dis 1986;4:71.
116. Perlman D, Ampel N, Schifman R, Cohn D, Patton C, Aquire M, Wang W, Blaser M. Persistent *Campylobacter jejuni* infections in patients with HIV. Ann Intern Med 1988; 108:540–546.
117. Siegal FP, Lopez C, Hammer GS, et al. Severe acquired immunodeficiency in male homosexuals manifested by chronic perianal ulcerative herpes simplex lesions. N Engl J Med 1981; 305:1439.
118. Quinnan GV, Masur H, Rook AH, et al. Herpesvirus infections in the acquired immunodeficiency syndrome. JAMA 1984;252:72.
119. Jacobson MA. Foscarnet therapy for AIDS-related opportunistic herpesvirus infections. In: Volberding P, Jacobson MA, eds. AIDS Clinical Review 1992. New York: Marcel Dekker; 1992:173–189.
120. Epstein E: Acyclovir for immunocompromised patients with herpes zoster. N Engl J Med 1983;309:1254.
121. Mintz L, Drew WL, Miner RC, et al. Cytomegalovirus infections in homosexual men. Ann Intern Med 1983; 99:326.
122. Macher AM, Reichert CM, Straus SE, et al. Death in the AIDS patient: Role of cytomegalovirus. N Engl J Med 1983;309:1454.
123. Knapp AB, Horst DA, Eliopoulos G, et al. Widespread cytomegalovirus gastroenterocolitis in a patient with the acquired immunodeficiency syndrome. Gastroenterology 1983; 85:1399.
124. Bachman DM, Rodrigues MM, Chu FC, et al. Culture-proven cytomegalovirus retinitis in a homosexual man with the acquired immunodeficiency syndrome. Ophthalmology 1982; 89:797.
125. Laurence J. AIDS Report: CMV infections in AIDS patients. Infections in Surgery 1986;7:603–610.
126. Tapper ML, Rotterdam HZ, Lerner CW, et al. Adrenal necrosis in the acquired immunodeficiency syndrome. Ann Intern Med 1984;100:239–241.
127. Masur H, Lane HC, Palestine A, et al. Effect of 9-(1,3-dihydroxy-2-propoxymethyl) guanine on serious cytomegalovirus disease in eight immunosuppressed homosexual men. Ann Intern Med 1986;104:41–44.
128. Koretz SH, Buhler WC, Brewin A, et al. Treatment of serious cytomegalovirus infection with 9-(1,3-dihydroxy-2-propoxymethyl) guanine in patients with AIDS and other immunodeficiences. N Engl J Med 1986; 314:801–805.

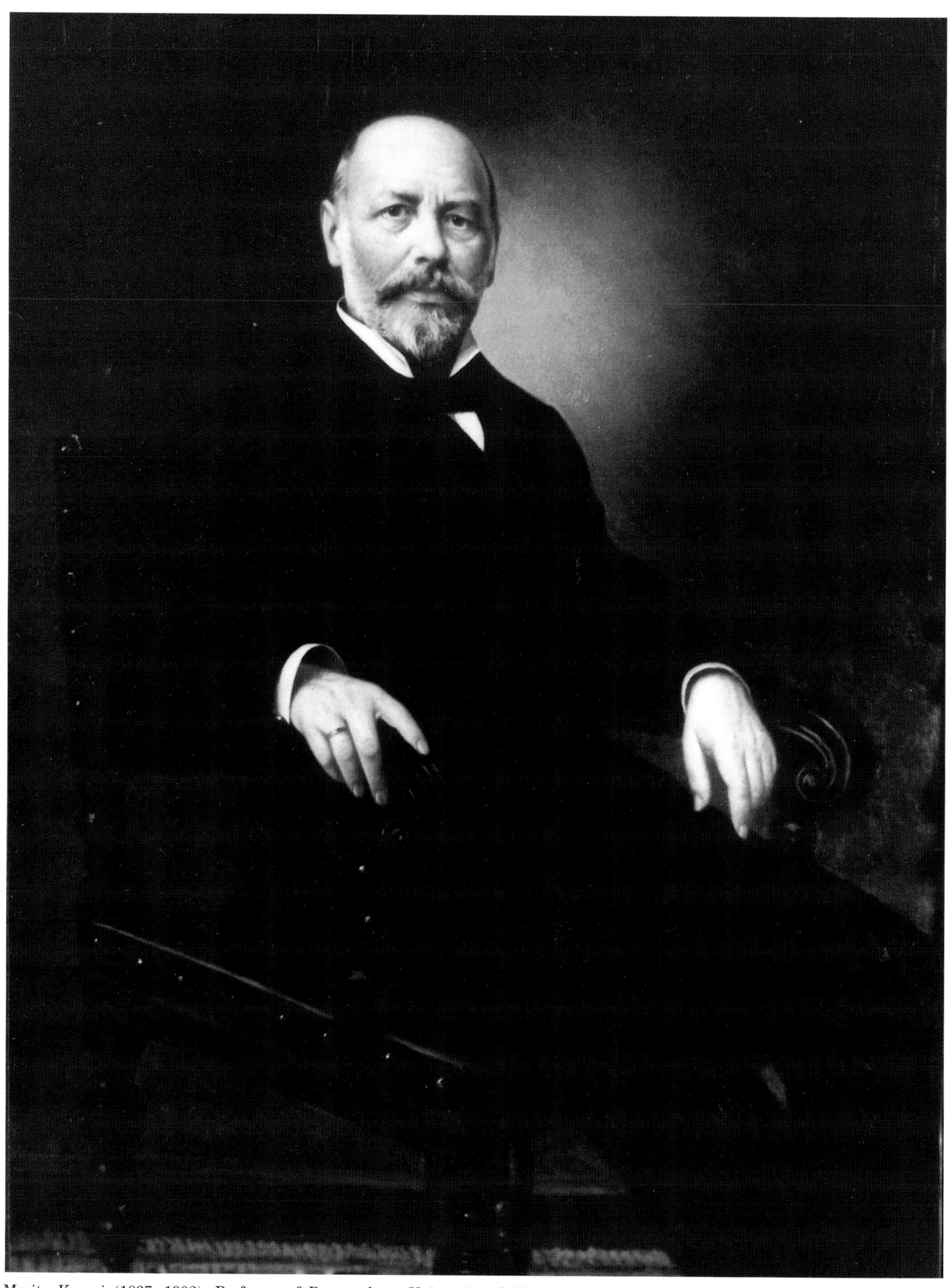

Moritz Kaposi (1837–1902), Professor of Dermatology, University of Vienna. (Courtesy of Professor Klaus Wolff, Department of Dermatology, University of Vienna, Vienna, Austria.)

CLINICAL MANIFESTATIONS AND HISTOPATHOLOGIC FEATURES OF CLASSIC, ENDEMIC AFRICAN, AND EPIDEMIC AIDS-ASSOCIATED KAPOSI'S SARCOMA

Aby Buchbinder
Yao-Qi Huang
Clay J. Cockerell
Alvin E. Friedman-Kien

3

Kaposi's sarcoma (KS) is a neoplasm with protean manifestations whose etiology, pathogenesis, and epidemiology suggest the use of the term *opportunistic neoplasm.* The syndrome of "multiple idiopathic pigmented sarcoma of the skin," first described by Moritz Kaposi in 1872, remains the best clinical description of this tumor in all its forms; and the description of lower extremity lesions in elderly Jewish eastern European or Italian males still stands exact in its precision to this day.[1] The form of KS originally described by Kaposi, designated as *classic KS,* is now known to be only one of multiple heterogenous types of KS present in various patient populations.

In the 1930s, KS was described in young black males and prepubescent children in Africa, with clinical characteristics that differed from classic KS, and this condition was found to be endemic in regions of equatorial Africa.[2,3] In the 1960s, with the development of renal transplantation and the iatrogenic immunosuppression induced in transplant recipients, yet another form of highly aggressive KS was described.[4–7] It was in the early 1980s, however, that KS emerged as a prevalent condition in the United States and around the world. Simultaneous reports from New York and California described a disseminated and aggressive form of KS among young homosexual men.[8–11] Subsequently, this latter form of KS, designated *epidemic KS,* was found to be one of the manifestations of the acquired immunodeficiency syndrome (AIDS), and became one of the defining conditions of AIDS. More recently, a relatively benign form of KS not associated with the human immunodeficiency virus (HIV) or with AIDS was described in this same population of sexually active young homosexual men, prompting a reevaluation of the locution epidemic KS as a synonym for AIDS-associated KS.[12]

The occurrence of all the various forms of KS in well-defined populations; the epidemiologic features about the transmission of KS; the role of cytokines, growth factors, oncogenes, and viral factors in the etiology of KS; the hypothesis of its multifocal onset; the association with immune regulation disorders; and the increasing prevalence of KS have made this opportunistic neoplasm the subject of active study.

CLASSIC KAPOSI'S SARCOMA

(Figures 3–1 to 3–22)

As mentioned previously, classic KS is a slow-growing neoplasm that occurs mostly in elderly men of Mediterranean or Jewish eastern European descent.[13] The male to female ratio is 10–15:1, and the majority of patients are between 50 and 80 years old at the onset of the disease.[13,14] The lesions characteristically appear symmetrically in the lower extremities, often on the ankles and soles. The lesions have a tendency to develop first as patches, with plaque and nodular lesions appearing later in the course of the illness. The lesions of classic KS take the appearance of purplish to violaceous patches or confluent macules. Lesions may appear simultaneously at various sites and are thought to represent multifocal foci of disease. The lesions are not usually painful, and pruritus is absent (Table 3–1).

After a period of years, the lesions often progress in size and number, with the coalescence of old lesions and the appearance of new lesions locally or in other regions of the body. Edema, sometimes due to impairment of lymphatic drainage, is a frequent problem that may result in severe clinical symptoms such as pain, difficulties in walking, ulceration with resulting bleeding, and secondary infections. Infrequently, the tumor may invade locally, causing destruction of underlying subcutaneous tissues and, rarely, bones. The same symptoms may also appear in the absence of edema.

After prolonged periods of time, KS lesions may appear in other, often distant, regions including distal cutaneous sites as well as in internal visceral organs and lymph nodes. These sites are often asymptomatic and are discovered incidentally or at necropsy.[15] The course of the disease after symptomatic progression has occurred is often more aggressive and rapid, necessitating the initiation of therapy.

No associated condition has been described with classic KS; however, with time, one third of patients will develop another malignancy, most frequently an intermediate or aggressive non-Hodgkin's lymphoma.[16] Familial cases are rare.[2,17] The onset of these tumors may precede the onset of KS. A single report of the presence of retroviral-like electron microscopic particles in some of the KS lesions examined from a cohort of patients with the classic form of KS in the Greek Peloponnesus has been published.[18]

An association with human leukocyte antigen (HLA)-DR5 has been reported, however, without reporting the distribution of this HLA type in control populations of the same ethnic background.[19,20]

The presence of immunologic abnormalities in patients with classic KS has been described in some reports,[5,21–24] but the excess of second primary malignancies and the lack of geographic restriction in the well-defined populations in which the syndrome appears suggest that genetic, infectious, or immunologic factors rather than environmental factors need to be studied as possible contributing etiologic factors. Furthermore, it is interesting to note that other severe immunodeficiency states such as the Wiskott-Aldrich syndrome are not associated with KS, although they are associated with an increased incidence of lymphomas.[25]

The treatment for classic KS varies with the stage and the symptoms. Asymptomatic lesions are best left untreated. When local therapy is deemed to be sufficient for palliation of symptoms, cryotherapy, local excision, local radiation, laser therapy, electrocautery, curettage, and intralesional injection with chemotherapeutic agents are all possible options. When internal organ involvement with KS becomes symptomatic, when large mucocutaneous lesions require treatment, or when progressive dissemination occurs, systemic chemotherapy may be used. Active agents used singly or in combination include nitrogen mustard, 5-fluorouracil, cyclophosphamide, doxorubicin hydrochloride (Adriamycin), vincristine, vinblastine, etoposide, or interferon-α and may be used singly or in combination.[26,27] Patients survive for a median of 8 to 13 years; KS is the actual cause of death in patients with classic KS in approximately 20% of patients.[14,28]

Text continued on page 43

TABLE 3–1. CLINICAL CHARACTERISTICS OF KAPOSI'S SARCOMA VARIANTS

Type	Predominant Mucocutaneous Lesions	Mucocutaneous Distribution	Lymph Node Involvement	Visceral Involvement	Behavior
Classic	Some patches, mostly plaques and nodules usually rounded	Usually confined to lower extremities; disseminated lesions; late in course of disease	Rare	Sometimes	Indolent—gradual increase in number of lesions often associated with lymphedema; visceral lesions occur late, often discovered at autopsy; survival—10 to 15 years
Endemic African					
1. Benign nodular	Papules and nodules	Multiple localized tumors, most commonly seen on lower extremities	Rare	Rare	Indolent, resembles classic type disease; survival—8 to 10 years
2. Aggressive	Large exophytic nodules and fungating tumor	Most often located on the extremities	Rare	Sometimes	Progressive development of multiple lesions with invasion and destruction of underlying subcutaneous tissues and bone; survival—5 to 8 years
3. Florid	Nodules	Widely disseminated	Sometimes	Sometimes	Rapidly progressive; locally aggressive and invasive, early visceral involvement; survival—3 to 5 years
4. Lymphadenopathic	Rarely manifests lesions	Minimal	Always	Frequent	Rapidly progressive; survival—2 to 3 years
Iatrogenic immunosuppression	Patches, plaques, and nodules	Usually localized to the extremities; rarely disseminated	Rare	Sometimes	Indolent; occasional tumor regression after immunosuppressive therapy is discontinued
Epidemic (HIV-associated)	Patches, plaques, nodules; often fusiform and irregular	Multifocal, widely disseminated, often symmetric; frequent oral lesions	Frequent	Frequent	Rapidly progressive; survival—2 months to 5 years (median: 18 months)
Epidemic (HIV-negative)	Small nodules, patches or plaques	Multifocal, often on extremities	Rare	Rare	Indolent, appears to be more benign than classic type

Revised from Friedman-Kien AE, ed. Color Atlas of AIDS. Philadelphia: WB Saunders; 1989:44.

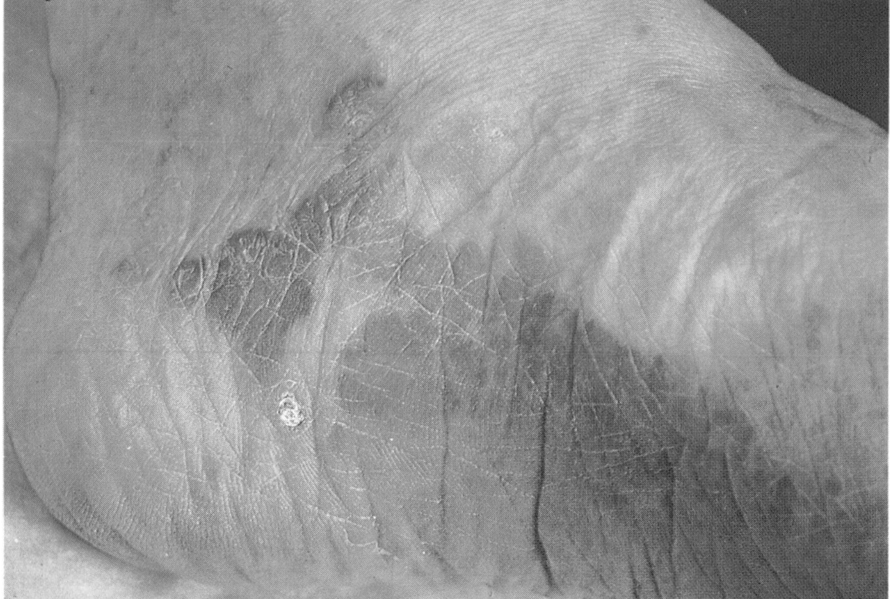

FIGURE 3–1. Classic Kaposi's sarcoma; patch stage
A 60-year-old man of eastern European origin with a large confluent pink patch-stage Kaposi's sarcoma lesion on the sole of the foot extending over the arch. This asymptomatic lesion had slowly increased in size over a 5-year period.

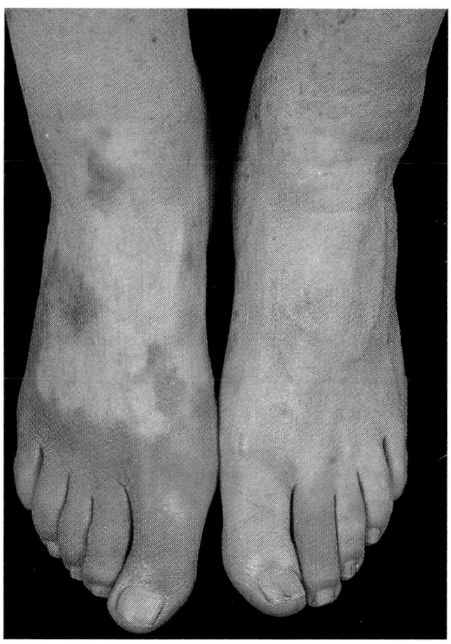

FIGURE 3–3. Classic Kaposi's sarcoma; patch stage
A large, asymptomatic, violaceous, flat, confluent lesion affecting all the toes of the left foot and several other macular lesions on the dorsum of the left foot and the right second toe. The lesions had been present for 4 years, gradually increasing in size and number.

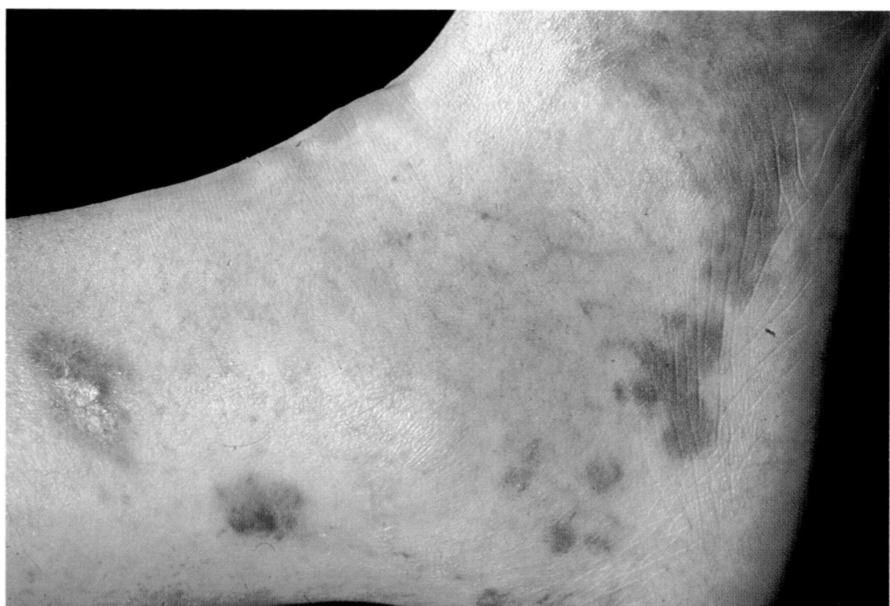

FIGURE 3–2. Classic Kaposi's sarcoma; patch stage
A 75-year-old Italian man with a large red-to-violet confluent flat lesion on the skin over the ankle with other macular and papular lesions developing on the lateral aspect of the foot.

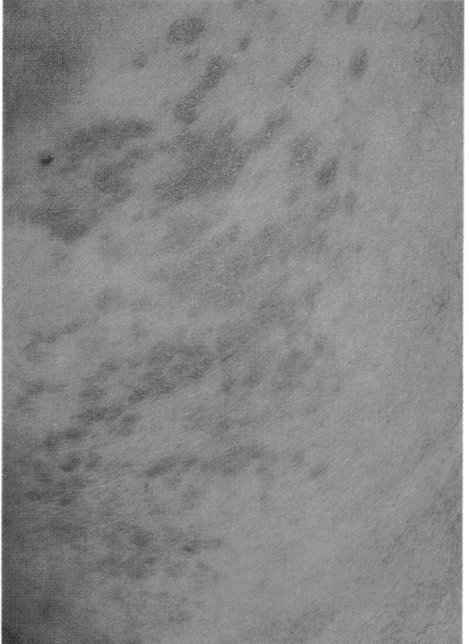

FIGURE 3–4. Classic Kaposi's sarcoma; patch-to-plaque stage
An 83-year-old man with Kaposi's sarcoma of several years' duration, who initially presented with lesions on the feet and slowly developed lesions on the lower legs and thighs. This close-up view of the upper thigh shows multiple small papules superimposed on confluent macular patch-stage lesions.

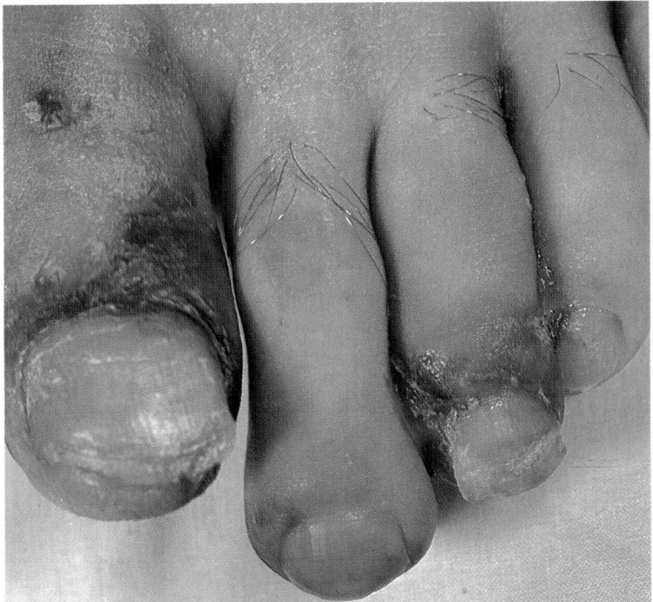

FIGURE 3–5. Classic Kaposi's sarcoma; plaque stage
Hyperpigmented purple indurated periungual lesions of Kaposi's sarcoma on the toes with some ulceration. These lesions could be mistaken for early gangrene, which can be seen in patients with peripheral vascular insufficiency.

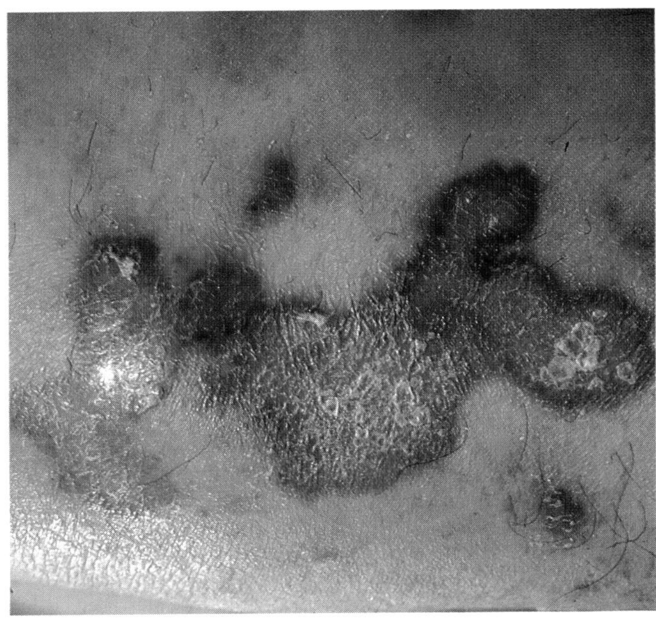

FIGURE 3–6. Classic Kaposi's sarcoma; plaque stage
Multiple, brown-to-purple serpiginous plaque-stage lesions of Kaposi's sarcoma with hyperpigmented borders, located on the lower extremity. Such lesions may occur in patients with long-standing disease.

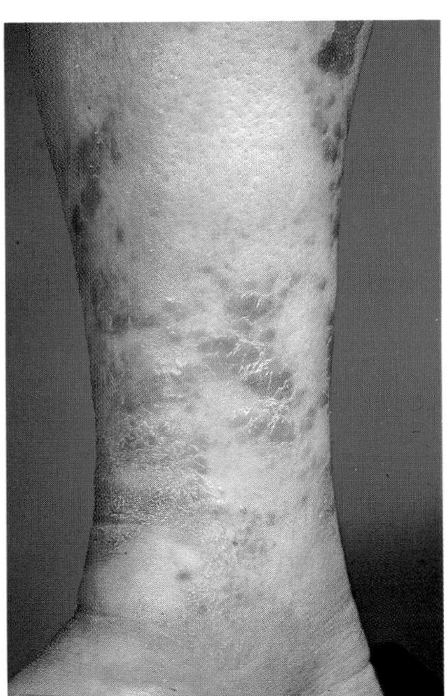

FIGURE 3–7. Classic Kaposi's sarcoma; plaque stage
Clusters of pink-to-violet plaque and papular tumors of long duration on the lower leg.

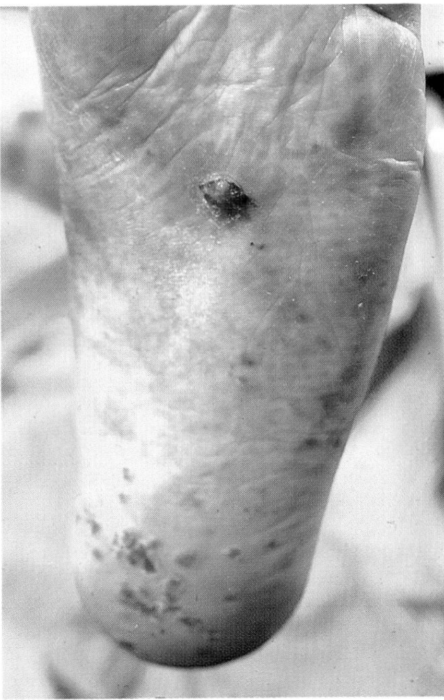

FIGURE 3–8. Classic Kaposi's sarcoma; nodular stage
There are multiple red and purple individual and clustered papular lesions of Kaposi's sarcoma on the heel of the foot. The isolated nodular tumor on the metatarsal region of the sole of the foot had been denuded following superficial trauma. Although these lesions look highly vascular, they do not bleed excessively when cut or bruised.

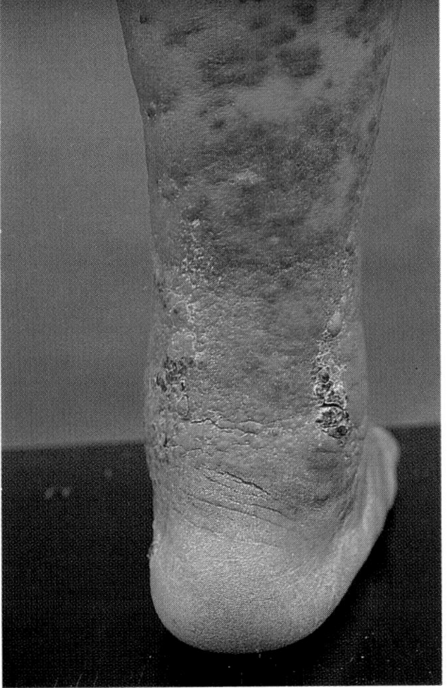

FIGURE 3–9. Classic Kaposi's sarcoma; plaque and nodular stage
Multiple pink-to-lavender plaques, papules, and nodules associated with chronic nonpitting edema. Some ulceration on the surface of tumor nodules is present on the ankle region.

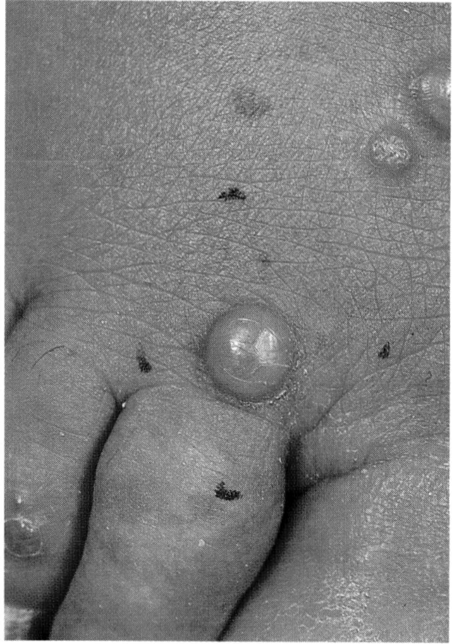

FIGURE 3–10. Classic Kaposi's sarcoma; nodular stage
Discrete, dome-shaped, pearly, opalescent nodules of Kaposi's sarcoma on the dorsum of the foot and the toes.

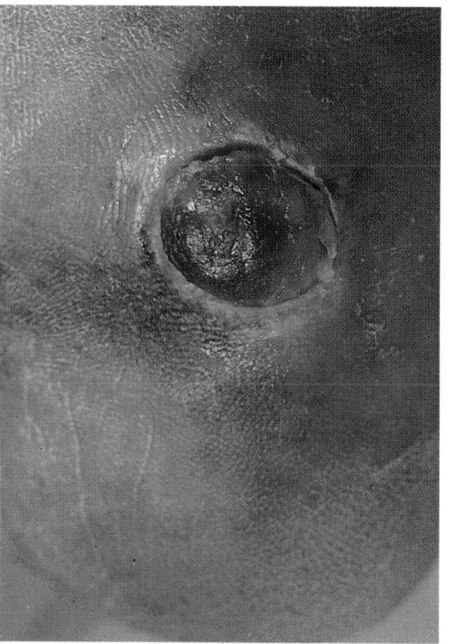

FIGURE 3–11. Classic Kaposi's sarcoma; nodular stage
A well-demarcated, round, nodular tumor on the sole of the foot near the lateral margin of the heel extruding through a collar of callous tissue. The surface of this tumor was denuded owing to friction while wearing shoes, a common complication seen with lesions in this location.

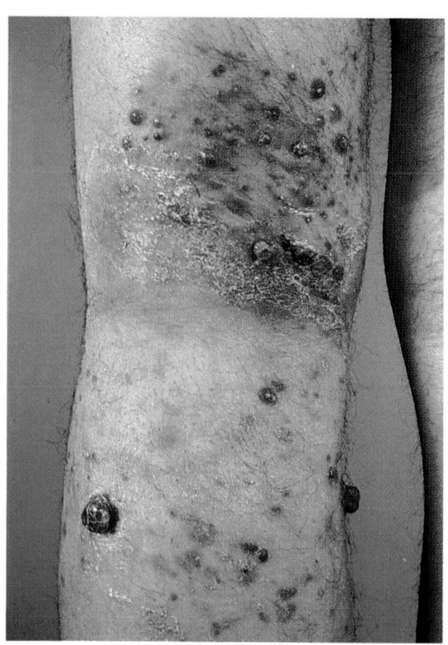

FIGURE 3–12. Classic Kaposi's sarcoma; nodular stage
Multiple deep purple to brown-black nodular tumors on the calf and popliteal fossa, associated with lymphedema.

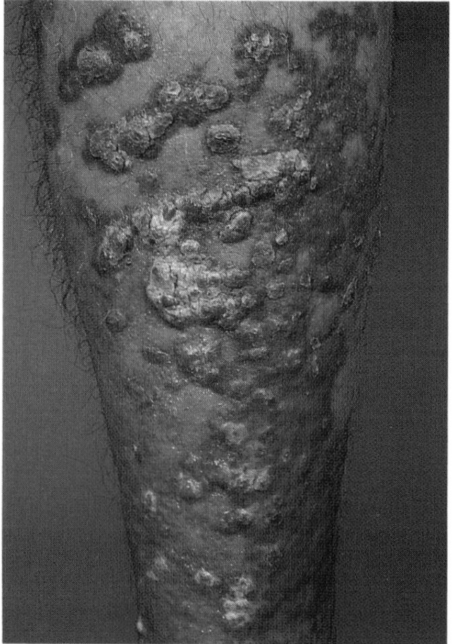

FIGURE 3–13. Classic Kaposi's sarcoma; nodular stage
Long-standing advanced disease on the lower extremity. Coalescing brown-to-violet plaque-to-nodular lesions of Kaposi's sarcoma with overlying adherent hyperkeratotic scales.

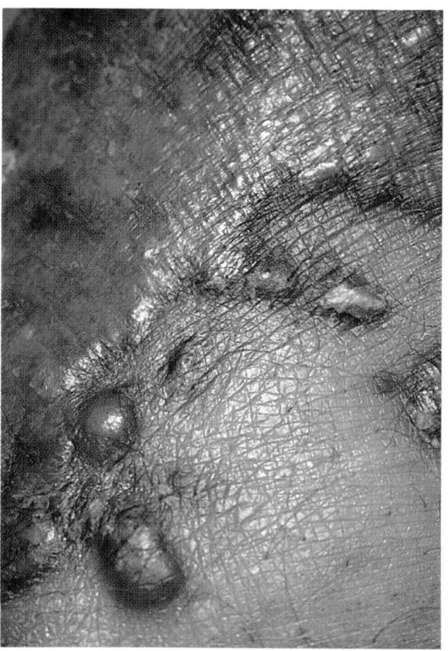

FIGURE 3–14. Classic Kaposi's sarcoma; nodular stage
A close-up view of a markedly indurated blue-to-purple plaque-stage lesion of Kaposi's sarcoma with well-demarcated border and evolving nodular elements.

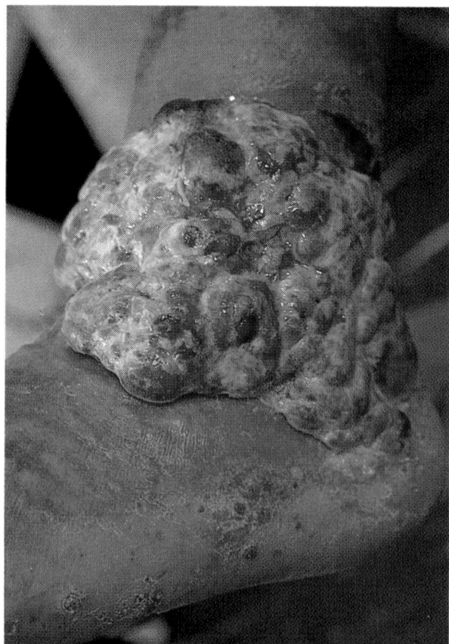

FIGURE 3–15. Classic Kaposi's sarcoma; nodular stage
A grumous, exophytic, fungating tumor of Kaposi's sarcoma on the ankle region of a patient who had his disease for 17 years. The local tumor invasion of the underlying subcutaneous muscle and bone observed in this case is unusual for the classic type of disease. The tumor regressed following local radiation treatment.

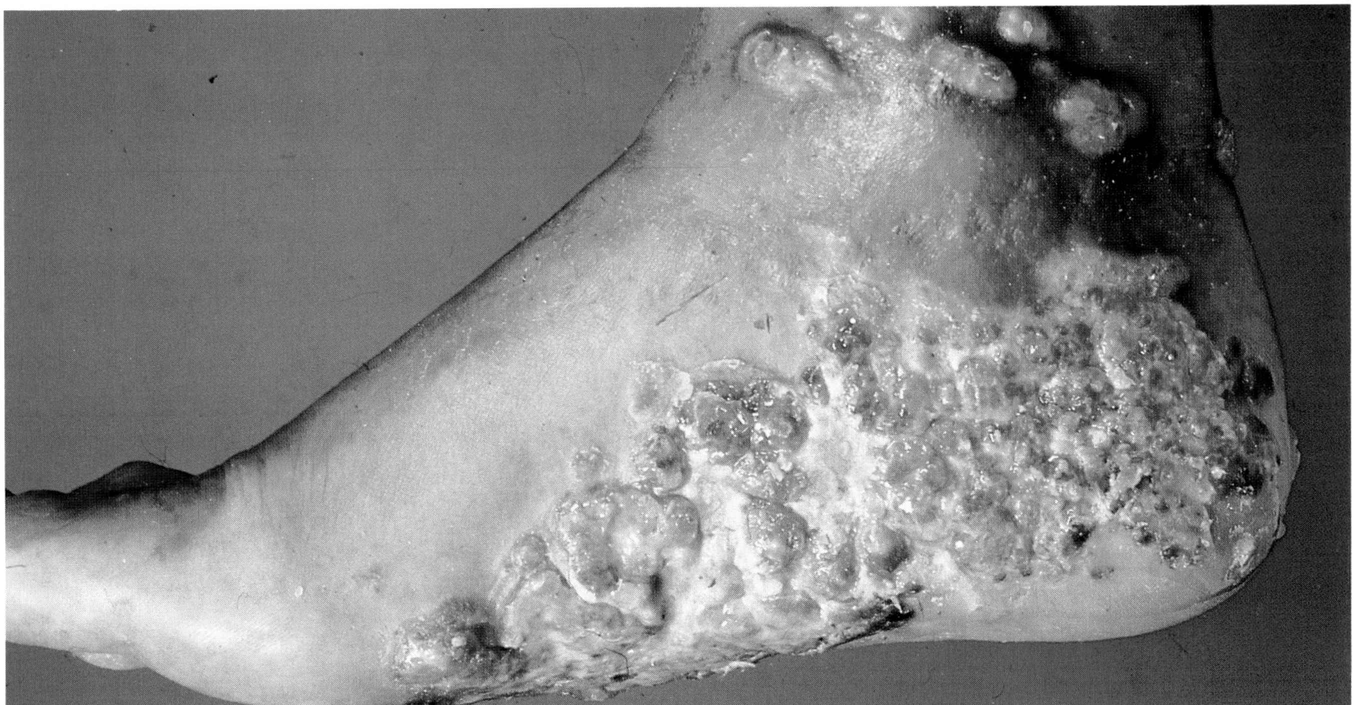

FIGURE 3–16. Classic Kaposi's sarcoma; nodular stage

A long-standing case of Kaposi's sarcoma affecting the lower extremity with ulceration of the tumor on the arch of the foot. There are rounded nodules extending over the ankle. These tumors responded very well to local radiation therapy.

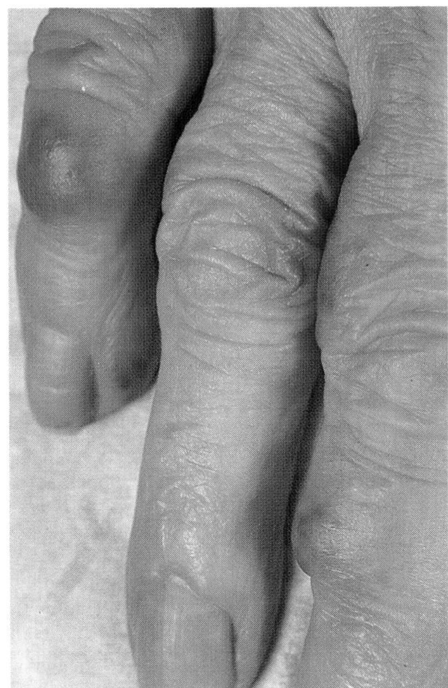

FIGURE 3–17. Classic Kaposi's sarcoma; nodular stage

Advanced, disseminated disease. Late-appearing, violet-colored nodular lesions of Kaposi's sarcoma on the fingers in a patient with disease on the lower extremities of several years' duration.

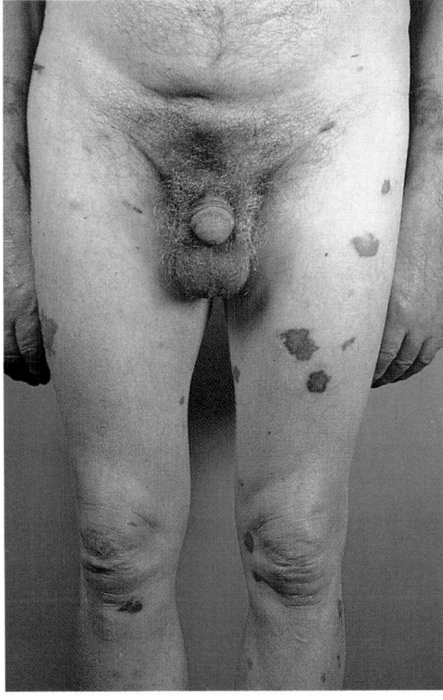

FIGURE 3–18. Classic Kaposi's sarcoma; plaque stage

An elderly Ashkenazic Jewish man who had Kaposi's sarcoma for 12 years with gradual development of multiple irregularly shaped, elevated plaque lesions ranging in color from red to deep purple, widely distributed over his body.

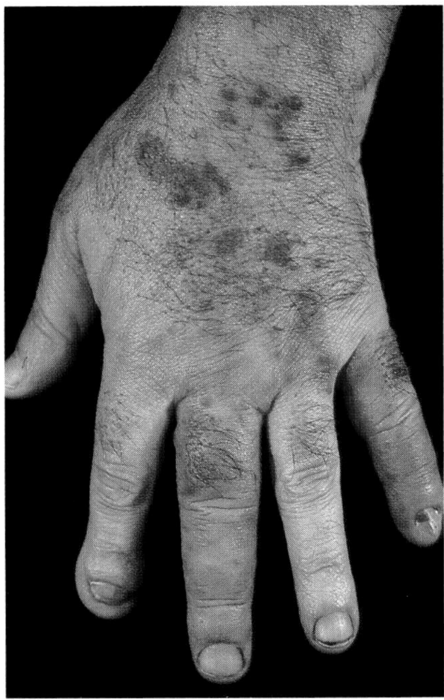

FIGURE 3–19. Classic Kaposi's sarcoma; patch, plaque, and nodular stage

Advanced, disseminated Kaposi's sarcoma, with purple macular, plaque, and papular lesions, which appeared simultaneously and late in the course of this patient's disease on the dorsum of the hand.

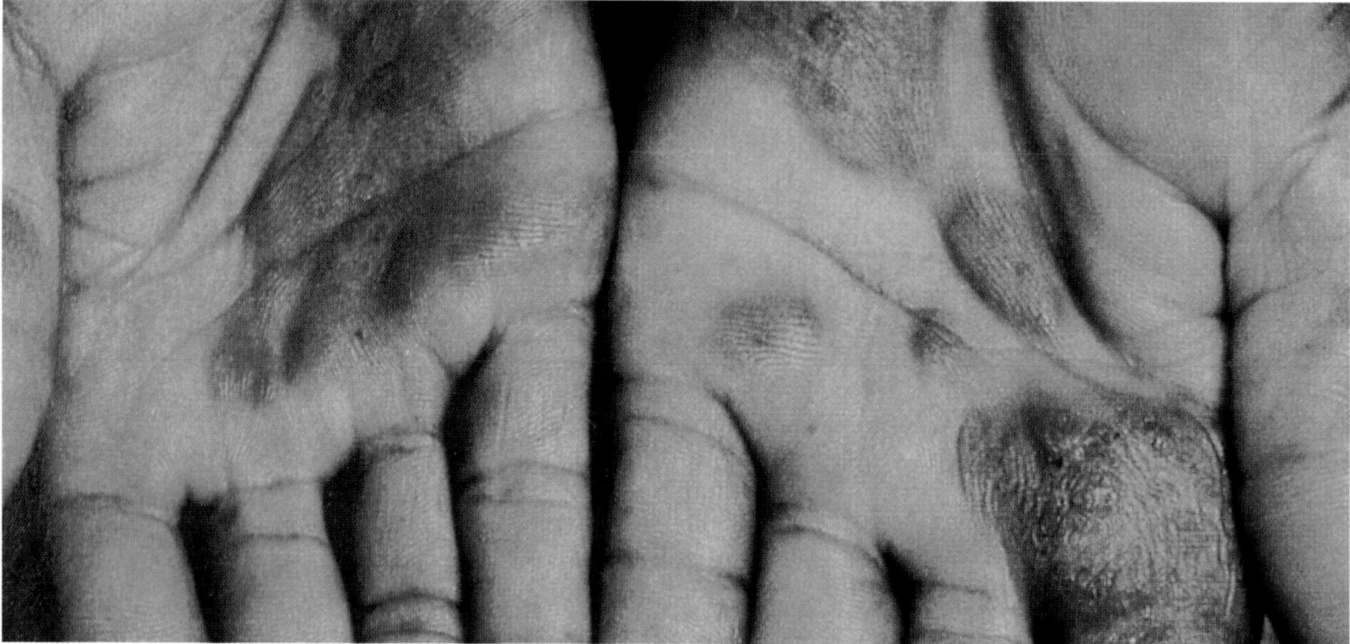

FIGURE 3–20. Classic Kaposi's sarcoma; plaque stage
Advanced disease with thickened violet-to-brown confluent plaques of Kaposi's sarcoma on the palms of both hands.

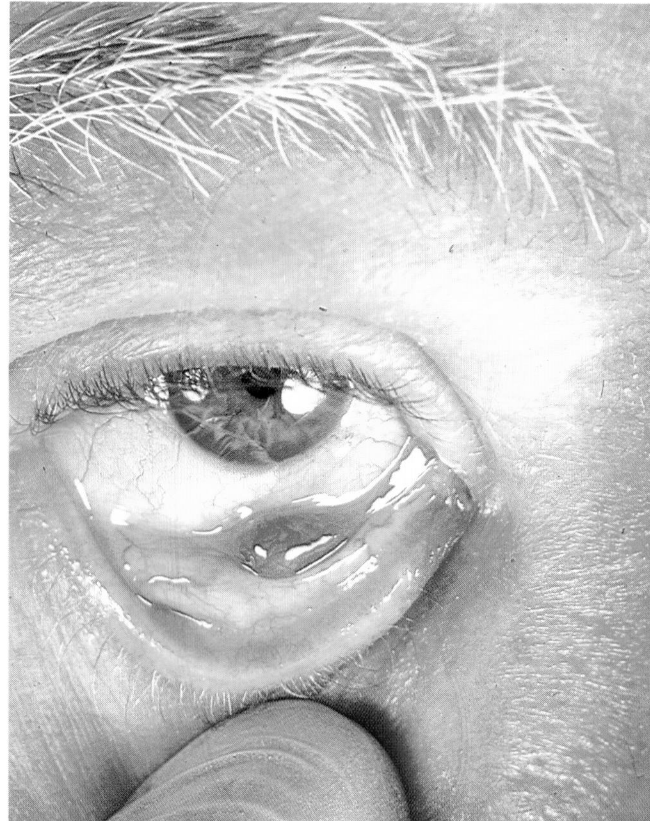

FIGURE 3–21. Classic Kaposi's sarcoma; nodular stage
An unusual red nodular tumor of Kaposi's sarcoma on the conjunctiva in an elderly patient with long-standing and widespread disease.

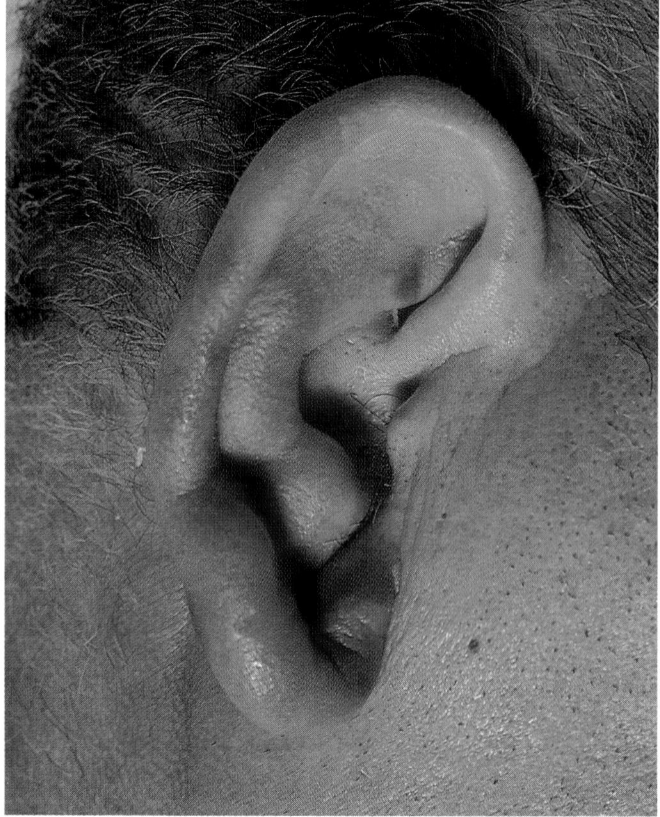

FIGURE 3–22. Classic Kaposi's sarcoma; nodular stage
A 53-year-old man with a Kaposi's sarcoma tumor affecting the earlobe and a few papular lesions on the other portions of the ear. The ear is an uncommon site of involvement in patients with the classic form of the disease.

KAPOSI'S SARCOMA IN AFRICA

(Figures 3–23 to 3–38)

In certain regions of sub-Saharan central Africa, KS represents up to 9% of all cancers.[2] In regions in which KS is so prevalent, it is referred to as *endemic African KS.* Four different forms of endemic African KS have been described that are distinguished on the basis of clinical features. Histologically, these forms of KS are indistinguishable from classic KS.

Endemic African KS was first described in the Bantu tribesmen of South Africa and was then recognized as being a prevalent condition in other sub-Saharan equatorial African countries including Zaire, Kenya, Uganda, Zimbabwe, Chad, and Gabon.[2,29] Interestingly, the incidence of KS in the Caucasian and Asian populations living in regions of endemic KS was found to be comparable to the incidence of classic KS in nonendemic regions.[30] As with classic KS, endemic KS is more prevalent in males who are otherwise healthy and have no systemic complaints. Spontaneous regressions of endemic KS lesions have been documented as is the case with classic KS (Table 3–2).[29]

Clinically, four forms of endemic KS are recognized (see Table 3–1).[31] They include a *benign nodular* form with papular or nodular lesions that appears most commonly in the extremities of males in their forties. This form of KS runs a benign course resembling classic KS with rare dissemination and with rare spontaneous regressions. A more malignant form of endemic KS, called *aggressive,* with larger exophytic fungating tumors that invade and destroy underlying tissues has also been described. Aggressive KS is also most commonly located on the extremities and is a slow, progressive disease. The third form of endemic African KS is termed *florid* and is a highly aggressive, rapidly progressive cancer that progresses rapidly and disseminates widely. Finally, a *lymphadenopathic* form of KS has been described that occurs mostly in prepubescent children, with KS lesions appearing predominantly in lymph nodes and with visceral dissemination but with minimal cutaneous lesions. This form of KS is highly malignant and is usually fatal within 1 or 2 years. All these four forms of KS occur with a higher prevalence in men.[32]

Although HIV infection may be endemic in regions in which endemic African KS is also prevalent, endemic KS is not caused by HIV.[33–35] Furthermore, endemic KS can be distinguished from HIV-associated KS on the basis of

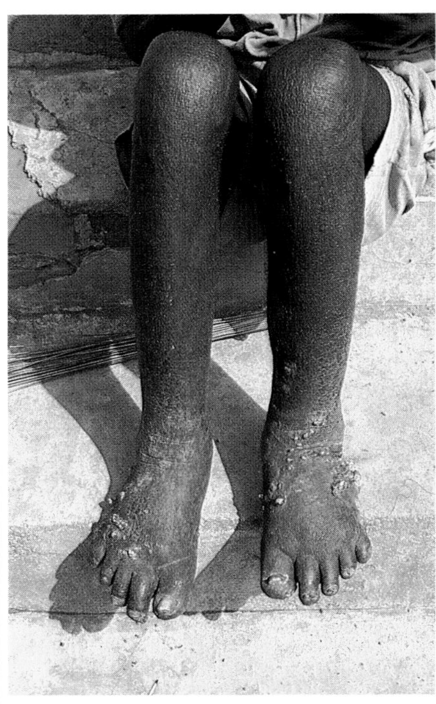

FIGURE 3–23. Endemic Kaposi's sarcoma (Africa); benign nodular type

TABLE 3–2. FEATURES OF KAPOSI'S SARCOMA PRESENT IN MORE THAN ONE TYPE OF THE SYNDROME

1. Male predominance
2. Association with human leukocyte antigen type
3. Multifocal onset of disease
4. Spontaneous regression of single lesions
5. Association with dysregulation of the immune system and lymphomas
6. Symmetric distribution
7. Absence of poor health or conditional symptoms
8. Association with human herpesvirus-8.

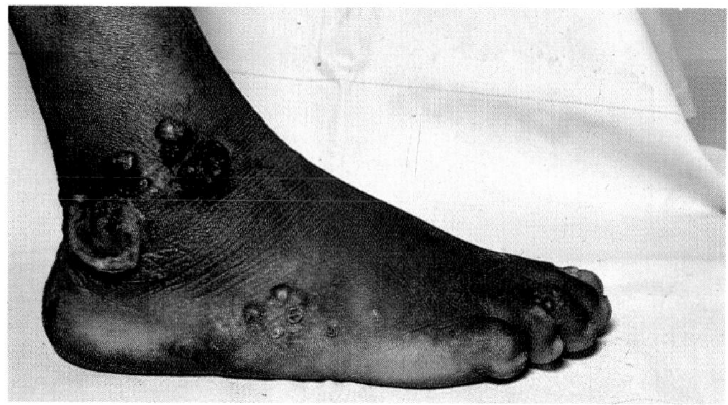

FIGURE 3–24. Endemic Kaposi's sarcoma (Africa); benign nodular type

There are multiple brown-to-black pearly tumor nodules seen on the lower extremity of this 36-year-old black African man with a large ulceration of the skin overlying the ankle region. The lesions were present for several years. (Courtesy of A. Templeton, MD, Chicago, and C. Olweny, MD, Makerere University Medical School, Kampala, Uganda.)

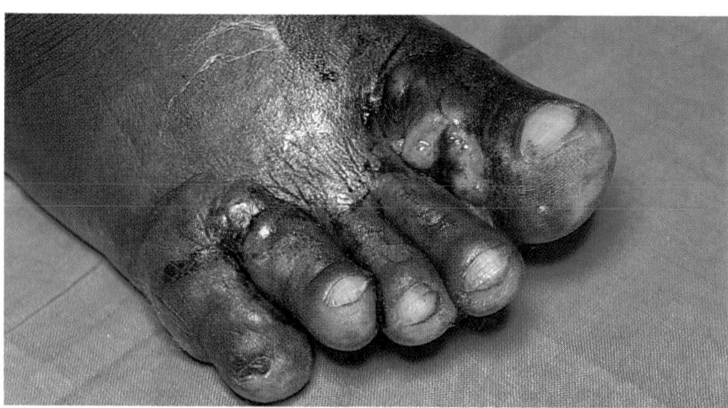

FIGURE 3–25. Endemic Kaposi's sarcoma (Africa); local aggressive type

A 27-year-old man who had his disease for 3 years. There is a denuded, ulcerated nodular tumor located on the great toe of his foot, which has locally invaded the subcutaneous tissues and bone. A similar tumor was present between the fourth and fifth toes on the same foot. (Courtesy of J. Ziegler, MD, San Francisco, and C. Olweny, MD, Makerere University Medical School, Kampala, Uganda.)

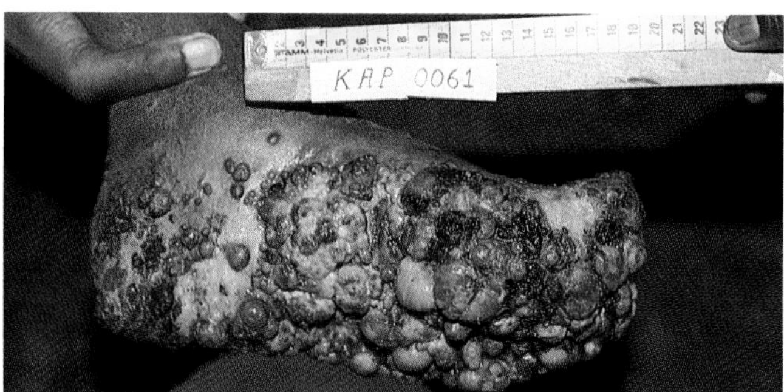

FIGURE 3–26. Endemic Kaposi's sarcoma (Africa); aggressive type

A 34-year-old man from Zaire with multiple and coalescent nodular tumors on the sole of the foot of 3 years' duration. The extensive involvement of the foot and toes included local invasion of the subcutaneous tissue and bone. The tumors vary from deep purple to black in color. The surfaces of several of the nodules are ulcerated. The patient's serum was found to be seronegative for HIV. (Courtesy of P. L. Gigase, MD, Antwerp, Belgium.)

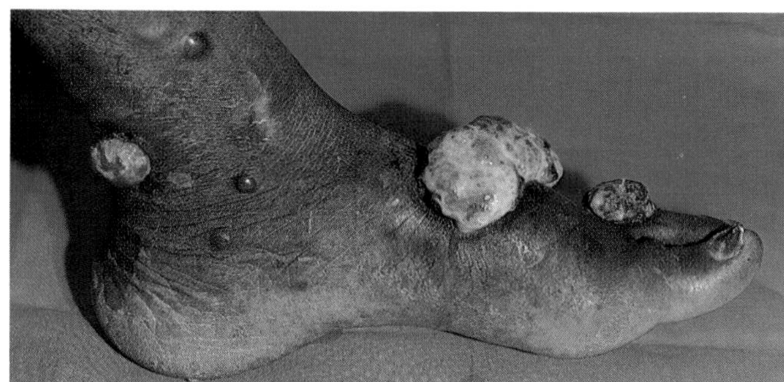

FIGURE 3–27. Endemic Kaposi's sarcoma (Africa); nodular aggressive type

Numerous large exophytic ulcerated tumors as well as smaller nonulcerated smooth nodules of Kaposi's sarcoma located on the lower leg and foot. (Courtesy of C. Olweny, MD, Makerere University Medical School, Kampala, Uganda.)

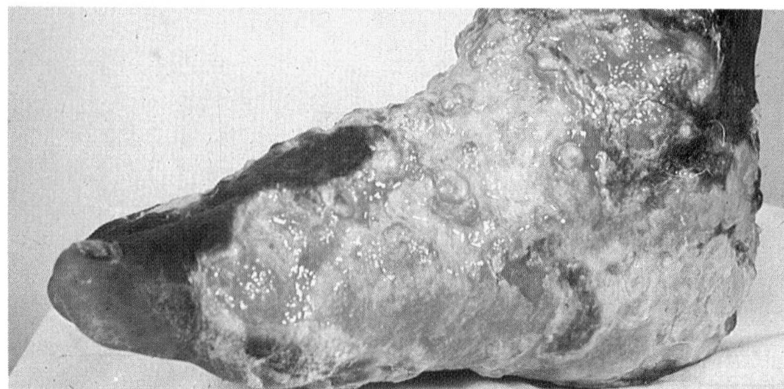

FIGURE 3–28. Endemic Kaposi's sarcoma (Africa); nodular aggressive type

A 43-year-old black African man with the locally aggressive and invasive form of Kaposi's sarcoma. There is extensive ulceration of the skin of the foot and invasion of the underlying bone and soft tissues. (Courtesy of C. Vogel, MD, Miami.)

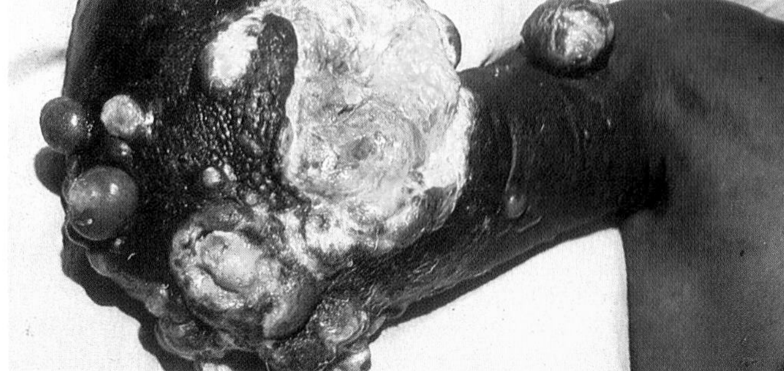

FIGURE 3–29. Endemic Kaposi's sarcoma (Africa); local aggressive type

Massive destructive locally invasive nodular lesions of Kaposi's sarcoma affecting the entire arm with a huge ulcerated mass occupying the antecubital fossa. Multiple large exophytic ulcerated and nonulcerated tumor nodules are present on the shoulder and arm. (Courtesy of C. Vogel, MD, Miami, and C. Olweny, MD, Makerere University Medical School, Kampala, Uganda.)

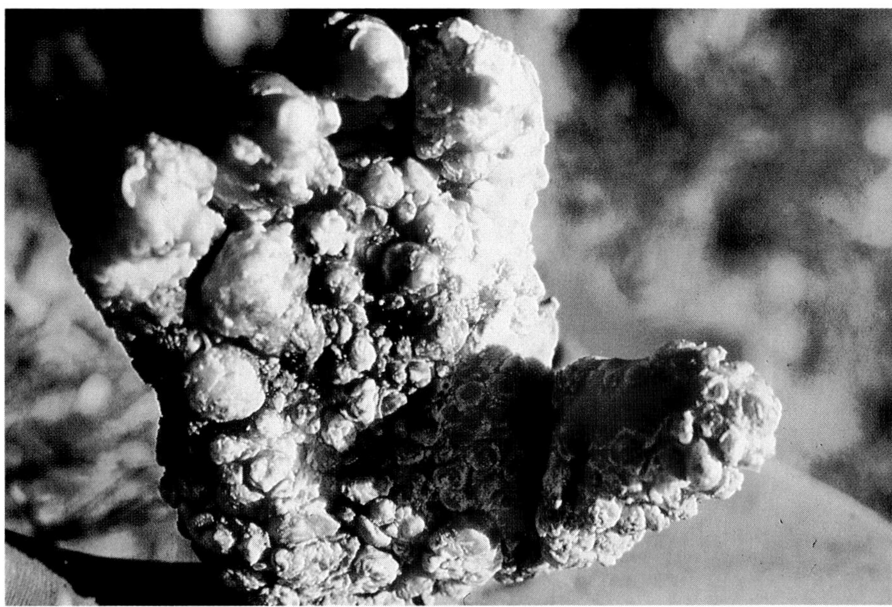

FIGURE 3–30. Endemic Kaposi's sarcoma (Africa); local aggressive type

The entire hand of this adult black man from Zaire is totally covered with multiple confluent nodular skin tumors, which had invaded and destroyed the subcutaneous tissue and bone, especially in the fingers. Such aggressive lesions are reported to respond to palliative radiation therapy; however, damage to the underlying tissue and bone is not reversible. (Courtesy of C. Vogel, MD, Miami.)

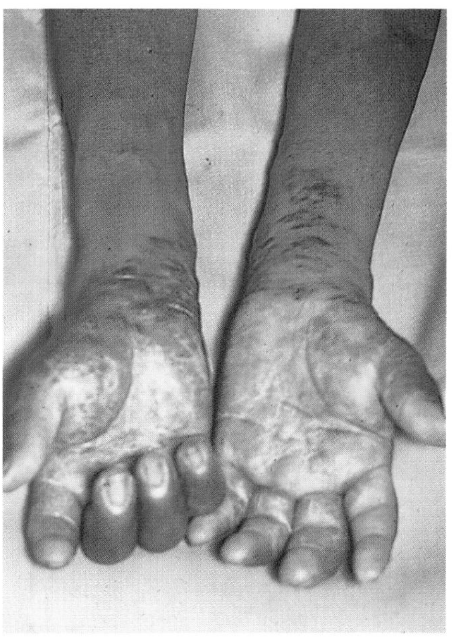

FIGURE 3–31. Endemic Kaposi's sarcoma (Africa); florid type

Multiple widely and rapidly disseminating nodules of Kaposi's sarcoma, seen on both forearms and palmar surfaces, on a 35-year-old black Ugandan. The tumor was found to infiltrate bone and soft tissues. The patient also had visceral involvement. (Courtesy of C. Olweny, MD, Makerere University Medical School, Kampala, Uganda.)

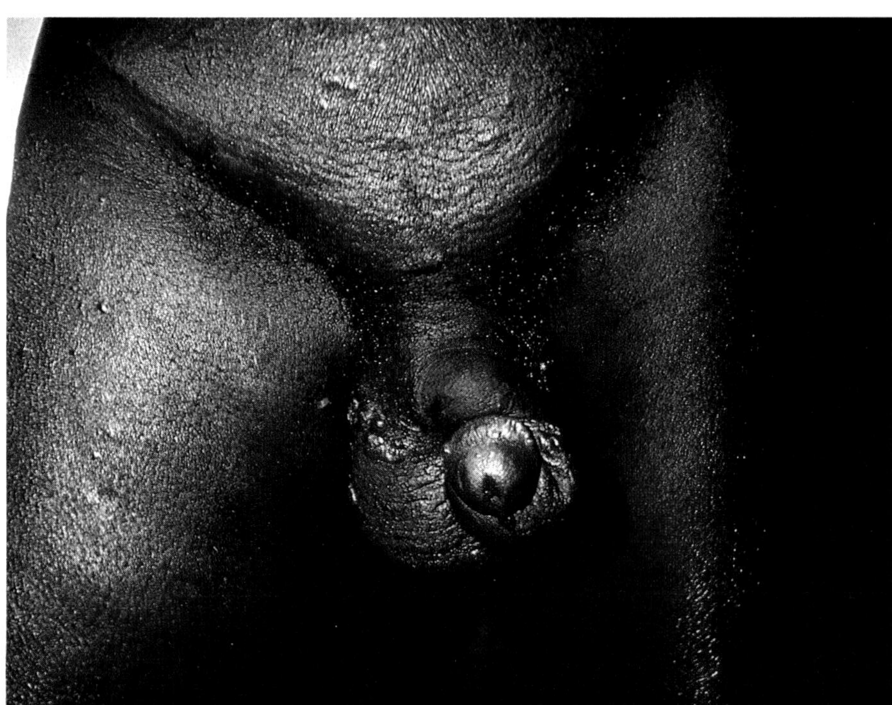

FIGURE 3–32. Endemic Kaposi's sarcoma (Africa); florid type

A 43-year-old black African man from Zaire with widespread Kaposi's sarcoma, including involvement of the inguinal nodes, first diagnosed in 1974. The disease ran a slowly progressive course. His serum HIV antibody status is unknown. (Courtesy of J. Ziegler, MD, San Francisco, and C. Olweny, MD, Makerere University Medical School, Kampala, Uganda.)

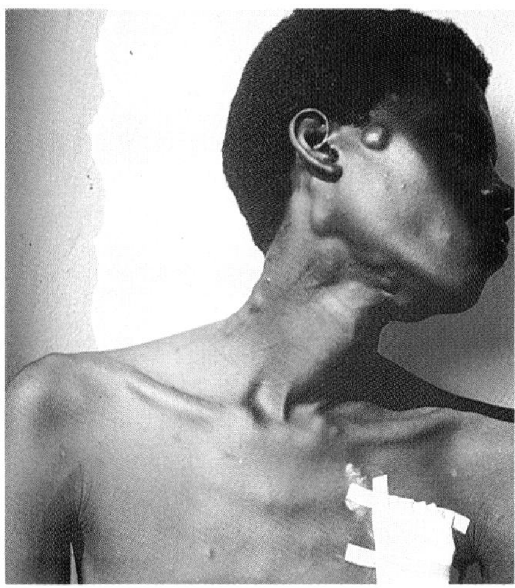

FIGURE 3–33. Endemic Kaposi's sarcoma (Africa); florid type

A 35-year-old black African man from Burundi with numerous cutaneous nodular lesions of Kaposi's sarcoma. The enlarged lymph nodes on his neck below the mandibular angle near his ear were infiltrated with Kaposi's sarcoma. Lymphadenopathic involvement is rarely seen in adults with this neoplasm. Although his clinical disease behaved like that seen in a patient with AIDS, this individual was seronegative to HIV (Courtesy of P. L. Gigase, MD, Antwerp, Belgium.)

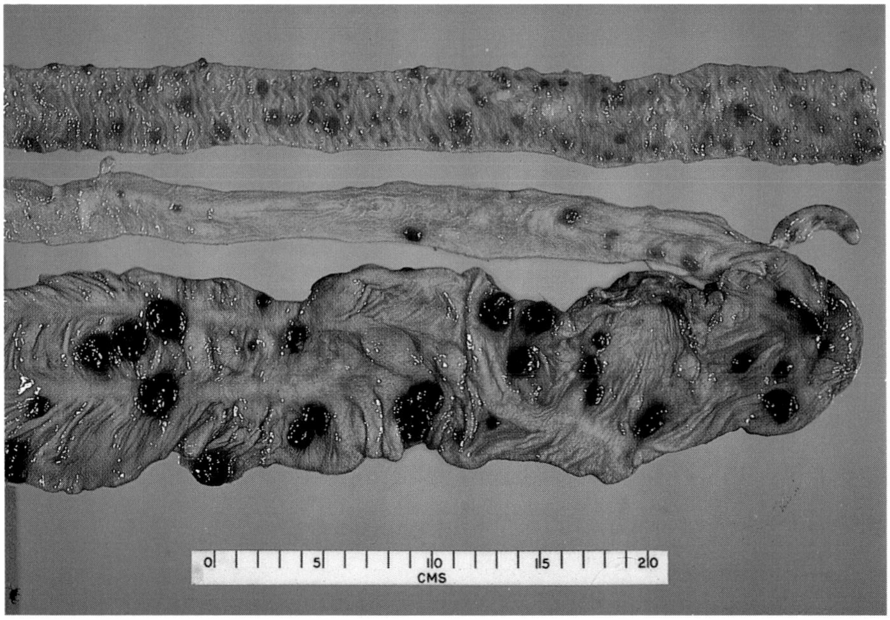

FIGURE 3–34. Endemic Kaposi's sarcoma (Africa); florid type

Gross pathologic specimen of the small and large intestines studded with red-to-black tumor nodules of Kaposi's sarcoma. (Courtesy of A. Templeton, MD, Chicago, and Makerere University Medical School, Kampala, Uganda.)

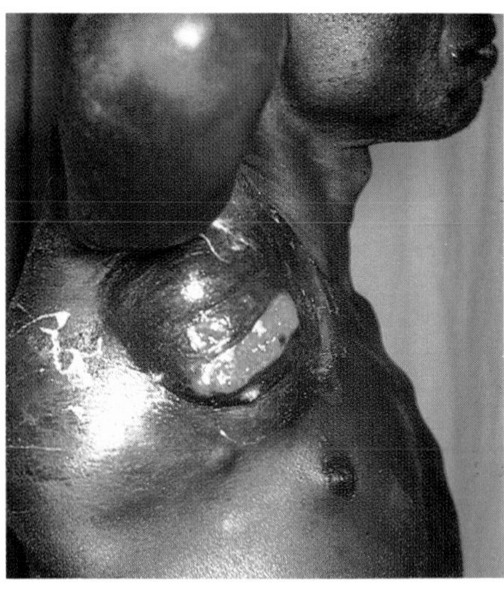

FIGURE 3–35. Endemic Kaposi's sarcoma (Africa); florid type

A black adult man with grossly enlarged axillary lymphadenopathy due to Kaposi's sarcoma. Lymph node involvement sometimes occurs in adults with the florid type of endemic disease but is more commonly seen in the pediatric population with the lymphadenopathic variety of Kaposi's sarcoma. (Courtesy of A. Templeton, MD, Chicago, and C. Olweny, MD, Makerere University Medical School, Kampala, Uganda.)

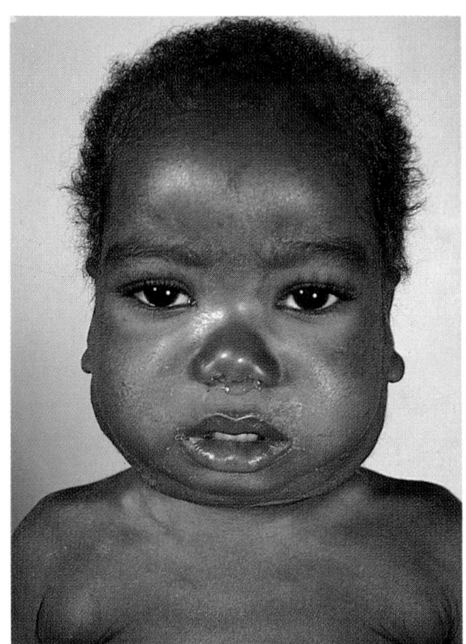

FIGURE 3–36. Endemic Kaposi's sarcoma (Africa); lymphadenopathic type

A 2-year-old boy with disseminated lymph node involvement with facial edema due to obstruction of lymphatic drainage. Also present is bilateral axillary adenopathy. The lymphadenopathic variety of the disease is seen primarily in children. Skin lesions are extremely uncommon in children with this form of the disease. (Courtesy of A. Templeton, MD, Chicago, and C. Olweny, MD, Makerere University Medical School, Kampala, Uganda.)

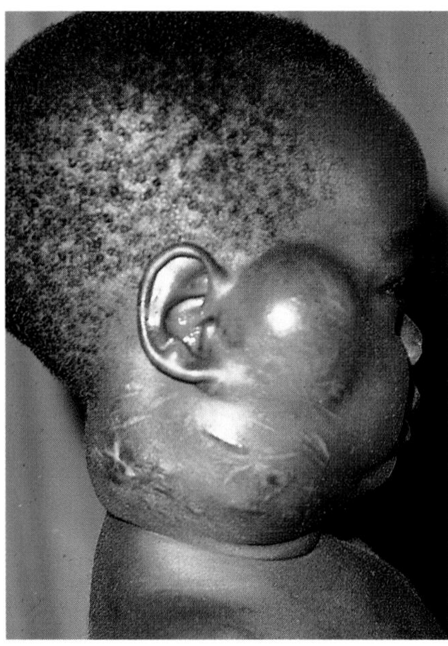

FIGURE 3–37. Endemic Kaposi's sarcoma (Africa); lymphadenopathic type

An 18-month-old boy with massive preauricular and cervical lymphadenopathy due to Kaposi's sarcoma. The lymphadenopathic form of the disease responds poorly to either chemotherapy or radiation therapy. (Courtesy of C. Olweny, MD, Makerere University Medical School, Kampala, Uganda.)

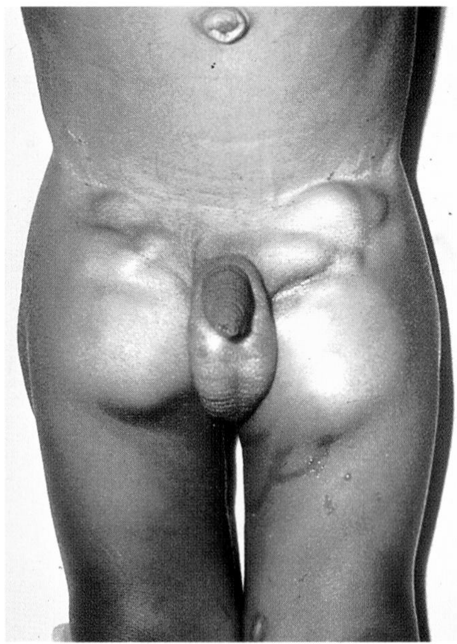

FIGURE 3–38. Endemic Kaposi's sarcoma (Africa); lymphadenopathic type

A 3-year-old black African boy with bilateral inguinal and femoral lymph node enlargement due to Kaposi's sarcoma. (Courtesy of C. Vogel, MD, Miami, and C. Olweny, MD, Makerere University Medical School, Kampala, Uganda.)

clinical features. Male and female patients are affected equally with AIDS-associated KS in equatorial Africa. These patients often have progressive mucocutaneous lesions, constitutional symptoms of weight loss and lymphadenopathy, and the development of oral candidiasis, oral hairy leukoplakia, and other infections, especially pneumonias.[33–35] African patients with AIDS-associated KS are infected with HIV.[34]

Treatment of endemic African KS is initiated when warranted by increasing symptoms or progression of lesions. Radiotherapy is effective in treating localized tumors.[36] When systemic therapy is necessary, cytotoxic drugs such as vincristine, actinomycin D, dacarbazine, bleomycin, razoxane, carmustine, and doxorubicin hydrochloride (Adriamycin) have been used singly or in combination.[36–38]

KAPOSI'S SARCOMA IN IATROGENICALLY IMMUNOSUPPRESSED PATIENTS

Case reports of KS appearing in patients with systemic lupus erythematosus,[39] with temporal arteritis,[40] or with lymphoproliferative disorders while on one or more immunosuppressive agents[17,41–44] has been described; however, the onset of organ transplantation with the ensuing need for prolonged immunosuppression brought to light the association of KS with iatrogenic immunosuppression. When the immunosuppressive therapy has been modified or discontinued, the KS has been found to regress in some of these cases.

As with classic KS, KS associated with iatrogenic immunosuppression appears more in male than in female patients, and the prevalence of KS in persons of Mediterranean or eastern European Jewish origin is excessive.[45–49] Furthermore, an excess of HLA-B5, HLA-B8, HLA-B18, and HLA-DR5 and a decreased frequency of HLA-A1 and HLA-B7 have been noted.[50] This HLA distribution is similar to that found in individuals of Italian, Greek, Jewish, and Arabic backgrounds.[50] In Saudi Arabia, KS is the most common tumor that develops after renal transplantation.[49]

The KS lesions in the setting of iatrogenic immunosuppression are indistinguishable from those of classic KS except that nodular forms predominate and early visceral involvement is frequent. Usually, lesions appear after approximately 20 months of immunosuppressive therapy and may appear anywhere on the skin.[47] Visceral involvement with widespread dissemination occurs in approximately 40% of cases, affecting mainly the gastrointestinal tract and the lungs (see Table 3–1).[40] The incidence of KS appears to be higher in patients receiving cyclosporin than in those receiving conventional immunosuppressive agents (e.g., corticosteroids) (10% vs 3%).[47]

The lesions of KS associated with iatrogenic immunosuppression regress with reduction or discontinuation of the immunosuppressive regimen in approximately one third of patients; however, the prognosis of transplant recipients who develop KS is poor.[46,47] If an aggressive or a rapidly progressive course is present, systemic chemotherapy may be necessary. This patient population is also at risk for the development of non-Hodgkin's lymphomas, often of multifocal nature.[51]

EPIDEMIC KAPOSI'S SARCOMA ASSOCIATED WITH AIDS

(Figures 3–39 to 3–110)

An epidemic incidence of Kaposi's sarcoma associated with the development of *Pneumocystis carinii* pneumonia in a restricted population of young sexually active homosexual men was the first evidence of the development of a heretofore undescribed disease, now known as AIDS.[8–11] The lesions of KS occurring with this new disease were histologically identical in appearance to those of the indolent classic form of KS, but the clinical behavior of the tumor was that of a highly aggressive and often disseminated tumor.

Epidemic KS associated with AIDS manifests almost exclusively in patients infected with HIV-1 whose risk factor for HIV-1 infection is sexual activity with male homosexuals. The majority of patients with AIDS-associated KS are thus sexually active homosexual males, with an average age of 37 years. Recipients of blood transfusions who have developed AIDS-associated KS have often received blood donated by patients who were sexually active homosexual men and who developed AIDS-associated KS before or after the donation of the blood.[52] The few women in the United States who developed AIDS-associated KS were frequently found to have had bisexual partners.[53,54] Studies investigating the role of inhaled amyl or butyl nitrites,[55,56] intestinal parasites,[57] cytomegalovirus infection,[58,59] hepatitis B infection,[60,61] fecal-oral contact,[62,63] and various sexual practices[52,56,60,62,64–67] have all been inconclusive in finding significant associations with the development of AIDS-associated KS in the at-risk population.

Text continued on page 53

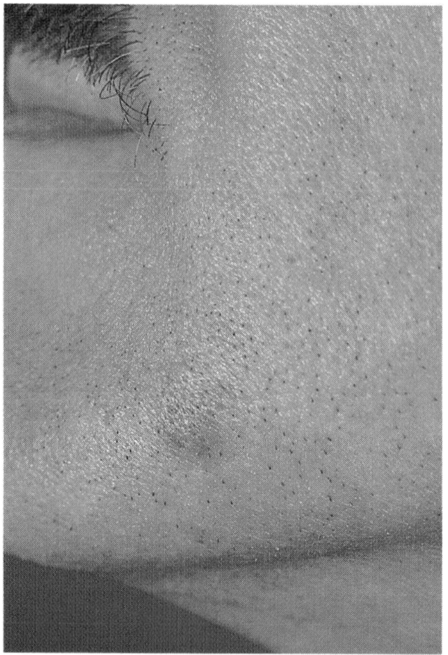

FIGURE 3–39. Epidemic Kaposi's sarcoma; patch stage

This totally asymptomatic faint pink macular lesion of Kaposi's sarcoma spontaneously appeared on the side of this patient's chin. Similar patch-stage lesions developed at distant sites on the patient's body at about the same time.

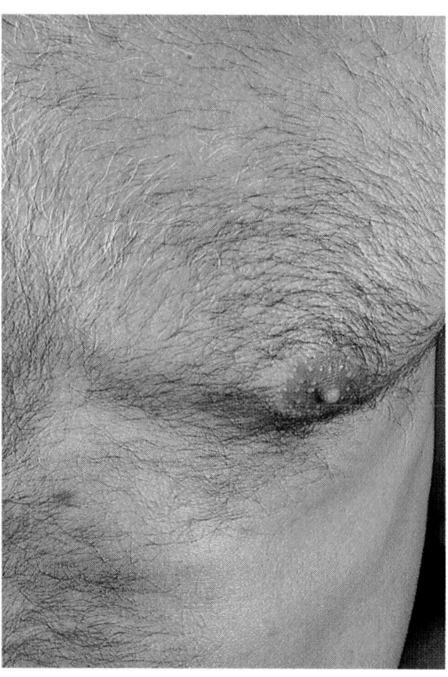

FIGURE 3–40. Epidemic Kaposi's sarcoma; patch stage

A 44-year-old otherwise healthy homosexual man with a single flat red macule of Kaposi's sarcoma on his lower chest.

FIGURE 3–41. Epidemic Kaposi's sarcoma; patch stage

An elongated flat lesion on the trunk, which varied in color from pink to red, was initially ignored because the patient thought that this "spot" represented a minor bruise. As this skin lesion became darker in color, other macules developed at distant sites. The patient sought medical attention at that time.

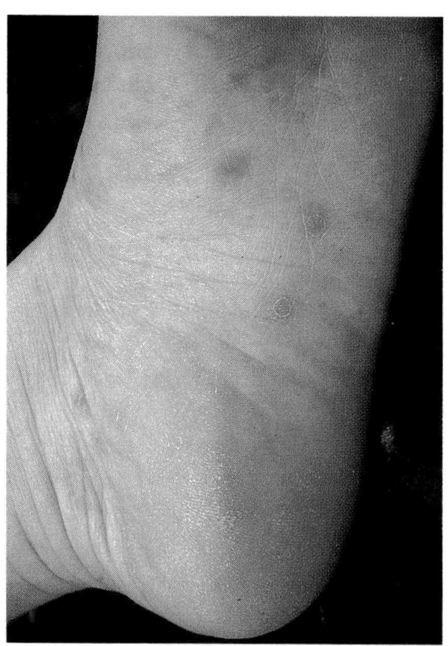

FIGURE 3–42. Epidemic Kaposi's sarcoma; patch stage

A 23-year-old homosexual man with multiple flat tawny-pink lesions on the sole and ankle of the foot. Initially, the lesions were thought to represent secondary syphilis. There were several other cutaneous lesions of a similar nature widely disseminated over the rest of his body.

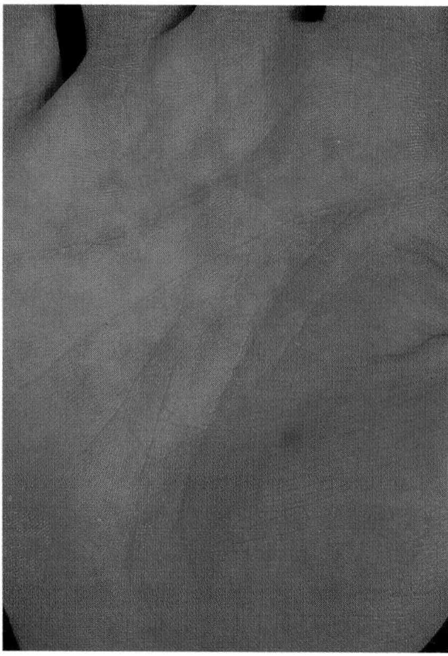

FIGURE 3–43. Epidemic Kaposi's sarcoma; patch stage

A single light-brown flat macular lesion on the palm of the hand. The biopsy confirmed the diagnosis of Kaposi's sarcoma.

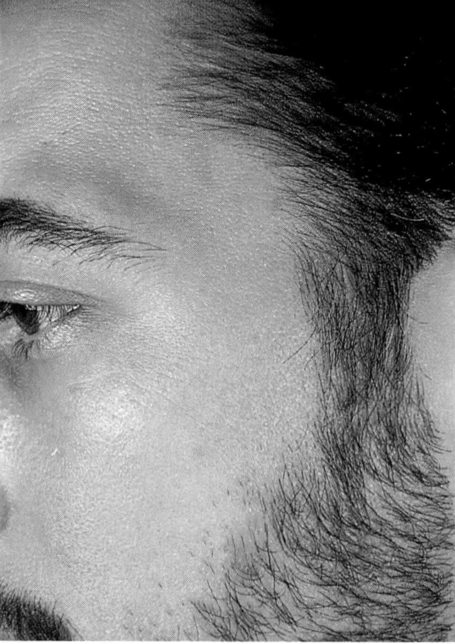

FIGURE 3–44. Epidemic Kaposi's sarcoma; patch stage

Multiple patch-stage lesions on the temple and bearded areas of the face. The lesions were slightly irregular in shape and widely dispersed over the rest of the body.

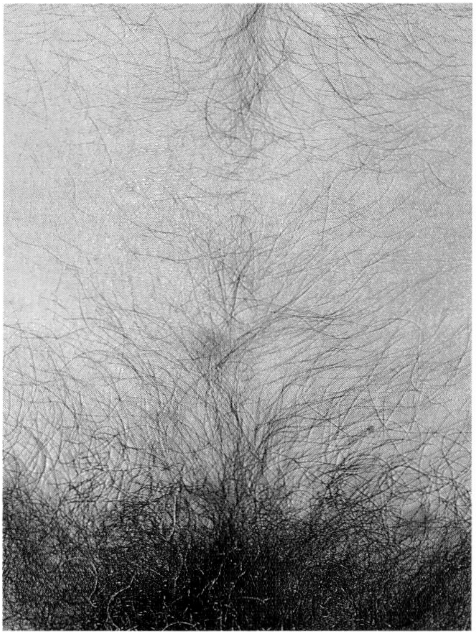

FIGURE 3–45. Epidemic Kaposi's sarcoma; patch stage

A 39-year-old homosexual man with multiple reddish macules on the lower abdomen and pubic region.

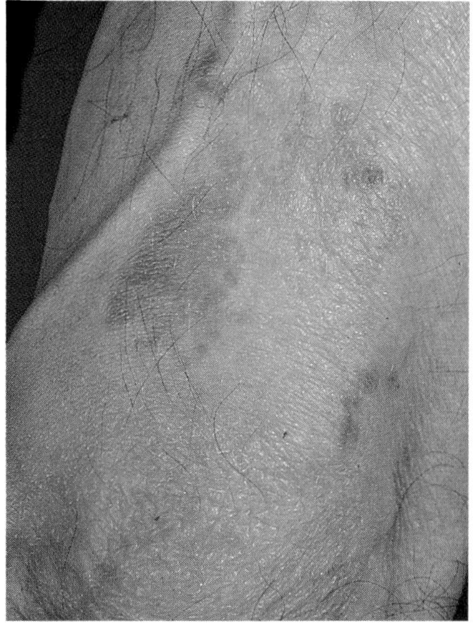

FIGURE 3–46. Epidemic Kaposi's sarcoma; patch stage

These red, flat, irregularly shaped lesions were initially mistaken for bruises. When additional lesions developed, a diagnosis of Kaposi's sarcoma was confirmed by biopsy.

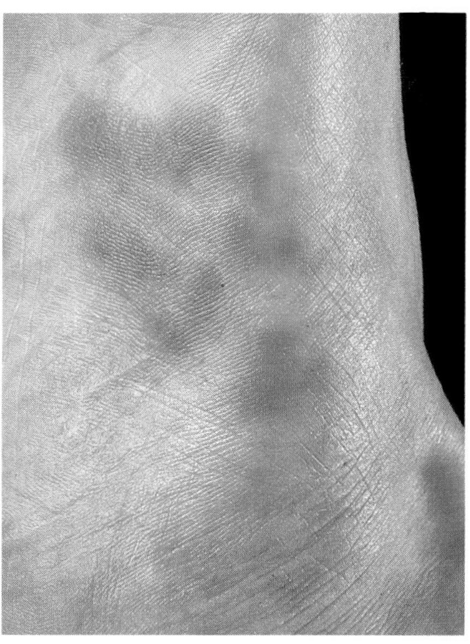

FIGURE 3–47. Epidemic Kaposi's sarcoma; patch stage

These tawny to pink coalescing macules on the ankle region were thought to be secondary to trauma. They were asymptomatic and were only diagnosed as Kaposi's sarcoma when the patient developed multiple other lesions on distant sites of his body.

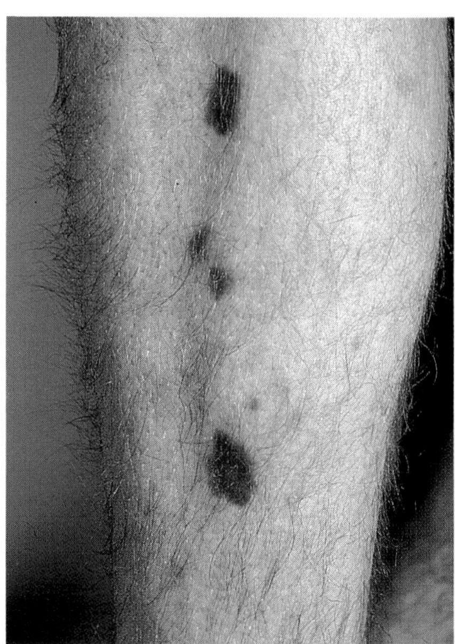

FIGURE 3–48. Epidemic Kaposi's sarcoma; patch stage

Several flat, blue-black macular lesions of Kaposi's sarcoma on the lower leg had been present for 2 years.

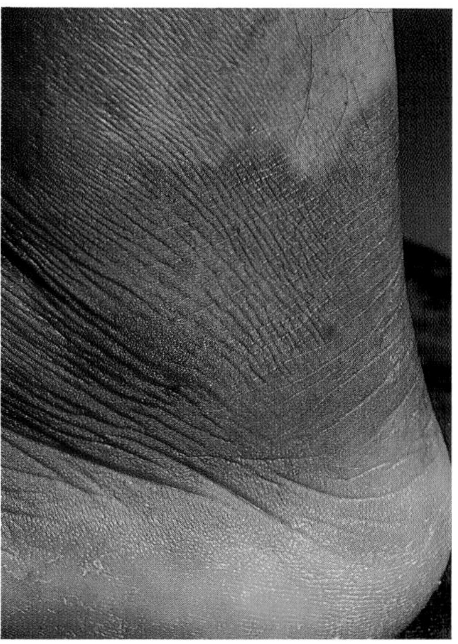

FIGURE 3–49. Epidemic Kaposi's sarcoma; patch stage

This large, asymptomatic, hyperpigmented patch of Kaposi's sarcoma on the ankle region of a mulatto homosexual man was ignored by the patient and remained undiagnosed for several months until the patient suddenly developed a life-threatening opportunistic infection with toxoplasmosis.

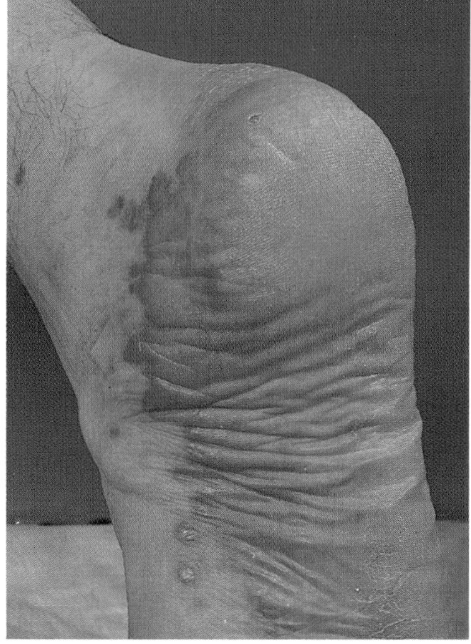

FIGURE 3–50. Epidemic Kaposi's sarcoma; patch stage

A large, pink, confluent, flat lesion of Kaposi's sarcoma, located on the sole of the foot extending from the heel. Numerous satellite lesions are also present on the ankle and at the border of this patch-stage lesion. This lesion, which had been present for several months, was initially thought to represent a tinea pedis infection that did not respond to topical antifungal medication. The diagnosis of Kaposi's sarcoma was confirmed by biopsy. This resembles the classic variety of the tumor (see Fig. 3–1).

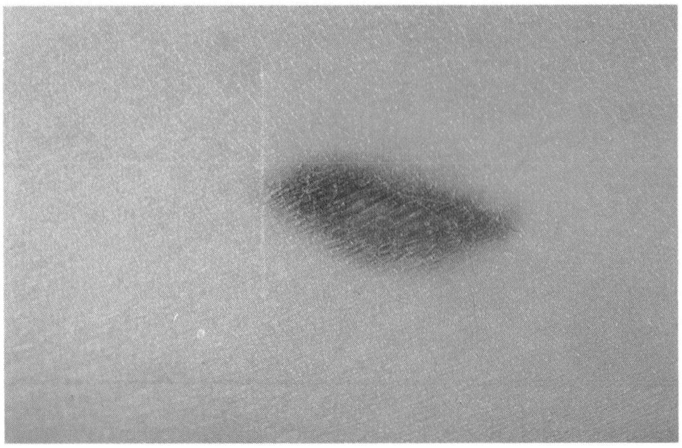

FIGURE 3–51. Epidemic Kaposi's sarcoma; patch-to-plaque stage
A close-up view of a violet-to-brown, hyperpigmented, elliptic, slightly indurated lesion on the trunk.

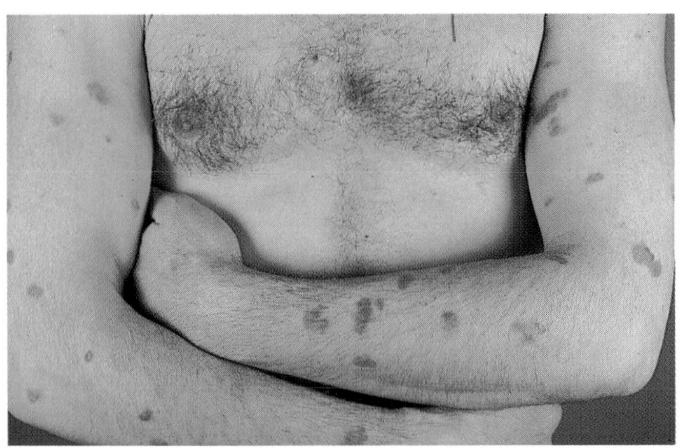

FIGURE 3–52. Epidemic Kaposi's sarcoma; plaque stage
Multiple elongated and irregularly shaped violet-to-brown plaque lesions of Kaposi's sarcoma on the upper extremities.

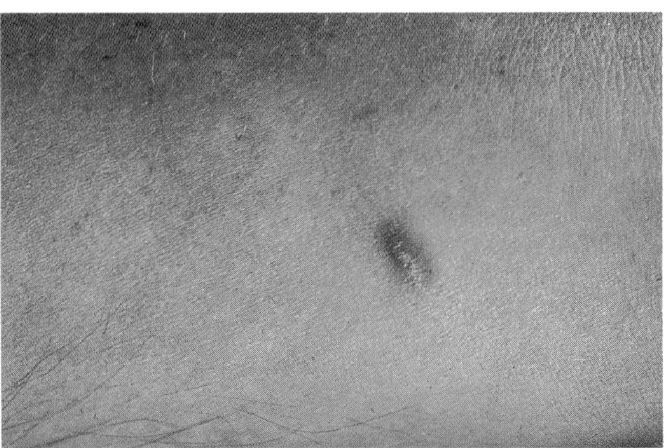

FIGURE 3–53. Epidemic Kaposi's sarcoma; plaque stage
A raised fusiform violaceous lesion on the upper arm of a patient who developed this lesion several months after experiencing his first bout of *Pneumocystis carinii* pneumonia.

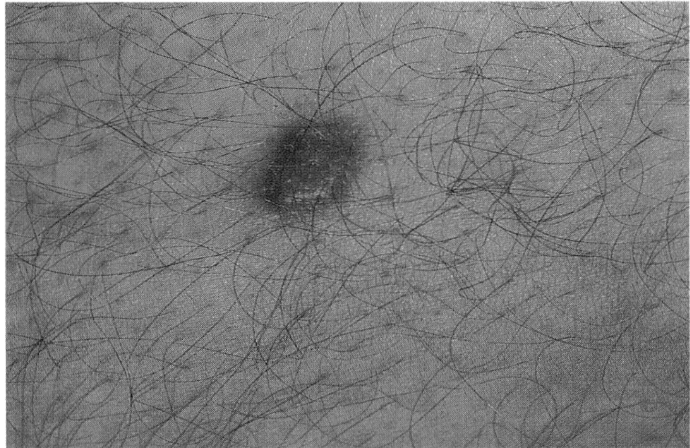

FIGURE 3–54. Epidemic Kaposi's sarcoma; plaque stage
An elevated red-to-brown polygonal lesion that became increasingly pigmented over several months, especially at the peripheral margin.

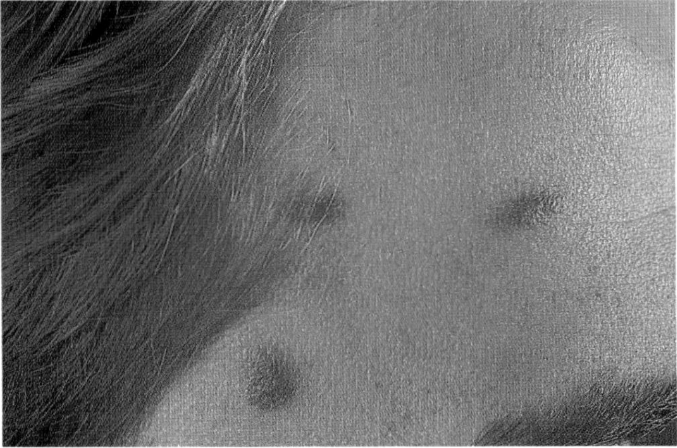

FIGURE 3–55. Epidemic Kaposi's sarcoma; plaque stage
Three ovoid, indurated, red-to-purple plaques found on the temple. The diagnosis of Kaposi's sarcoma was initially made in this patient several months earlier, when a lymph node biopsy was performed and proved to have foci of tumor.

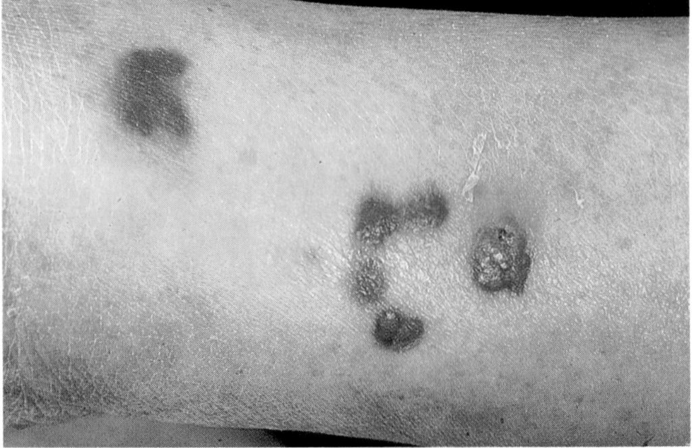

FIGURE 3–56. Epidemic Kaposi's sarcoma; plaque stage
Multiple dark brown-to-black lesions had been present on the skin of this patient's arm for approximately 8 months. These lesions resemble malignant melanoma.

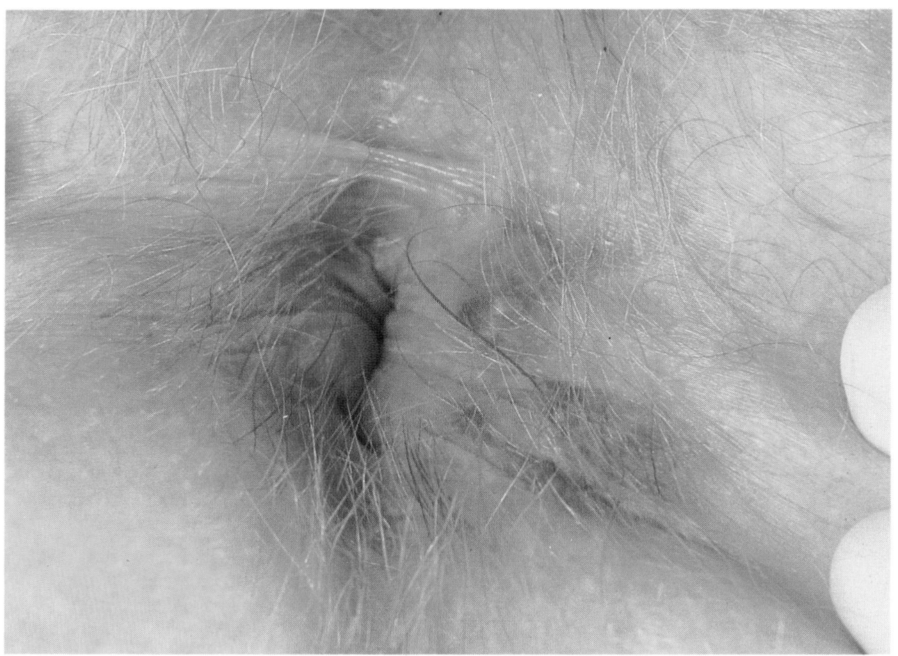

FIGURE 3–57. Epidemic Kaposi's sarcoma; plaque stage

A 40-year-old homosexual man with two lavender, irregularly shaped, asymptomatic plaque lesions of Kaposi's sarcoma on the right side of the perianal skin. The patient also had several other mucocutaneous lesions of Kaposi's sarcoma. On colonoscopy, nodules of Kaposi's sarcoma were also found.

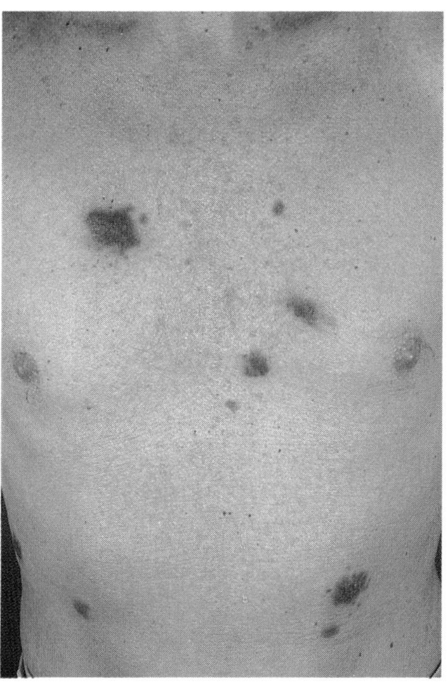

FIGURE 3–58. Epidemic Kaposi's sarcoma; plaque stage

Multiple large plaque lesions of Kaposi's sarcoma. Several of the lesions are surrounded by a yellowish halo similar to that observed in resolving bruises or ecchymoses of the skin. This halo is frequently observed associated with lesions of epidemic Kaposi's sarcoma.

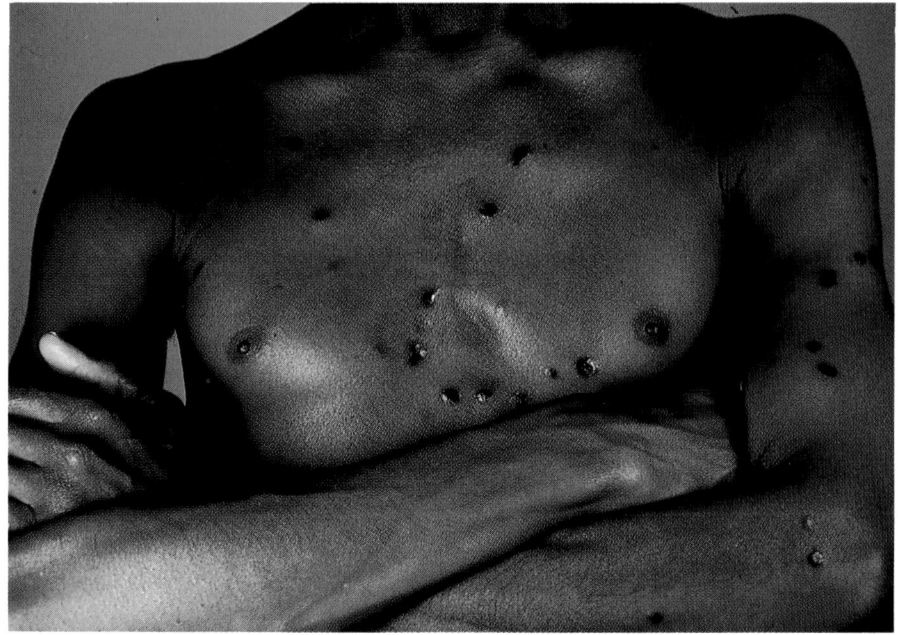

FIGURE 3–59. Epidemic Kaposi's sarcoma; plaque stage

This AIDS patient was an intravenous drug user who developed widely disseminated black papular skin lesions. Kaposi's sarcoma is uncommon in intravenous drug users with AIDS and is much more prevalent among the homosexual population at risk. In dark-skinned individuals, the lesions of Kaposi's sarcoma rapidly become hyperpigmented.

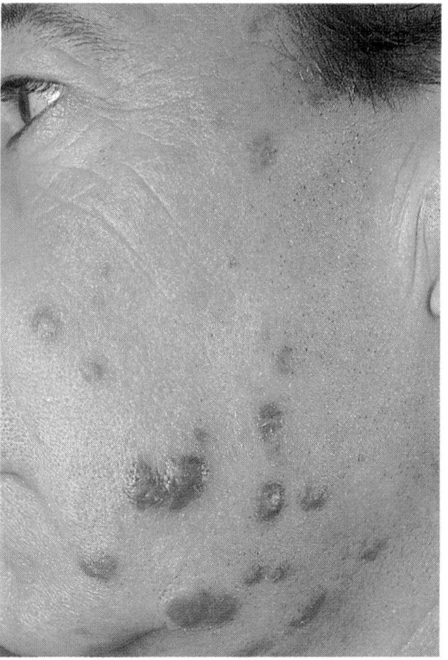

FIGURE 3–60. Epidemic Kaposi's sarcoma; plaque-to-nodular stage

A 60-year-old homosexual Hispanic man presented with patch and plaque lesions on his face, some of which were developing into nodules. With time, several of the lesions coalesced.

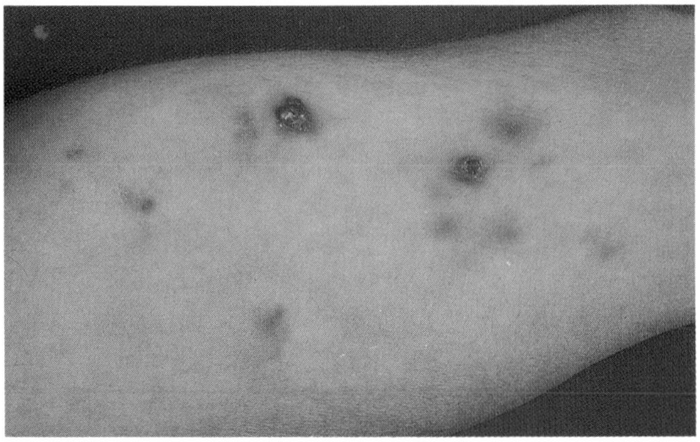

FIGURE 3–61. Epidemic Kaposi's sarcoma; patch, plaque, and nodular stages
Multiple cherry-red lesions of Kaposi's sarcoma in various stages (patch, plaque, and nodule) may appear concurrently in the same region. New lesions usually continue to develop during the course of the illness.

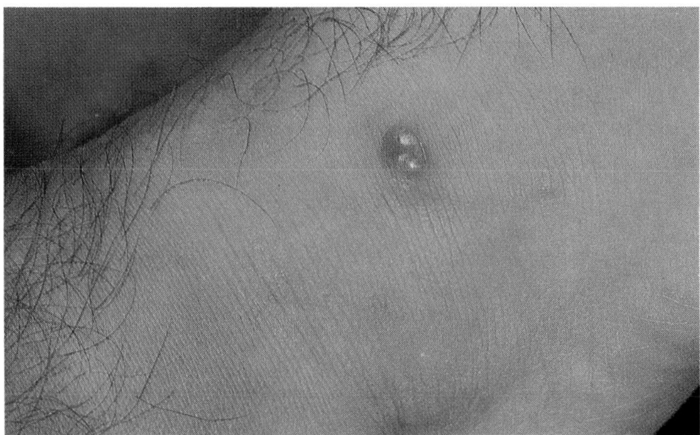

FIGURE 3–62. Epidemic Kaposi's sarcoma; nodular stage
A single, opalescent, pearl-like tumor nodule appeared in the skin of the antecubetal fossa of an otherwise asymptomatic 22-year-old HIV-seropositive homosexual man.

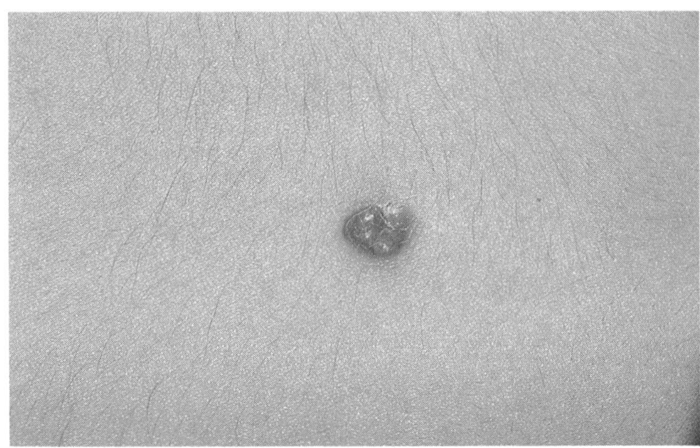

FIGURE 3–63. Epidemic Kaposi's sarcoma; nodular stage
An isolated, dark red, translucent, loculated, nodular skin tumor, which was the presenting lesion of Kaposi's sarcoma in this patient. This lesion could be mistaken for a basal cell carcinoma.

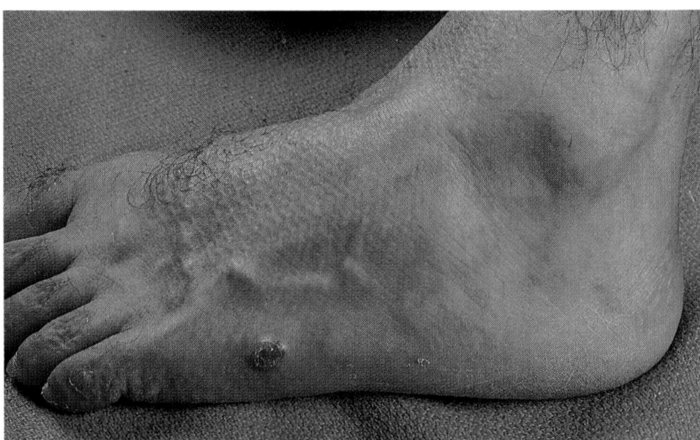

FIGURE 3–64. Epidemic Kaposi's sarcoma; nodular stage
A solitary extruding nodular tumor present on the lateral margin of the foot, which is reminiscent of the typical tumor often seen in patients with classic Kaposi's sarcoma.

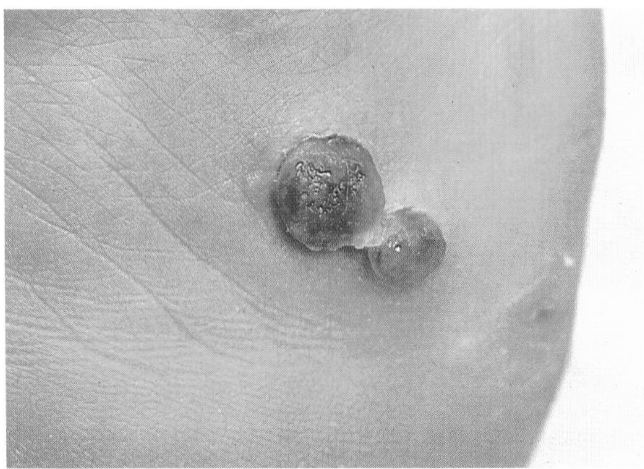

FIGURE 3–65. Epidemic Kaposi's sarcoma; nodular stage
Two adjacent nodular lesions, which appeared on the lateral margin of the heel below the ankle and within a month progressed from flat red macules to protruding nodules. The surfaces of these nodules are denuded.

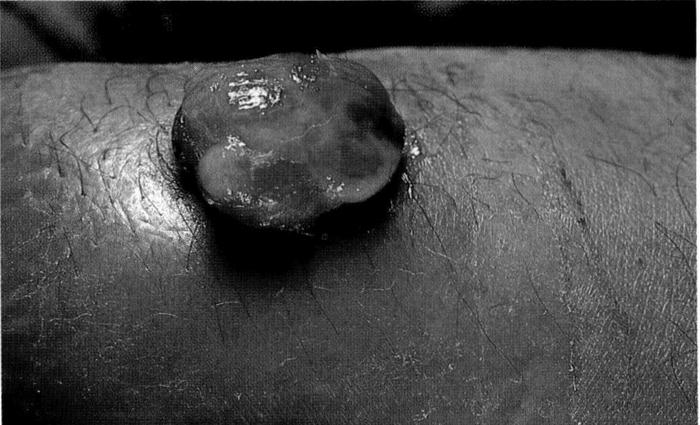

FIGURE 3–66. Epidemic Kaposi's sarcoma; nodular stage
A solitary tumor nodule located on the finger of a light-skinned black man with AIDS was one of many widespread lesions that developed over a 5-month period. The surfaces of such elevated lesions are prone to superficial trauma.

TABLE 3–3. ETIOLOGIC ASSOCIATIONS WITH KAPOSI'S SARCOMA

- Immunologic
  - Iatrogenic immune suppression used for:
    - Organ transplant recipients
    - Systemic lupus erythematosus
    - Temporal arteritis
  - Association with human leukocyte antigen subtype and ethnic background
- Infectious
  - Venereal disease
  - Cytomegalovirus
  - Papillomavirus
  - Retrovirus
- Growth factors
  - *Tat*-1
  - Interleukin-1β
  - Interleukin-6
  - Tumor necrosis factor-α
  - Oncostatin-M
  - Fibroblast growth factor-6
- Other
  - Inhalant amyl or butyl nitrites
  - Fecal-oral contact

In vitro studies have been plagued by the lack of knowledge about the cell of origin of KS as well as by the possible introduction of phenomena due to in vitro culture conditions.[68] Furthermore, the factors that are found to be important for the etiology of KS may not be the ones that play a role in promoting and enhancing the disease once it is established in vivo (Table 3–3). Recent investigations have suggested a possible role for a human papillomavirus-16 (HPV-16)–like virus in the etiology of KS and one for growth factors and their receptors in the development of AIDS-associated KS and in explaining the aggressive clinical course of AIDS-associated KS. Human papillomavirus-16–like sequences were detected in approximately 30% of classic and AIDS-related KS lesions but not in distant normal skin obtained from the same patient.[69] The further finding of such sequences by in situ hybridization in fresh specimens from AIDS-associated KS patients[70] implicates such an agent in the etiology of KS. Human papillomavirus-16 has already been linked to cervical cancer and to anal cancers, two conditions for which patients with HIV-1 infection are known to be at increased risk. Specifically, the population at risk for HIV-related anal cancer, namely, sexually active homosexual men, is the same as that at risk for AIDS-associated KS.[71]

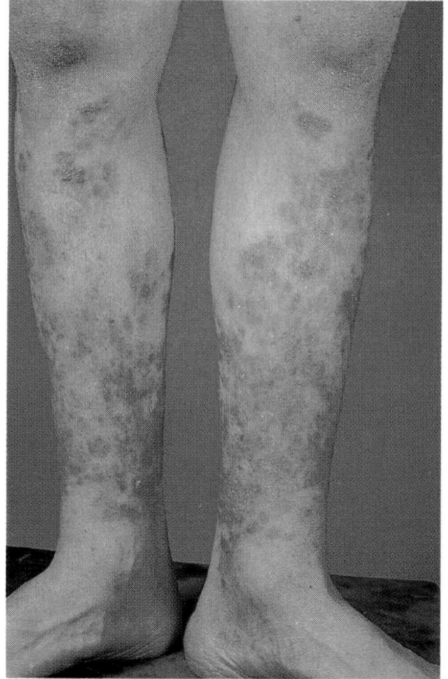

FIGURE 3–67. Epidemic Kaposi's sarcoma; plaque stage

A 35-year-old homosexual man with Kaposi's sarcoma primarily located on the lower extremities. As his disease progressed, new lesions developed in the same region, and the early discrete pink macules became confluent, indurated, and hyperpigmented. This distribution of lesions resembles the most frequent clinical presentation of classic Kaposi's sarcoma.

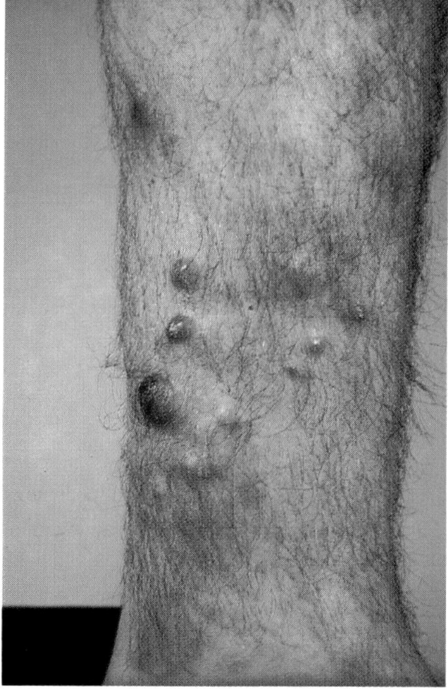

FIGURE 3–68. Epidemic Kaposi's sarcoma; nodular stage

A 47-year-old homosexual man of Italian extraction had multiple nodular lesions of Kaposi's sarcoma ranging in color from pink to brown on both lower extremities that had been present since 1980. The original diagnosis of classic Kaposi's sarcoma was changed to epidemic (AIDS-associated) Kaposi's sarcoma in 1982 when he developed *Pneumocystis carinii* pneumonia. A stored serum sample from 1979 was found to contain antibodies to HIV.

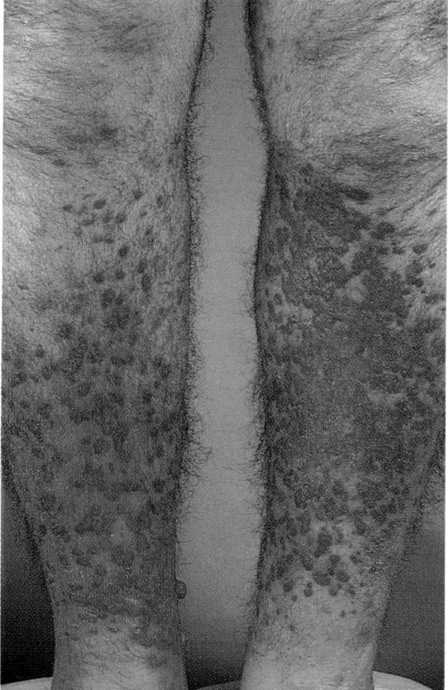

FIGURE 3–69. Epidemic Kaposi's sarcoma; plaque stage

This 39-year-old homosexual man of Mediterranean extraction developed multiple dark brown-to-purple plaque and nodular lesions predominantly located on the lower extremities, associated with chronic lymphedema. There is a subset of patients with epidemic Kaposi's sarcoma in whom the lesions tend to be localized to the lower extremities, a pattern that is similar to the typical classic variant of the disease (see classic pattern observed in Fig. 3–13).

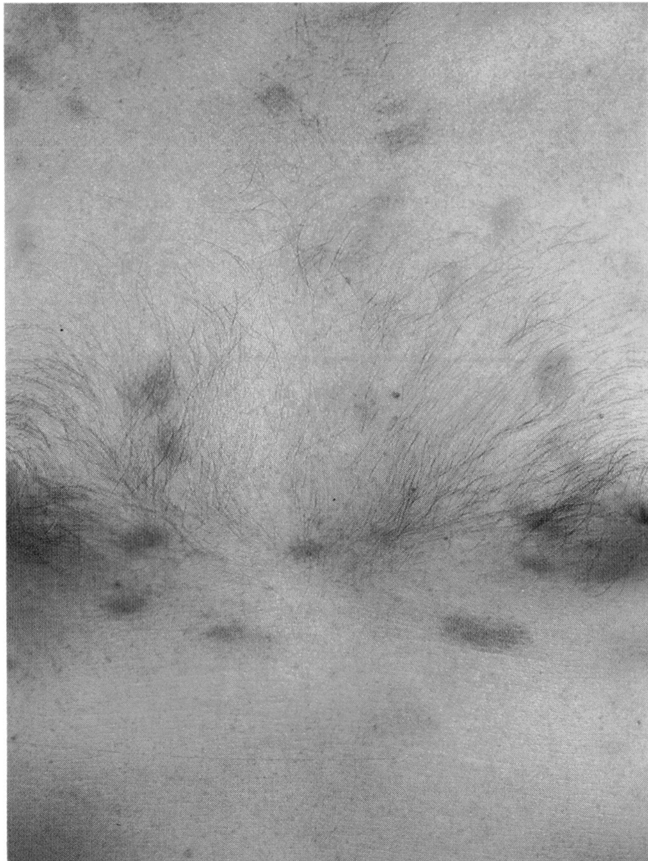

FIGURE 3–70. Epidemic Kaposi's sarcoma; patch-to-plaque stage

A 33-year-old homosexual man with bilateral dark pink to violet elongated lesions of Kaposi's sarcoma symmetrically and widely distributed over his entire body. The lesions resemble dabs of paint spattered on the skin surface. It is interesting to note that the lesions conform to the creases of the skin (lines of Langer).

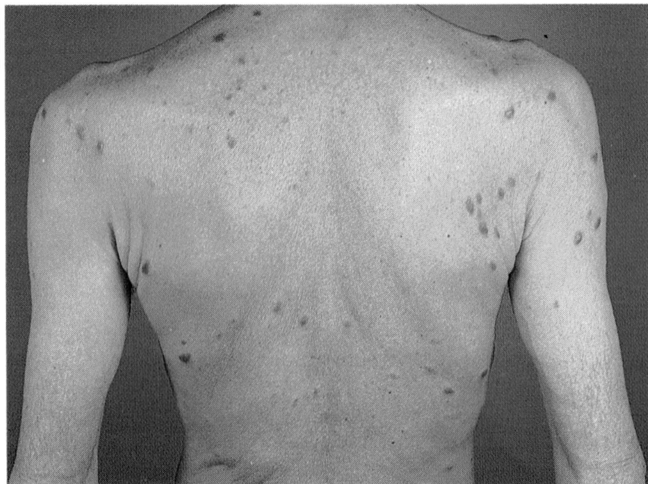

FIGURE 3–72. Epidemic Kaposi's sarcoma; plaque stage

A 58-year-old Hispanic homosexual man who was an intravenous drug user had multiple symmetric purple plaques, which developed rapidly over his trunk and extremities. Many of the lesions appear to follow the creases of the skin (lines of Langer).

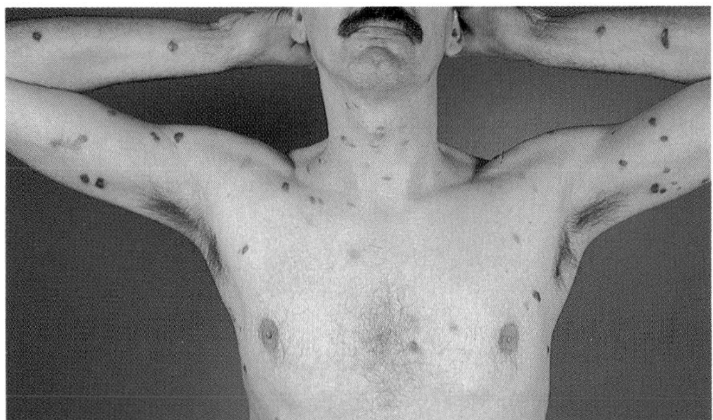

FIGURE 3–71. Epidemic Kaposi's sarcoma; plaque stage

A 41-year-old homosexual man with widespread, symmetric, cutaneous patches, plaques, and nodules of Kaposi's sarcoma that had been present for approximately 1 year. Some of the lesions have an elongated ovoid shape, and they vary in color from red to brown.

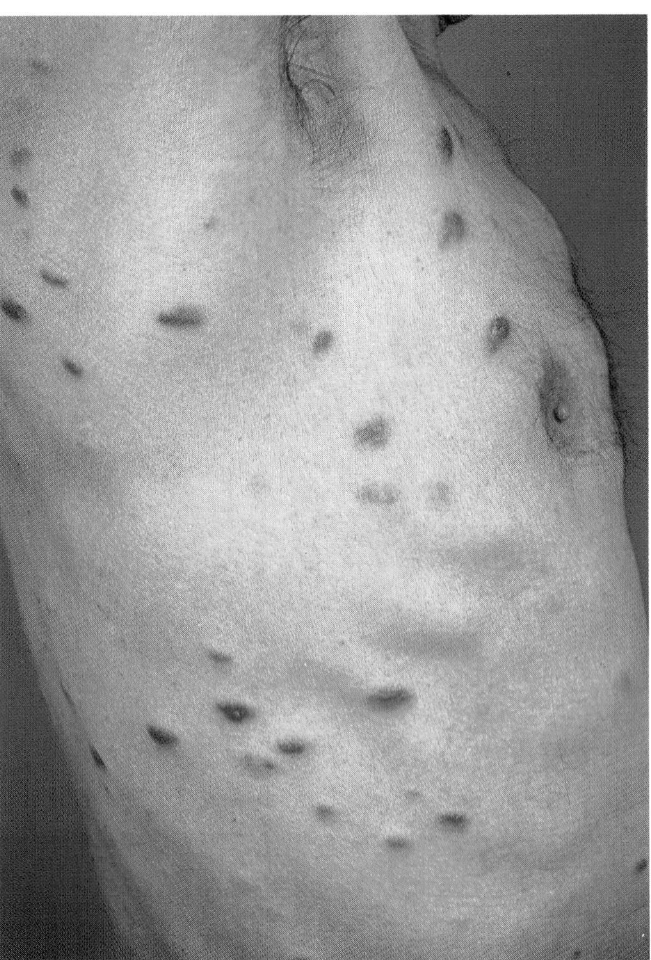

FIGURE 3–73. Epidemic Kaposi's sarcoma; plaque-to-nodular stage

Widely disseminated fusiform plaque lesions distributed symmetrically in a swirled pattern. They vary in color from dark red to violet. Some hyperpigmentation of the lesions is also evident.

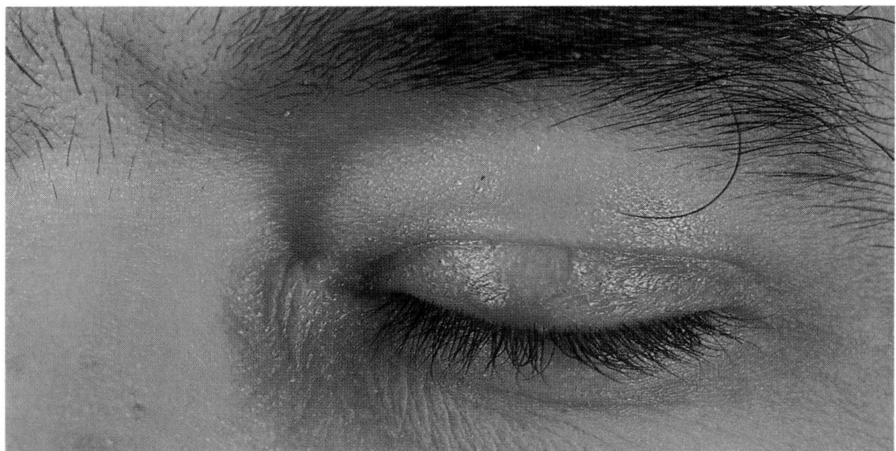

FIGURE 3–74. Epidemic Kaposi's sarcoma; plaque stage
A slightly indurated papular lesion on the upper eyelid of a patient with epidemic Kaposi's sarcoma. Initially, the lesion was thought to represent a stye and was examined by an ophthalmologist, who eventually performed a biopsy on the lesion when it did not respond to conventional therapy.

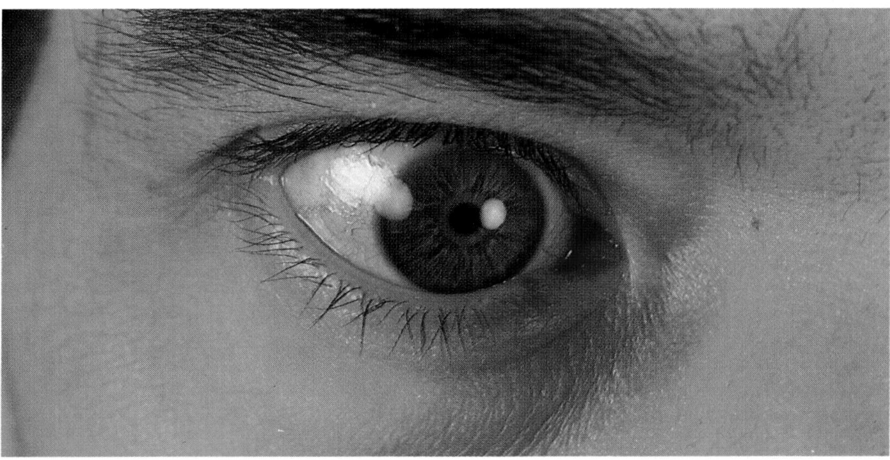

FIGURE 3–75. Epidemic Kaposi's sarcoma; patch stage
A linear red lesion on the lower eyelid margin of this bisexual male was one of many lesions present on the patient's skin. The lesion rapidly developed into a tumor nodule, which responded favorably to local radiation therapy.

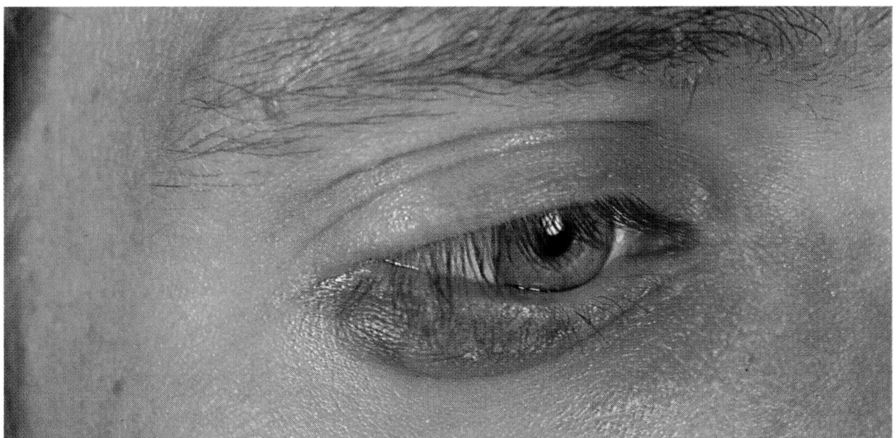

FIGURE 3–76. Epidemic Kaposi's sarcoma; plaque stage
Indurated violaceous lesion affecting the lateral lower eyelid.

In 1994, the DNA sequences of a novel herpesvirus-like agent were identified in AIDS-associated KS by representational difference analysis.[72] These unique sequences were found in more than 90% of AIDS-associated KS lesions examined. The sequences show some homology to the capsid and tegument protein genes of the γ-herpesviruses, herpesvirus saimiri and Epstein-Barr virus. Based on these similarities, the virus has been classified as new human herpesvirus: HHV-8. Furthermore, this virus has been detected in lesions obtained from different epidemiologic types of KS including the non–HIV-associated "classic" form of KS (CKS) seen in elderly men of eastern European Mediterranean background, the African endemic forms of KS, and that seen in HIV-negative homosexual men with KS.[73–76] HHV-8 has also been detected by polymerase chain reaction in some normal-appearing skin, peripheral blood mononuclear cells, and semen from some AIDS-associated KS patients.[72–75] The identified DNA sequences of the HHV-8 are well conserved in the various forms of KS, although some degree of sequence variation was found by single strand conformational polymorphism and sequencing.[73,74] These findings suggest that HHV-8 may play a role in the development of KS occurring in different populations.

In addition to KS, certain AIDS-related lymphomas and various skin lesions including basal cell carcinoma, squamous cell carcinoma, and actinic keratosis in iatrogenically immunosuppressed transplant recipients have also been shown to contain HHV-8 DNA.[81,82] The high degree of correlation (>90%) of HHV-8 presence with the various epidemiologic forms of KS suggests

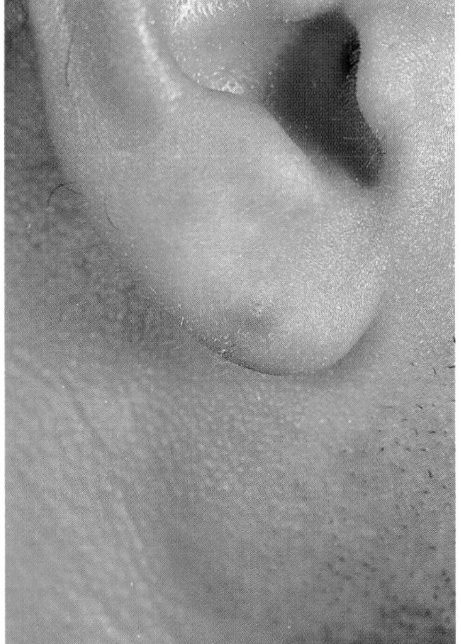

FIGURE 3–77. Epidemic Kaposi's sarcoma; nodular stage

A 29-year-old homosexual man with epidemic Kaposi's sarcoma. The patient presented with multiple faint macular lesions on his trunk and hard palate and this asymptomatic pink solitary nodule on the earlobe. Lesions on the ear have been reported rarely in the classic or endemic African forms of the disease.

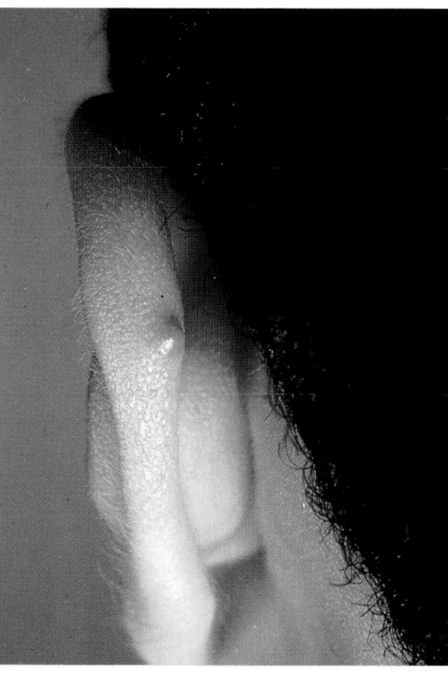

FIGURE 3–78. Epidemic Kaposi's sarcoma; nodular stage

A 30-year-old bisexual Hispanic man who was an intravenous drug user had a red tumor nodule on the pinna of the ear.

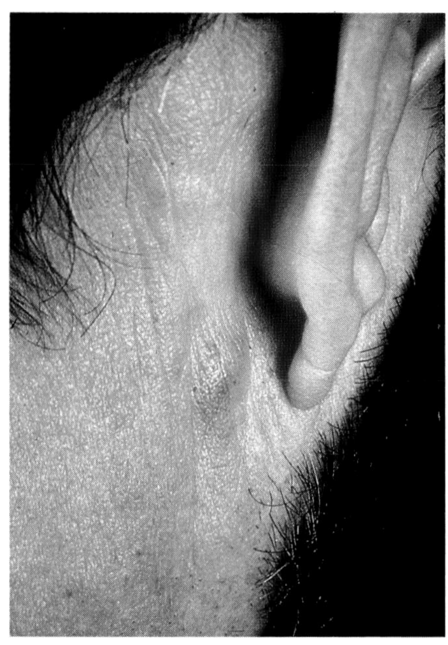

FIGURE 3–79. Epidemic Kaposi's sarcoma; nodular stage

A faint bluish posterior auricular skin nodule. This is a common, frequently overlooked site for Kaposi's sarcoma lesions to appear in patients with AIDS.

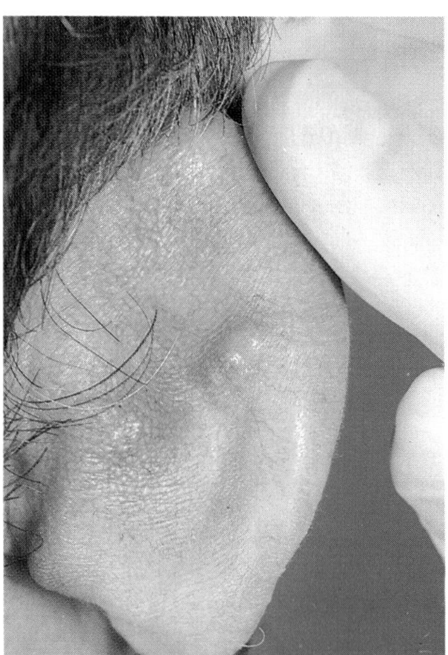

FIGURE 3–80. Epidemic Kaposi's sarcoma; nodular stage

Two opalescent bluish-colored asymptomatic nodules on the back of the ear.

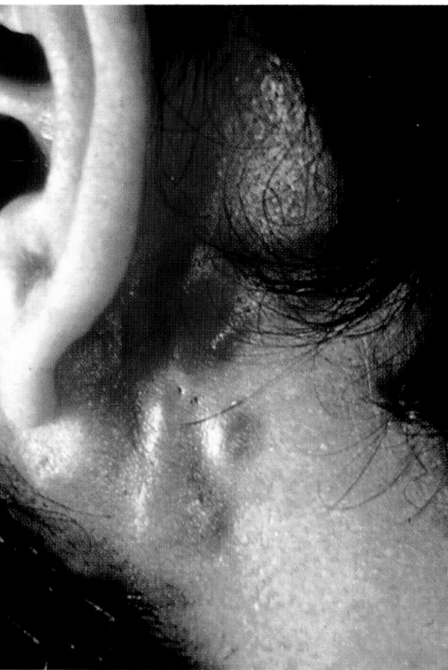

FIGURE 3–81. Epidemic Kaposi's sarcoma; plaque stage

A cluster of irregularly shaped, red, indurated plaques of Kaposi's sarcoma located behind the ear.

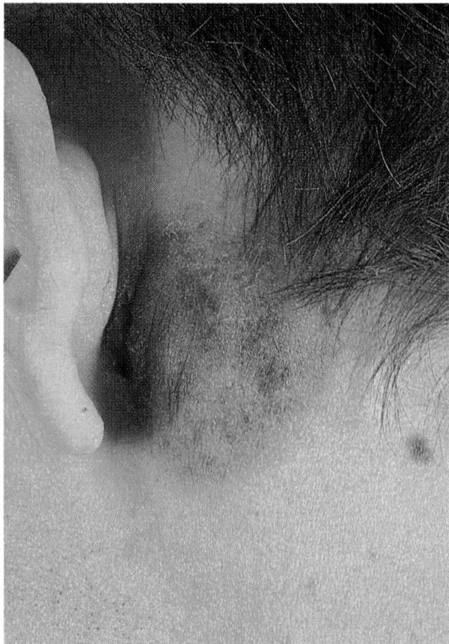

FIGURE 3–82. Epidemic Kaposi's sarcoma; patch stage

A large pink macular lesion with variegated pigmentation located behind the ear. This lesion resembles a superficial spreading melanoma. There is a small, brown, flat nevus just posterior to the tumor, which had been present since childhood.

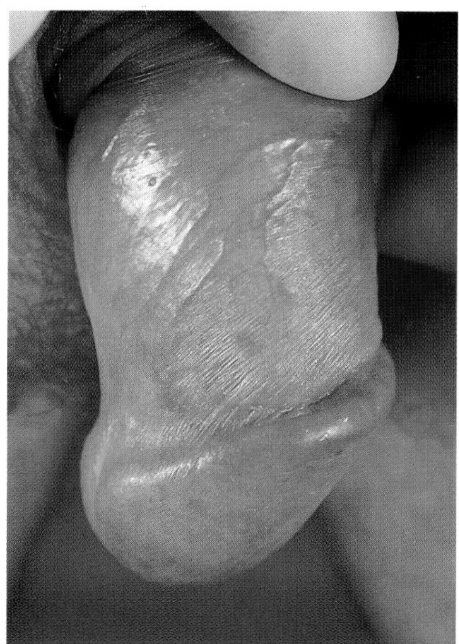

FIGURE 3–83. Epidemic Kaposi's sarcoma; patch stage

A 42-year-old Hispanic man with three asymptomatic faint red macules of Kaposi's sarcoma on the inner surface of the retracted foreskin.

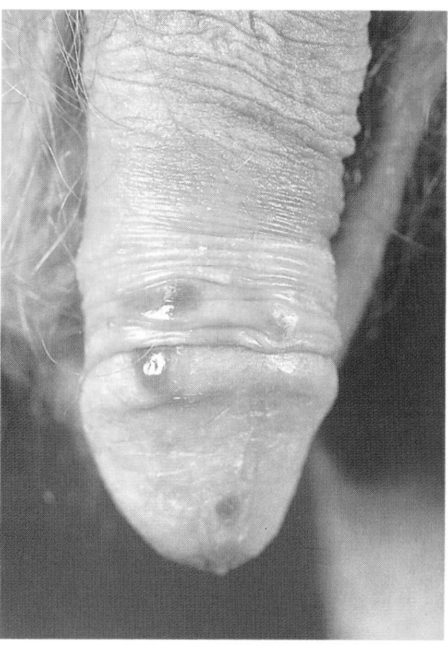

FIGURE 3–84. Epidemic Kaposi's sarcoma; plaque stage

Slightly indurated red papules seen on the inner aspect of the retracted foreskin and glans. These lesions resemble those of lichen planus or secondary syphilis.

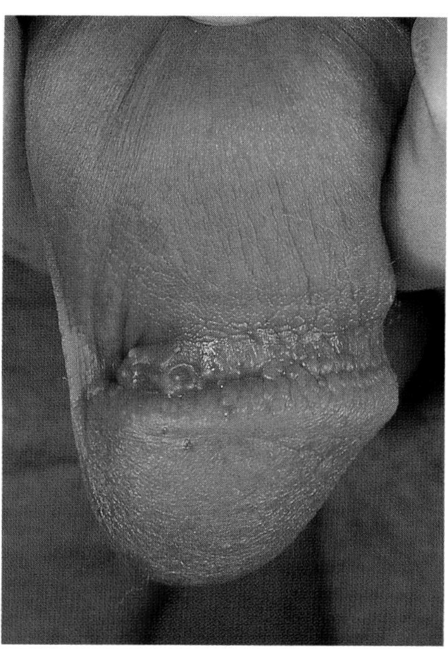

FIGURE 3–85. Epidemic Kaposi's sarcoma; nodular stage

Multiple red pinpoint and nodular lesions present along the coronal sulcus of the penis. The patient was initially thought to have condylomata acuminata. It was only after unsuccessful treatment with topical podophyllum that a biopsy was performed, which surprisingly revealed a diagnosis of Kaposi's sarcoma.

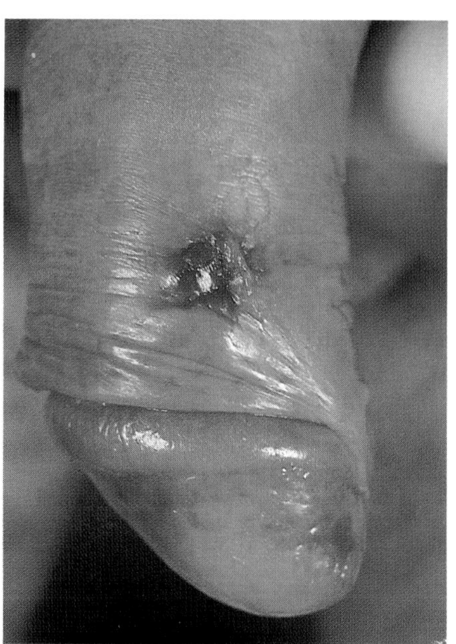

FIGURE 3–86. Epidemic Kaposi's sarcoma; nodular stage

A deep brown nodule of Kaposi's sarcoma on the lateral shaft of the penis. In addition, there is a purple macular lesion on the glans penis.

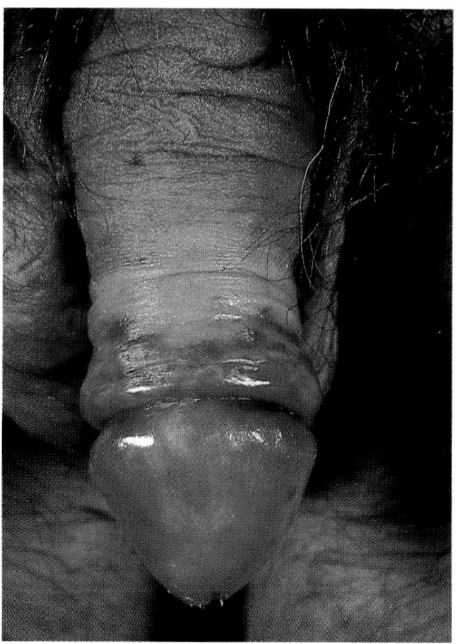

FIGURE 3–87. Epidemic Kaposi's sarcoma; advanced disease

A 37-year-old white man with an advanced infiltrative lesion of Kaposi's sarcoma that affected the entire glans and distal shaft of the penis. The lesion caused severe pain when the patient developed an erection and eventually caused urethral obstruction. On autopsy, the tumor was found to have invaded the corpus cavernosum.

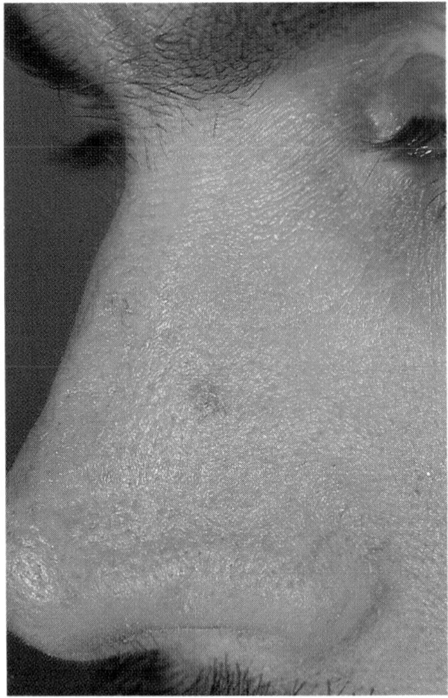

FIGURE 3–88. Epidemic Kaposi's sarcoma; patch stage

An isolated lavender macule of Kaposi's sarcoma on the side of the nose. Such early lesions could easily be overlooked or ignored by the patient and examining physician.

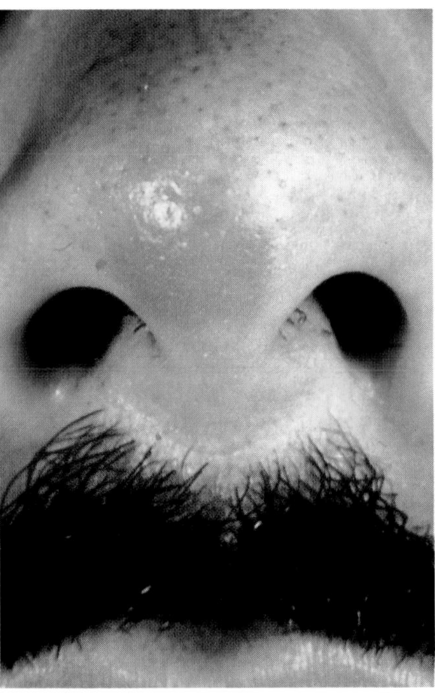

FIGURE 3–89. Epidemic Kaposi's sarcoma; patch stage

This erythematous patch-stage lesion on the nose of a 32-year-old homosexual man was originally thought to be the result of an insect bite.

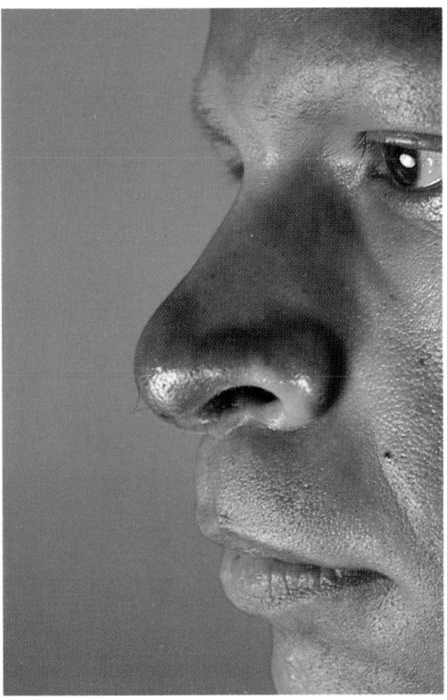

FIGURE 3–90. Epidemic Kaposi's sarcoma; patch stage

Large confluent hyperpigmented lesion of Kaposi's sarcoma in a mulatto homosexual man. Such lesions in dark-skinned individuals rapidly become hyperpigmented.

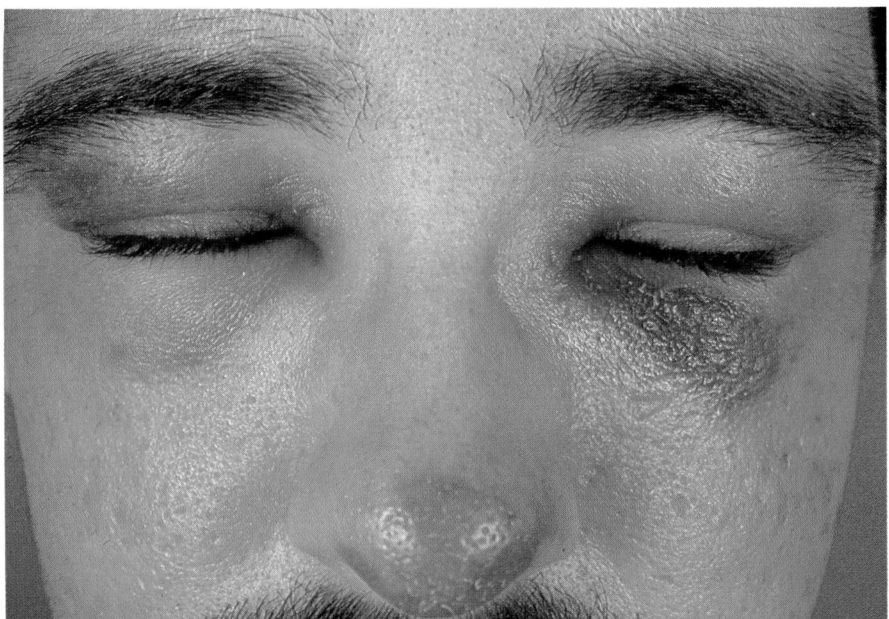

FIGURE 3–91. Epidemic Kaposi's sarcoma; advanced disease

Pink plaque-stage lesion on the skin of the tip of the nose that infiltrated into the nasal mucosa. The patient also has a large bluish purple macular lesion below his left eye and bilateral periorbital edema due to lymphatic obstruction, with yellowish discoloration.

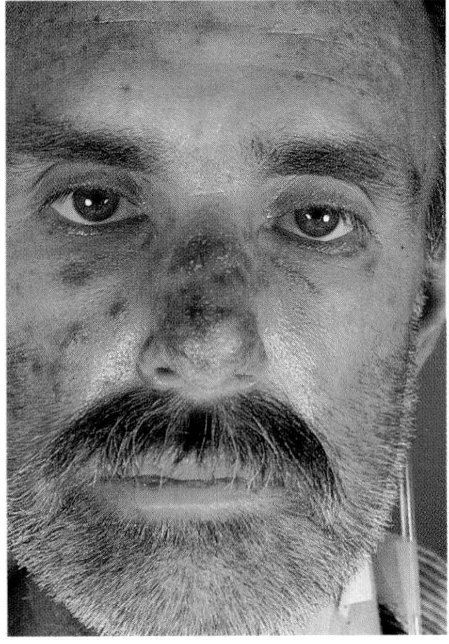

FIGURE 3–92. Epidemic Kaposi's sarcoma; advanced disease

A patient with widely disseminated mucocutaneous lesions of Kaposi's sarcoma. This picture illustrates infiltrative violaceous tumor involvement of the nose. Also note the tiny cherry-red tumor nodule on the inner canthus of the right eye.

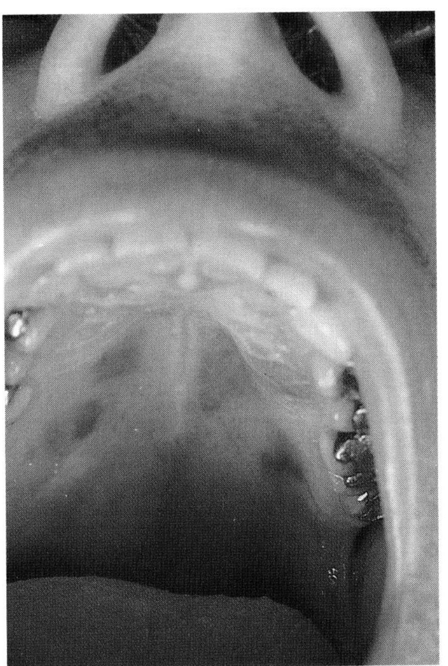

FIGURE 3–93. Epidemic Kaposi's sarcoma; patch stage
Several discrete asymptomatic violet macular lesions on the hard palate. Oral lesions, common in patients with epidemic Kaposi's sarcoma, are rarely reported in patients with classic or endemic African forms of this neoplasm.

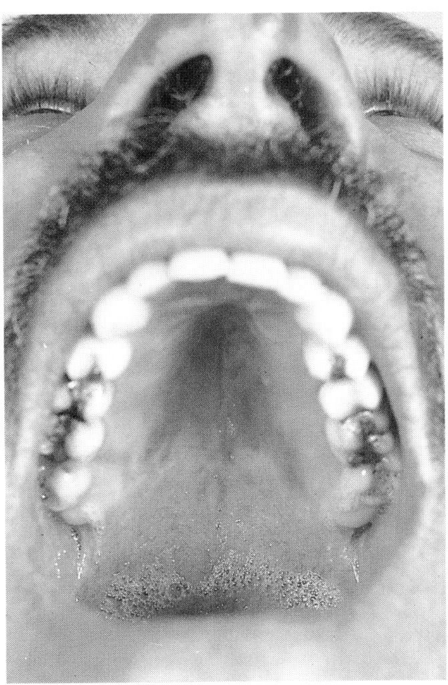

FIGURE 3–94. Epidemic Kaposi's sarcoma; patch stage
Large confluent macule of Kaposi's sarcoma on the hard palate. The macular lesions are almost always asymptomatic.

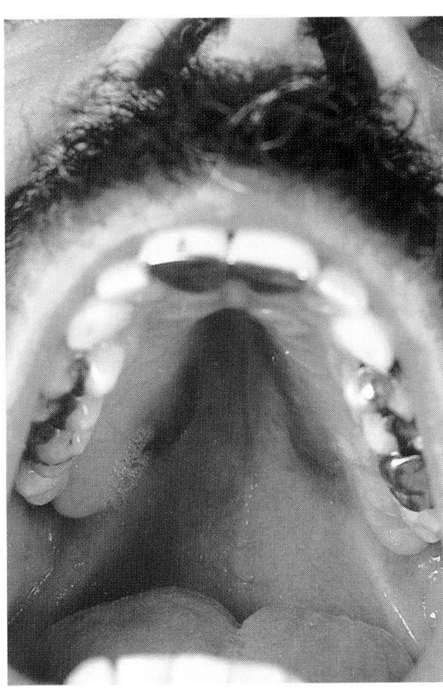

FIGURE 3–95. Epidemic Kaposi's sarcoma; plaque stage
Violet, symmetric indurated plaques of Kaposi's sarcoma on the hard palate of a homosexual man. These were among the earliest lesions to develop in this patient.

that KS may represent an "opportunistic" neoplasm and that this viral agent may play a significant role in the etiology or pathogenesis of KS, or both.

The presence of growth factors interleukin-1β,[83–85] basic fibroblast growth factor,[83,84] granulocyte-macrophage colony-stimulating factor,[83,84] interleukin-6 (IL-6),[84,86] tumor necrosis factor-α,[84,85] or fibroblast growth factor-6[87] in AIDS-associated KS–derived cell lines implies that such factors may play a role in the etiology of or the clinical course of the disease. Human immunodeficiency virus type 1 proviral sequences have not been detected in cells from KS tissues or in AIDS-associated KS–derived cell lines.[61] The transactivating factor Tat-1 has been found to double the growth of such KS cell lines in vitro.[88] Interleukin-6 has also been found to enhance the growth of AIDS-associated KS cell lines and to be present at elevated levels in KS lesions, and inhibition of IL-6 activity has been found to inhibit the growth-enhancing activity of IL-6.[86] Importantly, IL-6 levels have been found to be elevated in the serum and KS tissue of patients with AIDS,[89,90] and thus IL-6 may serve as an in vivo factor relevant to the clinical course of disease in AIDS patients. Interestingly, IL-6 has been shown to be important in the regulation of B-lymphocyte function and is a growth factor for hybridoma-plasmacytoma lines[91,92] and may play a role in the increased incidence of B-cell lymphomas in patients with AIDS. Oncostatin-M has been found to be an important KS-derived cell line growth factor present in the supernatant culture fluid of human T-cell lymphoma virus–infected cell cultures, but the role of such a factor in vivo remains to be elucidated.[93–95] Furthermore, the glycoprotein 130β subunit of the IL-6 receptor has been identified as part of the oncostatin-M receptor and has been shown to convert the leukemia inhibitory factor receptor into a high-affinity oncostatin-M receptor.[96] It has thus been suggested that differential expression of the alpha chain of the IL-6 or oncostatin-M receptor may be responsible for the differential effect of some cytokines in AIDS-associated KS–derived cell lines compared with those in their normal cell counterparts.[95–98]

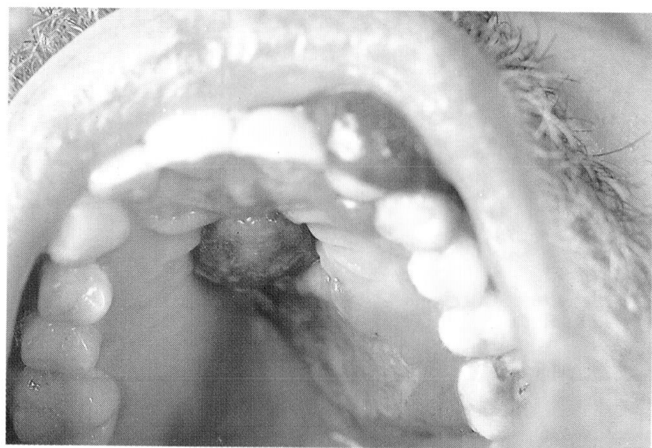

FIGURE 3–96. Epidemic Kaposi's sarcoma; nodular stage
Extensive Kaposi's sarcoma of the oral cavity with a large purple nodular tumor on the hard palate and a red gingival nodular lesion extending over the left incisor. Also present is a chronic oral ulcer on the mucosa of the hard palate due to herpes simplex virus.

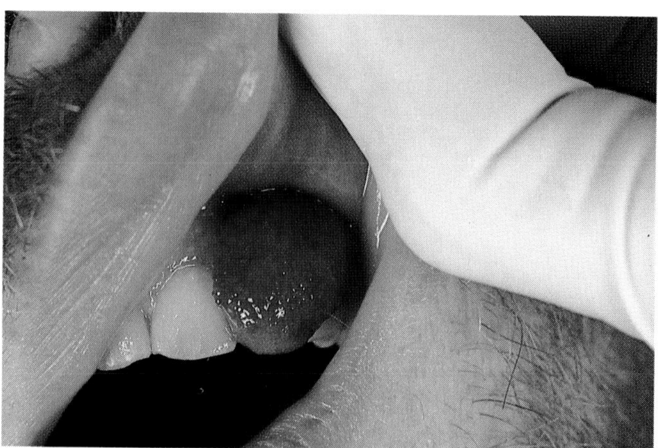

FIGURE 3–97. Epidemic Kaposi's sarcoma; nodular stage
A close-up view of the large, deep, red, stalactite-like tumor extending from the gingiva over the incisor tooth (also seen in Fig. 3–60).

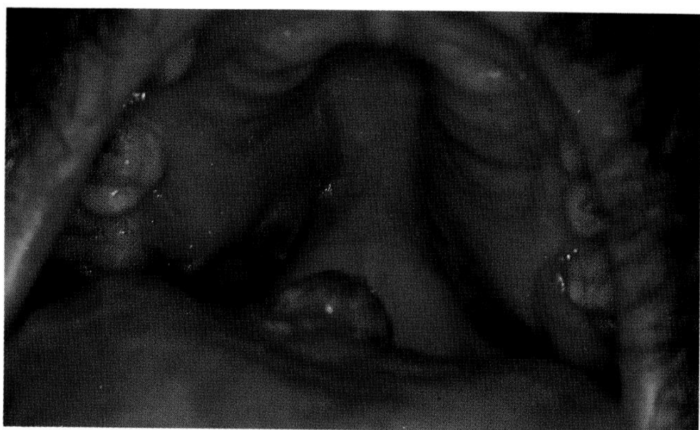

FIGURE 3–98. Epidemic Kaposi's sarcoma; nodular stage
Bilateral symmetric pink-to-purple nodular tumors on the hard palate. Also present is a nodular lesion on the tongue. Kaposi's sarcoma affecting the tongue has been reported rarely.

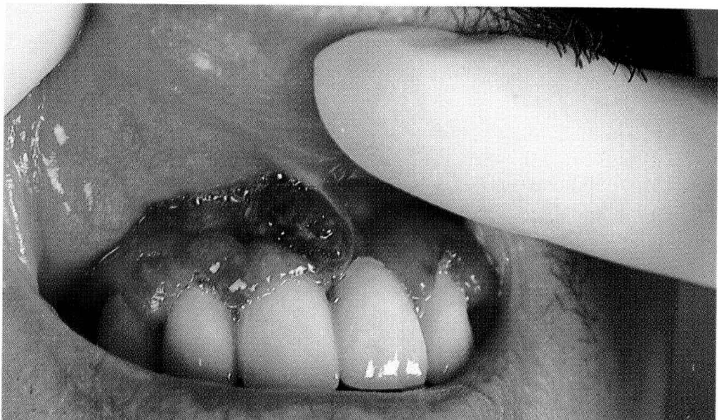

FIGURE 3–99. Epidemic Kaposi's sarcoma; nodular stage
Multiple nodular red and purple lesions of Kaposi's sarcoma affecting the gingiva extensively.

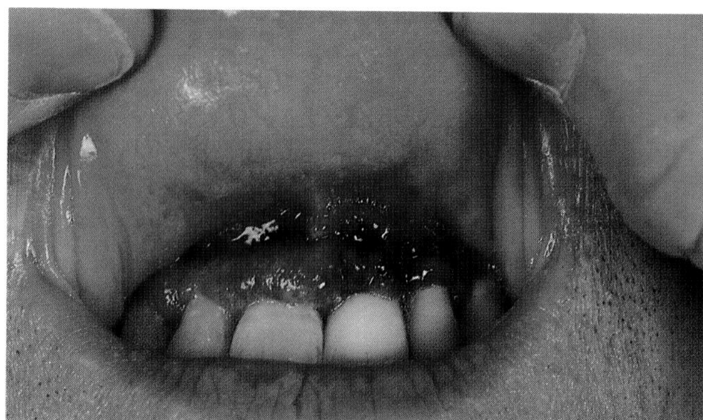

FIGURE 3–100. Epidemic Kaposi's sarcoma; nodular stage
Numerous hemorrhagic-appearing deep red lesions located on the lower gingiva and extending onto the labial mucosa.

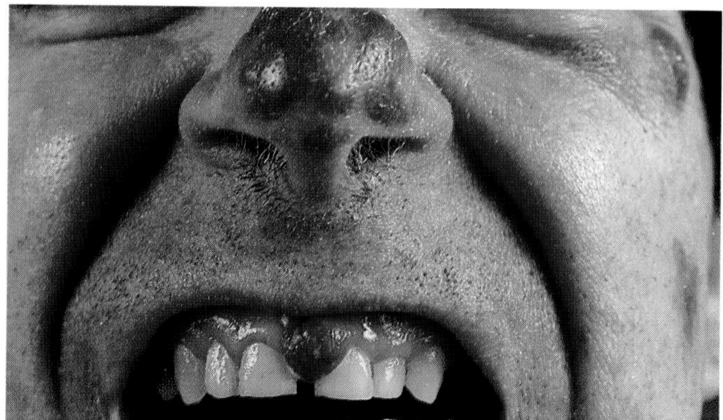

FIGURE 3–101. Epidemic Kaposi's sarcoma; plaque and nodular stages
A homosexual man with advanced-stage disease with widely disseminated deep purple plaque and nodular tumor lesions of the skin and oral mucosa.

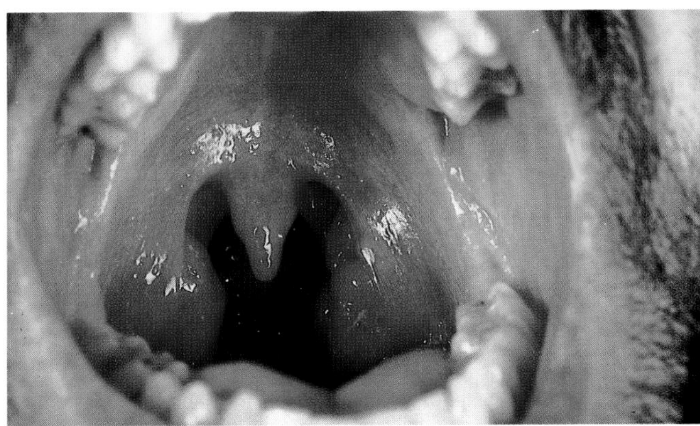

FIGURE 3–102. Epidemic Kaposi's sarcoma; nodular stage
Bilateral enlarged erythematous tonsils, found at tonsillectomy to be due to Kaposi's sarcoma. (Courtesy of N. Cohen, MD, New York University Medical Center.)

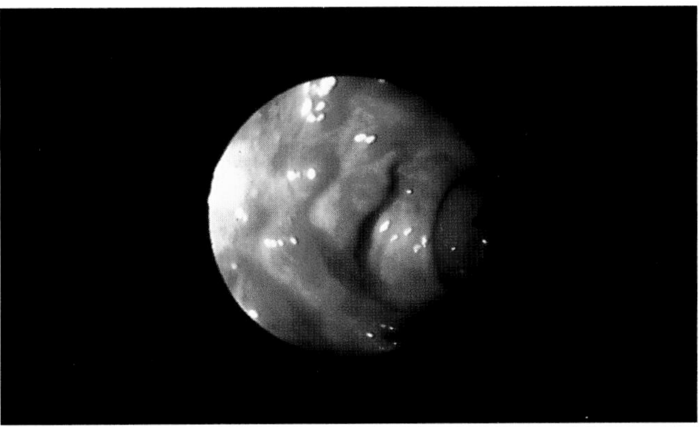

FIGURE 3–103. Epidemic Kaposi's sarcoma; nodular stage
Nodular lesions detected in the esophagus by endoscopy examination. At autopsy the patient was found to have numerous nodular lesions extending throughout the entire gastrointestinal tract. (Courtesy of L. Horowitz, MD, Department of Medicine, New York University Medical Center.)

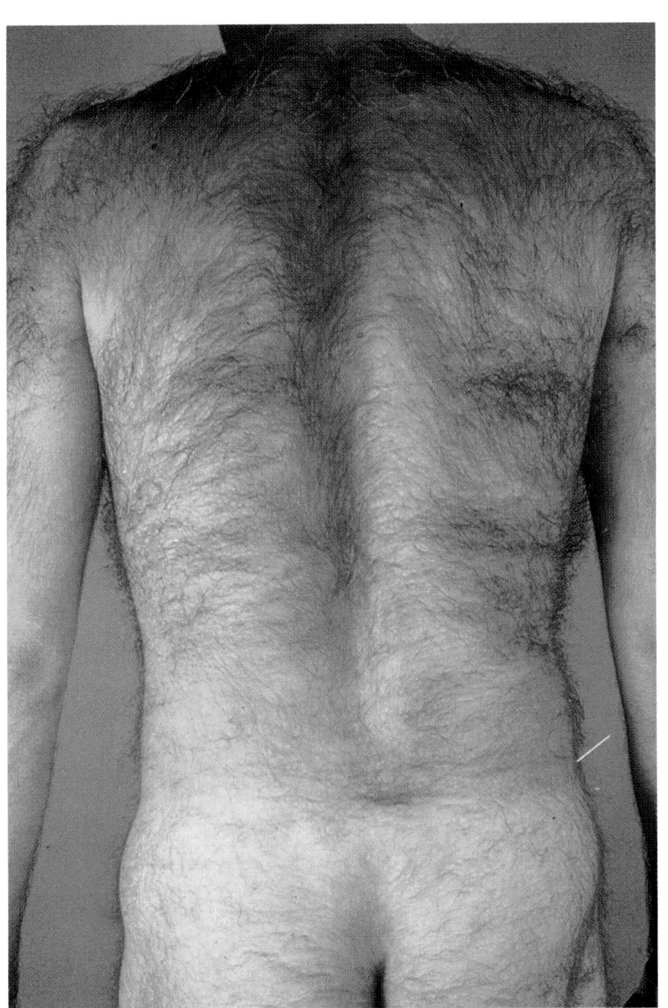

FIGURE 3–104. Epidemic Kaposi's sarcoma
This photograph is of the back of a 36-year-old homosexual man who was one of the earliest AIDS patients seen at New York University Medical Center in early 1981. He presented with only a few macular lesions of Kaposi's sarcoma on his face and oral mucosa. There were no lesions on his back at that time.

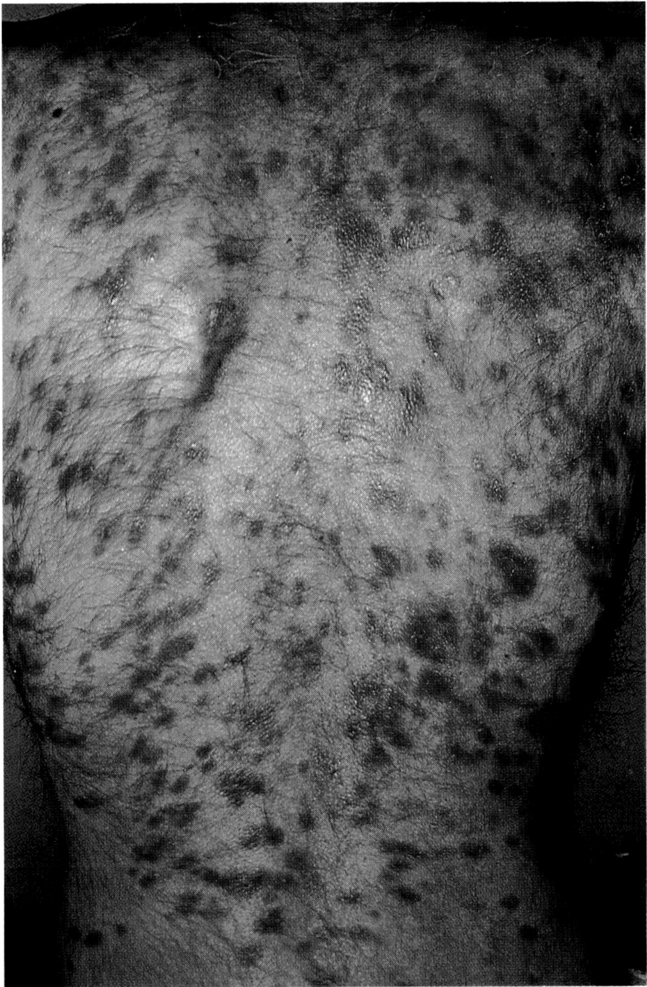

FIGURE 3–105. Epidemic Kaposi's sarcoma; plaque stage lesion
A follow-up photograph of the back of the same patient seen in Figure 3–104, taken 6 months later, illustrates the rapid development of widely disseminated purple plaques of Kaposi's sarcoma over his skin.

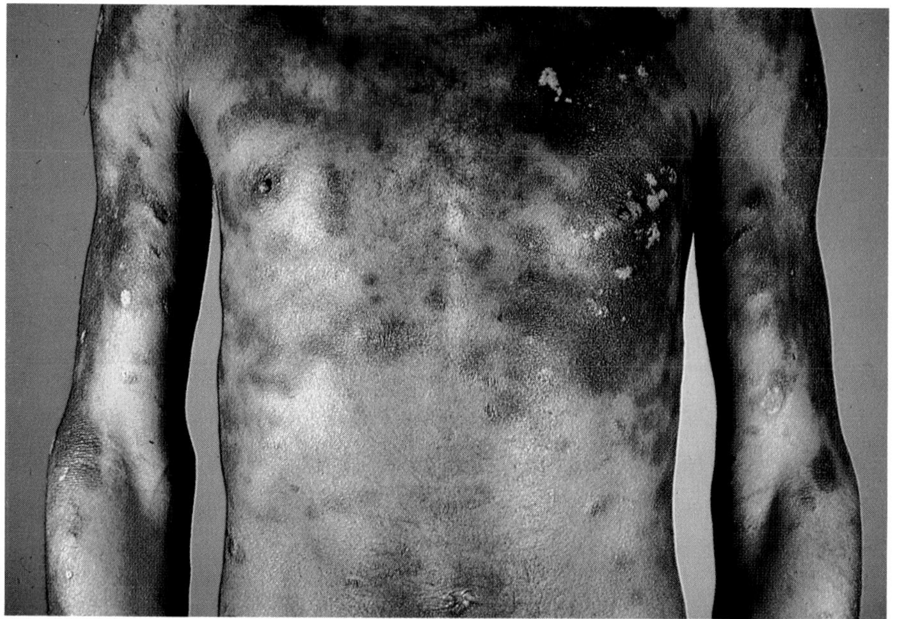

FIGURE 3–106. Epidemic Kaposi's sarcoma

A 31-year-old black man with extensive hyperpigmented confluent patch and plaque lesions of Kaposi's sarcoma on his trunk and upper extremities. Coincidentally, there are some hypopigmented areas representing long-standing vitiligo.

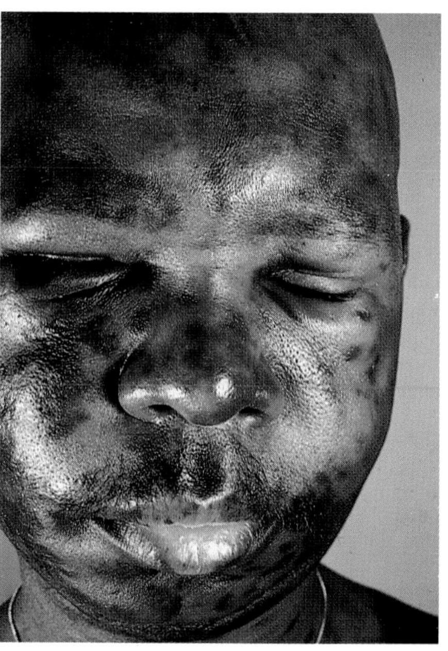

FIGURE 3–107. Epidemic Kaposi's sarcoma

The face of the same patient as in Figure 3–106. The large confluent lesions extended over his face and scalp were associated with marked facial edema due to invasive lymphatic obstruction.

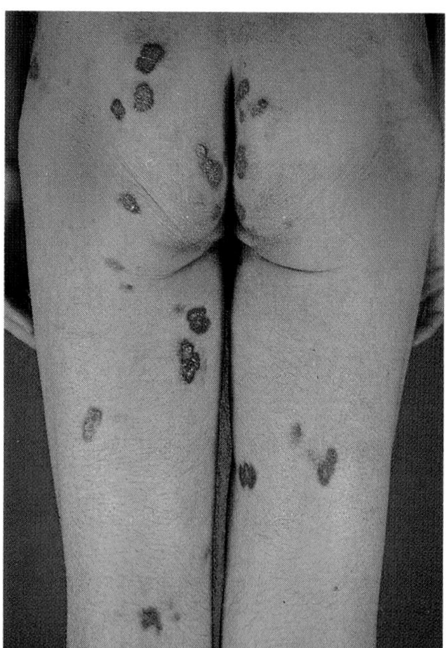

FIGURE 3–108. Epidemic Kaposi's sarcoma; plaque stage

A 24-year-old homosexual man with Kaposi's sarcoma of 2-years' duration. The patient is markedly cachectic following multiple opportunistic infections. There are widespread hyperpigmented purple-to-brown-black plaques on the lower extremities and buttocks, some with superficial surface erosions.

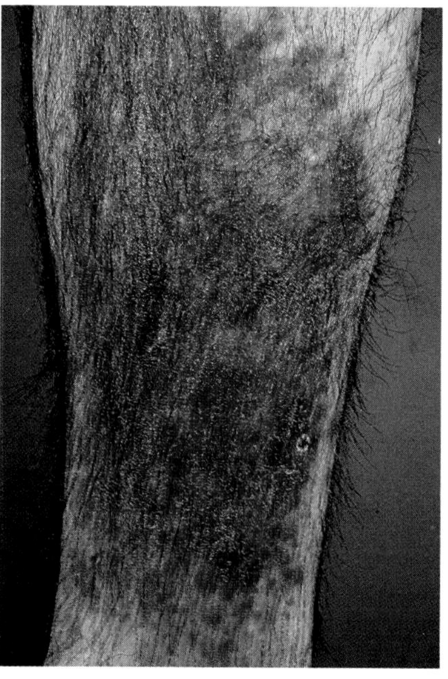

FIGURE 3–109. Epidemic Kaposi's sarcoma; plaque stage

A 37-year-old homosexual man with Kaposi's sarcoma for 2 years. As his disease progressed, macular and plaque-stage lesions increased in both size and number, coalescing to form this large, confluent, deep purple tumor involving a large area of the pretibial region.

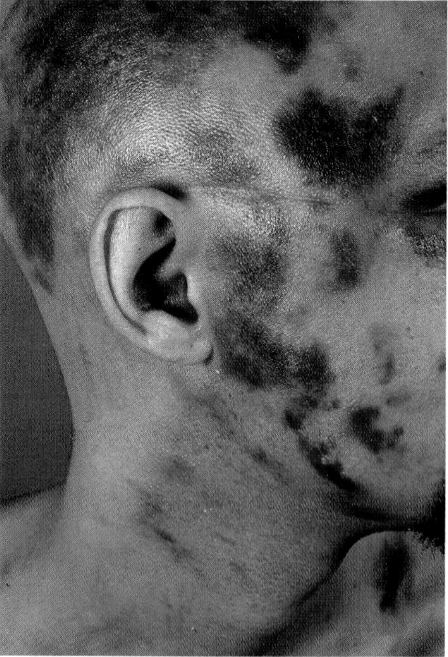

FIGURE 3–110. Epidemic Kaposi's sarcoma; plaque stage

Advanced disease with widespread, large deep purple-to-brown confluent plaque lesions of Kaposi's sarcoma on the head and neck in a 37-year-old homosexual man.

As was noted in studies of some endemic and transplant-associated lymphomas, early reports on patients developing AIDS-associated KS suggested an imbalance in the prevalence of HLA-DR5.[20,99] In more recent studies, such a phenomenon has not been found.[100] However, the linkage of HLA-DQw3 with cervical cancer,[101] the well-established link of HPV-16 with cervical cancer and with cervical dysplasia,[102] and the recognition of cervical cancer and dysplasia as AIDS- and HIV-1–related illnesses[103–106] suggests that the role of HLA type in the etiology of KS should be reevaluated. Also, the preliminary finding of circulating cells with KS-like features in patients with AIDS-associated KS[107] indicates that the multifocal nature of KS needs to be restudied.

The population of patients developing AIDS-associated KS has changed. An effective education program aimed at the prevention of HIV infection by sexual transmission in the gay community has resulted in dramatic decreases in the incidence of HIV infection as well as in the reduced incidence of KS in that population. Furthermore, patients with AIDS now survive longer owing to the earlier recognition, prevention, and treatment of the various opportunistic infections associated with AIDS. Thus, whereas AIDS-associated KS was often an early recognized manifestation of AIDS, often preceding the onset of opportunistic infections and often preceding the decrease in $CD4^+$ lymphocytes associated with the progressive immunodeficiency of AIDS, AIDS-associated KS now often appears as a late manifestation of the disease in patients who have been afflicted with multiple opportunistic infections and with profound reductions of their $CD4^+$ cell counts.[108–110]

Lesions of AIDS-associated KS appear as faint pink to purple or brownish-black patches, plaques, papules, or nodules anywhere on the skin or the oral mucosa. Unlike the distribution of lesions in classic KS, acral distribution is not a feature of AIDS-associated KS. The lesions usually begin as patches and evolve to the plaque and nodular stage. The lesions frequently appear in a symmetric distribution and may follow the creases of the skin (Langer's lines). Crops of lesions sometimes appear at one site. Occasionally, some lesions may regress spontaneously even as neighboring or distant sites of disease appear. With time, lesions may grow and coalesce. Local invasion of underlying tissue is uncharacteristic. Lesions on the lower extremities are often associated with edema, which may become severe. The cause of the edema is thought to be obstruction or invasion of local lymphatics or of more proximal lymph nodes in the inguinal region or pelvis. As with the other forms of KS, it is thought that new sites of disease arise independently and do not represent metastases from existing tumors. Histologic diagnosis of mucocutaneous tumors should be made by biopsy because many other pathologic conditions may resemble the lesions of KS. Although the tumor appears highly vascular clinically and under the microscope, biopsy rarely causes excessive bleeding unless an underlying blood vessel is cut. Furthermore, it is important to emphasize that even a biopsy-

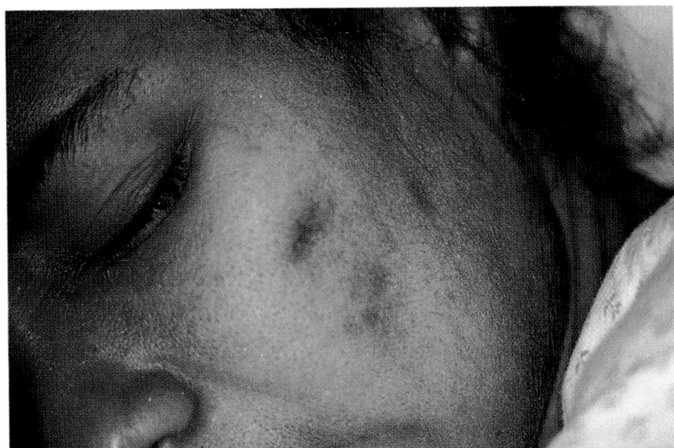

FIGURE 3–111. Epidemic Kaposi's sarcoma (Africa); patch stage

An HIV-seropositive black woman from Zaire, who developed widely disseminated red-to-purple macular lesions of Kaposi's sarcoma on her skin. (Courtesy of N. Clumeck, MD, Brussels, Belgium.)

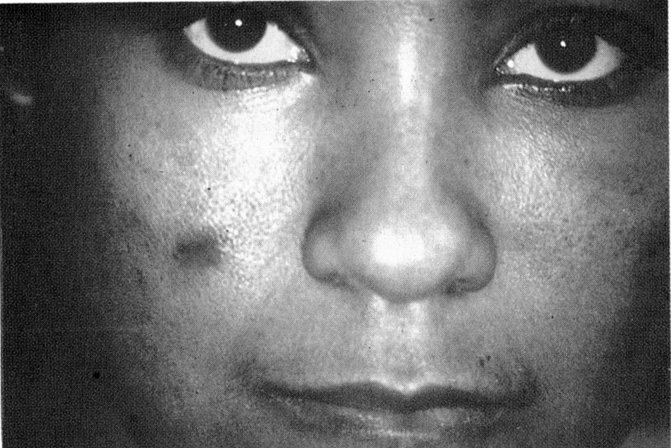

FIGURE 3–112. Epidemic Kaposi's sarcoma (Africa); plaque stage

The patient has a purple ovoid plaque of Kaposi's sarcoma on her left cheek. Other skin lesions were present, widely distributed over the rest of her body. (Courtesy of N. Clumeck, MD, Brussels, Belgium.)

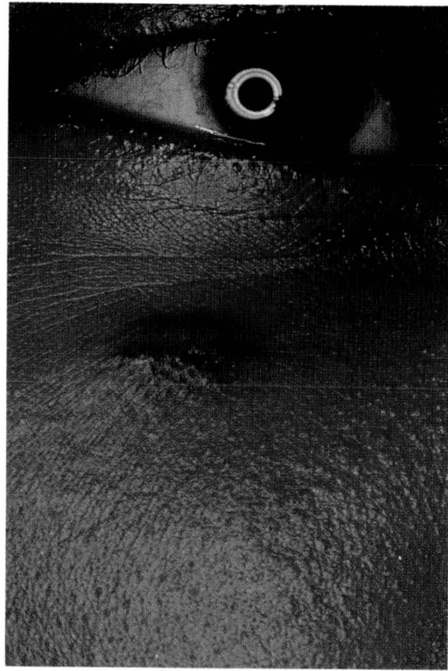

FIGURE 3–113. Epidemic Kaposi's sarcoma (Africa); plaque stage
A 27-year-old black woman from Zaire who sought medical attention in Brussels, Belgium, when she noted the development of asymptomatic purple-to-black nodules of Kaposi's sarcoma on her skin. The patient was found to have serum antibodies to HIV. Illustrated here is a lesion of Kaposi's sarcoma on her cheek, just below the eye. (Courtesy of N. Clumeck, MD, Brussels, Belgium.)

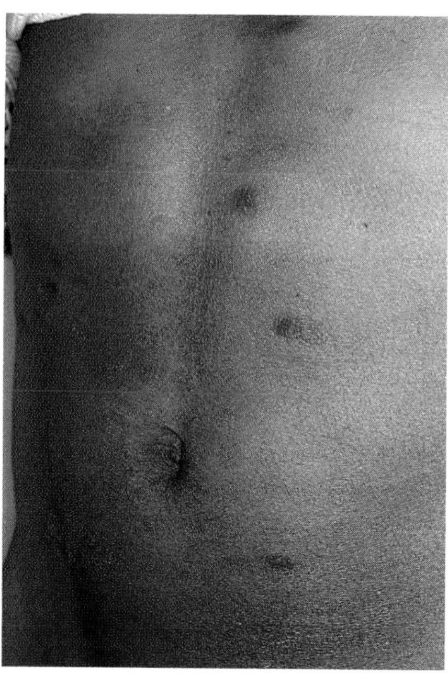

FIGURE 3–114. Epidemic Kaposi's sarcoma (Africa); plaque and nodular stage
Plaque and nodular lesions over the abdomen in this young black man from Zaire who was seropositive for HIV antibodies. There is considerable confusion between the incidence of the endemic form and the epidemic AIDS-associated varieties of Kaposi's sarcoma seen in Africa. (Courtesy of N. Clumeck, MD, Brussels, Belgium.)

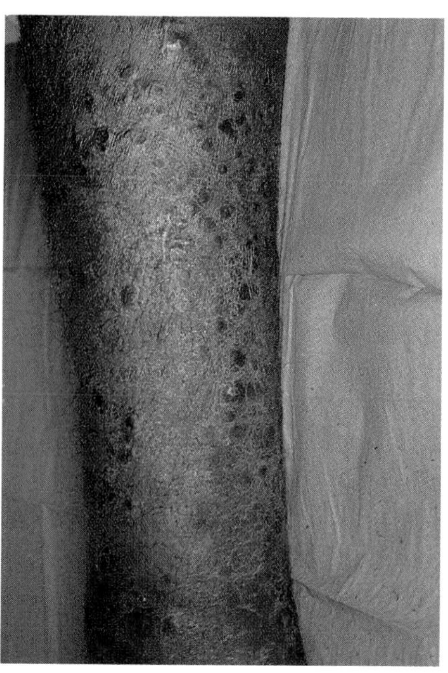

FIGURE 3–115. Epidemic Kaposi's sarcoma (Africa); plaque stage
A 37-year-old black man from central Africa with AIDS-associated Kaposi's sarcoma rapidly developed multiple dark brown-to-black plaque-stage lesions, which were widely disseminated over his body. During the fulminant course of his brief illness, he developed multiple opportunistic infections. (Courtesy of N. Clumeck, MD, Brussels, Belgium.)

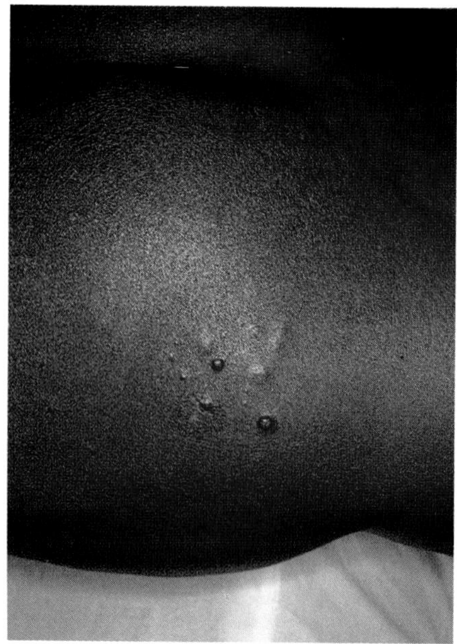

FIGURE 3–116. Epidemic Kaposi's sarcoma (Africa); nodular stage
A cluster of purplish-brown nodules on the side of the hip and buttock of this young black man from Zaire who was HIV antibody seropositive. (Courtesy of N. Clumeck, MD, Brussels, Belgium.)

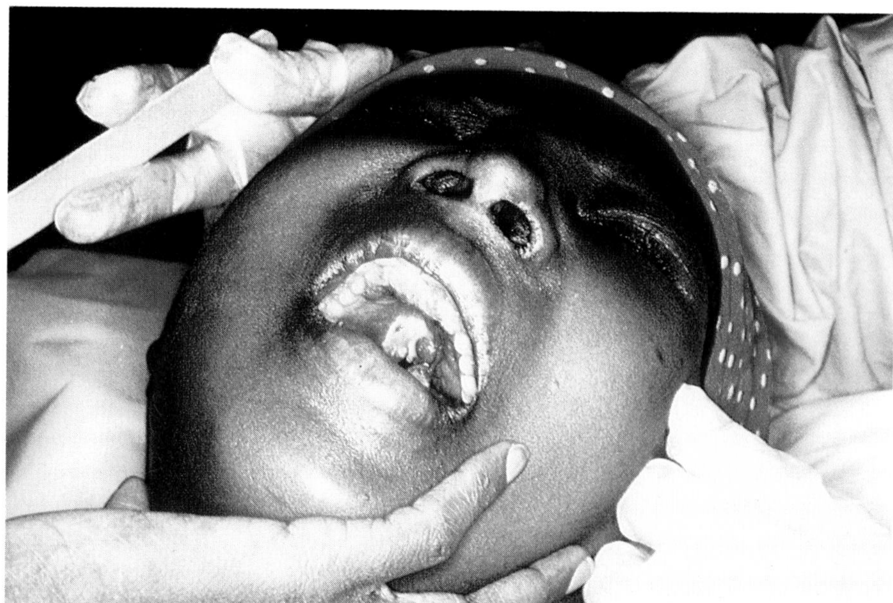

FIGURE 3–117. Epidemic Kaposi's sarcoma (Africa); nodular stage
A 36-year-old black woman with nodular tumors of Kaposi's sarcoma on the hard palate who had come from Zaire to Belgium for treatment. Other lesions were present on her skin as well. (Courtesy of N. Clumeck, MD, Brussels, Belgium.)

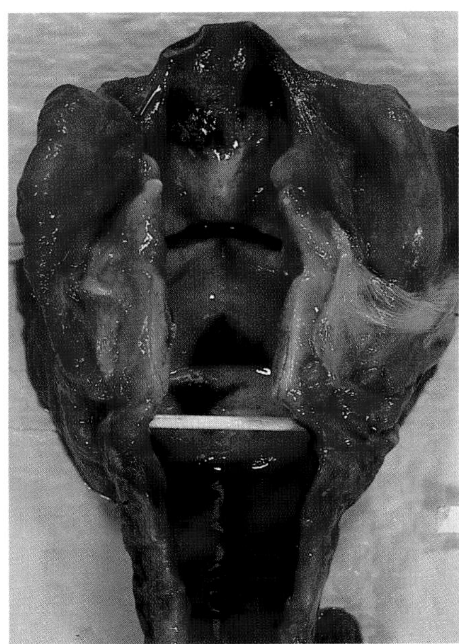

FIGURE 3–118. Autopsy, disseminated Kaposi's sarcoma

Autopsy specimen from a 47-year-old homosexual man with disseminated Kaposi's sarcoma and a history of multiple, recurrent opportunistic infections. Autopsy revealed extensive cutaneous Kaposi's sarcoma and visceral organ involvement, including tracheobronchial tree, liver, spleen, gastrointestinal tract, and lymph nodes. Multiple flat to slightly raised black hemorrhagic lesions of Kaposi's sarcoma were present in the supraglottic and infraglottic regions of the larynx and in the trachea. (Courtesy of John Li, MD, Northcentral Bronx Hospital, New York.)

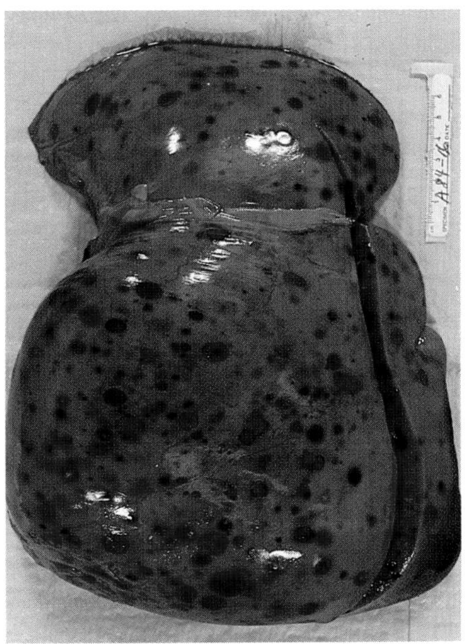

FIGURE 3–119. Autopsy, disseminated Kaposi's sarcoma

Autopsy of patient in Figure 3–117 shows an external view of the liver revealing numerous flat, red-purple areas of Kaposi's sarcoma in both lobes. (Courtesy of John Li, MD, Northcentral Bronx Hospital, New York.)

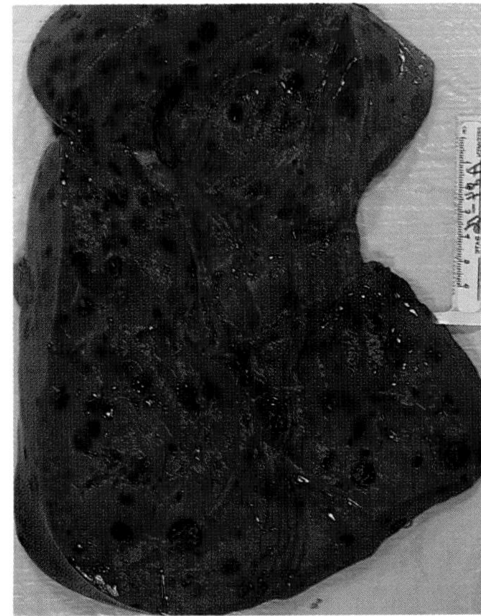

FIGURE 3–120. Autopsy, disseminated Kaposi's sarcoma

Cut surface view of the liver of the patient shown in Figure 3–117 shows the organ to be studded with hemorrhagic foci of Kaposi's sarcoma. (Courtesy of John Li, MD, Northcentral Bronx Hospital, New York.)

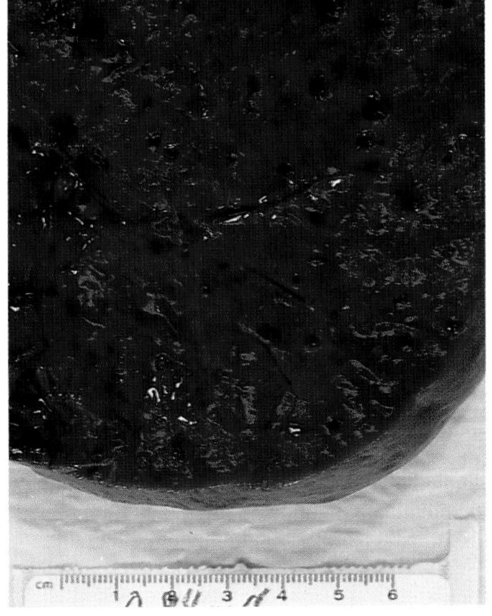

FIGURE 3–121. Autopsy, disseminated Kaposi's sarcoma

Cut surface of the spleen of the patient shown in Figure 3–117 revealing multiple nodules of Kaposi's sarcoma. (Courtesy of John Li, MD, Northcentral Bronx Hospital, New York.)

proven diagnosis of KS in an individual with risk factors for AIDS-associated KS does not necessarily imply infection with HIV because there are reported cases of young homosexual men with a mild form of KS who have no clinical or laboratory evidence of HIV infection. Therefore, serologic tests for antibodies to HIV must be performed before making a diagnosis of AIDS.

Visceral involvement with AIDS-associated KS is frequent and may occur in the absence of detectable cutaneous lesions.[111] The oral cavity is a common site of disease and is not infrequently the first site of AIDS-associated KS.[112,113] Kaposi's sarcoma can appear on the palate, the gingiva, the tongue, or the buccal mucosa. Symptoms such as pain, erosion, or interference with speech or eating may develop due to enlarging KS lesions, which may require treatment. The gastrointestinal tract is also a frequent site of disease, but in most cases these lesions are asymptomatic and are often only recognized at autopsy. However, symptoms of gastrointestinal KS lesions may be related to bleeding, ulceration, intussusception, or obstruction. The tumors arise from the submucosa and appear as deep red vascular nodules that may be ulcerated. As with cutaneous lesions, visceral KS tumors rarely bleed during biopsy unless underlying vessels are nicked. No predictor of visceral AIDS-associated KS exists, although 40% of patients with oral KS also have been found to have gastrointestinal involvement as well.[114] Survival does not appear to be affected by the presence of gastrointestinal KS.[113]

The respiratory tract may also be affected by KS, especially when widely disseminated tumor is present, and such tumors contribute to the death of patients in 25% of cases.[115–118] Other disease

TABLE 3–4. STAGING OF KAPOSI'S SARCOMA

Tumor extent
- Stage I: cutaneous, usually indolent
- Stage II: cutaneous, locally aggressive, with or without regional lymph nodes
- Stage III: generalized mucocutaneous and/or lymph node involvement*
- Stage IV: visceral

Symptomatic status
- A: asymptomatic
- B: systemic signs: >10% weight loss, temperature >100°F orally, of noninfectious origin and lasting >2 weeks

* Generalized means more than upper or lower extremities alone: includes minimal gastrointestinal disease defined as fewer than five lesions, <2 cm in combined diameter.
From Krigel R, Laubenstin L, Muggia F. Kaposi's sarcoma: A new staging classification. Cancer Treatment Rep 1983;67:531–534.

processes such as infections are often present simultaneously in the lungs of patients with AIDS-associated KS. The KS lesions may appear as nodular infiltrates in the lung or as pleural-based plaques, and pleural effusions may be present.[118–123] The diagnosis is frequently difficult, and bronchoscopic biopsy specimens are often nondiagnostic.[124–126] As is the case with KS and gastrointestinal lesions, KS that affects the pulmonary tract may appear in the absence of cutaneous lesions, and the presence of cutaneous or oral lesions does not predict pulmonary involvement with KS.

Tumors of AIDS-associated KS have been described at almost every site in autopsy series including the spleen, the liver, the bone, the central nervous system, and the urinary and genital tracts.[127–129] Tumors at these sites may cause symptoms due to compression or destruction of surrounding structures or to obstruction but are frequently asymptomatic and only discovered incidentally or at autopsy.

Treatment of AIDS-associated KS is individualized to the patient. Often, patients with AIDS-associated KS are also affected with or have been treated for one or more opportunistic infections or other opportunistic neoplasms. Their tolerance to chemotherapy and radiation therapy is thus decreased. Specifically, the oral cavity of patients with AIDS is highly sensitive to radiation, and treatment of oral lesions with radiation therapy causes remarkable discomfort, prolonged and severe painful mucositis, loosening of the teeth, and dryness of the mouth that interfere with eating and speech and results in secondary infections and malnutrition.[130] Local injections of chemotherapeutic agents such as vinblastine or even electrocauterization or cryotherapy can provide a good palliative effect. Tolerance to systemic myelosuppressive agents is also reduced owing to the HIV-related neutropenia frequently seen in patients with advanced AIDS, to infection of the bone marrow with atypical mycobacteria or various viruses, and to the concomitant treatment with other myelosuppressive drugs such as zidovudine or ganciclovir.

When cosmetic treatment of exposed lesions is required, the use of cosmetic camouflage has provided excellent results. If single lesions require treatment, cryotherapy, electrocautery, surgical excision, local radiation therapy, and intralesional injection with agents such as bleomycin, vinblastine, or interferon-α have provided good palliation.[131] When disseminated or aggressive disease is present, systemic therapy with one or more chemotherapeutic agents or with high-dose interferon-α may be required (Tables 3–4 and 3–5). The use of growth factors such as granulocyte colony-stimulating factor or of gran-

TABLE 3–5. STAGING OF KAPOSI'S SARCOMA (KS)

	Good Risk (All of the Following)	Poor Risk (Any of the Following)
Tumor (T)	Confined to skin and/or lymph nodes and/or minimal oral disease*	Tumor-associated edema or ulceration Extensive oral KS Gastrointestinal KS KS in other nonnodal viscera
Immune System (I)	CD4⁺ cells ≥200/μl	CD4⁺ cells <200/μl
Systemic Illness (S)	No history of opportunistic infection or thrush No "B" symptoms† Performance status ≥70 (Karnofsky)	History of opportunistic infection and/or thrush "B" symptoms present Performance status <70 Other HIV-related illness (e.g., neurologic disease, lymphoma)

* Minimal oral disease is nonnodular KS confined to the palate.
† "B" symptoms are unexplained fever, night sweats, >10% involuntary weight loss, or diarrhea persisting more than 2 weeks.
From Krown SE, Metroka C, Wernz JC. Kaposi's sarcoma in the acquired immunodeficiency syndrome: A proposal for uniform evaluation, response, and staging criteria. J Clin Oncol 1989;7:1201–1207.

ulocyte-macrophage colony-stimulating factor has been found to allow anemic or neutropenic AIDS-associated KS patients who otherwise would be prone to develop multiple life-threatening infections to receive myelosuppressive agents.[132–134] It is important to note that AIDS-associated KS is infrequently attributed as the direct cause of death in patients who are severely immunosuppressed and usually expire from one or more opportunistic infections. Treatment of AIDS-associated KS is usually palliative and rarely results in prolonged complete remissions. Active agents that have been used systemically include vincristine, vinblastine, bleomycin, etoposide, doxorubicin hydrochloride (Adriamycin), and 4′-epirubicin.[134–140] Such agents may be used as single drugs or in combination. Frequently, the response rate is higher when combinations are used than when agents are used singly.[141,142] Antiretrovirals such as zidovudine have been evaluated in combination with chemotherapy but are of questionable efficacy in altering the outcome of AIDS-associated KS.[143,144]

Interferon-α has also been found to be active against this disease and, in addition, may also act as an antiretroviral agent.[145–154] It has been used as part of chemotherapeutic regimens.[155,156] Newer experimental approaches to the treatment of AIDS-associated KS include the use of various new chemotherapeutic agents,[157] the employment of new delivery systems such as liposome-encapsulated daunorubicin that is supposed to preferentially target KS lesions,[158,159] and more recently the use of potential antiangiogenic agents.[160] Approaches such as the use of anti-sense oligonucleotides directed at the purported etiologic factors of KS such as HPV-16 or IL-6 may also emerge.

EPIDEMIC KAPOSI'S SARCOMA IN NON–HIV-INFECTED PATIENTS

Cases of KS appearing in young sexually active homosexual men who had no serologic or virologic evidence of HIV infection have been reported with increasing frequency.[161–164] These patients, all of whom are at behavioral risk for infection with HIV and most of whom have had sexual exposure to HIV-infected individuals, have been followed for a period of more than 3 years. They show no evidence of HIV infection by enzyme-linked immunosorbent assay (ELISA), Western blot, viral cultures of peripheral blood mononuclear cells, and polymerase chain reaction after repeated testing over a period of years.[12,154] Their CD4 cell counts, CD4 to CD8 ratios, and immunologic parameters all remain normal for years after the diagnosis of KS. No evidence for Tat-1 sequences in the clinical KS lesions was found by polymerase chain reaction.[165] It thus appears as if yet another form of epidemic KS is being recognized, with the characteristics of a sexually transmitted disease independent of HIV or AIDS (see Table 3–2).

The lesions of KS in this newly recognized syndrome may appear anywhere on the body. Patients present with one or a limited number of lesions that may have been present for months. The lesions appear as red to violaceous patches or plaques. Local treatment of these lesions has proved effective, and recurrence or dissemination of KS has not been described in this group of patients who usually have fewer than 10 lesions. Clinically, these patients have no other signs or symptoms other than the few small cutaneous lesions. It is essential that these patients be tested repeatedly for HIV to confirm that they do not have AIDS-associated KS, which is a more ominous condition. There appears to be no relation between this condition and the newly described non–HIV-associated CD4 lymphopenia.[166–168]

HISTOPATHOLOGIC FEATURES OF KAPOSI'S SARCOMA

IMPORTANCE OF ACCURATE DIAGNOSIS OF KAPOSI'S SARCOMA

It is important that KS be recognized and diagnosed with certainty for a number of reasons. Although most cases are readily recognized clinically, biopsies should be performed to establish the diagnosis microscopically in cases in which there is any doubt. Kaposi's sarcoma may, however, be the presenting sign of HIV infection and may be confused clinically with other processes. It is not uncommon that a biopsy specimen submitted as an angioma or other benign vascular lesion in a patient not thought to have HIV infection is subsequently shown to be KS associated with AIDS. In addition, some conditions may be confused with KS, both clinically and histologically. Many of these may have serious consequences if left untreated.

It is especially important that pathologists be aware of the numerous forms KS may take both in the skin and in visceral organs. Failure to recognize KS histologically may lead to patients going undiagnosed and untreated, leaving them vulnerable to opportunistic infections. However, overdiagnosis may lead to anxiety and severe psychological problems, even suicide.

In general, KS in HIV-infected individuals has similar histologic features to classic KS seen in elderly individuals. Clinically, the two conditions are quite distinct in distribution, rapidity of spread, and response to treatment. The HIV-associated KS is similar to both the KS that arises in other immunocompromised patients and to the epidemic African form of KS.

BIOPSY TECHNIQUE

To arrive at a precise histologic diagnosis of KS, it is important that a representative and adequate biopsy of a lesion be performed. Because this neoplasm manifests most commonly in the skin, punch or incisional biopsies are preferred methods of sampling KS lesions. Especially in early stages, KS tends to affect the reticular dermis more than the superficial papillary dermis; thus, a superficial biopsy may fail to be deep enough for a precise diagnosis to be made. On occasion, KS lesions may be associated with other vascular proliferations such as pyogenic granuloma or bacillary angiomatosis. A superficial biopsy may sample an area of granulation tissue rather than the neoplastic process and lead to failure to diagnose KS.

HISTOLOGIC STAGES OF KAPOSI'S SARCOMA

DIFFUSE VASCULAR PROLIFERATION

The very earliest histologic change of KS may not represent KS at all. One study has demonstrated a subtle proliferation of blood vessels in clinically unaffected skin of individuals with AIDS, a finding that may be the earliest manifestation of impending KS.[169] This may be a consequence of either a generalized viral infection involving endothelial cells in widespread fashion[170] or a circulating vascular proliferation factor that has yet to be identified.[171] Recently, HIV Tat protein has been suggested as such a proliferative factor (see earlier discussion). Such changes may be difficult to detect and may not always be noticeable.

PATCH-STAGE DISEASE (Figures 3–122 to 3–129)

The earliest recognizable form of Kaposi's sarcoma is early patch-stage disease. Clinically, skin lesions are usually characterized by small pinkish macules that can be difficult to recognize as KS. In general two histological patterns of patch-stage KS have been described.[172,173] In one type, there is an increased number of dilated vascular spaces with irregular shapes lined by thin, flattened endothelial cells. The vascular spaces are often difficult to appreciate, but when present, they appear to dissect between collagen bundles in the upper reticular dermis. Characteristically in this form, preexisting blood vessels and adnexal structures are surrounded by a vascular proliferation that may appear to protrude into vascular lumina. This has been referred to as the *promontory sign* (see Fig. 3–124). There is also an infiltrate of lymphocytes and plasma cells interstitially between vessels associated with extravasated erythrocytes and siderophages. The endothelial cells lining the bizarre blood vessels are either thin and spindle shaped or somewhat oval or round. Most of the endothelial cells show no evidence of mitoses or pleomorphism.[172,173]

The second pattern of patch-stage KS consists of a proliferation of spindle and oval endothelial cells almost exclusively around preexisting blood vessels of the upper reticular dermis. This has been referred to as "pseudogranulomatous" because the aggregations of plump endothelial cells surrounded by plasma cells and lymphocytes give a histologic appearance similar to that of interstitial granulomatous inflammation. Small vascular spaces and extravasation of erythrocytes are also observed. In addition to these two patterns, there may be overlap with features of both in the same specimen. Features common to both patterns include the presence of clefts lined with thin endothelial cells between collagen bundles. This correlates with the electron microscopic finding of pseudopodia of endothelial cells extending for long distances along collagen bundles.

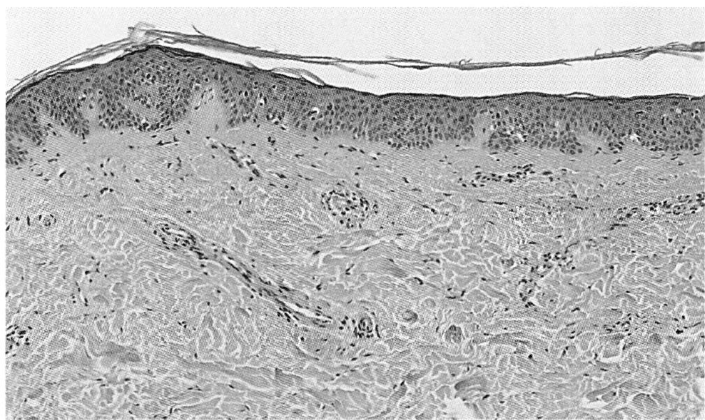

FIGURE 3–122. Early vascular proliferation; "prepatch" stage of Kaposi's sarcoma

At low magnification, minimal change is visible, although there is a slight proliferation of blood vessels in the dermis. Hematoxylin and eosin stain (original magnification ×40).

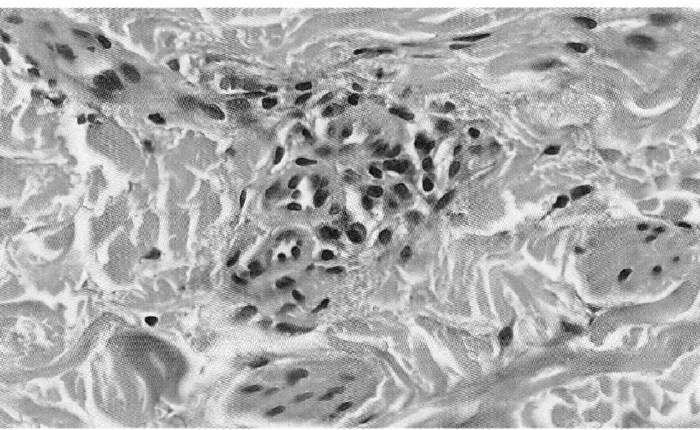

FIGURE 3–123. Early vascular proliferation

Higher magnification of specimen in Figure 3–122 demonstrates an early proliferation of slightly irregular vascular spaces surrounding preexisting round blood vessels. Note the few extravasated erythrocytes and plasma cells. Hematoxylin and eosin stain (original magnification ×400).

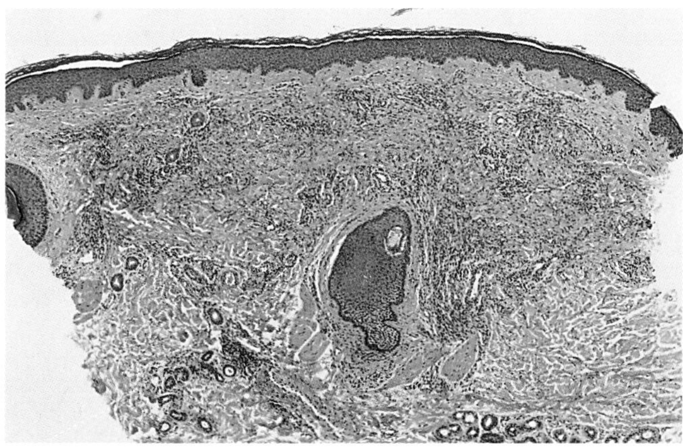

FIGURE 3–124. Kaposi's sarcoma; patch stage

At low magnification there is a diffuse infiltrative process that affects the reticular dermis and spares the papillary dermis. Hematoxylin and eosin stain (original magnification ×25).

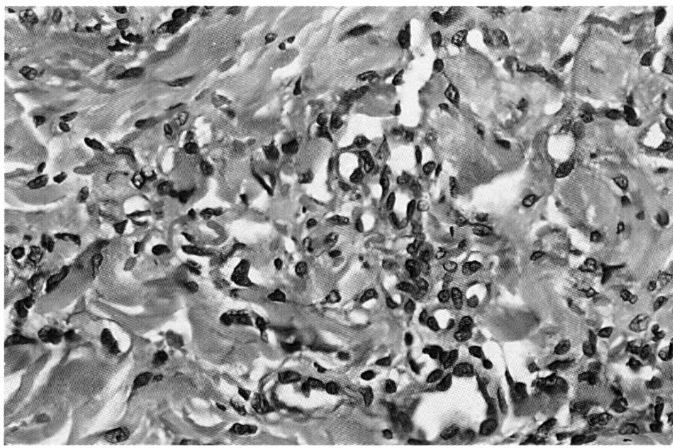

FIGURE 3–125. Kaposi's sarcoma, higher magnification; patch stage

There are irregular vascular spaces surrounding preexisting normal blood vessels diffusely in the dermis. The vessels are jagged and lined by plump endothelial cells. Note the extravasation of erythrocytes and scattered plasma cells. Hematoxylin and eosin stain (original magnification ×400).

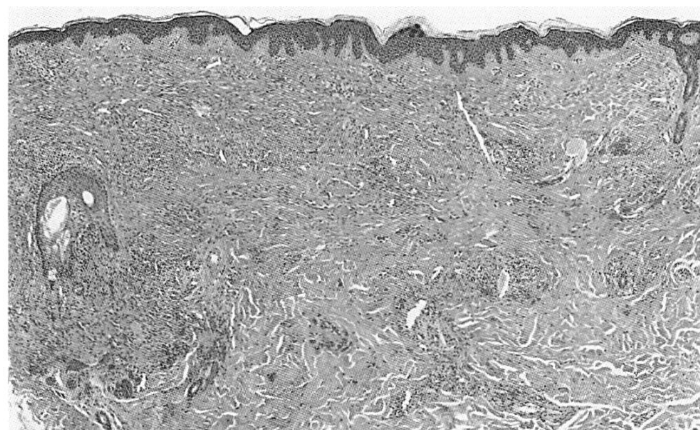

FIGURE 3–126. Kaposi's sarcoma; late patch, early plaque stage

There is a diffuse proliferation of spindle cells in the dermis. Small slit-like spaces can be appreciated at low magnification. Hematoxylin and eosin stain (original magnification ×25).

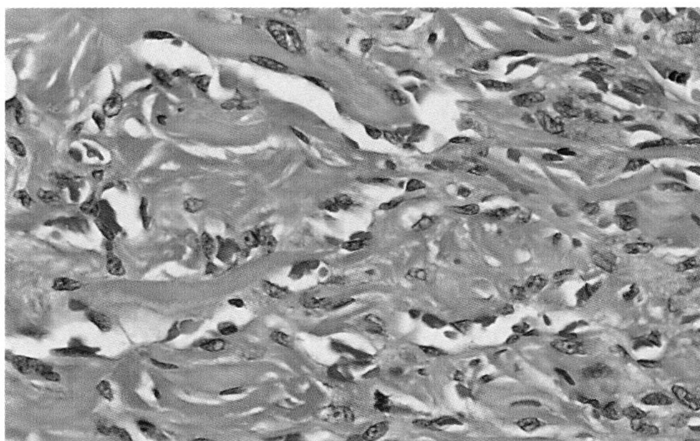

FIGURE 3–127. Kaposi's sarcoma; late patch, early plaque stage

The higher magnification reveals abundant, jagged, slit-like vascular spaces diffusely between and among collagen bundles in the dermis. Scattered mitotic figures are seen, and there are extravasated erythrocytes. Hematoxylin and eosin stain (original magnification ×400).

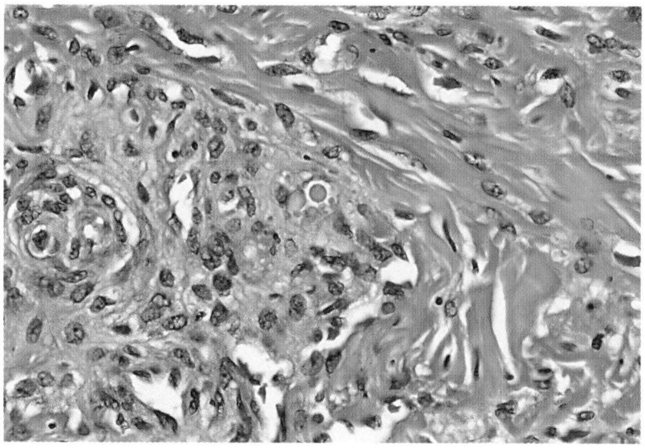

FIGURE 3–128. Kaposi's sarcoma; late patch, early plaque stage

In another area, there were more solid aggregations of plump endothelial cells. Note the presence of pale pink–staining hyaline globules, which are a clue to the diagnosis. These represent the degenerating erythrocytes. Hematoxylin and eosin stain (original magnification ×400).

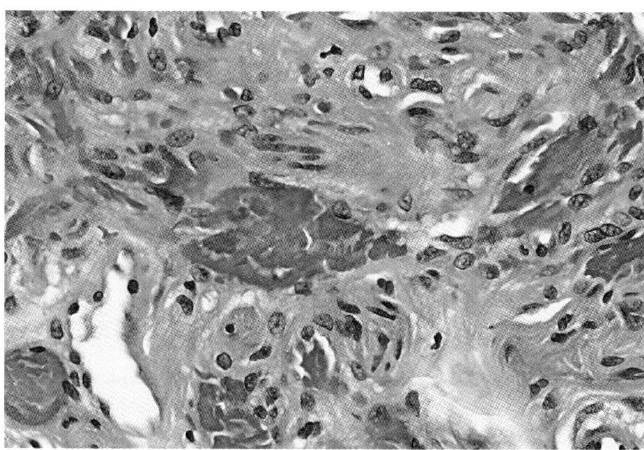

FIGURE 3–129. Kaposi's sarcoma; late patch, early plaque stage

Another clue to the diagnosis of Kaposi's sarcoma is the sludging of erythrocytes within irregular vascular spaces, which is depicted in this photograph. Note the absence of true thrombosis. Hematoxylin and eosin stain (original magnification ×400).

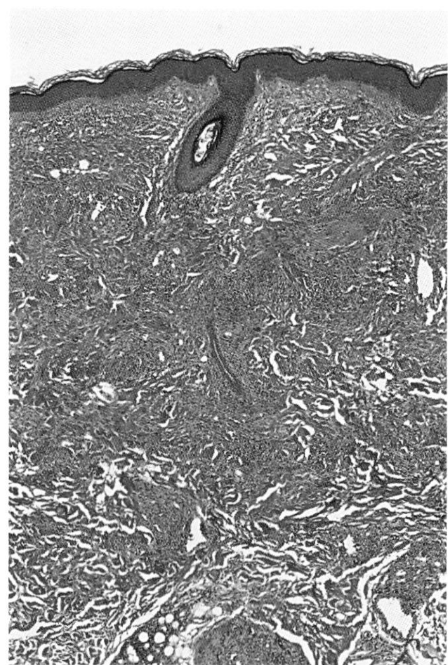

FIGURE 3–130. Kaposi's sarcoma; plaque stage

There is a diffuse spindle cell proliferation that affects the reticular dermis predominantly. Numerous jagged, irregular, slit-like vascular spaces are readily visualized at low magnification. Hematoxylin and eosin stain (original magnification ×25).

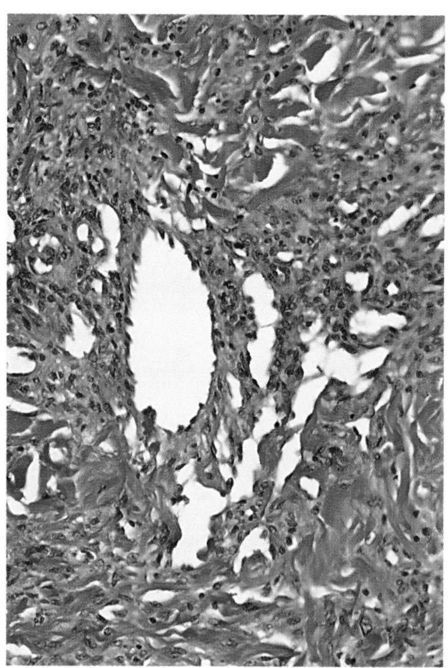

FIGURE 3–131. Kaposi's sarcoma; plaque stage

Higher magnification reveals a more densely cellular process comprising plump endothelial cells. Many irregular jagged vascular spaces are present and some surround preexisting vessels. Hematoxylin and eosin stain (original magnification ×300).

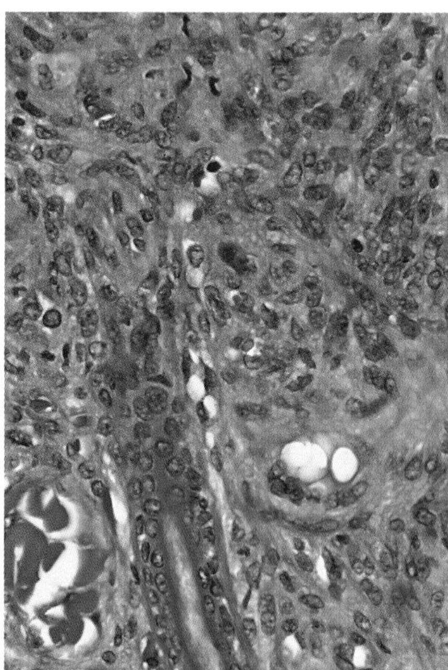

FIGURE 3–132. Kaposi's sarcoma; plaque stage

Higher magnification of a more cellular area demonstrates the cytologic features of the neoplastic cells. Note the plump spindle and round shape to the cells with abundant cytoplasm. There are also hyaline globules and extravasated erythrocytes. Hematoxylin and eosin stain (original magnification ×450).

PLAQUE-STAGE DISEASE
(Figures 3-130 to 3-132)

In time, the vascular proliferation may become more extensive and may spread to affect most of the reticular dermis as well as the upper subcutaneous fat. This more densely cellular variant of KS is clinically recognizable as either a papule or a plaque and histologically is referred to as the plaque stage.[173-175] The tendency of the abnormal vessels to be mostly interstitial or mostly perivascular is maintained, but the greater number of endothelial cells in the lesion results in a caricature of the patch stage. Blood vessels are very bizarre and jagged but thin walled. Occasionally, rounded thick-walled vessels may be seen admixed with the neoplastic vessels. Such vessels may represent preexisting plexuses or abnormal vessels altered by stasis when lesions are on the lower extremities. The inflammatory cell infiltrate in plaque lesions is more dense, and sometimes small nodules of plasma cells are seen throughout the lesion. Extravasated erythrocytes and siderophages may be numerous. Because of the abundant extravasation of erythrocytes, erythrophagocytosis may be seen. The breakdown products of phagocytosed erythrocytes take on a pinkish refractile appearance and have been referred to *hyalin globules*. Although they are not spe-

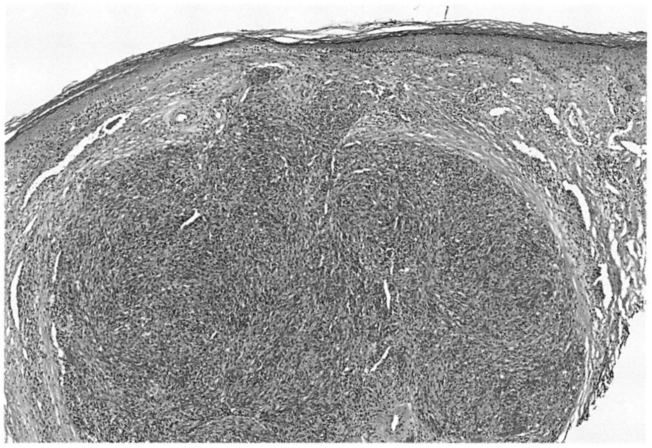

FIGURE 3-133. Kaposi's sarcoma; nodular stage
In the dermis is a circumscribed nodule composed almost wholly of spindle-shaped cells. Numerous erythrocytes are present within the lesion, and there are small vascular slits just visible at low magnification. Hematoxylin and eosin stain (original magnification ×25).

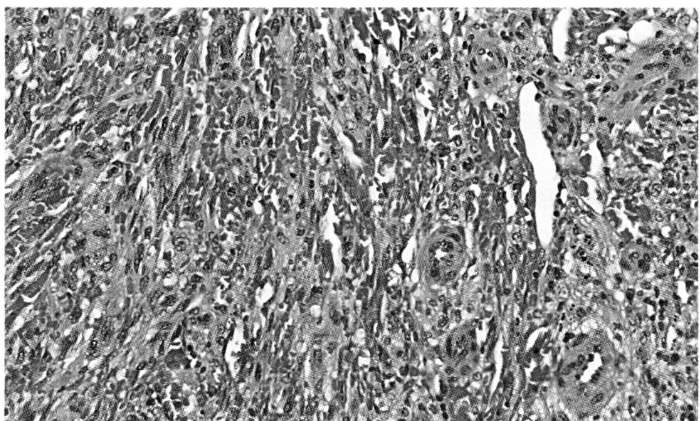

FIGURE 3-134. Kaposi's sarcoma; nodular stage
Higher magnification demonstrates the numerous erythrocytes and spindle cells to better advantage. Note siderophages and diffuse, slit-like vascular spaces. Hematoxylin and eosin stain (original magnification ×250).

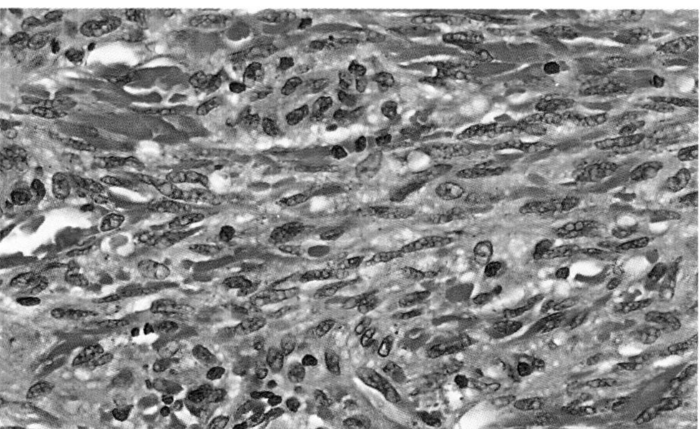

FIGURE 3-135. Kaposi's sarcoma; nodular stage
Still higher magnification of a different area reveals the spindle cell nature of the process. Although there are abundant extravasated erythrocytes and hyaline globules, the number of true vascular spaces has diminished greatly, which may cause confusion with other spindle cell neoplasms. Hematoxylin and eosin stain (original magnification ×400).

cific for KS, they are a helpful finding when the diagnosis is in question.[173–175]

NODULES AND TUMORS (Figures 3–133 to 3–135)

Nodules and tumors may develop either from patches and plaques or in some cases de novo. The nodular stage of KS is a spindle cell proliferation characterized by interweaving fascicles of spindle cells.[173–175] Extravasated erythrocytes are abundant between individual spindle cells. Careful examination shows that small slit-like and round spaces between individual fascicles of spindle cells represent vascular spaces. On occasion, the progression from a plaque to a nodule of KS is seen within the same specimen. Individual nodules may increase in size from a solitary focus or may develop as a consequence of coalescence of smaller aggregations of spindle cells. The neoplastic cells characteristically have elongated nuclei with somewhat vesicular chromatin and vacuolation of the cytoplasm. Atypia is a prominent feature in these lesions, and numerous mitotic figures and marked pleomorphism are commonly observed. Nodules may be located at any site within the skin including the papillary dermis and the subcutis, although the reticular dermis is affected most commonly.[176,177] In some cases, the lesions may be quite deeply situated and may be connected to underlying fascia, muscle, and even bone.[176,177] Occasionally, lesions may be pedunculated and surrounded by epithelial collarettes. Ulceration and zones of necrosis may be seen. Inflammatory infiltrates consist mostly of lymphocytes and plasma cells with other cells being present less frequently.

HISTOLOGIC VARIANTS

ANGIOMATOUS FORM (Figures 3–136 to 3–138)

In addition to the types of KS discussed previously, there are a number of histologic variants that may cause confusion in diagnosis. A not uncommon variant of KS is the so-called angiomatous form.[173] In this lesion are well-formed blood vessels that are somewhat irregular in size and shape and are usually aggregated. Vascular spaces are lined by thin, flattened endothelial cells rather than round or plump ones characteristically seen in angiomas. Such vascular spaces may be present in the middermis but may on occasion be associated with preexisting adnexal structures or normal-appearing blood vessels. In addition, it is not uncommon for the vascular spaces of angiomatous KS to be filled with erythrocytes. This condition is to be distinguished from thrombosis, which is a not uncommon finding in normal angiomas that have been traumatized. On occasion, the red blood cells within the lumina of angiomatous lesions of KS may assume an orange color (see Fig. 3–134). The reason for this is unclear. Despite these features, it may be quite difficult to distinguish an angiomatous KS lesion from a true angioma in some cases. As a general rule, careful evaluation of surrounding areas reveals features of patch- or plaque-stage KS, or both (see Fig. 3–134).[173]

TRAUMATIZED LESIONS

A KS lesion may be traumatized, resulting in a superimposed granulation tissue response. In such cases, a superficial biopsy may sample granulation tissue that may be erroneously interpreted either as a pyogenic granuloma or as granulation tissue. It is important to be aware that this phenomenon can occur and to mention in the pathology report that the biopsy was taken superficially and that the stated diagnosis may be a consequence of a sampling error. Only when deeper biopsies are done will the more characteristic features of KS be seen.

COEXISTING KAPOSI'S SARCOMA AND BACILLARY ANGIOMATOSIS

Lesions of KS and bacillary angiomatosis may occur in contiguity,[178] which may lead to confusion in diagnosis. Bacillary angiomatosis is characterized by lobular proliferations of round blood vessels with epithelioid endothelial cells, many of which protrude into vascular lumina.[179] An inflammatory cell infiltrate of numerous neutrophils is characteristically seen with scattered deposits of purplish granular material corresponding to colonies of bacteria. A Warthin-Starry stain reveals clumps of bacilli in the areas of angiomatosis.[179] No bacteria are seen in the KS areas.

RESOLVING LESIONS

Kaposi's sarcoma lesions that have undergone resolution as a result of therapy with x-irradiation, topical application of liquid nitrogen, or chemotherapy may have features that are not diagnostic of KS. Histologically, one sees abundant siderophages, dermal fibroplasia and sclerosis, and only scattered residual endothelial cells between collagen bundles. Soon after treatment, especially of nodules, there may be a dense inflammatory cell infiltrate with extensive necrosis of endothelial cells.[173]

EXTRACUTANEOUS KAPOSI'S SARCOMA

Extracutaneous KS may differ histologically and may have a slightly different developmental chronology than KS lesions in the skin. The most commonly affected sites other than the skin are the lymph nodes, the gastrointestinal tract, and the respiratory tract.[180] In lymph nodes the earliest changes are those that have been referred to as "hypervascular follicular hyperplasia."[181] Vascular channels within the node are prominent, increased in number, and associated with an increase in the number of plasma cells.[182]

In time, these areas may develop more classic findings of KS, namely, interweaving fascicles of spindle cells, vascular slits, and extravasation of erythrocytes with siderophages. In time, entire lymph nodes may be replaced by fully developed KS.[182,183]

The gastrointestinal tract is also commonly involved. Virtually the entire gastrointestinal tract from the oral cavity to the anus may be affected.[183] In general, the histologic findings are similar to those seen in the skin, although angiomatous features may be seen somewhat more commonly. Early lesions of KS may show simply dilated irregular blood vessels not easily recognizable as KS.[183] Similar findings have been reported in early lesions of the pulmonary parenchyma as well.[183]

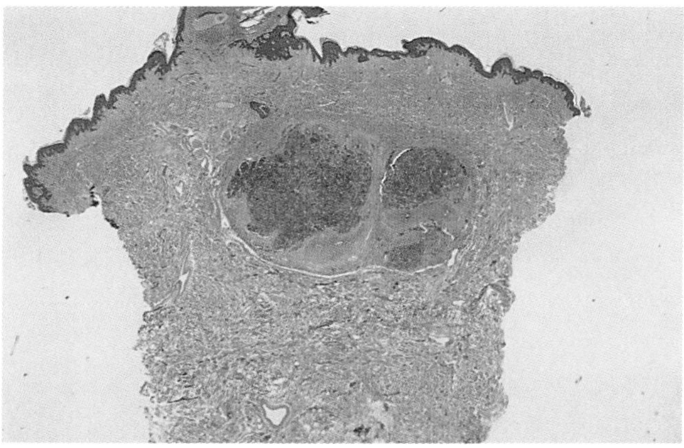

FIGURE 3–136. "Angiomatous" Kaposi's sarcoma
Low magnification demonstrates a circumscribed vascular proliferation in the mid-reticular dermis. Hematoxylin and eosin stain (original magnification ×20).

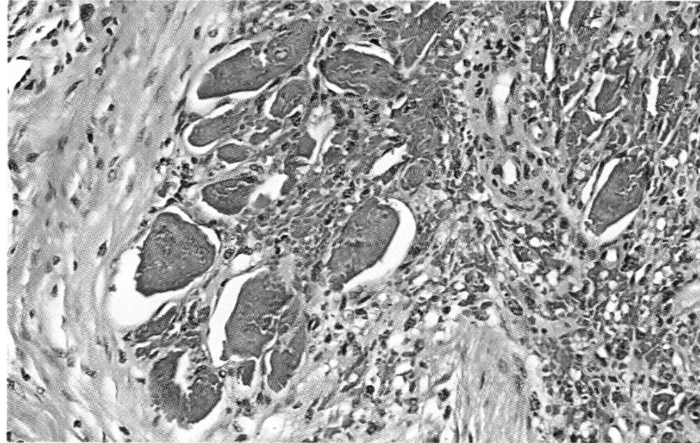

FIGURE 3–137. "Angiomatous" Kaposi's sarcoma
Higher magnification demonstrates irregularly shaped blood vessels filled with erythrocytes. There are also numerous extravasated erythrocytes and siderophages. Note the somewhat orange color to the red cells that have sludged within the vascular spaces. Hematoxylin and eosin stain (original magnification ×250).

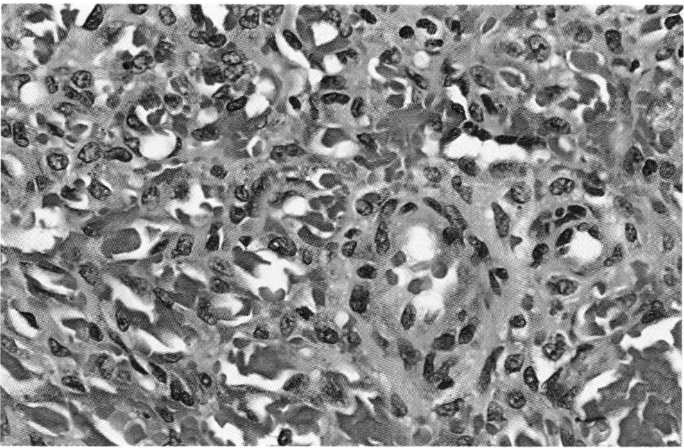

FIGURE 3–138. "Angiomatous" Kaposi's sarcoma
In another area of the proliferation, there were more irregular jagged vascular spaces, some of which surrounded preexisting round normal blood vessels. In this area, the diagnosis of Kaposi's sarcoma can be made with greater confidence. Hematoxylin and eosin stain (original magnification ×400).

HISTOLOGIC SIMULATORS OF KAPOSI'S SARCOMA

Kaposi's sarcoma may simulate a number of different processes in the skin, both inflammatory and neoplastic.[184] Conversely, KS may be simulated by a number of different entities. If the criteria outlined earlier are applied carefully, it is unlikely that confusion in diagnosis will result.

ANGIOMA

Probably the most common simulator of KS is an angioma. Clinically such lesions are vascular in appearance, and in patients at risk for HIV infection, KS will be the most likely clinical diagnosis proffered. Histologically, angiomas are almost always associated with plump, round endothelial cells, which line vascular lumina.[173,174] Such vessels may be located superficially without a tendency to involve deeper vessels such as the midvascular plexus and usually have no tendency to be centered around preexisting blood vessels or adnexal structures. Furthermore, the pattern of an angioma is usually homogeneous, whereas progression from patch to nodular stages may be seen in a given lesion of KS.[173]

BACILLARY ANGIOMATOSIS

Bacillary angiomatosis occasionally may be confused with KS, but the two do not simulate each other histologically with great frequency. Bacillary angiomatosis is characterized by a lobular proliferation of round blood vessels with thick plump ("epithelioid") endothelial cells.[179] Numerous neutrophils are commonly seen in densely cellular lesions, a finding almost never seen in KS. Finally, silver stains such as Warthin-Starry stain for bacteria readily distinguish the two in the majority of cases.[179]

ACROANGIODERMATITIS

Severe stasis changes, especially those that have evolved to acroangiodermatitis, may be confused clinically with KS.[184] Histologically, this lesion is readily distinguished from plaque-stage KS because individual blood vessels are thick walled, round, and lined with plump endothelial cells. No tendency to the formation of bizarre, jagged blood vessels that surround preexisting ones is seen.[173] When stasis changes are superimposed on lesions of KS, the vascular changes of stasis mentioned earlier are seen in the superficial portion of the specimen with the more characteristic features of patch- and plaque-stage KS present beneath.[173]

ANGIOSARCOMA

Rarely, KS may simulate angiosarcoma and vice versa. In general, the endothelial cells lining the neoplastic vascular spaces of angiosarcoma are large, strikingly pleomorphic, and atypical. Aggregations of neoplastic endothelial cells may be present freely within lumina of vascular spaces, a finding not seen in KS.[173,174] Almost never are angiosarcomas lined by thin, typical-appearing endothelial cells.

SPINDLE CELL NEOPLASMS

Other spindle cell neoplastic processes may mimic KS, especially nodule- and tumor-stage lesions, particularly if they are examined using high magnification primarily. Kaposi's sarcoma lesions are almost always associated with vascular slits and usually contain numerous extravasated erythrocytes. Careful searches for signs of differentiation in other spindle cell neoplasms usually help to distinguish them from KS. For example, the presence of melanin and evidence of cornification distinguishes spindle cell melanomas and spindle cell carcinomas, respectively, from KS.[173] Nevertheless, in some cases, the similarity between spindle cell neoplasms and KS may be so great as to require the performance of immunoperoxidase studies. Most cases of KS stain positively for vascular-associated antigens such as *Ulex europaeus,*[174] although some lesions may not stain positively. Cells that stain positive for factor XIIIa are also present.

INFLAMMATORY DERMATOSES

On occasion, inflammatory conditions may simulate KS. Granuloma annulare, especially the interstitial form, may be associated with perivascular infiltrates of epithelioid cells and lymphocytes, simulating a patch-stage lesion of KS with a "pseudogranulomatous" appearance.[173] Careful evaluation reveals the epithelioid cells to represent histiocytes. Furthermore, the absence of plasma cells in the infiltrate is another clue that such a lesion is not KS. Necrobiosis lipoidica may simulate patch-stage lesions of KS, but the degree of sclerosis and the presence of fibrin and degenerated collagen within the centers of areas of palisaded granulomatous inflammation are not characteristic of KS.[173] Early patch-stage lesions of KS may simulate persistent purpuric dermatitis.[173] Careful evaluation of such lesions will reveal the vascular spaces lined by the thin endothelial cells.

DERMATOFIBROMA AND SCAR

Fibroblastic proliferations such as dermatofibromas and scars may either simulate KS or be simulated by it.[173] Once again, inspection of the vessels within a dermatofibroma reveals them to be round and thick walled and associated with an inflammatory infiltrate of histiocytes, many of which may be multinucleated. The characteristic change of epidermal hyperplasia overlying a dermatofibroma is yet another clue to the diagnosis. Scars may be associated with a vascular proliferation, which is usually composed of round endothelial cells. Such vascular proliferations in scars are also associated with abundant, newly formed, basophilic collagen.

NEWLY DESCRIBED VASCULAR PROLIFERATIONS

Several newly described vascular proliferations have been described within the last several years, some of which may have both clinical and histologic similarity to KS. Microvenular hemangioma, described in 1991 by Hunt and colleagues, is clinically characterized by a reddish-purple papule or plaque that is usually on the proximal extremities and often in a young individual.[185] Histologically, the lesion is characterized by a diffuse proliferation of slightly irregular blood vessels lined by plump endothelial cells. Usually, minimal if any inflammatory infiltrate is seen, and the number of slit-like jagged irregular vessels is less than that in plaque-stage KS with which it may be confused.

Targetoid hemosiderotic hemangioma is a lesion that is characterized clinically by a small papular angiomatous lesion surrounded by a brownish dark area that represents extravasation of erythrocytes with secondary breakdown, resulting in a "hemosiderotic" appearance. The usual location is on the trunk or extremity. Histologically, there is a proliferation of rounded blood vessels in the dermis that form small lobular aggregations associated with extravasated erythrocytes and abundant siderophages. Most patients who develop this lesion are middle aged.

Tufted angioma is a lesion often seen in children that may be painful. Large reddish-to-purple patches and plaques with scattered papules develop and gradually increase in size. Most are located on the proximal extremities, especially the thigh. Histologically, there is a diffuse proliferation of rounded vessels that assume the appearance of small "tufts" of blood vessels that resemble a glomerulus of a nephron.

Glomeruloid vascular proliferations may develop in association with hyperviscosity states such as hyperglobulinemia. Clinically, these may appear as small reddish areas or papules, usually on acral sites. Small, rounded vascular proliferations bearing similarity to glomeruli are present in the dermis, usually in the deeper dermis or upper subcutis. Careful inspection of lumina in these areas often reveals deposits of pinkish hyaline material that is the protein present in the circulation in excess.

Multinucleate cell angiohistiocytoma (angioblastoma of Nakagawa) manifests clinically as reddish-brown papules of the thigh of middle-aged women most commonly. Histologically, there is a subtle proliferation of small, rounded vessels in the dermis with admixed multinucleated cells with features of histiocytes.

MISCELLANEOUS CONDITIONS

Other conditions that have been reported occasionally to mimic KS include pyogenic granuloma, spindle and epithelioid cell nevus (Spitz's nevus), and pseudolymphoma.

ADDITIONAL POINTS

Although KS develops most commonly in patients at risk for HIV infection, recent evidence indicates that KS may occur in individuals who are not infected with HIV but have risk factors for it.[12] In such patients KS has a clinical appearance similar to that of classic KS. The recognition of this phenomenon has raised speculation that KS may be caused by a virus unrelated to HIV.[170] Human papillomavirus-16 DNA may be demonstrated in a significant percentage of HIV-associated KS lesions.

References

1. Kaposi M. Idiopatiches multiples pigment sarcom der Haut. Arch Dermatol Syphil 1872;4:265–272.
2. Oettle AG. Geographic and racial differences in the frequency of Kaposi's sarcoma as evidence of environmental or genetic causes. Acta Union Int Contra Cancrum 1962;18:330–363.
3. Davies JNP, Loethe F. Kaposi's sarcoma in African children. Acta Union Int Contra Cancrum 1962;19:349–399.
4. Penn I. Kaposi's sarcoma in organ transplant recipients. Transplantation 1979;27:8–11.
5. Harwood AR, Osoba D, Hofstader SL, Goldstein MB, Cardella CJ, Holecek MJ, Kunynetz R, Giammarco RA. Kaposi's sarcoma in recipients of renal transplants. Am J Med 1979;67:759–765.
6. Myers BD, Kessler E, Levi D. Kaposi's sarcoma in kidney transplant recipients. Arch Intern Med 1974; 133:307–311.
7. Gatti RA, Good RA. Occurrence of malignancy in immunodeficiency diseases: A literature review. Cancer 1971;28:89.
8. Friedman-Kien AE, Laubenstein L, Marmor M, et al. Kaposi's sarcoma and *Pneumocystis* pneumonia among homosexual men—New York and California. MMWR 1981;30:250–252.
9. Friedman-Kien AE. Disseminated Kaposi's sarcoma in young homosexual men. J Am Acad Dermatol 1981; 4:468–470.
10. Gottlieb MS, Schroff R, Schanker HM, et al. *Pneumocystis carinii* pneumonia and mucosal candidiasis in previously healthy homosexual men: Evidence of a new acquired cellular immunodeficiency. N Engl J Med 1981;305:1425.
11. Hymes KB, Cheung T, Greene JB, Prose NS, Marcus A, Ballard H. Kaposi's sarcoma in homosexual men—A report of eight cases. Lancet 1981:598.
12. Friedman-Kien AE, Saltzman BR, Cao YZ, Nestor MS, Mirabile M, Li JJ, Peterman TA. Kaposi's sarcoma in HIV-negative homosexual men (letter). Lancet 1990;335:168–169.
13. Rothman S. Remarks on sex, age and racial distribution of Kaposi's sarcoma and on possible pathogenic factors. Acta Union Int Contra Cancrum 1962;18:326–329.
14. Safai B, Good R. Kaposi's sarcoma—A review and recent developments. CA Cancer J Clin 1981;31:2–12.
15. Reynolds WA, Winkelmann RK, Soule EH. Kaposi's sarcoma: A clinicopathological study with particular reference to its relationship to the reticuloendothelial system. Medicine 1965;44:419–433.
16. Safai B, Mike V, Giraldo G, et al. Association of Kaposi's sarcoma with secondary primary malignancies: Possible etiopathogenic implications. Cancer 1980;45:1472–1479.
17. Bronson DM. Immunosuppressive therapy. In: Gottlieb G, Ackerman AB, eds. Kaposi's Sarcoma: A Text and Atlas. Philadelphia: Lea & Febiger; 1988:241–253.
18. Rappersberger K, Tschachler E, Zonzits E, Gillitzer R, Hatzakis A, Kaloterakis A, Mann DL, Popow-Kraupp T, Biggar RJ, Berger R, et al. Endemic Kaposi's sarcoma in human immunodeficiency virus type 1-seronegative persons: Demonstration of retrovirus-like particles in cutaneous lesions. J Invest Dermatol 1990;95:371–381.
19. Contu L, Cerimele D, Carcassi C, et al. Immunogenetic and immunologic study on classic Kaposi's sarcoma. IRCS Med Sci 1984;12:891–892.
20. Pollack MS, Safai B, Myskowski PI, Gold JW, Pandey J, Dupont B. Frequency of HLA and GM immunogenetic Kaposi's sarcoma. Tissue Antigens 1983;21:1–8.
21. Master SP, Taylor JF, Kyalwazi SK, Ziegler JL. Immunological studies in Kaposi's sarcoma. BMJ 1970;1:600–603.
22. Taylor JF, Ziegler JL. Delayed cutaneous hypersensitivity reactions in patients with Kaposi's sarcoma. Br J Cancer 1974;30:312–318.
23. Dobozy A, Husz S, Hunyadi J, Berko G, Simon N. Immune deficiencies and Kaposi's sarcoma (letter). Lancet 1973;2:625.
24. Marinig C, Fiorini G, Boneschi V, Melotti E, Brambilla L. Immunologic and immunogenetic features of primary Kaposi's sarcoma. Cancer 1985;55:1899–1901.
25. Filipovich AH, Zerbe D, Spector BD, Hersy JH. Lymphomas in persons with naturally occurring immunodeficiency disorders. In: McGrath IT, O'Connor GT, Ramot B, eds. Pathogenesis of Leukemias and Lymphomas: Environmental Influences. New York: Raven Press; 1984:225–234.
26. Muggia FM. Treatment of classical Kaposi's sarcoma: A new look. In: Friedman-Kien AE, Laubenstein LJ, eds. The Epidemic of Kaposi's Sarcoma and Opportunistic Infections. New York: Masson Publishing; 1984:57.
27. Alecu M, Ghyka G, Halalau F, Calugaru A, Coman G. Intralesional human leukocyte interferon treatment in the non-AIDS related Kaposi's sarcoma. Med Interne 1990;28:61–67.
28. Cox FH, Helwig EB. Kaposi's sarcoma. Cancer 1959;12:289.
29. Loewthe F, Murray JF. Kaposi's sarcoma: Autopsy findings in the African. Acta Union Int Contra Cancrum 1962;18:429–451.
30. Hood AF, Farmer ER, Weiss RA. Kaposi's sarcoma. Johns Hopkins Med J 1980;151:222–230.
31. Friedman-Kien AE, Ostreicher R, Saltzman B. Clinical manifestations of classical, endemic African, and epidemic AIDS-associated Kaposi's sarcoma. In: Friedman-Kien AE, ed. Color Atlas of AIDS. Philadelphia: WB Saunders; 1989:11–48.
32. Slavin G, Cameron HM, Forbes C, Mitchell RM. Kaposi's sarcoma in East African children: A report of 51 cases. J Pathol 1970;100:187.
33. Bayley AC. Occurrence, clinical behavior and management of Kaposi's sarcoma in Zambia. In: Beral V, Jaffe HW, Weiss RA, eds. Cancer, HIV, and AIDS. Plainview, NY: Cold Spring Harbor Laboratory Press; 1991:53–71.
34. Bayley AC, Downing RG, Cheingsong-Popov R, Tedder RS, Dalgleish AG, Weiss RA. HTLV-III serology distinguishes atypical and endemic Kaposi's sarcoma in Africa. Lancet 1985;1:359–361.
35. Bayley AC. Aggressive Kaposi's sarcoma in Zambia. Lancet 1984;1:1318.
36. Olweny CLM. Epidemiology and clinical features of Kaposi's sarcoma in tropical Africa. In: Friedman-Kien AE, Laubenstein LJ, eds. The Epidemic of Kaposi's Sarcoma and Opportunistic Infections. New York: Masson Publishing; 1984:25–40.
37. Vogel CL. Management of Kaposi's sarcoma. Chemotherapy I. In: Olweny CLM, Hutt MSR, Owor R, eds. Antibiotics and Chemotherapy. Basel: Karger; 1981:82–87.
38. Olweny CLM. Management of Kaposi's sarcoma. Chemotherapy II. In: Olweny CLM, Hutt MSR, Owor R, eds. Antibiotics and Chemotherapy. Basel: Karger; 1981:88–95.
39. Klein MB, Pereira FA, Kantor I. Kaposi's sarcoma complicating systemic lupus erythematosus treated with immunosuppression. Arch Dermatol 1974;110:602.
40. Leung F, Fam AG, Osoba D. Kaposi's sarcoma complicating corticosteroid therapy for temporal arteritis. Am J Med 1981;71:320–322.
41. Kinlen LJ. Immunosuppressive therapy and cancer. Cancer Surv 1982; 1:565–583.
42. Klepp O, Dahl O, Stenwig JT. Association of Kaposi's sarcoma and prior immunosuppressive therapy. Cancer 1978;42:2626–2630.
43. Gange RW, Wilson-Jones E. Kaposi's sarcoma and immunosuppressive therapy: An appraisal. Clin Exp Dermatol 1978;3:314.
44. Kapadia SB, Krause JR. Kaposi's sarcoma after long-term alkylating agent therapy for multiple myeloma. South Med J 1977;70:1011–1013.
45. Frances C, Farge D, Boisnic S. Syndrome de Kaposi des transplantes. J Mal Vasc 1991;16:163–165.

46. Bismuth H, Samuel D, Venancie P, Menouar G, Szekely AM. Development of Kaposi's sarcoma in liver transplant recipients: Characteristics, management and outcome. Transplant Proc 1991;23:1438–1439.
47. Penn I. The changing pattern of posttransplant malignancies. Transplant Proc 1991;23:1101–1103.
48. Alamartine E, Berthoux F. Complications carcinologiques après transplantation rénale. Presse Med 1991;20: 891–895.
49. Qunibi W, Akhtar M, Sheth K, Ginn HE, Al-Furayh O, DeVol EB, Taher S. Kaposi's sarcoma: The most common tumor after renal transplantation in Saudi Arabia. Am J Med 1988;84:225–232.
50. Brunson ME, Balakrishnan K, Penn I. HLA and Kaposi's sarcoma in solid organ transplantation. Hum Immunol 1990;29:56–63.
51. Cleary ML, Sklar J. Lymphoproliferative disorders in cardiac transplant recipients are multiclonal lymphoma. Lancet 1984;2:489–493.
52. Beral V, Peterman TA, Berkelman RL, Jaffe HW. Kaposi's sarcoma among persons with AIDS: A sexually transmitted infection? Lancet 1990;335:123–128.
53. Benedetti P, Greco D, Figoli F, Tirelli U. Epidemic Kaposi's sarcoma in female AIDS patients—A report of 23 Italian cases. AIDS 1991;5: 466–467.
54. Lassoued K, Clauvel JP, Fegueux S, Matheron S, Gorin I, Oksenhendler E. AIDS-associated Kaposi's sarcoma in female patients. AIDS 1991;5:877–880.
55. Haverkos HW. Nitrite inhalant abuse and AIDS-related Kaposi's sarcoma. J Acquir Immune Defic Syndr 1990;3(suppl 1):47–50.
56. Haverkos HW. The search for cofactors in AIDS, including an analysis of the association of nitrite inhalant abuse and Kaposi's sarcoma. Prog Clin Biol Res 1990;325:93–102.
57. Abrams DI. The relationship between Kaposi's sarcoma and intestinal parasites among homosexual males in the United States. J Acquir Immune Defic Syndr 1990;3(suppl 1): 44–46.
58. Andersen CB, Karkov J, Bjerregaard B, Visfeldt J. Cytomegalovirus infection in classic, endemic and epidemic Kaposi's sarcoma analyzed by in situ hybridization. APMIS 1991;99:893–897.
59. Hashimoto H, Muller H, Muller F, Schmidts HL, Stutte HJ. In situ hybridization analysis of cytomegalovirus lytic infection in Kaposi's sarcoma associated with AIDS: A study of 14 autopsy cases. Virchows Arch A Pathol Anat Histopathol 1987;411:441–448.
60. Marmor M, Friedman-Kien AE, Zolla-Pazner S, Stahl RE, Rubinstein P, Laubenstein L, William DC, Klein RJ, Spigland I. Kaposi's sarcoma in homosexual men: A seroepidemiologic case-control study. Ann Intern Med 1984;100:809–815.
61. Salahuddin SZ, Nakamura S, Biberfeld P, Kaplan MH, Markham PD, Larsson L, Gallo RC. Angiogenic properties of Kaposi's sarcoma-derived cells after long-term culture in vitro. Science 1988;242:430–433.
62. Beral V, Bull D, Darby S, Weller I, Carne C, Beecham M, Jaffe H. Risk of Kaposi sarcoma and sexual practices associated with faecal contact in homosexual or bisexual men with AIDS. Lancet 1992;335:632–635.
63. Darrow WW, Peterman TA, Jaffe HW, Rogers MF, Curran JW, Beral V. Kaposi's sarcoma and exposure to faeces. Lancet 1992;339:685.
64. Marmor M, Friedman-Kien AE, Laubenstein L, Byrum RD, William DC, D'onofrio S, Dubin N. Risk factors for Kaposi's sarcoma in homosexual men. Lancet 1982;1:1083–1107.
65. Beral V. Epidemiology of Kaposi's sarcoma. In: Beral V, Jaffe H, Weiss R, eds. Cancer, HIV, and AIDS. Plainview, NY: Cold Spring Harbor Laboratory Press; 1991;5–22.
66. Beral V, Bull D, Jaffe H, Evans B, Gill N, Tillett H, Swerdlow AJ. Is risk of Kaposi's sarcoma in AIDS patients in Britain increased if sexual partners came from United States or Africa? [published erratum appears in BMJ 1991 302(6779):752]. BMJ 1991;302:624–625.
67. Haverkos HW, Drotman DP, Morgan WM. Kaposi's sarcoma in patients with AIDS: Sex, transmission mode, and race. Biomed Pharmacother 1990;44:461–466.
68. Sturzl M, Brandstetter H, Roth WK. Kaposi's sarcoma: A review of gene expression and ultrastructure of KS spindle cells in vivo. AIDS Res Hum Retroviruses 1992;8:1753–1763.
69. Huang YQ, Li JJ, Rush MG, Poiesz BJ, Nicolaides A, Jacobson M, Zhang WG, Coutavas E, Abbott MA, Friedman-Kien AE. HPV-16-related DNA sequences in Kaposi's sarcoma. Lancet 1992;339:515–518.
70. Nickoloff BJ, Huang YQ, Li JJ, Friedman-Kien AE. Immunohistochemical detection of papillomavirus antigens in Kaposi's sarcoma. Lancet 1992;339:548–549.
71. Palefsky JM. Human papillomavirus-associated anogenital neoplasia and other solid tumors in human immunodeficiency virus-infected individuals. Curr Opin Oncol 1991;3:881–885.
72. Chang Y, Cesarman F, Pessin MS, Lee F, Culpepper JC, et al. Identification of new human herpes virus-like DNA sequences in AIDS-associated Kaposi's sarcoma. Science 1994;266:1865–1869.
73. Huang YQ, Li JJ, Kaplan MH, Poiesz B, Katabira E, et al.: Human herpes virus-like nucleic acid in various forms of Kaposi's sarcoma. Lancet 1995;345:759–761.
74. Moore PS, Chang Y. Detection of herpesvirus-like DNA sequences in Kaposi's sarcoma in patients with and those without HIV infection. New Engl J Med 1995;332:118–128.
75. Dupin N, Grandadam M, Calvez V. Herpesvirus-like DNA sequences in patients with Mediterranean Kaposi's sarcoma. Lancet 1995;345:761–762.
76. Schalling M, Ekman M, Kaaya E, Linds A, Biberfeld P. A role for a new herpesvirus (KSHV) in different forms of Kaposi's sarcoma. Nature Med 1995;1:767–768.
77. Ambroziak JA, Blackbourn DJ, Hermdier BG, et al. Herpes-like sequences in HIV-infected and uninfected Kaposi's sarcoma patients. Science 1995;268:582–583.
78. Collandre H, Ferris S, Gran O, et al. Kaposi's sarcoma and new herpesvirus. Lancet 1995;345:1043.
79. Boshoff C, Whitby D, Hatziioannou T, et al. Kaposi's sarcoma associated herpesvirus in HIV negative Kaposi's sarcoma. Lancet 1995;345:1043–44.
80. Lebbe C, Cremoux PD, Rybojad M, et al. Kaposi's sarcoma and new herpesvirus. Lancet 1995;345:1180.
81. Cesarman E, Chang Y, Moore PS, Said JW, Knowles DM. Kaposi's sarcoma-associated herpesvirus-like DNA sequences in AIDS-related body-cavity-based lymphomas. New Engl J Med 1995;32:1186–1191.
82. Rady PL, Yen A, Rollefson JL, Orengo I, Bruce S, et al.: Herpesvirus-like DNA sequences in non-Kaposi's sarcoma skin lesions of transplant patients. Lancet 1995;345:1340–1342.
83. Ensoli B, Nakamura S, Salahuddin SZ, Biberfeld P, Larsson L, Beaver B, Wong-Staal F, Gallo RC. AIDS–Kaposi's sarcoma–derived cells express cytokines with autocrine and paracrine growth effects. Science 1989;243:223–226.
84. Corbeil J, Evans LA, Vasak E, Cooper DA, Penny R. Culture and properties of cells derived from Kaposi sarcoma. J Immunol 1991;146:2972–2976.
85. Hober D, Haque A, Wattre P, Beaucaire G, Mouton Y, Capron A. Production of tumor necrosis-factor-α and interleukin-1 in patients with AIDS. Clin Exp Immunol 1989;78:329–333.
86. Miles SA, Rezai AR, Salazar-Gonzalez JF, Vander Meyden M, Stevens RH, Logan DM, Mitsuyasu RT, Taga T, Hirano T, Kishimoto T, et al. AIDS Kaposi sarcoma–derived cells produce and respond to interleukin 6. Proc Natl Acad Sci U S A 1990;87:4068–4072.
87. Huang YQ, Li JJ, Nicolaides A, Zhang WG, Friedman-Kien AE. Fi-

broblast growth factor 6 gene expression in AIDS-associated Kaposi's sarcoma. Lancet 1992;339:1110–1111.

88. Ensoli B, Barillari G, Salahuddin SZ, Gallo RC, Wong-Staal F. Tat protein of HIV-1 stimulates growth of cells derived from Kaposi's sarcoma lesions of AIDS patients. Nature 1990;345:84–86.
89. Breen E, Rezai A, Nakajima K. Infection with HIV is associated with elevated IL-6 levels and production. J Immunol 1990;144:480–484.
90. De Wit R, Raasveld MH, ten Berge RJ, van der Wouw PA, Bakker PJ, Veenhof CH. Interleukin-6 concentrations in the serum of patients with AIDS-associated Kaposi's sarcoma during treatment with interferon-alpha. J Intern Med 1991;229:539–542.
91. Kishimoto T, Hirano T. Molecular regulation of B lymphocyte response. Ann Rev Immunol 1988;6:485–512.
92. Kishimoto T, Akira S, Taga T. Interleukin-6 and its receptor: A paradigm for cytokines. Science 1992;258:593–597.
93. Nakamura S, Salahuddin SZ, Biberfeld P, Ensoli B, Markham PD, Wong-Staal F, Gallo RC. Kaposi's sarcoma cells: Long term culture with growth factor from retrovirus-infected $CD4^+$ T cells. Science 1988;242:426–430.
94. Nair BC, DeVico AL, Nakamura S, Copeland TD, Chen Y, Patel A, O'Neil T, Oroszlan S, Gallo RC, Sarngadharan MG. Identification of a major growth factor for AIDS-Kaposi's sarcoma cells as oncostatin M. Science 1992;255:1430–1432.
95. Miles SA, Martinez-Maza O, Rezai A, Magpentay L, Kishimoto T, Nakamura S, Radka SF, Linsley PS. Oncostatin M as a potent mitogen for AIDS–Kaposi's sarcoma–derived cells. Science 1992;255:1432–1434.
96. Gearing DP, Comeau MR, Friend DJ, Gimpel SD, Thut CJ, McGourty J, Brasher KK, King JA, Gillis S, Mosley B. The IL-6 signal transducer, gp130; and oncostatin M receptor and affinity converter for the LIF receptor. Science 1992;255:1434–1437.
97. Brown TJ, Rowe JM, Liu JW, Shoyab M. Regulation of IL-6 expression by oncostatin-M. J Immunol 1991;147:2175–2180.
98. Miles SA. Pathogenesis of human immunodeficiency virus–related Kaposi's sarcoma. Curr Concepts Oncol 1992;4:875–882.
99. Friedman-Kien AE, Laubenstein LJ, Rubinstein P. Disseminated Kaposi's sarcoma in homosexual men. Ann Intern Med 1982;96:693–700.
100. Rubenstein P, Rothman WM, Friedman-Kien A. Immunologic and immunogenetic findings in patients with epidemic Kaposi's sarcoma. Antibiot Chemother 1984;32:87–98.
101. Wank R, Thomssen C. High risk of squamous cell carcinoma of the cervix for women with HLA-DQw3. Nature 1991;352:723–725.
102. Koutsky LA, Holmes KK, Critchlow CW, Stevens CE, Paavonen J, Beckmann AM, De Rouen TA, Galloway DA, Vernon D, Kiviat NB. A cohort study of the risk of cervical intraepithelial neoplasia grade 2 or 3 in relation to papillomavirus infection. N Engl J Med 1992; 327:1272–1278.
103. Laga M, Icenogle JP, Marsella R, Manoka AT, Nzila N, Ryder RW, Vermund SH, Heyward WL, Nelson A, Reeves WC. Genital papillomavirus infection and cervical dysplasia: Opportunistic complications of HIV infection. Int J Cancer 1992;50:45–48.
104. Marte C, Kelly P, Cohen M, Fruchter RG, Sedlis A, Gallo L, Ray V, Webber CA. Papanicolaou smear abnormalities in ambulatory care sites for women infected with the human immunodeficiency virus. Am J Obstet Gynecol 1992;164:1232–1237.
105. Schafer A, Friedmann W, Mielke M, Schwartlander B, Koch MA. The increased frequency of cervical dysplasia-neoplasia in women infected with the human immunodeficiency virus is related to the degree of immunosuppression. Am J Obstet Gynecol 1991;164:593–599.
106. Vermund SH, Kelly KF, Klein RS, Feingold AR, Schreiber K, Munk G, Burk RD. High risk of human papillomavirus infection and cervical squamous intraepithelial lesions among women with symptomatic human immunodeficiency virus infection. Am J Obstet Gynecol 1991;165:392–400.
107. Feigal EG, Looney DJ, Poeschla E, Badel P, Wong-Staal F. Kaposi sarcoma–like cells (KSLC) obtained from peripheral blood of patients with Kaposi's sarcoma (abstract). Proc Am Soc Clin Oncol 1991;10:33.
108. Gompels MM, Hill A, Jenkins P, Peters B, Tomlinson D, Harris JR, Stewart S, Pinching AJ, Munro AJ. Kaposi's sarcoma in HIV infection treated with vincristine and bleomycin. AIDS 1992;6:1175–1180.
109. Peters BS, Beck EJ, Coleman DG, Wadsworth MJ, McGuinness O, Harris JR, Pinching AJ. Changing disease patterns in patients with AIDS in a referral center in the United Kingdom. BMJ 1991; 302:203–207.
110. Haverkos HW, Friedman-Kien AE, Drotman DP, Morgan WM. The changing incidence of Kaposi's sarcoma among patients with AIDS. J Am Acad Dermatol 1990;22:1250–1253.
111. Friedman-Kien AE, Saltzman BR. Clnical manifestations of classical, endemic African, and epidemic AIDS-associated Kaposi's sarcoma. J Am Acad Dermatol 1990;22:1237–1250.
112. Bernal A, Del Junco GW, Gibson SR. Endoscopic and pathologic features of gastrointestinal Kaposi's sarcoma: A report of four cases in patients with the acquired immunodeficiency syndrome. Gastrointest Endosc 1985;31:74–77.
113. Friedman SL, Wright TL, Altman DF. Gastrointestinal Kaposi's sarcoma in patients with acquired immunodeficiency syndrome. Gastroenterology 1985;89:102–108.
114. Saltz RK, Kurtz RC, Lightdale CJ, Myskowski P, Cunningham-Rundles S, Urmacher C, Safai B. Kaposi's sarcoma. Gastrointestinal involvement, correlation with skin findings and immunologic function. Dig Dis Sci 1984;29:817–823.
115. Ognibene FP, Steis RG, Macher AM. Kaposi's sarcoma causing pulmonary infiltrates and respiratory failure in the acquired immunodeficiency syndrome. Ann Intern Med 1985;102: 471–475.
116. Meduri GU, Stover DE, Lee M, Myskowski PL, Caravelli JF, Zaman MB. Pulmonary Kaposi's sarcoma in the acquired immunodeficiency syndrome. Am J Med 1986;81:11–18.
117. Nash G, Fligiel S. Kaposi's sarcoma presenting as pulmonary disease in acquired immunodeficiency syndrome. Diagnosis by lung biopsy. Hum Pathol 1984;15:999–1001.
118. Touboul JL, Mayaud CM, Fouret P, Akoun GM. Pulmonary lesions of Kaposi's sarcoma. Intra-alveolar hemmorrhage and pleural effusion. Ann Intern Med 1985;103:808.
119. Kaplan LD, Hopewell KC, Jaffe H, Goodman PC, Bottles K, Volberding PA. Kaposi's sarcoma involving the lung in patients with the acquired immunodeficiency syndrome. J Acquir Immune Defic Syndr 1988;1:23–30.
120. Davis DS, Henschke CI, Chamides BK, Wescott JL. Intrathoracic Kaposi's sarcoma in AIDS patients: Radiographic-pathologic correlation. Radiology 1987;163:495–500.
121. Gill PS, Akil B, Colletti P, Rarick M, Loureiro C, Bernstein-Singer M, Krailo M, Levine AM. Pulmonary Kaposi's sarcoma: Clinical findings and results of therapy. Am J Med 1989;87:57–61.
122. Naidich DP, Tarres M, Garay SM, Birnbaum B, Ryback BJ, Schinella R. Kaposi's sarcoma: CT-radiographic correlation. Chest 1989;96:723–728.
123. Savit CJ, Schwartz AM, Rockoff SD. Kaposi's sarcoma of the lung in AIDS: Radiologic-pathologic analysis. AJR 1987;148:25–28.
124. Murray JF, Felton CP, Garay SM. Pulmonary complications of the acquired immunodeficiency syndrome. N Engl J Med 1984;310:1682–1688.
125. McKenna RJ, Campbell A, McMurtrey MJ, Mountain CF. Diagnosis for interstitial lung disease in patients with acquired immunodeficiency syndrome (AIDS): A prospective compari-

son of bronchial lavage, transbronchial lung biopsy, and open lung biopsy. Ann Thorac Surg 1986;41:318–321.
126. Zibrak JD, Silvestri RC, Costello P, Marlink R, Jensen WA, Robins A, Rose RM. Bronchoscopic and radiographic features of Kaposi's sarcoma involving the respiratory system. Chest 1990;90:476–479.
127. Reichert CM, O'Leary TJ, Levens DL, Simrell CR, Macher AM. Autopsy pathology in the acquired immunodeficiency syndrome. Am J Pathol 1983;112:357–382.
128. Guarda LA, Luna MA, Smith JL Jr, Mansell PW, Gyorkey F, Roca AN. Acquired immune deficiency syndrome: Postmortem findings. Am J Clin Pathol 1984;81:549–557.
129. Welch K, Finkbeiner W, Alpers CE. Autopsy findings in the acquired immunodeficiency syndrome. JAMA 1984;252:1152–1154.
130. Cooper JS, Fried PR. Oral radiotherapy in patients having AIDS. Arch Otolaryngol 1987;113:327–328.
131. Serfling U, Hood AF. Local therapies for cutaneous Kaposi's sarcoma in patients with acquired immunodeficiency syndrome. Arch Dermatol 1191;127;1479–1481.
132. Scadden DT, Bering HA, Levine JD, Bresnahan J, Evans L, Epstein C, Groopman JE. GM-CSF as an alternative to dose modification of the combination zidovudine and interferon-alpha in the treatment of AIDS-associated Kaposi's sarcoma. Am J Clin Oncol 1991;14(suppl 1):40–44.
133. Scadden DT, Bering HA, Levine JD, Bresnahan J, Evans L, Epstein C, Groopman JE. Granulocyte-macrophage colony-stimulating factor mitigates the neutropenia of combined interferon alfa and zidovudine treatment of acquired immune deficiency syndrome–associated Kaposi's sarcoma. J Clin Oncol 1991;9:802–808.
134. Gill PS, Bernstein-Singer M, Espina BM, Rarick M, Magy F, Montgomery T, Berry MS, Levine A. Adriamycin, bleomycin and vincristine chemotherapy with recombinant granulocyte-macrophage colony-stimulating factor in the treatment of AIDS-related Kaposi's sarcoma. AIDS 1992;6:1477–1481.
135. Shepherd FA, Burkes RL, Paul KE, Goss PE. A phase II study of 4′epirubicin in the treatment of poor-risk Kaposi's sarcoma and AIDS. AIDS 1991;5:305–309.
136. Caumes E, Guermonprez G, Katlama C, Gentilini M. AIDS-associated mucocutaneous Kaposi's sarcoma treated with bleomycin. AIDS 1992;6:1483–1487.
137. Lassoued K, Clauvel JP, Katlama C, Janier M, Picard C, Matheron S. Treatment of the acquired immunodeficiency syndrome–related Kaposi's sarcoma with bleomycin as a single agent. Cancer 1990;66:1869–1872.
138. Gelmann E, Longo D, Lane JC, Fauci AS, Masur H, Wesley M, Preble OT, Jacob J, Steis R. Combination chemotherapy of disseminated Kaposi's sarcoma in patients with the acquired immunodeficiency syndrome. Am J Med 1987;82: 456–462.
139. Laubenstein LJ, Kriegel RL, Odajnyk CM, Hymes KB, Friedman-Kien A, Wernz JC, Muggia FM. Treatment of epidemic Kaposi's sarcoma with etoposide or a combination of doxorubicin, bleomycin and vinblastine. J Clin Oncol 1984;2:1115–1120.
140. Mintzer DM, Real FX, Jovino L, Krown SE. Treatment of Kaposi's sarcoma and thrombocytopenia with vincristine in patients with the acquired immunodeficiency syndrome. Ann Intern Med 1985;102:200–202.
141. Gill PS, Rarick M, McCutchan JA, Slater L, Parker B, Muchmore E, Bernstein-Singer M, Akil B, Espina BM, Krailo M, et al. Systemic treatment of AIDS-related Kaposi's sarcoma: Results of a randomized trial. Am J Med 1991;90:427–433.
142. Gill PS, Rarick MU, Espina B, Loureiro C, Bernstein-Singer M, Akil B, Levine AM. Advanced acquired immune deficiency syndrome–related Kaposi's sarcoma. Results of pilot studies using combination chemotherapy. Cancer 1990;65:1074–1078.
143. Kovacs J, Deyton L, Davey R, Falloon J, Zunich K, Lee D, Metcalf JA, Bigley JW, Sawyer LA, Zoon KC, et al. Combined zidovudine and interferon-alpha therapy in patients with Kaposi's sarcoma and the acquired immunodeficiency syndrome (AIDS). Ann Intern Med 1989;111:280–287.
144. Lane HC, Falloon J, Walker RE, Deyton L, Kovacs JA, Masur H, Banks S, Kirk LE, Baseler MW, Salzman NP, et al. Zidovudine in patients with human immunodeficiency virus (HIV) infection and Kaposi's sarcoma. A phase II randomized, placebo-controlled trial. Ann Intern Med 1989;111:41–50.
145. Fischl MA. Antiretroviral therapy in combination with interferon for AIDS-related Kaposi's sarcoma. Am J Med 1991;90:2S–7S.
146. Fischl MA, Uttamchandani RB, Resnick L, Agarwal R, Fletcher MA, Patrone-Reese J, Dearmas L, Chidekel J, McCann M, Myers M. A phase I study of recombinant human interferon-alpha 2a or human lymphoblastoid interferon-alpha n1 and concomitant zidovudine in patients with AIDS-related Kaposi's sarcoma. J Acquir Immune Defic Syndr 1991; 4:1–10.
147. Mitsuyasu RT. Interferon alpha in the treatment of AIDS-related Kaposi's sarcoma. Br J Haematol 1991;79(suppl 1):69–73.
148. Sawyer LA, Metcalf JA, Zoon KC, Boone EJ, Kovacs JA, Lane HC, Quinnan GV Jr. Effects of interferon-alpha in patients with AIDS-associated Kaposi's sarcoma are related to blood interferon levels and dose. Cytokine 1990;2:247–252.
149. Evans LM, Itri LM, Campion M, Wyler-Plant R, Krown SE, Groopman JE, Goldsweig H, Volberding PA, West SB, Mitsuyasu RT, et al. Interferon-alpha 2a in the treatment of acquired immunodeficiency syndrome–related Kaposi's sarcoma. J Immunother 1991;10:39–50.
150. Rozenbaum W, Gharakhanian S, Navarette MS, De Sahb R, Cardon B, Rouzioux C. Long-term follow-up of 120 patients with AIDS-related Kaposi's sarcoma treated with interferon alpha-2a. J Invest Dermatol 1990;95:161S–165S.
151. Shepperd FA, Evans WK, Garvey B, Read SE, Klein M, Fannin MM, Coates R. Combination chemotherapy and alpha-interferon in the treatment of Kaposi's sarcoma associated with acquired immune deficiency syndrome. Can Med Assoc J 1988;139:635–639.
152. Safai B, Bason M, Friedman-Birnbaum R, Nisce L. Interferon in the treatment of AIDS-associated Kaposi's sarcoma: The American experience. J Invest Dermatol 1990;95: 166S–169S.
153. Volberding PA, Mitsuyasu RT, Golando JP, Spiegel RJ. Treatment of Kaposi's sarcoma with interferon alfa-2b (Intron-A). Cancer 1987;59:620–625.
154. Lane HC, Feinberg J, Davey V, et al. Antiretroviral effects of interferon-alpha in AIDS-associated Kaposi's sarcoma. Lancet 1986;2:1218–1222.
155. Gill PS, Rarick MU, Bernstein-Singer M, Espina BM, Jones B, Montgomery T, Sharma D, Rasheed S, Levine AM. Interferon-alpha maintenance therapy after cytotoxic chemotherapy for treatment of acquired immunodeficiency syndrome–related Kaposi's sarcoma. J Biol Response Mod 1990;9;512–516.
156. Krown SE, Gold JW, Niedzwiecki D, Bundow D, Flomenberg N, Gansbacher B, Brew BJ. Interferon-alpha with zidovudine: Safety, tolerance, and clinical and virologic effects in patients with Kaposi sarcoma associated with the acquired immunodeficiency syndrome (AIDS) [published erratum appears in Ann Intern Med 1990;113(4):334]. Ann Intern Med 1990;112:812–821.
157. Bulfill JA, Grace WR, Astrow AB. Phase II trial of prolonged, low-dose oral VP-16 in AIDS-related Kaposi's sarcoma (abstract). Proc Am Soc Clin Oncol 1992;11:47.
158. Presant CA, Blayney D, Proffitt RT, Turner AF, Williams LE, Nadel HI, Kennedy P, Wiseman C, Gala K, Crossley RJ, et al. Preliminary re-

port: Imaging of Kaposi sarcoma and lymphoma in AIDS with indium-111-labelled liposomes. Lancet 1990;335:1307–1309.
159. Presant CA, Scolaro M, Kennedy P, Blayney DW, Flanagan B, Lisak J, Presant J. Liposomal daunorubicin as tumor-targeted chemotherapy: Initial clinical results in Kaposi's sarcoma (abstract). Proc Am Soc Clin Oncol 1992;11:46.
160. Nakamura S, Sakurada S, Salahuddin SZ, Osada Y, Tanaka NG, Sakamoto N, Sekiguchi M, Gallo RC. Inhibition of development of Kaposi's sarcoma-related lesions by a bacterial cell wall complex. Science 1992;255:1437–1440.
161. Afrasiabi R, Mitsuyasu R, Nashanian P. Characterization of a distinct subgroup of high risk persons with Kaposi's sarcoma and good prognosis who present with normal T4 cell number and T4:T8 ratio and negative HTLV-III/LAV serologic test results. Am J Med 1986;81:969–973.
162. Archer CB, Spittle MF, Smith NP. Kaposi's sarcoma in a homosexual—10 years on. Clin Exp Dermatol 1989;14:233–236.
163. Garcia-Muret MP, Pujol RM, Puig L, Moreno A, de Moragas JM. Disseminated Kaposi's sarcoma not associated with HIV infection in a bisexual man. J Am Acad Dermatol 1990;23:1035–1038.
164. Marguart EH, Engst R, Oehlschlaegel G. An 8-year history of Kaposi's sarcoma in an HIV-negative bisexual man (letter). AIDS 1991;5:346–348.
165. Huang YQ, Buchbinder A, Li JJ, Nicolaides A, Zhang WG, Friedman-Kien AE. Absence of *Tat* sequences in tissues of HIV negative patients with epidemic Kaposi's sarcoma. AIDS 1992;6:1139–1142.
166. Laurence J, Siegal FP, Schattner E, Gelman IH, Morse S. Acquired immunodeficiency without evidence of infection with human immunodeficiency virus types 1 and 2. Lancet 1992;340:273–274.
167. Centers for Disease Control and Prevention. Unexplained $CD4^+$ T-lymphocytopenia depletion in persons without evident HIV infection—United States. MMWR 1992;41:541–545.
168. Kessler H, Duncan R, Blok T, et al. Update: $CD4^+$ lymphocytopenia in persons without evident HIV infection—United States. MMWR 1993; 41:578–580.
169. Ruszczak Z, da Silva AM, Orfanos CE. Angioproliferative changes in clinically noninvolved, perilesional skin in AIDS-associated Kaposi's sarcoma. Dermatologica 1987;175:270–279.
170. Dictor M, Jarplid B. The cause of Kaposi's sarcoma: An avian retroviral analog. J Am Acad Dermatol 1988; 18:398–402.
171. Salahuddin SZ, Nakamura S, Biberfeld P, Kaplan MH, Markham PD, Larsson L, Gallo RC. Angiogenic properties of Kaposi's sarcoma-derived cells after long-term culture in vitro. Science 1988;242:430–433.
172. Ackerman AB. Subtle clues to conventional microscopy: The patch stage of Kaposi's sarcoma. Am J Dermatopathol 1979;1:165–172.
173. Gottlieb GJ, Ackerman AB. Kaposi's Sarcoma; A Text and Atlas. Philadelphia: Lea and Febiger; 1988:29–113.
174. Lever WF, Schaumburg-Lever G. Histopathology of the Skin. 6th ed. Philadelphia: JP Lippincott, 1983: 636–640.
175. Santucci M, Pimpinelli N, Moretti S, Giannotti B. Classic and immunodeficiency-associated Kaposi's sarcoma. Arch Pathol Lab Med 1988;112:1214–1220.
176. Safai B, Johnson KG, Myskowski PL, Koziner B, Yang SY, Cunningham-Rundles S, Godbold JH, Dupont B. The natural history of Kaposi's sarcoma in the acquired immunodeficiency syndrome. Ann Intern Med 1985;103:744–750.
177. Muggia FM, Lonberg M. Kaposi's sarcoma and AIDS. Med Clin North Am 1986;70:139–154.
178. Berger TG, Tappero JW, Kaymen A, LeBoit PE. Bacillary (epithelioid) angiomatosis and concurrent Kaposi's sarcoma in acquired immunodeficiency syndrome. Arch Dermatol 1989;125:1543–1547.
179. Cockerell CJ, Le Boit PE. Bacillary angiomatosis: A newly characterized, pseudoneoplastic, infectious, cutaneous vascular disorder. J Am Acad Dermatol 1990;22:501–512.
180. Niedt GW, Schinella RA. Acquired immunodeficiency syndrome: Clinicopathologic study of 56 autopsies. Arch Pathol Lab Med 1985;109:727–734.
181. Lubin J, Rywlin AM. Lymphoma-like lymph node changes in Kaposi's sarcoma. Arch Pathol 1971;92:338.
182. Amazon K, Rywlin AM. Subtle clues to the diagnosis by conventional microscopy: Lymph node involvement in Kaposi's sarcoma. Am J Dermatopathol 1979;1:173.
183. Amazon K, Rywlin AM. Systemic manifestations. In: Gottlieb GJ, Ackerman AB, eds. Kaposi's Sarcoma: A Text and Atlas. Philadelphia: Lea & Febiger, 1988:113–129.
184. Hennessey NP, Friedman-Kien AE. Clinical simulators of the lesions of Kaposi's sarcoma. In: Friedman-Kien AE, ed. Color Atlas of AIDS. Philadelphia: WB Saunders; 1989:49–71.
185. Hunt SJ, Santa Cruz DJ, Barr RJ. Microvenular hemangioma. J Cutan Pathol 1991;18(4):235–240.

Bibliography

Barbanti-Brodano G, Pagnani M, Viadana P, Beth-Giraldo E, Giraldo G. BK virus DNA in Kaposi's sarcoma. Antibiot Chemother 1987;38:113–120.

Centers For Disease Control. Revision of the case definition of acquired immunodeficiency syndrome for national reporting United States. MMWR 1985;34:373–375.

Chachoua A, Krigel RL, Lafleur F, Ostreicher R, Speer M, Laubenstein L, Wernz J, Rubenstein P, Zang E, Friedman-Kien AE. Prognostic factors and staging classification of patients with epidemic Kaposi's sarcoma. J Clin Oncol 1989;7:774–780.

Drew ML, Mills J, Hauer LB, Miner RC, Rutherford GW. Declining prevalence of Kaposi's sarcoma in homosexual AIDS patients paralleled by fall in cytomegalovirus transmission. Lancet 1988;1:66.

Grody WW, Lewin KJ, Naeim F. Detection of cytomegalovirus DNA in classic and epidemic Kaposi's sarcoma by in situ hybridization. Hum Pathol 1988;19:524–526.

Longo DL, Steis RG, Lane HC, Lotze MT, Rosenberg SA, Preble O, Masur H, Rook AH, Fauci AS, Jacob J. Malignancies in the AIDS patient: Natural history, treatment strategies and preliminary results. In: Selikoff IJ, Teirstein AS, Hirschman SZ, eds: Acquired Immune Deficiency Syndrome. Ann N Y Acad Sci 1984;437:421–429.

McDougall JK, Olson KA, Smith PP, Collier AC. Detection of cytomegalovirus and AIDS-associated retrovirus in tissues of patients with AIDS, Kaposi's sarcoma and persistent lymphadenopathy. Antibiot Chemother 1987;38:99–112.

Rappersberger K, Tschachler E, Zonzits E, Gillitzer R, Hatzakis A, Kaloterakis A, Mann DL, Popow-Kraupp T, Biggar RJ, Berger R. Endemic Kaposi's sarcoma in human immunodeficiency virus type 1 seronegative persons: Demonstration of retrovirus-like particles in cutaneous lesions. J Invest Dermatol 1990;95:371–381.

Taylor J, Afrasiabi R, Fahey JL, Korns E, Weaver M, Mitsuyasu R. Prognostically significant classification of immune changes in AIDS with Kaposi's sarcoma. Blood 1986;67:666–671.

CUTANEOUS MANIFESTATIONS OF HIV INFECTION

■■■■■■■■

Clay J. Cockerell
Alvin E. Friedman-Kien

4

The diagnosis and management of human immunodeficiency virus (HIV) infection has evolved dramatically since the initial recognition of the acquired immunodeficiency syndrome (AIDS). Because early diagnosis and prevention of opportunistic infections, as well as treatment of HIV infection itself have become significant priorities, individuals infected with HIV now survive longer. Issues related to the quality of life of these patients have thus begun to assume greater importance.

Cutaneous disorders may serve as initial clues either to the diagnosis of HIV infection itself or to the existence of serious underlying infectious diseases. They are also often the sources of severe morbidity, both physical and psychological.

VIRAL INFECTIONS

VIRAL ILLNESSES INDUCED BY HIV-1

Infection with HIV-1, the most common human immunodeficiency virus strain to cause HIV infection, induces several different clinical syndromes. The earliest manifestation is the acute exanthem of HIV infection. During this stage of the infection, HIV is widely disseminated, seeding lymphoid organs and other body sites.[1] Within 1 to 3 months, there is an immune response to HIV that results in dramatic decline of the viremia.[1]

Human immunodeficiency virus type 1 may induce a number of other conditions directly. With gradual depletion of $CD4^+$ cell numbers, patients become profoundly immunocompromised and develop AIDS.[1] Opportunistic infections caused by viruses, bacteria, fungi, and protozoa ensue, all of which are eventually life threatening. In addition, HIV-1 itself may induce direct effects on tissues and visceral organs. Gastrointestinal disease may be associated with chronic diarrhea and malabsorption—so-called HIV-associated enteropathy.[2] Infection of microglial cells in the brain by HIV may lead to dementia or to a number of other central nervous system lesions that have been described, including HIV encephalopathy, polyradiculopathy, meningitis, and nemaline rod myopathy.[3,4] Direct infection of stem cells and precursor cells in the bone marrow leads to bone marrow suppression with potential development of pancytopenia.[5] Anti-HIV antibodies lead to idiopathic thrombocytopenic purpura, and infection of the uveal tract can lead to retinopathy.[6,7] The muscles may be affected by a polymyositis-like syndrome as well as myocarditis.[8,9] In childhood, HIV-1 infection may induce premature thymic involution with subsequent profound immunodepression.[10] In addition, HIV-related nephropathy may lead to chronic renal failure.[11]

VIRAL ILLNESSES INDUCED BY HIV-2

Human immunodeficiency virus type 2, the other pathogenic human retroviral lentivirus, was first noted in 1985 in West Africa and was originally named human T lymphotropic virus type 4 (HTLV-IV).[12,13] This virus causes an acquired immune deficiency syndrome virtually identical to that induced by HIV-1, although there is a longer incubation period for the development of AIDS following HIV-2 infection.[14] Outcome among HIV-2 infected patients may be slightly better as the degree of immunodeficiency may be less. Modes of transmission of this virus are similar to those for HIV-1, although HIV-2 may spread more slowly by heterosexual transmission.[15] Both viruses are similar in structure, although there are genetic differences. The incidence of HIV-2 infection has not attained the epidemic proportions of that of HIV-1.

ACUTE EXANTHEM OF HIV INFECTION

Definition

The acute reaction associated with HIV seroconversion refers to an acute viral prodrome associated with a cutaneous eruption that corresponds to the acute infection with HIV-1.[16]

Epidemiology

The acute exanthem associated with HIV-1 seroconversion is usually characterized as a benign, often subclinical, disorder that has been reported to occur in 10 to 50% of all newly diagnosed cases of HIV infection.[16–19] In a study of a population of individuals with occupationally acquired HIV infection, however, it was observed in 81%, indicating that the reaction occurs more frequently than originally thought.[20] The incubation period ranges from 3 to 6 weeks and varies with the route of infection, being shorter with hematogenous transmission and with larger viral inocula.[16–19]

Clinical Manifestations

Patients develop a sensation of malaise and soon thereafter develop fever that can be as high as 38.9°C (102°F) or, occasionally, higher. Night sweats, pharyngitis, fatigue, lymphadenopathy, and a fine morbilliform eruption that affects the trunk, chest, back, and upper arms develops within one to several days (Fig. 4–1)[16,17] The cutaneous eruption is similar to that seen with other viral illnesses or drug hypersensitivity reactions. The entire syndrome generally lasts for 4 to 5 days and usually resolves with complete recovery. Patients are highly infectious during this time, and although the $CD4^+$ count may remain perfectly normal, it may fall to as low as 200 cells/mm^3. In one study, the mean $CD4^+$ cell count at the time of presentation was 495 with a range of 178 to 1082 cells/mm^3.[21] A severe form of acute HIV infection may develop with persistent HIV p24 antigenemia, recurrent viremia, rapid decline in $CD4^+$ cell numbers, and accelerated disease progression.[21] Systemic manifestations include pneumonitis, esophagitis, meningitis, abdominal pain, and melena. Skin manifestations that may be seen include urticaria, perlèche, palatal and esophageal ulcers, enanthemata, and candidiasis.[21,22] Herpesvirus infections may also supervene.[21] The prognosis for patients with HIV infection who suffer from prolonged symptomatic primary HIV infection is significantly poorer than for those who are asymptomatic or who have a mild primary infection. Seventy-eight percent of those with a prolonged primary HIV infection progress to Centers for Disease Control and Prevention (CDC) group IV at 3 years compared with 10% of patients who are asymptomatic or who have only a mild primary infection.[23]

Pathogenesis

The pathogenesis of the development of the acute prodrome of HIV infection has not been fully elucidated but is thought to correspond to widespread infection of cells with HIV. This most likely leads to release of cytokines and inflammatory mediators that result in expression of disease. Immunocytochemistry has revealed that most of the infiltrating cells in skin lesions are $CD4^+$ T cells with an admixture of $CD8^+$ cells.[24]

Histopathology

Histologic evaluation of skin biopsies taken from the morbilliform eruption demonstrates an infiltrate consisting primarily of lymphocytes with occasional plasma cells around blood vessels of the superficial vascular plexus.[24] There is also slight spongiosis, and occasional individually necrotic keratinocytes may be seen in the epidermis. These findings are similar to those observed in other viral exanthemata as well as in morbilliform drug eruptions.

Laboratory Findings

Although no specific laboratory findings other than a demonstration of specific evidence of HIV infection can be found (such as the presence of HIV p24 antigen or antibodies directed to HIV), an elevated erythrocyte sedimentation rate, leukopenia, and cerebrospinal fluid lymphocytic pleocytosis may be observed. In the case of fulminant acute HIV infection, laboratory findings of profound immunosuppression as alluded to earlier may be demonstrated.[23]

Differential Diagnosis

The differential diagnosis includes other viral exanthemata such as those caused by parvovirus, measles, and rubella. Drug eruptions, too, may cause similar eruptions and must be excluded, especially as HIV-infected patients may be under treatment with numerous medications.

Diagnosis

The diagnosis of the acute HIV exanthem is based on the presence of a characteristic clinical picture in an individual with risk factors for the development of HIV infection. Blood tests that reveal either positive anti-HIV antibody titers by the enzyme-linked immunosorbent assay (ELISA) method and Western blot assay or circulating p24 antigen are confirmatory. Other possible viral disorders should be excluded by obtaining acute and convalescent viral titers.

Treatment

Zidovudine and other antiviral agents have been administered to patients with the acute HIV viral exanthem without repeatable success.[1,25,26]

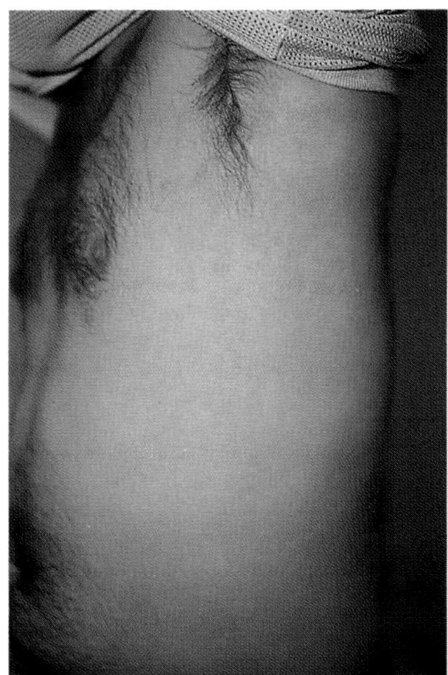

FIGURE 4–1. Acute seroconversion reaction of HIV infection

This is generally manifest as a widespread morbilliform eruption that is of short duration.

HERPESVIRUS INFECTIONS

Definition

Herpesvirus infection refers to infection by one of the different viruses of the herpesvirus family. Some of these include human herpesvirus types 1 and 2 (herpes simplex virus [HSV-1, HSV-2]), type 3 (varicella-zoster virus), type 4 (Epstein-Barr virus), type 5 (cytomegalovirus [CMV]), and type 6.

Incidence

Herpesvirus infections are commonly encountered in patients infected with HIV and may be seen in up to 20 to 50% of patients at some point during the course of HIV infection.[27] Depending on the degree of immunodeficiency, the likelihood of a patient developing one of these eruptions can approach 95%, as in the case of CMV infection when $CD4^+$ counts fall below 100 cells/mm^3.[28] The prevalence of infection with these viruses ranges from 20 and 40% for HSV to virtually 100% for varicella-zoster virus, Epstein-Barr virus, and CMV.[29]

Pathogenesis

Herpesviruses are all enveloped, double-stranded DNA viruses that characteristically cause latent or persistent infections that may last for the lifetime of the host. Transmission of HSV occurs by mucous membrane contact that leads to a primary mucocutaneous infection. Accompanying this, the virus travels along axons to nerve cell bodies in the dorsal root ganglion, where latency is established. On reactivation, HSV is transported to mucocutaneous sites via efferent nerves. Actively replicating virus in the epithelium leads to the characteristic vesicular lesions. Latent virus may be found not only in the nervous system, but also in the reticuloendothelial system, as well as in other tissues such as the skin. All of these viruses have a tropism for epithelial cells, with which they fuse. Following fusion, viral DNA becomes incorporated into the host genome, which leads to the formation of new viruses. All produce characteristic cytopathic effects in infected cells that can be recognized microscopically. Primary infections tend to be more severe and prolonged, whereas recurrent disease is usually localized. Immunocompromised hosts may develop severe primary infections that may be life threatening.[30]

Herpes simplex virus type 1 is the most common cause of oral herpetic infection, but HSV-2 is the most common etiologic agent for anogenital herpes infections. It is well documented that genital ulcerations are risk factors for the acquisition of HIV infection.[31,32] Given that HSV-2 is the most common cause of genital ulcerations in the United States and Europe, it is a potential serious risk factor for the development of HIV infection. In addition to serving as a risk factor for the development of HIV infection, HSV and HIV have important interactions that may have serious implications for patients with HIV infection. In vitro, HSV can potentiate HIV replication independent of HSV replication because HSV produces an early protein that results in enhanced HIV gene expression and replication. This phenomenon is a result of intracellular transactivation of HIV.[33] It has been suggested that the presence of herpes zoster is predictive of a progression from HIV infection to AIDS,[34] but whether this is a true risk factor or an artifact has been called into question. Several studies have shown that herpes zoster is not a reliable clinical marker for rapid progression to AIDS after adjustment for $CD4^+$ cell numbers.[35–37]

Clinical Manifestations

Herpes Simplex Virus. Oral, labial, and genital HSV infections are commonly seen in immunocompetent patients and may be well localized in HIV-infected individuals who are relatively immunocompetent. These are manifest as painful grouped vesicles on an erythematous base that rupture and become crusted (Fig. 4–2). Healing is usually complete in less than 2 weeks. Once significant immune suppression supervenes, lesions caused by HSV may become progressive and may be manifest by chronic ulcerative mucocutaneous lesions that last for longer than 1 month.[38] Tender, painful, ulcerative lesions of the penis, perianal area, and lip are quite characteristic, although other manifestations include perioral lesions and chronic ulcerative lesions on the glabrous skin such as that of the digits.[39] Lesions that are untreated may continue to enlarge dramatically and become quite deeply situated and extremely painful. Other lesions may appear verrucous and hyperplastic. Epithelial sites other than mucocutaneous ones may be affected, including the cornea, tracheobronchial tree, and esophagus, as well as visceral sites such as the lung, pericardium, liver, and brain.[40,41]

Varicella-Zoster Virus. Between 8 and 13% of patients who develop AIDS have a history of prior herpes zoster infection.[34] It generally appears within 2 to 7 years following seroconversion, often while the patient is asymptomatic. It may precede the development of oral thrush and oral hairy leukoplakia by more than 1 year. As mentioned before, varicella-zoster, like other minor cutaneous infections in HIV-infected hosts, is thought by many to be predictive of progression from HIV infection to AIDS, having

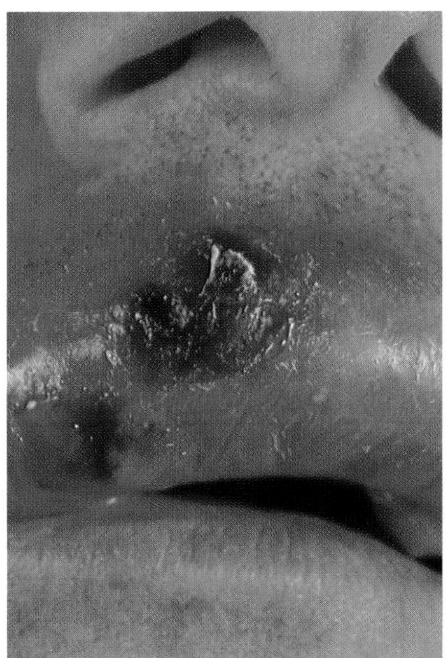

FIGURE 4–2. Herpes simplex ulcers
Herpes simplex infections may be persistent and result in chronic necrotizing ulcers.

been associated with progression in 23% at 2 years, 46% at 4 years, and 73% at 6 years. The virus exists in a dormant state in a dorsal root ganglion that becomes infected during prior varicella infection. With activation, the virus progresses down nerves of a solitary dermatome leading to the characteristic zosteriform distribution of painful, tense vesicles in the skin (Fig. 4–3). In addition to zoster, HIV-infected individuals may develop varicella that most commonly follows a benign course. However, in some cases, it may be associated with pulmonary involvement that may be fatal.[42] If an HIV-infected patient is exposed to varicella-zoster virus for the first time, careful consideration should be given to the use of varicella-zoster immunoglobulin, prophylactic acyclovir, or possibly, the newly released varicella vaccine.

Complications tend to be more significant in HIV-infected immunocompromised patients than in their immunocompetent counterparts (Fig. 4–4). Second episodes of varicella, repeat zoster infections, and multidermatomal forms may occur. Zoster may develop in children shortly after a course of primary varicella,[43] and recurrent episodes of zoster have been documented in 5 to 23% of HIV-infected hosts, usually in those with advanced immunodeficiency. Dissemination of virus with development of blisters over large areas of the skin may develop concomitant with the characteristic zosteriform group of vesicles.[44,45] Postherpetic neuralgia after typical zoster seems to be more com-

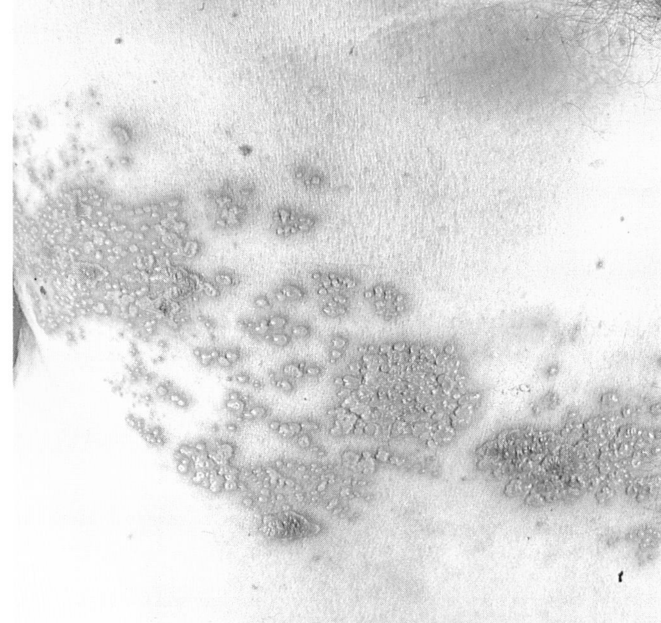

FIGURE 4–3. Herpes zoster
Painful vesicles on an erythematous base in a dermatomal distribution is virtually pathognomonic for this condition caused by the varicella zoster virus. This infection may be a harbinger that the patient may later develop bona fide AIDS.

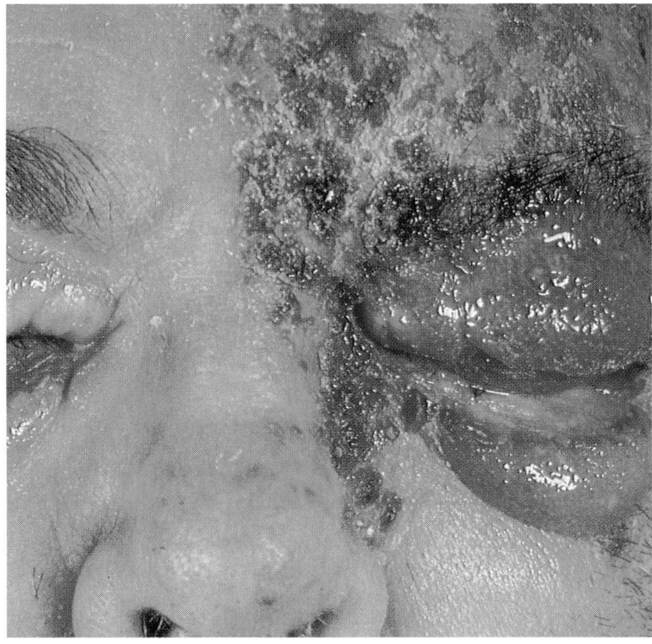

FIGURE 4–4. Herpes zoster
Infections may be severe and fulminant in immunocompromised patients.

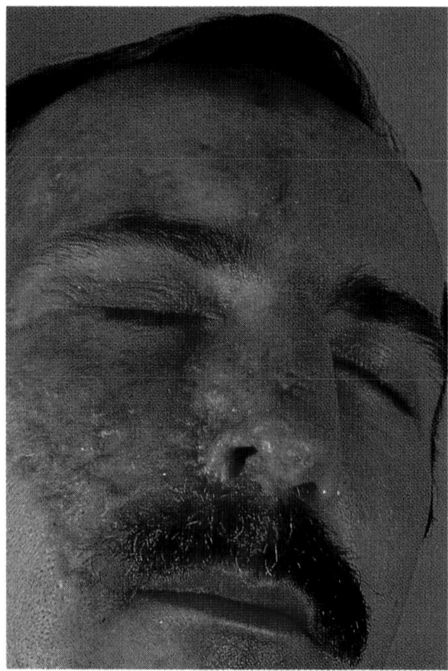

FIGURE 4–5. Herpes zoster
Severe residual scarring of the face occurring as a sequela to herpes zoster. This complication is more frequent in patients with AIDS.

mon in HIV-infected patients. This is manifest as persistent, severe pain in an affected dermatome that is often resistant to all forms of therapy. Crusted, punched-out ulcerations that leave painful atrophic scars may also be associated with postherpetic neuralgia (Fig. 4–5).[46,47] Generally, these lesions develop a thick overlying eschar and are remarkable for the lack of surrounding erythema. They occur most commonly on the buttocks and lower extremities but may be disseminated. Chronic verrucous lesions may also be seen that are often resistant to therapy with acyclovir.[48]

Cytomegalovirus. Up to 90% of patients with AIDS may develop acute active CMV infection at some point during their illness; it is the most common cause of serious opportunistic viral infection in patients with AIDS.[28] Fifty percent of all AIDS patients have CMV viremia, which leads to clinical manifestations of retinitis and gastroenteritis. Serious CMV retinitis may occur in between 5 and 10% of patients and is found in 30% of AIDS patients at autopsy.[49] Esophagitis and colitis as well as a proctocolitis may develop in 5 to 10%.[2] In the skin, CMV may assume a number of different clinical manifestations, including ulcerations, keratotic verrucous lesions, palpable purpuric papules, and diffuse ulcerations.[3,4] Vesicular, bullous, and generalized morbilliform eruptions as well as hyperpigmented indurated plaques and a generalized bullous toxic epidermal necrolysis-like eruption associated with CMV hepatitis have been reported.[5,6] Most patients with CMV perianal ulcerations have ongoing CMV proctocolitis, and these ulcers most likely represent contiguous spread to the skin from the gastrointestinal tract (Fig. 4–6).[7] Many patients have combined herpes simplex and CMV infections (Figs. 4–7 through 4–9).[8]

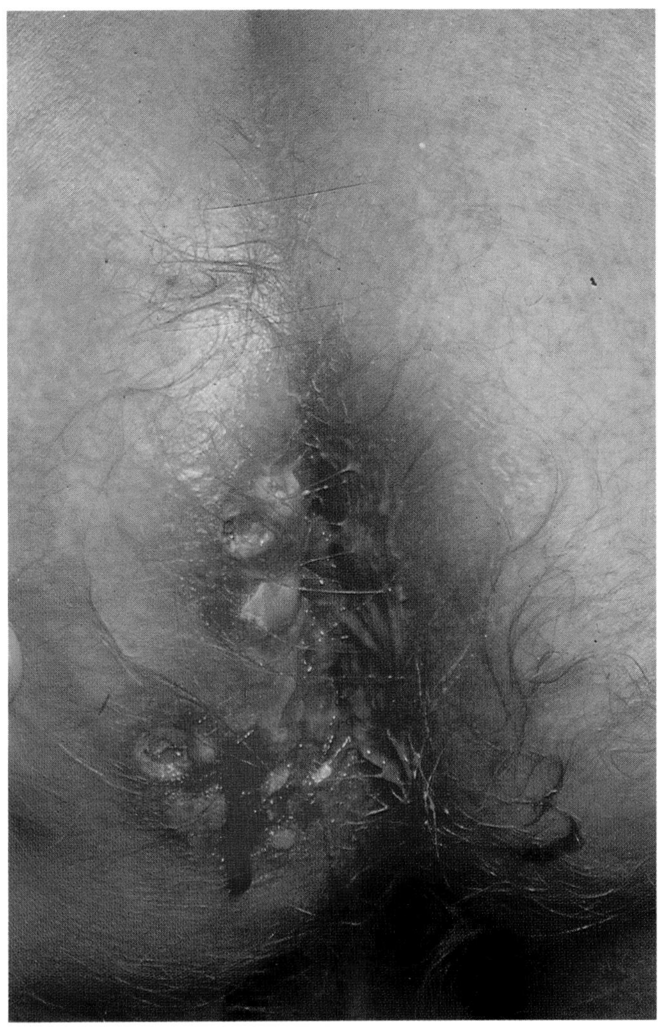

FIGURE 4–6. Combined herpesvirus and cytomegalovirus ulcerations

Necrotizing nonhealing perianal ulcerations in this case were due to herpesvirus and infection with cytomegalovirus in a patient with AIDS.

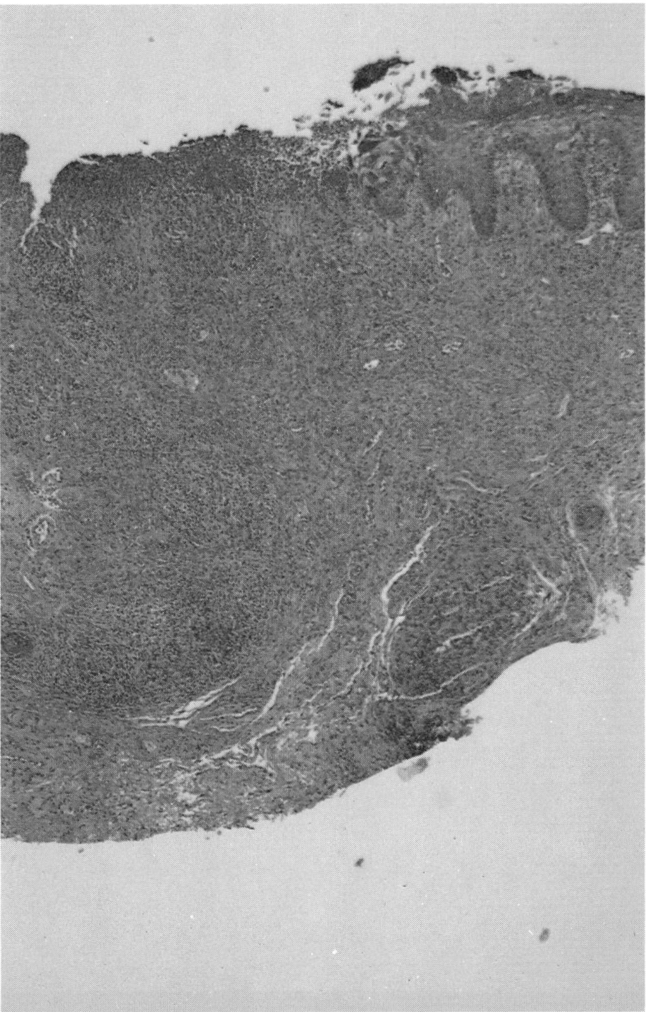

FIGURE 4–7. Combined herpesvirus and cytomegalovirus ulcerations

This punch biopsy taken from near a mucous membrane shows an ulceration with a dense inflammatory cell infiltrate.

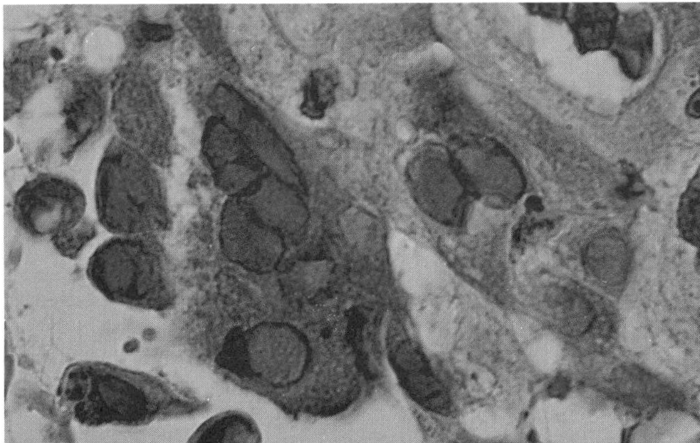

FIGURE 4–8. Combined herpesvirus and cytomegalovirus infection

Higher magnification at the surface of the ulcer shows multinucleated giant cells of herpes simplex virus infection.

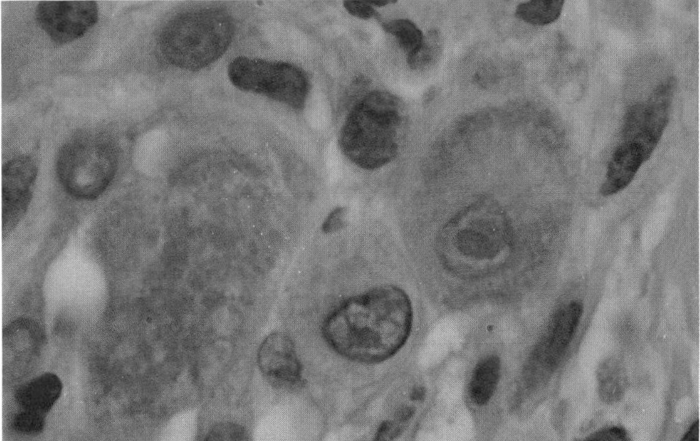

FIGURE 4–9. Combined herpesvirus and cytomegalovirus ulcerations

An area taken from beneath the ulceration shows giant fibroblasts with intranuclear and intracytoplasmic purplish inclusion bodies of cytomegalovirus. Thus, there were two infectious agents within one skin lesion.

Oral Hairy Leukoplakia (Epstein-Barr Virus). Epstein-Barr virus selectively infects cells of the B-lymphocyte lineage and certain types of squamous epithelia. The majority of adults have been previously infected with the virus and harbor it in the latent phase. Primary Epstein-Barr virus infection is manifested as infectious mononucleosis. After primary replication in the oropharyngeal epithelium, virion entry into the B-cell system provides a means for long-term viral carriage and serves to disseminate the infection to other sites. With advanced immunodeficiency in HIV-infected patients, Epstein-Barr virus replication occurs once again, leading to either oral hairy leukoplakia, Burkitt's lymphoma, or Epstein-Barr virus–associated large cell lymphoma.

Oral hairy leukoplakia is manifest as one or more whitish plaques, usually on the lateral margins of the tongue, that are virtually always seen in individuals who are immunocompromised (Figs. 4–10 and 4–11). The surface of the plaques may be smooth, corrugated, or remarkably folded and may be so thick that hair-like projections appear. Clinically, oral hairy leukoplakia may mimic other white lesions of the mucous membranes, including true premalignant leukoplakia as well as candidiasis.[9] Characteristically, the lesion may not be rubbed off with a tongue depressor which is a helpful finding in distinguishing it from candidiasis, with which a patient may be concomitantly infected. These lesions are asymptomatic and cause little problem, although they may occasionally become quite verrucous and lead to dysphagia. The incubation period from primary HIV infection to the detection of oral hairy leukoplakia varies from 5 to 10 years, and the presence of oral hairy leukoplakia correlates with moderate to advanced immunodeficiency.[10] It has also been correlated with progression from HIV infection to AIDS, as 48% of patients with oral hairy leukoplakia develop AIDS by 16 months and 83% by 31 months.[11]

Histopathology

Herpes simplex and varicella-zoster virus infections characteristically are manifest by an intraepidermal acantholytic vesicular dermatitis associated with characteristic cytopathic effects in epithelial cells (see Fig. 4–8). There is margination of the chromatin with ballooning nuclear degeneration associated with pinkish intracytoplasmic and intranuclear inclusions known as Cowdry bodies. Cells float freely within a vesicle space and are associated with a variable amount of inflammatory infiltrate in the dermis that consists of lymphocytes, histiocytes, eosinophils, neutrophils, and plasma cells. Careful inspection of dermal inflammatory infiltrates demonstrates perineural and intraneural inflammation associated with degeneration of nerves.[12] In patients who are severely immunocompromised who develop infection with either herpes simplex or varicella-zoster virus, extensive cytonecrosis of the epidermis occurs that is associated with abundant viral infection of keratinocytes.[13] Often a complete syncytium of infected keratinocytes is seen that is associated with involvement of follicles and adnexal structures. In some lesions, there may be extensive ulceration so that the herpetically infected cells cannot be visualized. In these cases, special immunoperoxidase stains and DNA probes may be useful in detecting viral antigens that may not be visible with routine microscopy. Skin lesions caused by both viruses appear identical histologically.

Cytomegalovirus infection characteristically is manifest by infection of fibroblasts and endothelial cells in the dermis that is associated with overlying ulceration. Cutaneous epithelial cells are generally not infected, although gastrointestinal epithelium may be affected. Individual cells are enlarged to several times their normal diameter and contain purplish intracytoplasmic and intranuclear inclusions with a somewhat crystalline shape (see Fig. 4–9). There is a variable amount of inflammatory infiltrate in the dermis. It is important to ensure that a mixed viral infection is not present, as it is not uncommon to see both HSV and CMV within the same section.

Oral hairy leukoplakia is manifest by marked epithelial hyperplasia with a verrucous corrugated appearance (Fig. 4–12).[14] Individual keratinocytes are altered dramatically, with ballooning degeneration giving rise to extensive pallor (Fig. 4–13). Minimal inflammation is seen in the lamina propria. The differential diagnosis includes other ballooning degenerative lesions of the mouth, including chronic maceration and white sponge nevus. Electron microscopy as well as DNA in situ hybridization can be used to demonstrate viral particles in the epithelium, especially in the upper rather than the lower portions.[15,50]

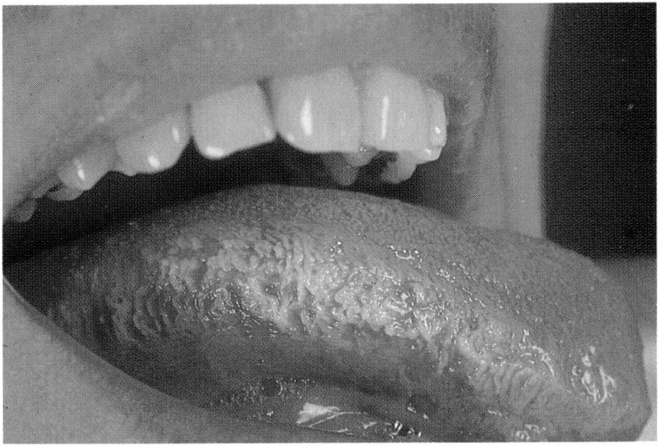

FIGURE 4–10. Oral hairy leukoplakia

A whitish verrucous corrugated plaque commonly seen on the lateral surfaces of the tongue is characteristic of this condition caused by the Epstein-Barr virus. When scraped with a tongue blade or other instrument, the lesion does not wipe away.

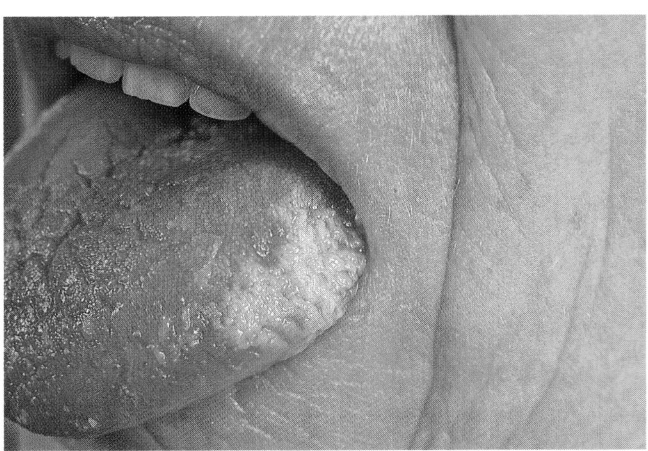

FIGURE 4–11. Another example of oral hairy leukoplakia

In this case, the patient was a woman who had received blood transfusions.

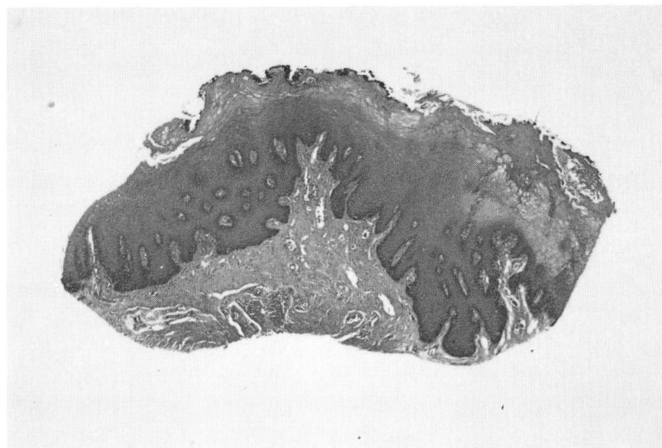

FIGURE 4–12. Punch biopsy of oral hairy leukoplakia

Note the epidermal hyperplasia and pallor of the uppermost portion of the epithelium.

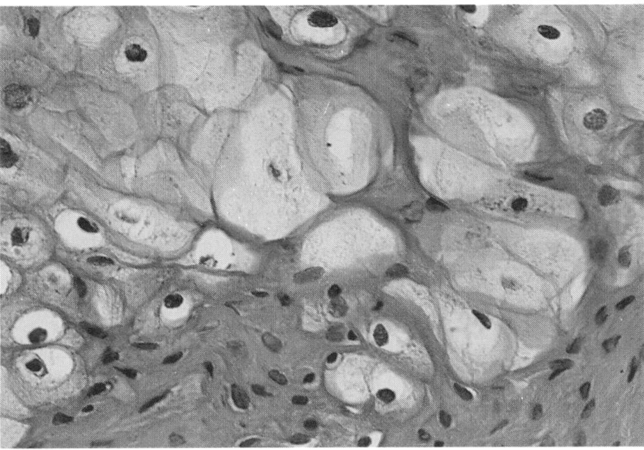

FIGURE 4–13. Oral hairy leukoplakia

Marked ballooning of keratinocytes responsible for pallor seen at lower magnification. The extensive ballooning degeneration is characteristic of oral hairy leukoplakia.

Laboratory Findings

In general, no characteristic laboratory findings are associated with these infections, although patients with primary Epstein-Barr virus infection show B-cell proliferation and exaggerated T-cell responses. Most patients with CMV infection have $CD4^+$ cell counts of less than 200 cells/mm^3, as do patients with severe HSV and varicella-zoster infections. Zoster and oral hairy leukoplakia may occur in patients who are more immunocompetent. In one study, the mean $CD4^+$ cell number of patients with oral hairy leukoplakia was 390.[51]

Differential Diagnosis

Clinically, the differential diagnosis of herpesvirus infections includes other chronic ulcerative conditions such as aphthous ulcerations, ulcerative opportunistic atypical mycobacterial and deep fungal infections, and traumatic ulcers. Verrucous lesions may mimic a number of different conditions, including epithelial neoplasms and infections associated with pseudocarcinomatous hyperplasia. Cytomegalovirus also must be distinguished from ulcerative conditions and from vasculitis when purple-red papules are present in the skin. Oral hairy leukoplakia must be distinguished from hypertrophic candidiasis as well as from true histologic leukoplakia and squamous cell carcinoma, leukokeratosis oris, white sponge nevus, verruca vulgaris, lichen planus, mucous patches of syphilis, and other white lesions of the mucous membranes.

Diagnosis

Diagnosis is made on the basis of culture, smears, biopsy, and clinical appearance of lesions. Tzanck preparations usually reveal the presence of multinucleated giant cells of HSV or varicella-zoster virus infection. As mentioned earlier, microscopic examination of scrapings will be negative for hyphae, which therefore excludes the diagnosis of candidiasis in lesions of oral hairy leukoplakia. Involvement of the inferolateral surface of the tongue is also characteristic of oral hairy leukoplakia and aids in its distinction from other processes. Electron microscopy and DNA probe analysis may also be useful in identifying virally infected cells. Immunoperoxidase stains for CMV, HSV, and varicella-zoster virus are commercially available and can increase the speed and the sensitivity of detection of these agents.

Treatment

Herpesvirus infections are treated with acyclovir at doses that range from 200 to 1000 mg orally every 4 hours while the patient is awake or Famciclovir, 500 mg orally every 8 hours for zoster. Resistant cases require treatment with intravenous foscarnet sodium or vidarabine.[52,53] On occasion, patients with seemingly resistant varicella-zoster or HSV infection may be suffering from atrophic gastritis, which prevents absorption of acyclovir, so that a change to intravenous administration may be effective. Other helpful measures may include local care with cool compresses or sitz baths, topical anesthetics such as 2–5% lidocaine gel or ointment, and pramoxine ointment or lotion. A newly released agent, Emla (eutectic mixture of local anesthetics), may also be helpful in relieving pain when applied topically under occlusion. Herpes zoster may be associated with acute pain that may respond to treatment with narcotics or even nonsteroidal anti-inflammatory agents. A more serious complication is postherpetic neuralgia that results as a consequence of neural inflammation and infection with fibrosis around nerves and leads to secondary neural compromise. Treatment consists of managing the underlying viral infection with high doses of acyclovir as well as attempting to block the chronic pain that is produced following its resolution. In general, topical agents are rarely helpful, although capsaicin and Emla cream have been effective in some patients. Amitriptyline, carbamazepine (Tegretol), nerve blocks, Triavil, biofeedback, hypnosis, and fentanyl patches are other measures that have been reported to be effective in some cases. Cytomegalovirus requires treatment with ganciclovir (dihydroxy propoxymethyl guanine [DHPG]).[54] In cases of painful perianal ulcerations, compresses and topical anesthetics may be required.

Oral hairy leukoplakia often requires no treatment but may respond to treatment with acyclovir at the dosage of 200 to 400 mg five times a day; topical podophyllum resin, either 20% in alcohol applied two to three times daily or 25% in tincture of benzoin applied in the office for 5 minutes and then removed; or application of topical isotretinoin (Retin A) gel. Local destructive measures may also be beneficial.[55,56]

HUMAN PAPILLOMAVIRUS INFECTIONS

Definition

Human papillomavirus (HPV) infection refers to infections with viruses of the subfamily Papillomavirinae (family Papovaviridae). The viruses are small, double-stranded DNA viruses that are 50 to 55 nanometers in diameter. Characteristically, infection with HPV causes squamous epithelial proliferation. At least 60 types of HPV have now been recognized using DNA hybridization technology.

Incidence

Human papillomavirus infection is an extremely prevalent disorder and is one of the most common viral infections of humans. One study of college-aged women in a major university revealed that 46% were infected with HPV.[57] One percent of college students examined in one university were shown to have clinical evidence of condylomata acuminata, whereas 16% showed evidence of HPV infection using colposcopy, exfoliative cytology, or sensitive methods to detect HPV antigens or HPV DNA.[58] The annual incidence of condylomata acuminata has been reported as high as 106.5 per 100,000 or about 0.1% of the entire population.[59] Men and women are affected similarly, with a ratio of 1.0 : 1.4, and the median age of infection with anogenital HPV is 22 to 25 years. In HIV-infected individuals, HPV infection is even more prevalent. In one study, anogenital warts were demonstrated in 20% of HIV-infected homosexual men and 27% of homosexual men with AIDS.[60] Using more sensitive studies, 48% of HIV-negative homosexual men and 54% of homosexual men with AIDS were shown to have evidence of HPV infection.[61] Human papillomavirus types 16 and 18 are the most common viral isolates from anogenital condylomata.

Pathogenesis

Human papillomaviruses are transmitted by close, repeated contact that is often sexual in nature. The virus has a tropism for squamous epithelium and enters the cells of the basal cell layer probably through microscopic abrasions following exposure. The incubation period for condyloma acuminatum varies from 3 weeks to 8 months, averaging 2.8 months.[62] Following internalization, the virus enters the nucleus, where it either leads to productive infection or undergoes latency. Transcription of HPV takes place primarily in basal cells, whereas virion production occurs in more differentiated layers of the epithelium so that only the surface contains infectious viral particles.[63–65] Infectious viral particles are released with desquamated cells that are shed from skin or mucous membranes. Because of its tendency to produce latent infections, irrespective of whether clinical lesions develop, the virus usually remains in a quiescent state for the life of the host.

In addition to causing verrucae and papillomas, HIV infection may cause development of carcinoma. Human papillomavirus proteins bind p53, a tumor suppressor gene product that leads to unregulated cell growth and neoplasia (see Neoplasia).[66] Cell-mediated immunity plays an important role in controlling HPV infection,[67,68] and patients with depressed cell-mediated immunity are predisposed to develop multiple HPV-induced lesions, including neoplasms.[69,70] Furthermore, HIV *tat* protein transactivates HPV, which leads to increased HPV expression.[71,72]

Different HPV types tend to cause different clinical lesions, although there is significant overlap. Cutaneous nongenital lesions such as plantar, common, or flat warts are caused most commonly by HPV types 1, 2, 3, and 4. Epidermodysplasia verruciformis may be caused by a number of different viruses. The benign form of the condition, which is associated with minimal malignant potential, is induced by HPV types 3 and 10, whereas those that form with malignant potential are caused by HPV types 5 and 8. Mucosal lesions that affect either the genital, oral, or laryngeal epithelia are also caused by a variety of different viruses. Human papillomavirus types 6 and 11 generally induce benign lesions, whereas types 16, 18, 31, and 33 are associated with the potential for malignancy, especially types 16 and 18. In one study in Europe, HPV types 6 and 11 were the most common types detected from condylomata,[73,74] but in a later study of American patients, HPV types 16 and 18 were the most common in isolates, and combined infections were quite common.[61] This has serious implications given the oncogenic potential of these viruses. Bowenoid papulosis lesions are caused almost exclusively by HPV types 16 and 18, with 16 being the most common.[75]

Clinical Manifestations

Verruca vulgaris lesions are skin-colored to reddish verrucous hyperkeratotic papules or plaques that may occur on any surface of the skin (Fig. 4–14). Glabrous skin is commonly affected, especially around the fingers and on the extremities, although the face and head and neck area are also frequent sites of involvement. Individual small blackish bleeding points are often seen, which correspond to dilated blood vessels and intraepidermal hemorrhage. Patients with HIV infection, especially those who are immunocompromised, may present with multiple verruca vulgaris lesions, especially in periungual locations. Multiple plantar warts, including mosaic warts, may develop that may lead to pain with walking. Extensive flat and filiform warts on the bearded area of the face manifest by small verrucous papules are also seen in HIV-infected individuals and may be the first sign of HIV infection (Figs. 4–15 and 4–16).

Human papillomavirus in men can affect the penis, urethra, scrotum, and perianal, anal, and rectal area. Condyloma acuminatum is usually recognized as soft, sessile tumors with surfaces that range from smooth to very rough with finger-like projections. Perianal condylomata are usually roughened and cauliflower-like, whereas penile lesions are often smooth and papular. Exuberant cauliflower-like plaques of condylomata acuminata that affect the perianal region as well as flexural areas such as the axillae and angles of the mouth also may be seen (Fig. 4–17). Extensive perianal condylomata may lead to difficulty with defecation and secondary constipation. Penile condylomata are usually 3 to 5 mm in diameter and often occur in groups of three to four. These lesions usually cause no symptoms, but occasionally patients complain of pruritus, irritation, or bleeding as a result of trauma. Although classic condyloma acuminatum is easily recognized, a second type of HPV-induced lesion known as a flat, keratotic plaque may be more difficult to detect. These lesions project only slightly above the normal epithelium, have a rough surface, and may be somewhat pigmented. Subclinical HPV infection is common in men and manifests as diffuse foci of epithelial hyperplasia that are invisible in routine examination.[76] Subclinical HPV infection as well as intraurethral condylomata may serve as a major reservoir for HPV in the population, although it is not known whether HPV can be transmitted from men with subclinical infection to sexual partners. Treatment failure in women may represent, in some cases, reinfection by a male sexual partner with one of these occult forms of HPV infection.

In women, the spectrum of clinical disease induced by HPV may be quite broad. Classic exophytic lesions of condyloma acuminatum of the external genitalia are generally readily recognized, although detection of other forms of HPV infection requires colposcopic and sigmoidoscopic examination. Vulvar condylomata acuminata appear as soft, whitish, sessile tumors with papular or fine, finger-like projections. They are seen most commonly in moist areas such as the introitus and labia.[77] Vaginal condylomata acuminata are seen in one third of women with vulvar condylomata. Generally multiple lesions are present.[78] Vaginal discharge, pruritus, and postcoital bleeding may occur, although most vaginal condylomata are asymptomatic. Several patterns of subclinical vaginal HPV infection are identifi-

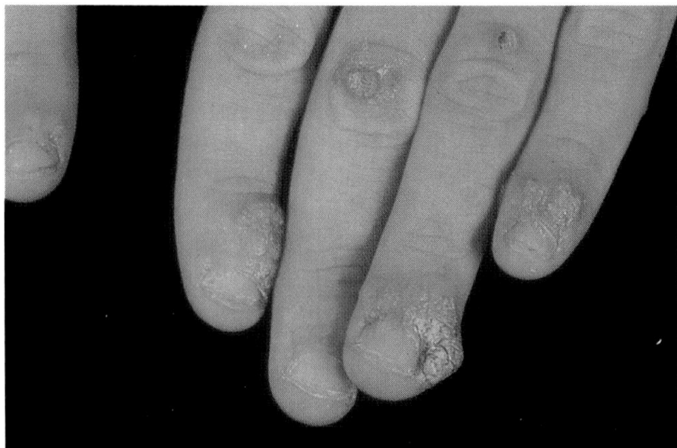

FIGURE 4–14. Verruca vulgaris lesions

Hyperkeratotic verrucous papules that coalesce, especially in the periungual area, may pose a therapeutic as well as a cosmetic problem in the AIDS patient.

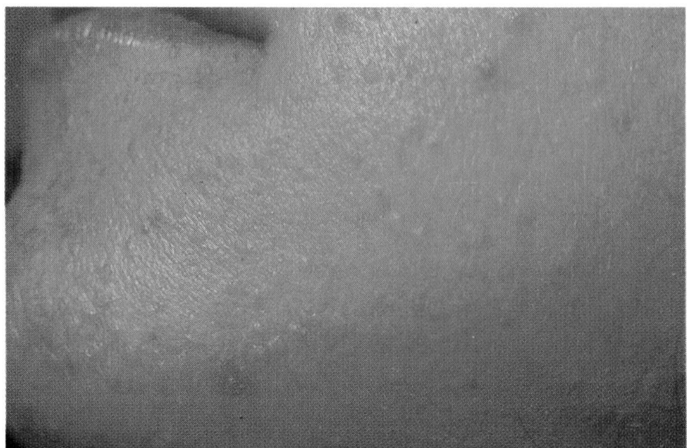

FIGURE 4–15. Verrucae plana

Myriad skin-colored flat warts can occasionally be seen in patients with AIDS. Such lesions are virtually impossible to eradicate.

able via acetic acid staining of the vaginal mucosa followed by colposcopic examination. These include elongated vaginal papillae analogous to individual fronds of condylomata, acetowhite epithelium appearing as sharply-defined flat, whitish patches and reverse punctation appearing as multiple tiny acetowhite white spots on the vaginal walls. Cervical condylomata occur in 20% of women with HPV infection in other areas of the genital tract.[78] They usually appear as papillary epithelial projections in the cervical transformation zone and in the squamous epithelium on colposcopic examination.

Bowenoid papulosis may appear identical to condyloma acuminatum but usually manifests as small, brown, flat-topped papules that affect the genital and perigenital area (Fig. 4–18). The condition is seen in both sexes but is more common in men. Lesions may become confluent and hyperplastic, and in some cases there may be progression to fully developed squamous cell carcinoma. The shaft of the penis is affected more commonly than the glans.

Epidermodysplasia verruciformis has been reported in patients with HIV infection and consists of a widespread papular eruption of reddish to skin-colored, flat, wartlike lesions that affect mostly the sun-exposed areas of the skin (Fig. 4–19).[79,80] We recently evaluated a patient with a widespread erythroderma that on biopsy showed features of diffuse HPV infection.

Verrucous carcinoma manifests as a large verrucous plaque or tumor, most commonly in the perianal location, and has also been reported in patients with HIV infection (see subsequent discussion).

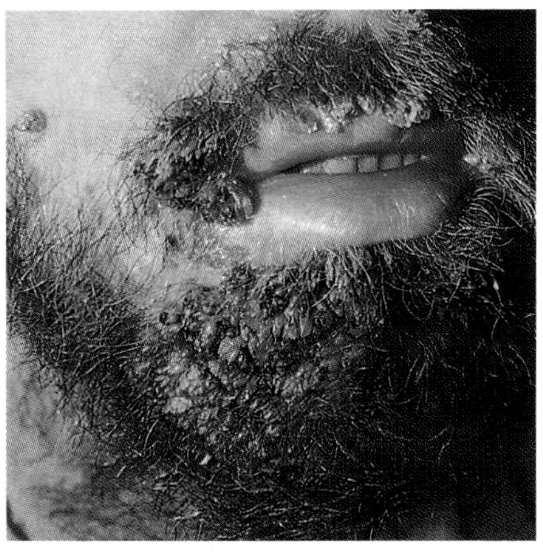

FIGURE 4–16. Human papillomavirus infection
Extensive human papillomavirus infection of the beard in a patient with AIDS. Occasionally, these infections become extremely severe, causing significant cosmetic deformity, as seen here.

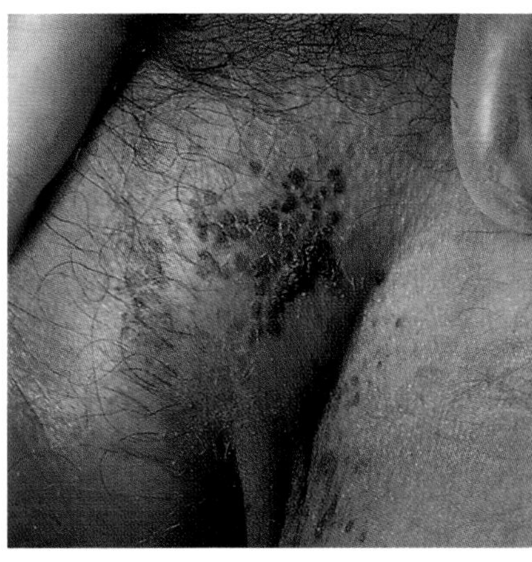

FIGURE 4–18. Bowenoid papulosis
There are multiple brown flat-topped papules in the genital area. Histopathologically, these reveal changes of squamous cell carcinoma in situ.

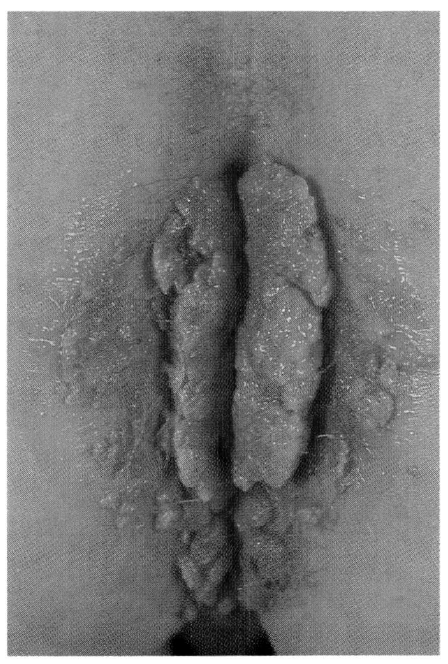

FIGURE 4–17. Condylomata acuminata
Multiple vegetating coalescing condylomata acuminata in the perianal area of a patient with AIDS. When this is extensive, problems with anal blockage may occur.

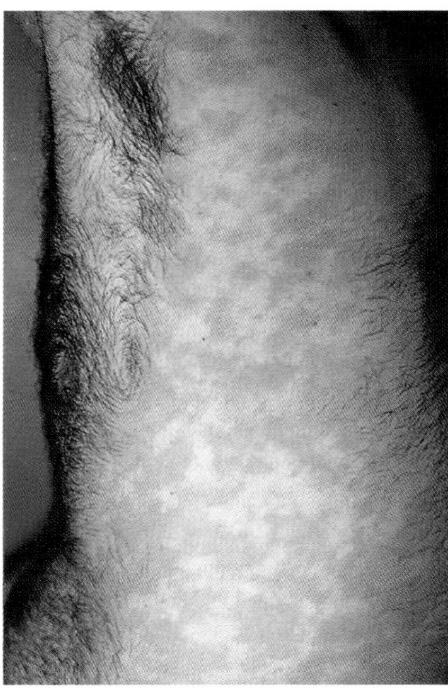

FIGURE 4–19. Epidermodysplasia verruciformis in AIDS
This is a manifestation of a widespread human papillomavirus infection that is associated with the development of squamous cell carcinoma.

Histopathology

Verruca vulgaris lesions are characterized by marked epidermal hyperplasia with acanthosis, papillomatosis, dilated blood vessels in the papillary dermis, intraepidermal hemorrhage, and parakeratosis. Condylomata acuminata are usually manifest as dome-shaped papular lesions with acanthosis and koilocytosis. Lesions are usually gently papillated rather than being digitated. More florid examples of condylomata acuminata may be associated with extensive papillomatosis and digitation. Bowenoid papulosis has the architectural features of a condyloma but histologically shows changes of atypical keratinocytic proliferation and features of squamous cell carcinoma in situ (Figs. 4–20 and 4–21). Verrucous carcinoma has histologic features similar to large condylomata acuminata except lesions extend deeply, often with epithelial components in the soft tissues and muscularis. Lesions of epidermodysplasia verruciformis appear similar to flat verrucae except that atypical keratinocytic changes may be present that are suggestive of evolving carcinoma in situ.

Laboratory Findings

In general, routine laboratory findings are noncontributory in these cases, although patients with extensive disease often are found to have $CD4^+$ cell numbers lower than 500 cells/mm^3.[81]

Differential Diagnosis

The differential diagnosis of HPV infection includes other benign epithelial neoplasms, including seborrheic keratoses, pyogenic granulomata, nevi, and other various keratoses and acanthomata. Condylomata acuminata may have features similar to condylomata lata of syphilis, whereas Bowenoid papulosis and verrucous carcinoma may mimic benign HPV-induced counterparts. Erosive HPV-induced cervicitis may appear similar to other forms of chronic cervicitis.

Diagnosis

The diagnosis of clinical HPV-induced lesions is based on clinical features in the context of histopathologic findings. It is important to perform biopsies in any cases that could conceivably represent manifestations of a malignant HPV-induced condition. In difficult cases, immunoperoxidase stains for HPV antigens, DNA in situ hybridization, as well as the polymerase chain reaction can be performed to increase the sensitivity of diagnosis (see later discussion).

The acetowhite test is a technique that can be used to detect the presence of subclinical HPV infection of the glabrous skin or of the mucous membranes. On the skin, the technique consists of the application of dilute acetic acid, usually by placing an acetic acid–soaked gauze onto the skin of the penis, scrotum, or both. Three percent acetic acid is used, and the area is soaked generally for approximately 5 minutes and then examined either directly or under magnification. A shiny white or grayish-white appearance of the skin occurs as the result of the acetic acid causing swelling and maceration of virally induced epithelial hyperplasia, which generally has enhanced permeability and increased glycogen content. Most benign HPV-induced lesions are shiny and white, but intraepithelial neo-

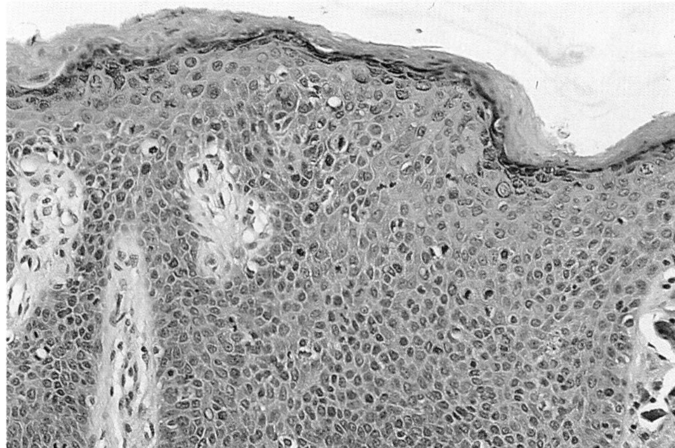

FIGURE 4–20. Histopathology of bowenoid papulosis
There is acanthosis of the epithelium with papillomatosis. There is also disordered epithelial maturation. Hematoxylin and eosin stain (original magnification ×50).

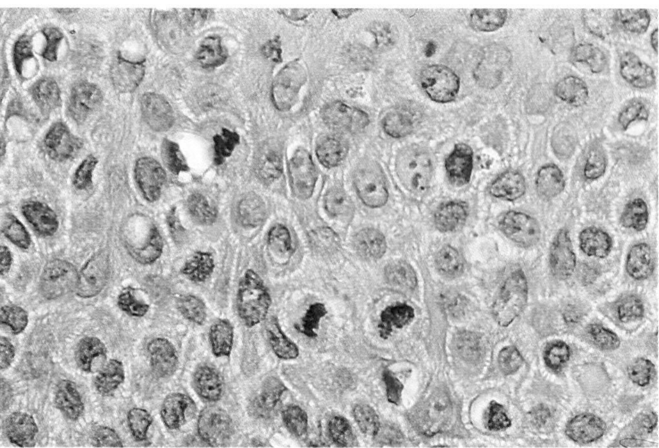

FIGURE 4–21. Bowenoid papulosis histology
Higher magnification demonstrates the abundant mitotic figures and cytologic atypia. Hematoxylin and eosin stain (original magnification ×400).

plasms tend to be duller gray or dull white. Microscopic evaluation of acetowhite lesions reveals epithelial hyperplasia and usually koilocytic changes in nuclei. The presence of viral particles or viral DNA can be demonstrated by using more sensitive techniques. In women, acetowhite epithelium is one form of subclinical vaginal HPV infection that appears as sharply defined flat whitish patches, whereas reverse punctation appears as multiple tiny acetowhite spots on the vaginal walls. Subclinical cervical HPV infection also may be detected by acetowhite highlighting which demonstrates a snow-white lesion with an irregular outline and a jagged, angular border with feathered margins. Staining with quarter-strength Lugol's iodine is another technique that can be used in conjunction with colposcopy, as staining is diminished in areas of fully developed carcinoma in situ.

Exfoliative cytology as well as histology can be quite valuable in diagnosing HPV infection. Cells with enlarged, vacuolated nuclei and perinuclear clear areas in the cytoplasm are known as a koilocytes. These cells are highly characteristic of HPV infection, and their presence is generally regarded as diagnostic.[82] Many HPV-infected tissues did not exhibit koilocytosis, however, so that cytologic and histologic specimens that do not show this change cannot be assumed to be free of papillomavirus. Electron microscopy can be used to identify HPV particles in some tissue specimens.[74] Immunohistochemistry using an antibody to shared papillomavirus structural protein is another simple way to detect the presence of HPV. Antisera to HPV proteins are coupled with horseradish peroxidase or biotin and used to stain tissue sections. Although the method is more sensitive than routine histologic staining, it fails to identify many infected tissues, especially when evolving neoplasia is present,[76] and, unfortunately, currently available papillomavirus antesera do not distinguish reliably among different HPV types. The most commonly used test for detecting and typing HPV is a Southern blot assay. In this assay, DNA is extracted from a tissue specimen and cut into specific fragments, which are then separated according to size. The separated fragments are transferred to a solid-membrane support that is then exposed to labeled, cloned DNA of a known type of HPV. If HPV DNA is present, the labeled probe binds to the membrane and can be detected. The method is quite specific and can detect levels as low as one HPV DNA molecule per 10 cells or fewer. Another commonly used method is the tissue in situ hybridization assay.[83] In this procedure, a tissue section is mounted on a microscopic slide and is exposed to a labeled HPV DNA probe. After treatment to detect the binding of the labeled DNA, the slide is examined microscopically for evidence of HPV DNA. One final technique commonly used to identify HPV DNA sequences is the polymerase chain reaction.[84] In this technique, bacterial enzymes are used to amplify a small segment of HPV DNA and can be utilized on paraffin-embedded tissue.[85] The sensitivity of the polymerase chain reaction assay is about one HPV genome per cell.[86] A combination utilizing in situ hybridization and polymerase chain reaction testing has been described.[87] In this method, multiple primer sets are used to generate DNA fragments with overlapping sequences. These are then amplified in situ. The in situ amplification allows direct assessment of viral expression in tissue samples, including smears.

Treatment

Treatment of HPV-induced lesions revolves around measures that result in diminution of clinical lesions, destruction of premalignant or malignant lesions, reduction of symptoms, and minimization of transmission to uninfected individuals. Successful therapy depends on the ability of the host's immune status to keep viral infection in check. Frequent recurrences are probably a consequence of reactivation of latent HPV infection, and therapy often must be extended to include normal-appearing tissue. Unfortunately, no treatment has been shown to eradicate HPV entirely.

Treatment of verruca vulgaris generally consists of destructive measures such as application of topical chemicals such as salicylic or trichloroacetic acid, cryotherapy with liquid nitrogen, or surgery. Condyloma acuminatum lesions are usually treated by applying podophyllum resin. Podophyllum resin is derived from two plants: *Podophyllum peltatum,* a North American variety, and *Podophyllum emodi,* an Indian species. These plants contain compounds that arrest mitosis in metaphase. Following the application of podophyllum resin, an acute inflammatory reaction occurs that is accompanied by intracellular and intercellular edema, mitotic arrest, and cell death over the next 24 hours. The usual strength is a 10 to 50% resin in tincture of benzoin. The tincture is applied directly to lesions by a physician or an assistant in an office outpatient session with instructions for the patient to wash it off in 4 to 6 hours. Although generally normal areas of the skin are avoided, in some cases of extensive disease, larger areas such as the entire penile shaft may be "painted" with the resin. Treatments are administered weekly until resolution or until significant reduction of the number of lesions ensues. At that point, secondary destruction with liquid nitrogen cryosurgery or surgical destruction may be performed. Although generally safe, complications of severe necrosis and scarring in the anogenital area, fistula in ano, dermatitis, balanitis, and phimosis may develop, especially if the substance is left on the skin or mucosa for long periods of time.[88] Systemic reactions rarely occur.[89,90]

Podofilox (Condylox; Oclassen, Ventura, Calif.), the active ingredient in podophyllum resin, applied twice a day for 3 days per week for 3 to 4 weeks is a regimen that is often quite effective and can be used by the patient at home, but recurrence is common and adjunctive destructive measures are often required.[91] Liquid nitrogen cryotherapy applied either with a cotton-tipped applicator or a hand-held spraying device for about 10 to 30 seconds to yield a 15- to 30-second thaw time is also effective treatment for these lesions but is associated with the complications of pain, blistering, and ulceration.[92] Electrodesiccation and curettage and carbon dioxide laser vaporization have also been performed, but care must be taken to avoid adverse consequences of infectious HPV and, possibly, HIV in the laser plume.[93,94] Verruca plantaris lesions are generally treated with topical 40% salicylic acid plaster applied daily with paring of hyperkeratotic areas, although intralesional bleomycin and liquid nitrogen therapy have also been used. Verruca plana and verruca filiformis are treated commonly with tretinoin (Retin-A) 0.05% cream or 0.01% gel applied daily and increased two to three times per day depending on the amount of irritation that can be tolerated. Topical 5-fluorouracil cream (Efudex) may be applied once or twice per day and may be used in combination with tretinoin. Light electrodesiccation and liquid nitrogen application may be used as an adjunct. Bowenoid papulosis is generally treated by electrodesiccation and curettage, although liquid nitrogen cryodestruction is also usually effective. Verrucous carcinoma requires excisional surgery although treatments with iontophoresis of chemotherapeutic agents has been described and is a promising alternative.

Interferon also may be used to treat condyloma acuminatum successfully. The dosage is approximately 1 million units three times weekly intralesionally for 8 to 12 weeks. The frequency of visits and expense are generally prohibitive for this form of therapy except in selected instances.[95] Parenteral interferon has also been used at doses of 2 million units intramuscularly for 10 days with good responses, although fever, myalgias, and headaches may supervene. Subcutaneous interferon may be useful as adjunctive therapy, as it may enhance the immune response to HPV. Although topical 5-fluorouracil may be utilized for treatment of HPV-induced anogenital malignancies, it is generally not recommended for use of nonmalignant HPV infections.

POXVIRUS INFECTIONS

Poxviruses are the largest of the animal viruses, and of these, two have been reported to infect HIV-seropositive patients, specifically molluscum contagiosum and vaccinia. These are complex DNA viruses, which replicate in the cytoplasm and are especially adapted to epidermal cells.

Incidence

Molluscum contagiosum develops in 10 to 20% of patients with AIDS.[96] Most patients who develop severe molluscum contagio-

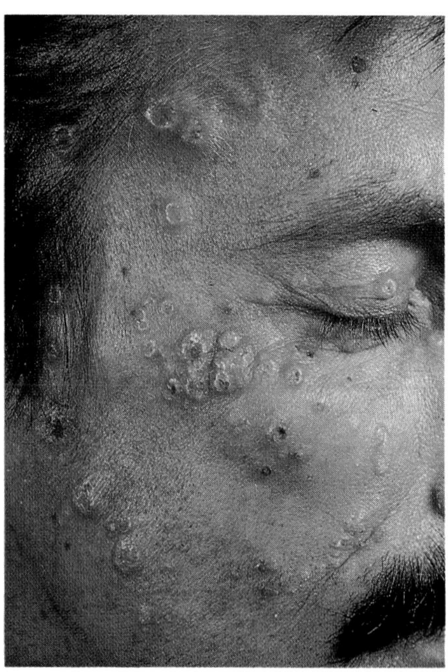

FIGURE 4–22. Molluscum contagiosum
Numerous large umbilicated waxy papules of molluscum contagiosum are seen on the face of this patient with AIDS. They have coalesced to form crusted plaques. They may be seen on other body parts as well.

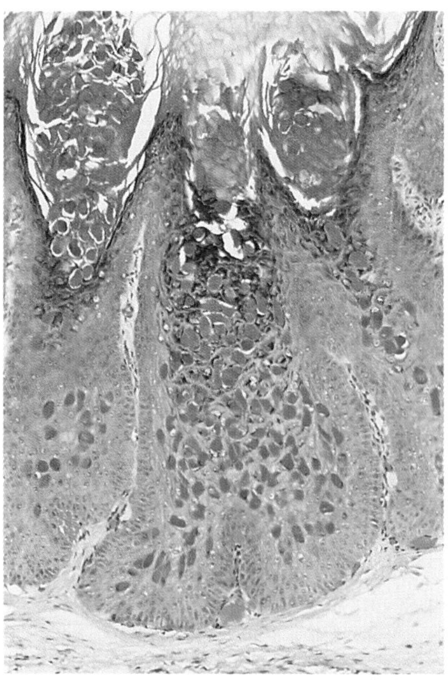

FIGURE 4–23. Histopathology of molluscum contagiosum
There is an exoendophytic papule, which results in the typical umbilicated appearance of the lesions seen clinically. Molluscum bodies can be visualized at scanning magnification. Hematoxylin and eosin stain (original magnification ×40).

sum are severely immunocompromised at the time of infection with $CD4^+$ cell counts of less than 200 to 250 cells/mm^3. Vaccinia virus infection occurs only sporadically in patients who have been occupationally exposed or are accidental hosts. One case was reported in a military recruit who received a smallpox vaccine.[97]

Pathogenesis

Molluscum contagiosum is spread by direct contact and has a tropism for epidermal epithelium. The virus replicates in the cytoplasm and eventually completely fills it with viral particles known as molluscum or Henderson-Patterson bodies. These compress the nucleus to the periphery of the cell, which subsequently ruptures so that adjacent cells become infected. The epithelium of follicles is preferentially infected, which coalesces to form the characteristic waxy umbilicated papule.

Vaccinia causes similar infection, except that rather than filling the nucleus with molluscum bodies, prominent vacuolar (ballooning) degeneration develops within cells. Prominent inflammation and, eventually, scarring occur.

Clinical Manifestations

Molluscum contagiosum infection is characterized by dome-shaped umbilicated translucent 2- to 4-mm papules that develop on any part of the body but preferentially affect the genital areas and the face, especially around the eyes. Lesions may number in excess of 100, and individual lesions may become gigantic, greater than 1 cm in diameter.[98] Large plaques composed of many smaller lesions ("agminate" form) occur rarely in immunocompetent hosts but are seen not infrequently in immunocompromised individuals (Fig. 4–22). Individual lesions have a tendency to affect follicles and are therefore umbilicated, containing a central keratinous plug. In some cases, molluscum contagiosum infection may induce a localized dermatitis known as *molluscum dermatitis.*[99] Most lesions resolve spontaneously within 6 to 12 months in immunocompetent hosts. In HIV-infected patients, however, lesions may develop rapidly, that is, over 2 to 4 weeks, and may persist for months to years.

Vaccinia lesions are characterized by tense umbilicated vesicles and pustules that are similar to those described in other patients with widespread disseminated vaccinia infection. Patients are usually clinically ill with fever and acute toxic symptoms associated with viremia.

Pathogenesis

The pathogenesis of molluscum contagiosum infection is thought to be related to an epidermal growth factor–like polypeptide that is induced by infection with the virus.[100] The virus first enters basilar keratinocytes and leads to an increase in cell turnover that extends to the suprabasilar layer and finally into the prickle cell layer. Cellular proliferation produces lobulated epidermal growth, which compresses the dermal papillae until they appear as fibrous septa between pear-shaped lobules with apices that extend to the surface of the epidermis. In spite of basal cell infection with the virus, the basal cell layer remains intact. The incubation period is variously estimated from 14 days to 6 months.

Histopathology

There is a characteristic dome-shaped papule with a central crater that arises as a consequence of coalescence of numerous follicles and adnexal structures infected by the molluscum virus (Fig. 4–23). Identification of the characteristic molluscum body, a 25-micrometer structure manifest as a pinkish, hyaline-like, oval structure within the cytoplasm of suprabasilar keratinocytes or floating free within the central crater, is pathognomonic (Fig. 4–24). They are usually present in large numbers near the surface of the center of fully developed lesions. Most molluscum lesions are associated with minimal inflammation, but when they rupture into the dermis, there may be a pronounced inflammatory infiltrate. Some of the lymphocytes in the dermis may assume atypical features that have been likened to Reed-Sternberg cells.[101]

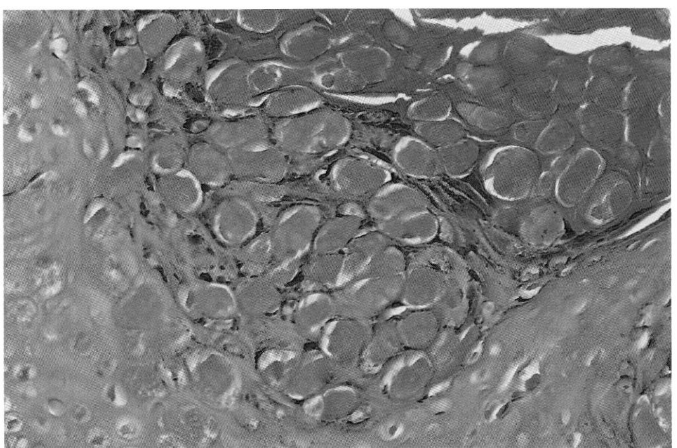

FIGURE 4–24. Molluscum contagiosum

Higher magnification of molluscum contagiosum reveals the purplish homogenous bodies that are characteristic of the viral infection. Hematoxlyin and eosin stain (×400).

Vaccinia infection manifests with a dense inflammatory cell infiltrate in the dermis that is associated with prominent intraepidermal ballooning degeneration, reticular alteration, and edema of the papillary dermis.

Laboratory Findings

Specific antibodies may be found in up to 80% of patients with molluscum contagiosum. As mentioned previously, most patients with extensive molluscum contagiosum associated with HIV infection have $CD4^+$ counts below 250 cells/mm^3.

Differential Diagnosis

In patients with HIV infection, waxy umbilicated lesions of cryptococcosis, cutaneous pneumocystosis, and other infectious disorders may appear similar to those of molluscum contagiosum; a biopsy is often necessary to exclude more serious infections. Solitary molluscum lesions may resemble pyogenic granuloma, keratoacanthoma, or basal cell carcinoma and may occasionally be difficult to define. Vaccinia infection may appear similar, if not identical, to other poxvirus infections such as milker's nodule and orf. Sweet's disease, bullous pyoderma gangrenosum, and polymorphous light eruption may have similar clinical features.

Diagnosis

Application of a small amount of liquid nitrogen or ethyl chloride will highlight the central umbilication of individual lesions, a finding that strongly suggests the diagnosis. In most cases, the diagnosis is readily established on the basis of clinical appearance or by histologic evaluation of a skin biopsy specimen or a smear of contents of a papule, or both. Vaccinia infection is diagnosed on the basis of the clinical appearance of the eruption in the context of a history of exposure to the causative agent. Virtually all cases develop in patients who have had occupational exposure or who have been vaccinated for smallpox recently.

Treatment

Treatment of molluscum contagiosum is generally carried out by using destructive measures. Cryotherapy is the usual method of treatment and may be successful, especially if done every 1 to 2 weeks until lesions have resolved. Lesions are sprayed with liquid nitrogen for 5 to 10 seconds to yield a 15- to 20-second thaw time. Although the method is generally safe, dyspigmentation may develop in dark-skinned individuals, so patients should be informed about this complication before treatment. Unfortunately, discontinuation of therapy is often associated with recurrence. Electrosurgery, application of topical keratolytic preparations, application of cantharidin, and removal by currette are other effective therapies. Tretinoin cream 0.025% may be applied to decrease the tendency to recurrence. Experimentation with wax stripping and application of salicylic acid pastes have also been attempted with moderate success.

Vaccinia infection may respond to treatment with semithiocarbazone, although treatment is generally ineffective. Unfortunately, the condition is associated with a high mortality rate.

OTHER VIRAL INFECTIONS

Several other viral infections have been reported to develop with increased frequency in patients with HIV infection. Parvovirus B19, which is the cause of erythema infectiosum (fifth disease), has been reported to cause an exanthem in patients with HIV infection and to lead to persistent and occasionally fatal aplastic anemia.[102] The major target for the human parvovirus is the bone marrow erythroid progenitor cell. The exanthem and polyarthralgia that result in fifth disease are a result of antigen-antibody immune complexes and develop as bone marrow recovery is under way. In patients with immune deficits, however, persistent infection causing severe chronic anemia has been reported. An adenovirus has been noted to have caused an unusual palisaded granulomatous inflammatory dermatitis in one patient with AIDS.[103] Although in most patients the disorder resolves without incident, fatal pneumonia has been noted. Coxsackie and enteroviruses may also lead to morbilliform or vesicular eruptions that may be florid.

Measles is a highly contagious childhood infection caused by the measles virus, a paramyxovirus, and is manifest clinically by fever, coryza, cough, conjunctivitis, enanthema, Koplik's spots, and an exanthem. Measles has been reported sporadically in patients with HIV infection with variable courses. Although most patients recover uneventfully, a 4-year-old child with AIDS developed a measles eruption associated with giant cell pneumonitis that proved fatal. The patient had never received measles immunization.[104] Others have noted atypical-appearing exanthems associated with pneumonitis and encephalitis as well as more characteristic-appearing eruptions. Treatment consists of intravenous ribavirin and gamma globulin.[105]

BACTERIAL INFECTIONS

DEFINITION

Bacterial folliculitis, impetigo, bacillary epithelioid angiomatosis, botryomycosis, *Pseudomonas* infections, streptococcal axillary lymphadenitis, mycobacterial infections, syphilis, and other venereal diseases are some of the bacterial infections that may develop in patients with HIV infection. These disorders may be localized or may be widespread, affecting many organs. There may be a number of different clinical morphologic findings, many of which may be quite nondescript. For this reason, it is important that skin biopsies and cultures be performed in an immunocompromised patient in whom a skin lesion develops that could represent a manifestation of a serious bacterial infectious disease.

EPIDEMIOLOGY

Most banal bacterial infections such as folliculitis and impetigo are caused by *Staphylococcus* and *Streptococcus,* organisms commonly encountered in immunocompetent hosts. *Staphylococcus aureus* is the most common cutaneous and systemic bacterial pathogen in HIV-infected adults. The initial site of colonization with *S. aureus* is the nares. A nasal carriage rate of approximately 50% has been observed in HIV-infected hosts, which is twice that of HIV-seronegative homosexual and heterosexual men.[106] Multiple breaks in the skin from needle sticks, dermatoses, and immunodeficiency are risk factors for the development of *S. aureus* infection. Up to 83% of patients with AIDS may suffer from some form of *S. aureus* infection at some point during the course of HIV disease.[107] Infection with *Pseudomonas* species is also seen with some frequency in patients who are HIV infected, and up to 8% of all cases of bacteremia in patients with AIDS are due to these organisms.[108] Aggressive *Haemophilus influenzae* infection of the head and neck has also been observed.[109] Approximately 50 cases of bacillary angiomatosis, a condition caused by rickettsia-like organisms of the genus *Bartonella* (formerly *Rochalimaea*), have been reported.

Virtually any of the mycobacteria may induce skin lesions in up to 10% of patients with systemic mycobacterial infections. Extrapulmonary disease is commonly found in patients with AIDS. *Mycobacterium avium-intracellulare* has been isolated from the skin in patients with blood cultures that are positive for the same organism, and mycobacterium haemophilum has also been documented to cause skin lesions.[110–112] This is of importance as the latter organism is more difficult to culture than other *Mycobacteria,* requiring supplementation of media with blood use and other growth factors. Infection with *Mycobacterium bovis* following bacille Calmette-Guérin vaccination in a patient with HIV infection has also been reported.[113] Leprosy has been observed only rarely in patients with HIV infection, the reason for which remains unknown.

Syphilis is common in patients with HIV infection, and of all reported cases of syphilis, 25% develop in HIV-infected hosts.[114] Venereal diseases are also encountered commonly in HIV-infected individuals. Lymphogranuloma venereum, chancroid, granuloma inguinale, and *Neisseria gonorrhoeae* infection all may develop and may be more severe as a consequence of immunocompromise.

Pathogenesis

Although it has been recognized for many years that CD4$^+$ cell counts are lowered in patients with HIV infection, additional immunologic abnormalities have been recognized and have been shown to be important. Dysfunctions in the B-cell arm of the immune response as well as in neutrophils and macrophages have been described.[115–117] HIV-infected patients may be neutropenic because of myelosuppression from medications and bone marrow infections such as those caused by *M. avium-intracellulare.* Furthermore, patients in later stages of HIV infection suffer from defective neutrophil chemotaxis as well as a decrease in the late stage oxidative burst, with consequent diminished killing of *S. aureus.*[118] Indwelling venous catheters that are commonly placed in patients with HIV infection serve as portals of entry for infection and are a risk for systemic infection with bacteria and other pathogens.[119] Elevated serum IgE levels are also associated with *S. aureus* infections and may play a role in the alteration of the immune system, leading to defective eradication of organisms.[120]

Although immunocompromise predisposes patients to the development of colonization and infection by bacterial microorganisms, it also predisposes to recrudescence or reactivation of latent infections. *Mycobacterium tuberculosis* frequently produces infection in HIV-positive patients, probably as a result of reinfection or reactivation of preexisting infectious foci. An increasing number of infections with strains resistant to antituberculous medications have been reported, often with devastating consequences. Syphilis, too, has been shown to be associated with reactivation of presumed previously killed organisms in patients having prior disease treated with recommended antibiotic regimens.

Bacillary angiomatosis is a bacterial infection caused by organisms of the genus *Bartonella,* specifically *Bartonella quintana* and *Bartonella henselae.* An endocarditis has been associated in one case with *Bartonella elizabethae.*[121] The pathogenesis is not completely known but it has been postulated that either a vasoproliferative factor is produced by the bacterium itself or is induced to be formed by the host as a consequence of bacterial infection.

Clinical Manifestations

In HIV-seropositive patients, mucocutaneous manifestations of bacterial infections may manifest multiple different morphologic features. Pustules, ulcers, cellulitis, nodules, papules, and panniculitis may all be encountered. Clinical appearances may be quite nondescript and may mimic other disorders.

FOLLICULITIS, ABSCESSES, FURUNCLES, IMPETIGO, AND RELATED INFECTIONS

Folliculitis generally appears as widely distributed acneiform papules and pustules. Lesions may be pruritic and excoriated. Although in most cases infections are confined to the skin, occasionally sepsis may develop. In some cases, the bacterial density may increase significantly as a consequence of immunodepression leading to botryomycosis or ecthyma.[122] These disorders appear as nondescript verrucous papules or as necrotizing ulcerations, respectively. Soft tissue and deeply seated bacterial infections such as cellulitis, pyomyositis, deep soft tissue abscesses, and necrotizing fasciitis may also develop in HIV-infected hosts.[123] These generally manifest as diffuse, red, warm, tender areas in the skin. There is often extreme toxemia associated with deeper infections such as these, so that early recognition is essential. Streptococcal axillary lymphadenitis is a diffuse, painful swelling of lymph nodes in the axillae that is usually bilateral.[124] When incised, copious pustular drainage is noted. Impetigo appears as localized or widespread edematous crusted areas of the skin associated with yellowish surface crusts (Figs. 4–25 and 4–26). Although impetigo is seen most commonly on the face and shoulders, in patients with HIV infection it is seen more often in the axillary, inguinal, and other intertriginous locations. The infection usually begins with painful red macules that may develop superficial vesicles that rupture, oozing serous and purulent fluid that contains potentially infective HIV. A characteristic honey-colored surface crust usually forms, and satellite lesions may develop. In some cases, intact bullae and pustules may be observed.

S. aureus may be manifest as a wide range of cutaneous infections in HIV-infected individuals in addition to those mentioned earlier (Fig. 4–27). Secondary infection of scabies, spongiotic dermatitis, herpetic ulcers, Kaposi's sarcoma, and molluscum contagiosum have all been described. Botryomycosis is most commonly caused by *S. aureus* and represents a manifestation of extension of staphylococcal folliculitis with the formation of bacterial colonies in the dermis.[125,126] Clinically, this often appears as a nondescript papule or plaque in the skin that may be surrounded by pustules on the trunk, neck, or extremities. An atypical plaque-like staphylococcal folliculitis has been described in patients with HIV infection.[127] It manifests as violaceous plaques up to 10 cm in diameter with superficial pustules and crusts occurring in the groin, axilla, or scalp. Nonmenstrual toxic shock syndrome, most commonly associated with the use of nasal packing, infected wounds, or surgical sites, has also been reported in patients with advanced HIV infection.[128,129] Patients present with fever, shock, diffuse cutaneous erythema, and conjunctival injection with subsequent desquamation. Recurrent episodes of pyoderma-associated fever, hypotension, and erythroderma may also supervene. This is caused by a toxin-producing variant of *S. aureus.* A similar eruption has been reported that is caused by *Streptococcus pyogenes* and is known as the toxic strep syndrome.

Folliculitis, otitis externa, and ecthyma gangrenosum, both primary and secondary to septicemia, may be caused by *Pseudomonas aeruginosa* as well as *Pseudomonas cepacia* that may be acquired from hot tub use.[130,131] The clinical manifestations of these disorders when caused by *Pseudomonas* species appear similar to those caused by other pyogenic bacteria, namely, firm erythematous nodules as papulopustules with necrosis, so that cultures are essential in making this distinction.[132]

A condition with features similar to Job's syndrome has been described in patients with HIV disease that manifests as recurrent staphylococcal abscesses associated with markedly increased serum IgE levels and diminished polymorphonuclear leukocyte chemotaxis.[133] Chronic diffuse dermatitis associated with elevated serum IgE levels and eosinophilia

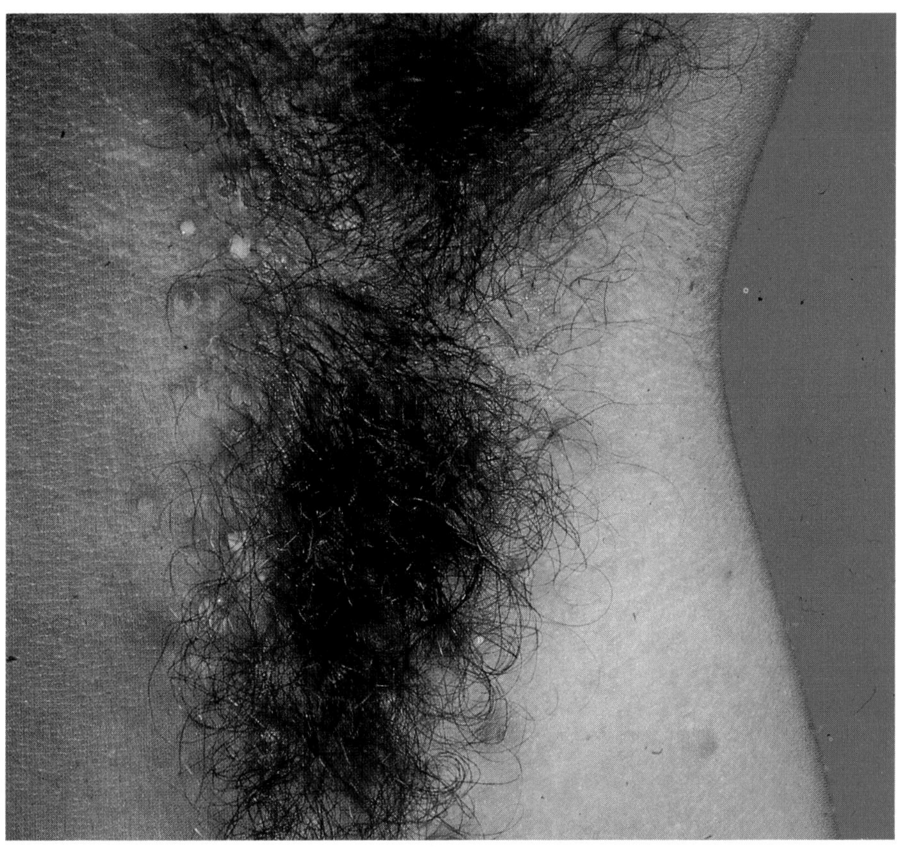

FIGURE 4–25. Impetigo
This infection may be widespread and fulminant in patients with HIV infection or AIDS.

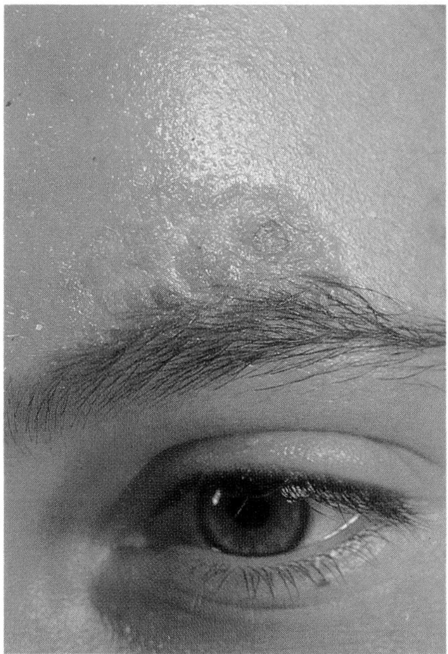

FIGURE 4–26. Impetigo
The characteristic erosion covered by a honey-colored crust is pictured here.

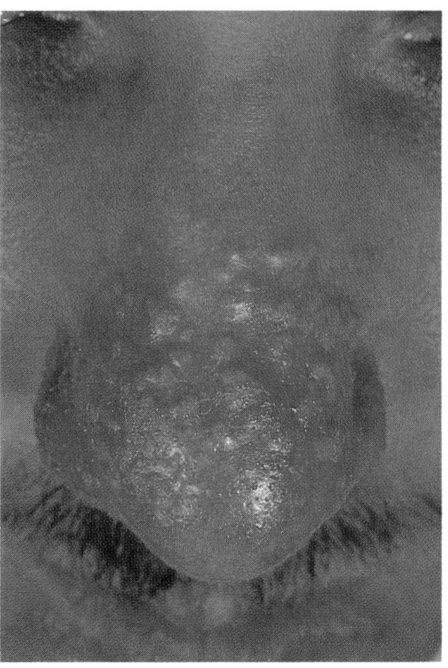

FIGURE 4–27. Pyoderma
A severe pyoderma as pictured here may be seen in patients with HIV infection or AIDS. Many different bacterial organisms can cause this clinical syndrome.

associated with recurrent *S. aureus* and *Candida albicans* infection have also been observed.[134]

H. influenzae cellulitis, which manifests as diffuse erythema and edema often on the head and neck area, may develop in patients with HIV infection.[109] This infection may be aggressive with a greater tendency to become disseminated or to affect deeper soft tissues and vital structures. Infections with *Streptomyces, Nocardia,* and *Actinomyces* appear as thickened verrucous plaques or as chronic draining sinuses.[135] One HIV-infected patient developed infection due to *Actinomyces naeslundii,* which was manifest as diffuse facial swelling following extraction of teeth.[136] Deep-seated abscesses caused by *Rhodococcus equi* have been observed on multiple occasions.[137] *Corynebacterium diphtheriae* may cause bullous lesions that ulcerate and became covered with a grayish pseudomembrane.[138] One case was associated with systemic toxemia and cardiac dysfunction. Infections caused by "diphtheroids" may lead to pustular folliculitis-like lesions, whereas salmonellosis may be associated with an eruption of faint pink macules on the skin.[139] Multiple infectious agents may be found within a given skin lesion in patients with HIV infection and AIDS. Mixed infections with pyogenic bacteria and acid-fast bacilli as well as viruses and fungi have been reported.

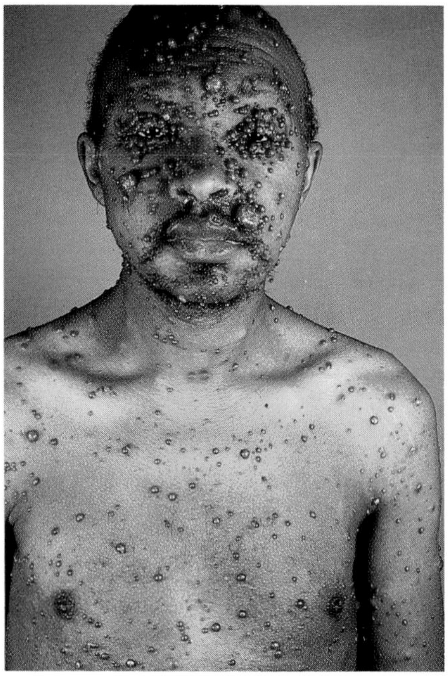

FIGURE 4–28. Bacillary angiomatosis
This rare and unusual vascular proliferation is sometimes seen in patients with AIDS or HIV infection. It is distinct from Kaposi's sarcoma.

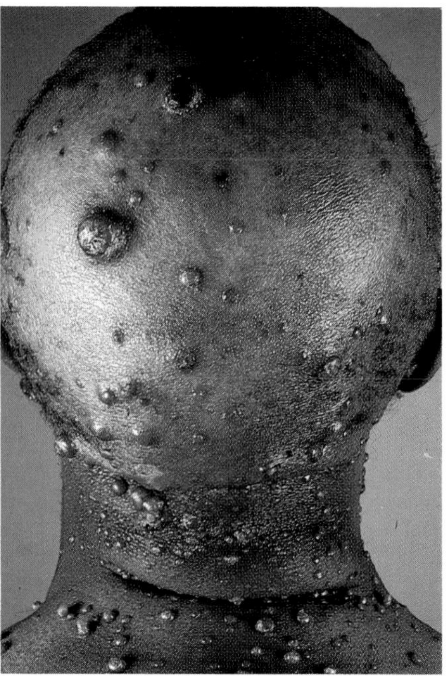

FIGURE 4–29. Bacillary angiomatosis
In contradistinction to the lesions of Kaposi's sarcoma, these lesions are friable and pedunculated. This condition is caused by bacteria of the genus *Bartonella*.

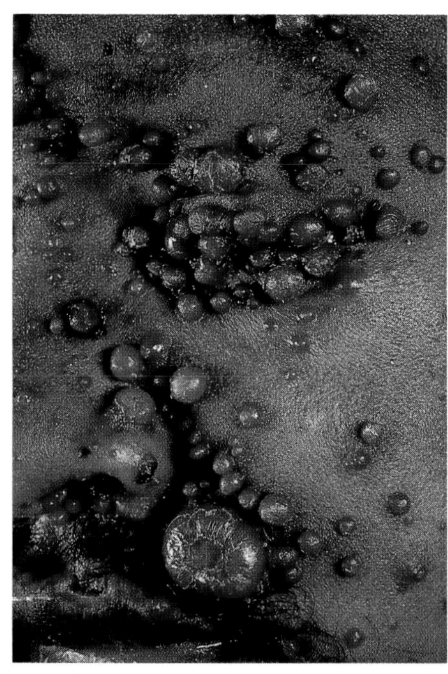

FIGURE 4–30. Bacillary angiomatosis
Close-up view demonstrating the dome-shaped sessile and pedunculated papules and nodules of bacillary angiomatosis.

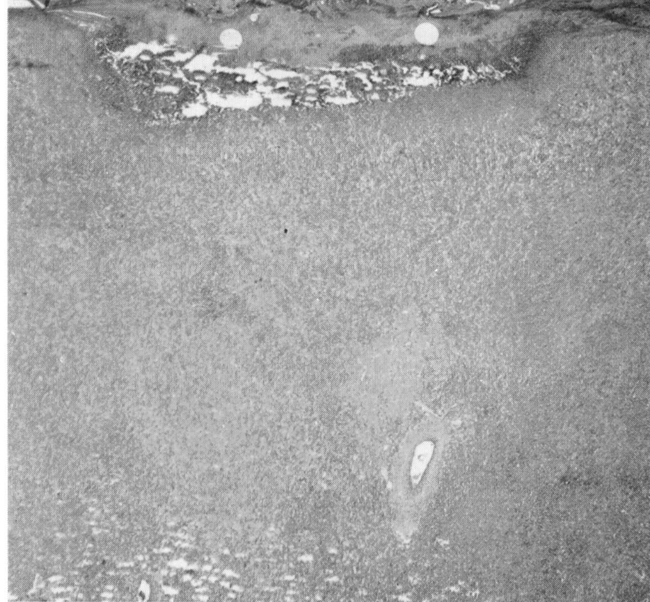

FIGURE 4–31. Bacillary angiomatosis
Histologic photomicrograph of bacillary angiomatosis. There is a vascular proliferation characterized by pale-staining cells surrounding vascular spaces. Note the presence of numerous neutrophils throughout the lesion.

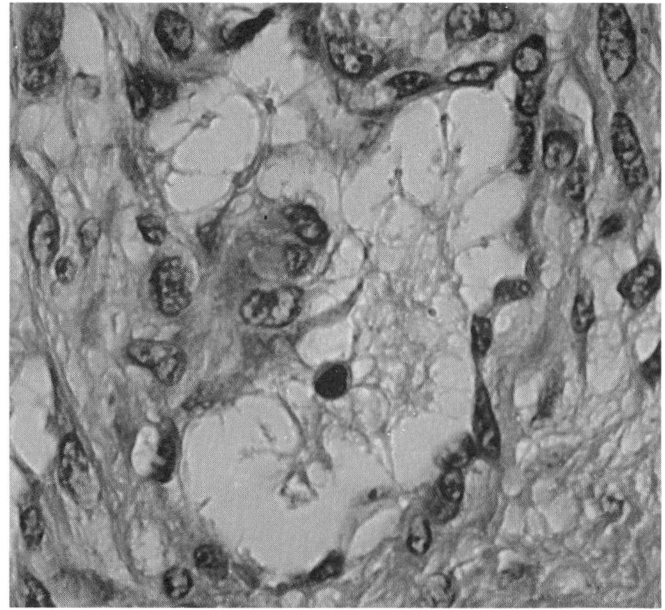

FIGURE 4–32. Bacillary angiomatosis
High magnification reveals the cells to have cuboidal shapes with abundant pale-staining cytoplasm. Plump endothelial cells protrude into the lumen of the vessel. This appearance is distinct from that of Kaposi's sarcoma.

BACILLARY ANGIOMATOSIS

There are a number of different clinical manifestations of cutaneous disease in bacillary angiomatosis (Figs. 4–28 through 4–33). Cutaneous vesicular lesions are the most common, and of these, small, pinpoint reddish to purple papules are the earliest lesions. These may assume an appearance similar to that of pyogenic granulomata and are seen in two thirds of patients with cutaneous disease.[140–142] They range in number from one to several thousand and in size from 1 mm to several centimeters. Lesions may ulcerate, be covered by a crust, or both. The second most common skin lesion is the subcutaneous nodule that occurs in approximately 50% of patients with skin lesions. It may be located deeply in the subcutis and extend to affect soft tissue and bone.[143] Two cases of deep-seated skeletal muscle pyomyositis have been reported.[144] When bone is involved, lesions are generally osteolytic in nature. Nondescript crusted ulcerations, plaques, and cellulitis may also be seen in 5 to 10% of patients.[145] Viscera may be affected either as disseminated vascular lesions or as bacillary peliosis hepatis. Although virtually every organ system may be affected, the liver and spleen are the most common sites of involvement. Liver disease may develop in patients without skin lesions and is usually manifest by elevated levels of circulating liver enzymes. Patients with bacillary angiomatosis may develop fever, weight loss, and night sweats.[146] These symptoms usually resolve with institution of antibiotic therapy.

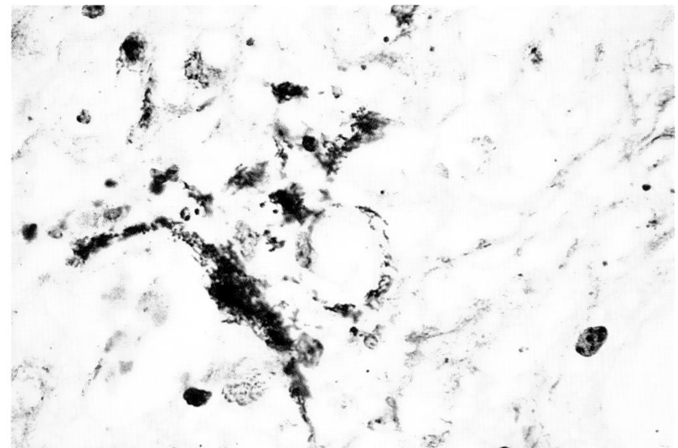

FIGURE 4–33. Bacillary angiomatosis, Warthin-Starry stain
There are numerous irregular masses of darkly staining bacteria, which represent *Bartonella* species. Warthin-Starry stain (original magnification ×400).

MYCOBACTERIAL INFECTIONS

Mycobacterial skin lesions may assume a number of different appearances (Figs. 4–34 and 4–35). Small papules and pustules that resemble folliculitis, atopic dermatitis-like eruptions, localized cutaneous abscesses, suppurative lymphadenitis, nonspecific ulcerations, palmar and plantar hyperkeratoses, and sporotrichoid nodules all have been reported.[147–149] Tuberculous lymphadenitis in particular is a characteristic finding of disseminated tuberculosis in intravenous drug users with AIDS and manifests as suppurative draining lymph nodes in the neck, axillae, or groin.[150] *Mycobacterium marinum* may cause classic swimming pool granulomata in patients with HIV disease and may manifest as verrucous nodules, often with a sporotrichoid distribution. Most reported cases behave in a relatively indolent fashion and demonstrate good response to appropriate antibiotic therapy. *M. haemophilum* is a ubiquitous bacterium that may cause cutaneous infections in AIDS patients. Lesions may take the form of painful erythematous papules and nodules on the distal extremities and ears.[148]

SYPHILIS

Syphilis may occur in a number of forms in patients with HIV infection, ranging from classic papulosquamous forms with involvement of the palms and soles and mucous membranes to unusual forms that may defy diagnosis (Figs. 4–36 through 4–39). Unusual manifestations of syphilis in these patients include rapid progression from the primary chancre to gummatous tertiary lues in a matter of months, lues maligna (syphilis with vasculitis), sclerodermiform lesions, rupial verrucous plaques, extensive oral ulcerations, keratoderma, deep cutaneous nodules, rubeoliform eruptions, and widespread gummata.[151–153] Central nervous system disease has been noted more frequently and with greater severity in patients with HIV infection, and painful meningovascular syphilis has developed following the presumed adequate treatment of secondary syphilis.[154]

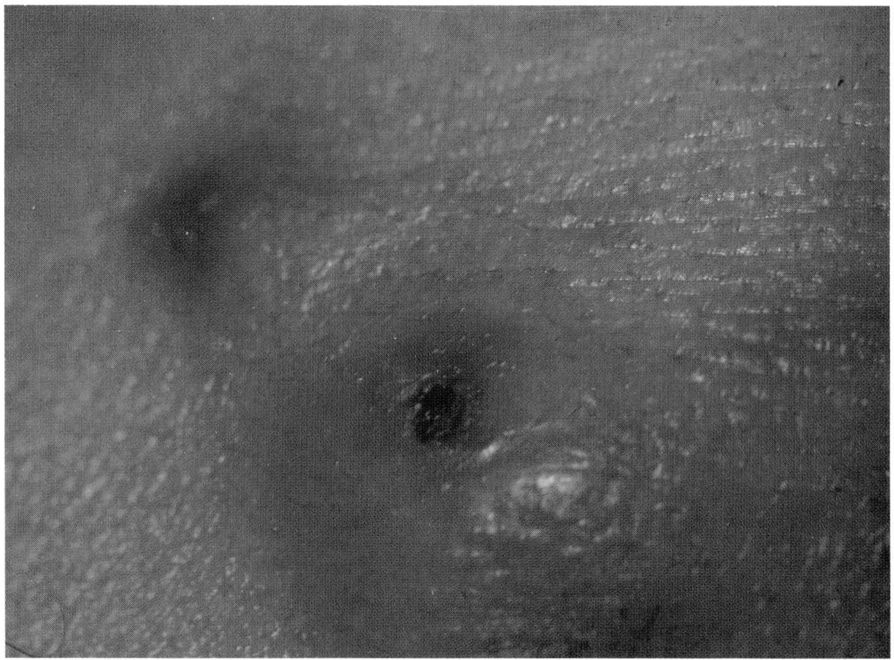

FIGURE 4–34. Cutaneous acid-fast bacterial infection

Individual acneiform crusted papules present on the trunk and extremities clinically had a very nondescript appearance but histologically revealed myriad acid-fast bacilli. In this case, the organism was *Mycobacterium tuberculosis*.

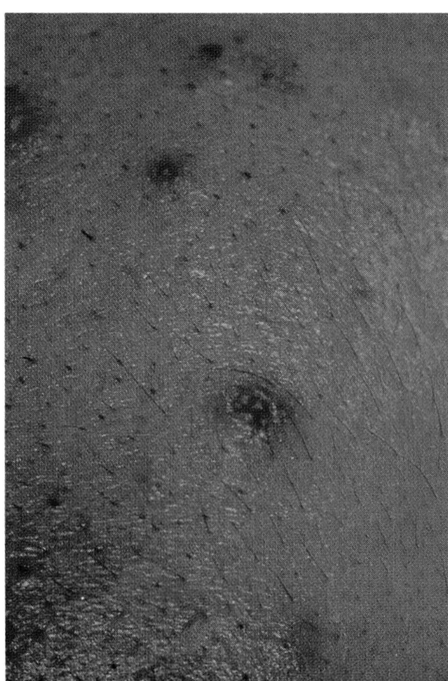

FIGURE 4–35. Cutaneous acid-fast bacterial infection

Another example of the relatively nondescript nature of these lesions. This is distinct from the usual clinical appearance of cutaneous tuberculosis.

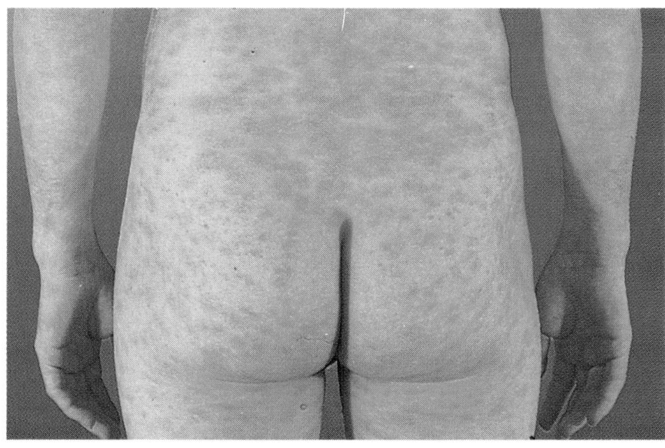

FIGURE 4–36. Secondary syphilis

Widespread eruption of reddish-brown papules with scales is characteristic of this condition. In patients with HIV infection, it may be more florid and may be associated concomitantly with a lesion of tertiary syphilis.

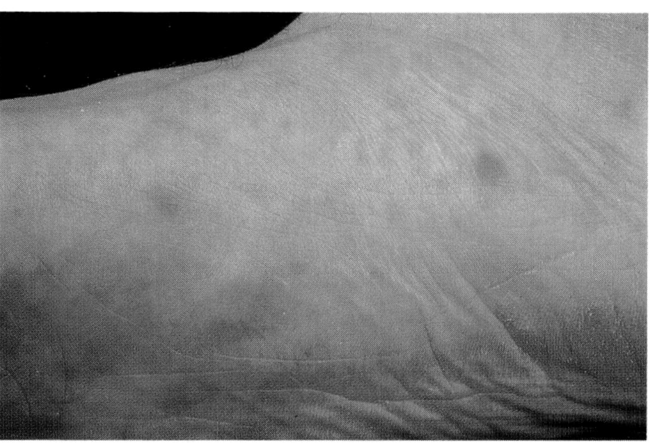

FIGURE 4–37. Secondary syphilis

Characteristic reddish-brown papules on the soles. Such lesions on occasion have been mistaken for Kaposi's sarcoma.

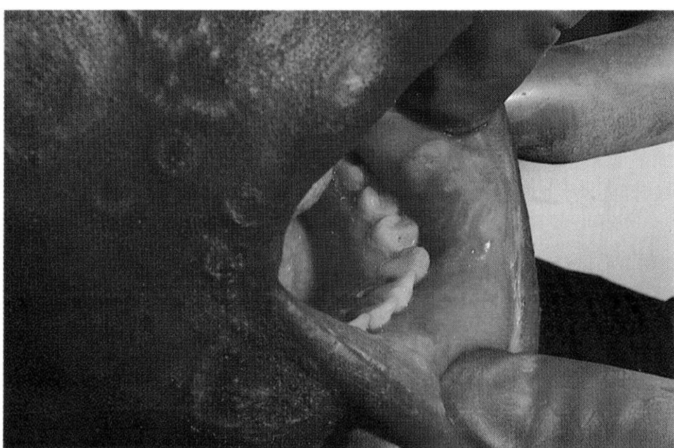

FIGURE 4–38. Mucous patches of secondary syphilis

Notice the annular configuration of the lesions on the skin and the whitish, erosive plaques present on the labial mucosa. Such lesions are teeming with spirochetes.

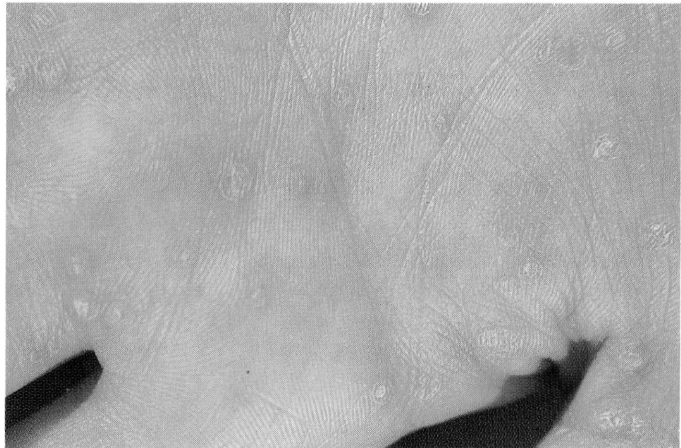

FIGURE 4–39. Secondary syphilis

Close-up view of papules of secondary syphilis to demonstrate the scaling and slight crusting present on the surface.

OTHER VENEREAL DISEASES

Granuloma inguinale caused by *Calymmatobacterium granulomatis* may develop in HIV-infected individuals. Generally, this disorder manifests as vegetating lesions on the penis associated with pseudo-bubos in the inguinal crease. Lymphogranuloma venereum, although relatively uncommon in HIV-infected individuals, has also been reported more recently. Patients develop generalized lymphadenopathy accompanied by vulvar or penile edema with ulcerations and erosions. In addition, nonspecific genital ulcerations, from which a number of bacteria may be isolated, may be observed, the precise etiology of which may remain unclear. Chancroid is a common sexually transmitted disease in some parts of the world, and it has been increasing in incidence in the United States. The causative organism is a gram-negative coccobacillus, *Haemophilus ducreyi*. Cases have been reported in patients with HIV infection, especially in Africa. One case manifested as a nonhealing penile lesion of 4 months' duration with ulcerations on the knee, leg, and foot.[155] Gonocococcemia with oligoarticular gonococcal arthritis of the hips and sternoclavicular joints also may develop in these patients.[156]

Histopathology

Histopathologic findings of folliculitis generally include collections of neutrophils within infundibula of hair follicles and a mixed perifollicular inflammatory cell infiltrate. When rupture of follicles occurs, there is often a perifollicular granulomatous infiltrate with fibrosis. Botryomycosis is characterized by a diffuse inflammatory cell infiltrate in the dermis associated with colonies of gram-positive bacteria that form grains in the skin. These generally appear bluish-purple in hematoxylin and eosin–stained sections. Ecthyma is manifested histologically as a deep ulcer that often extends to the subcutaneous fat, with extensive degeneration of dermal collagen. There is a mixed inflammatory cell infiltrate of neutrophils, eosinophils, and histiocytes.

Histopathologic findings in bacillary angiomatosis are characterized by a lobular proliferation of capillaries associated with enlarged epithelioid-appearing endothelial cells (see Figs. 4–31 and 4–32). The background stroma is usually edematous in superficial lesions and more compact in deeper ones. Neutrophils and leukocytoclasis are often seen in the interstitium between vessels. The presence of neutrophils within lesions is a valuable finding that permits distinction from ulcerated pyogenic granulomas that may have similar histologic features although neutrophils are present primarily under areas of ulceration. Granular amphophilic aggregates are characteristically seen adjacent to vessels, often in association with neutrophils, which represent masses of *Bartonella* organisms. These appear black after staining with the Warthin-Starry stain (see Fig. 4–33). Electron microscopy is confirmatory. Although the diagnosis can usually be made on the basis of microscopic examination of routine hematoxylin and eosin–stained tissue sections, atypia of endothelial cells may be marked on occasion, causing histologic confusion with angiosarcoma.

The histopathology of cutaneous syphilis is usually similar to that in immunocompetent hosts, demonstrating the characteristic superficial and deep psoriasiform lichenoid pattern of inflammation associated with plasma cells and histiocytes. However, unusual histologic findings have been seen, including vasculitis as well as very sparse inflammatory infiltrates with minimal numbers of plasma cells and abundant spirochetes (Figs. 4–40 through 4–42).

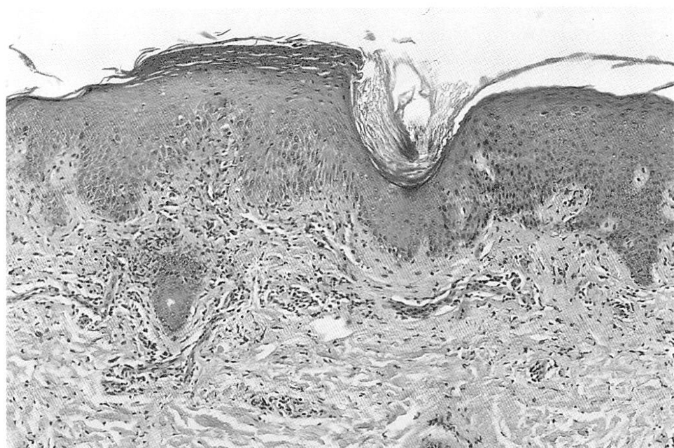

FIGURE 4–40. Syphilis

Syphilis may have many different patterns microscopically. In this case, there are slight psoriasiform hyperplasia with parakeratosis and a sparse infiltrate of inflammatory cells in the dermis. Hematoxylin and eosin stain (original magnification ×40).

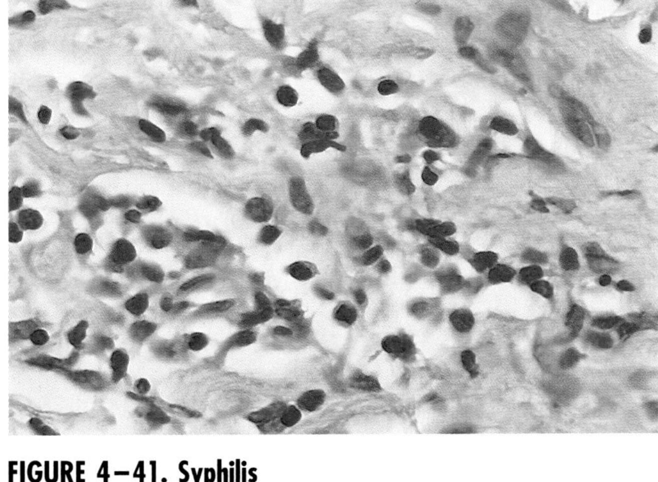

FIGURE 4–41. Syphilis

Higher magnification of syphilis reveals an infiltrate of lymphocytes and scattered plasma cells around blood vessels, which were a clue to the diagnosis. Hematoxylin and eosin stain (original magnification ×400).

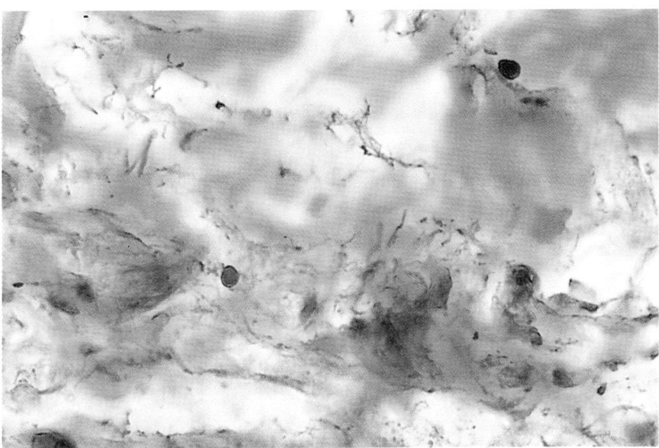

FIGURE 4–42. Syphilis

Starry stain revealed innumerable spirochetes. This patient had very low titers of circulating antibody to *Treponema pallidum.* Warthin-Starry stain (original magnification ×400).

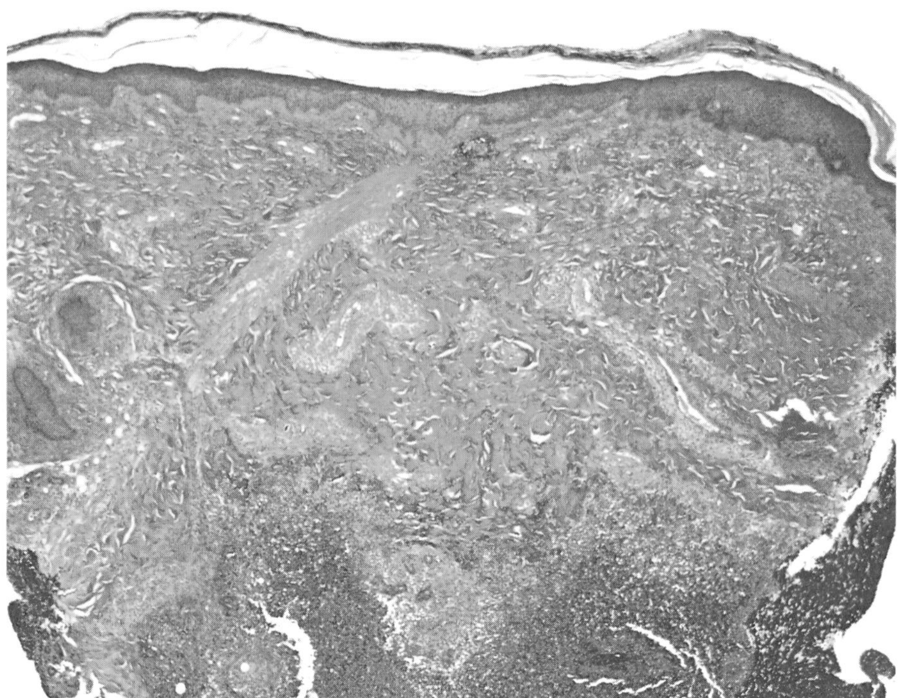

FIGURE 4–43. Abscess

There is a diffuse dermatitis present in the depths of the specimen consisting of numerous neutrophils and some histiocytes. These are the features of an abscess.

Cutaneous mycobacterial infections may assume classic patterns of suppurative granulomatous infiltrates in the dermis associated with pseudocarcinomatous hyperplasia, although other unusual patterns may be observed, including dense areas of suppuration with minimal granulomatous infiltrate (Figs. 4–43 and 4–44).

Laboratory Findings

In pyogenic bacterial infections, laboratory findings may be similar to what would be expected in an immunocompetent host with a similar bacterial infection. In the setting of immunocompromise, however, patients may suffer from serious systemic bacterial infections yet not mount significant elevations in white blood cell counts or demonstrate characteristic "left shifts." Patients with syphilis may be truly seronegative on serologic tests for syphilis despite the presence of demonstrable spirochetes in biopsy speci-

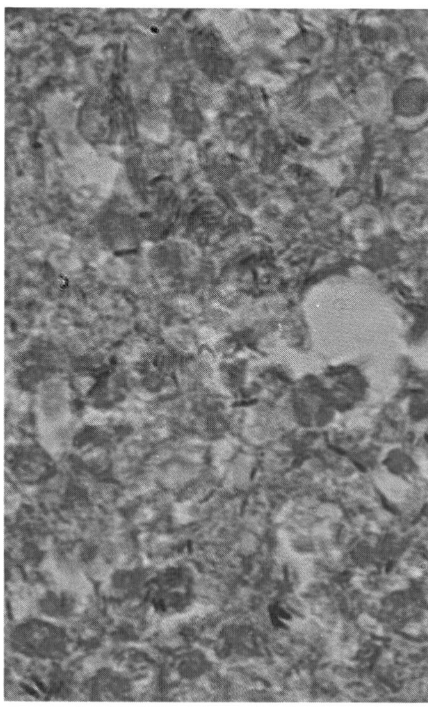

FIGURE 4–44. *Mycobacterium tuberculosis* infection

Stains for mycobacteria revealed innumerable acid-fast bacilli. These proved to be *M. tuberculosis,* but *Mycobacterium avium-intracellulare* may produce identical clinical and histologic features.

mens. Seronegativity may be due to a prozone phenomenon, a consequence of improperly diluted very high antibody titers, or a consequence of true absence of antibody. Patients with bacillary angiomatosis usually have $CD4^+$ cell counts of less than 250 cells/mm^3, although they do not generally demonstrate characteristic laboratory findings. The white blood cell count may be elevated in immunocompetent patients but is most often slightly depressed in HIV-infected individuals. Results of serologic tests for anti-*Bartonella* antibody are usually positive by the time the clinical diagnosis has been made. *Bartonella henselae* can be isolated from blood if lysis centrifugation blood cultures are used and plated on freshly prepared chocolate agar or other supplemented media at 35°C in 5% carbon dioxide–humidified atmosphere or at 30°C in air for 14 days. *Bartonella quintana* can be isolated from cutaneous lesions by cocultivation with an endothelial cell monolayer.[157,158]

In attempting to isolate *M. haemophilum,* researchers find that results of routine mycobacterial cultures are often negative because the organism has unique growth requirements. It grows only when the culture is kept at low temperatures and supplemental iron is added in the form of hemolyzed red blood cells.

Differential Diagnosis

The differential diagnosis of bacterial folliculitis includes eosinophilic pustular folliculitis, a condition not associated with bacterial infection, as well as other forms of folliculitis such as those induced by atypical mycobacteria or fungi. Ecthyma may appear similar to other forms of ulcerations, including those induced by septic processes and factitial ones. Botryomycosis may be simulated by conditions that develop verrucous papules in the skin, including many other infectious disorders. The differential diagnosis of deep soft tissue infections includes diffuse superficial cutaneous infections such as cellulitis and erysipelas. Streptococcal axillary lymphadenitis must be distinguished from hidradenitis suppurativa and other causes of suppurative lymphadenitis, such as cat-scratch disease and tuberculous lymphadenitis. Bullous impetigo may appear similar to superficial pemphigus or pustular psoriasis.

Skin lesions caused by *M. haemophilum* may closely mimic those of Kaposi's sarcoma, which may lead to inappropriate treatment of this infection as Kaposi's sarcoma. Lack of response to treatment of presumed Kaposi's sarcoma is an indication for the performance of a skin biopsy. Cutaneous lesions induced by other atypical mycobacteria may be quite nondescript and may simulate folliculitis, chronic ulceration, or inflammatory panniculitis.

Bacillary angiomatosis must be differentiated from other vascular lesions that develop in patients with HIV infection, especially Kaposi's sarcoma. Generally, the lack of macular and plaque lesions or the presence of lesions oriented along skin lines is helpful in making this distinction. Histopathologic findings are also distinct.

Syphilis may have protean manifestations in patients with HIV infection just as it may in immunocompetent hosts. The list of diseases that may be simulated includes many other bacterial and fungal infections as well as connective tissue disorders, Kaposi's sarcoma, and lymphoma.

Diagnosis

Diagnosis of these infections is generally made on the basis of clinical findings and the results of smears, biopsies, and cultures. Whenever the possibility exists that a mucocutaneous lesion in an HIV-infected individual could be secondary to dissemination of a serious bacterial infection such as that due to a mycobacterium, skin biopsies should be performed for histologic evaluation and microbiologic cultures. A battery of special stains is usually required, and, in some cases, immunoperoxidase stains for acid-fast bacilli may increase speed and sensitivity of diagnosis. Smears of pustules that show neutrophils may help distinguish bacterial folliculitis from eosinophilic pustular folliculitis. Just as with skin biopsies, these smears should be stained with Gram's stain as well as with periodic acid–Schiff and acid-fast stains to ensure that more serious infections are not missed. Cultures, complement fixation studies, and the polymerase chain reaction are techniques that also may be used to assist in the rapid diagnosis of these infections. In cases of syphilis, although serologic testing is generally reliable, it must be remembered that in HIV-infected patients with active syphilis, Venereal Disease Research Laboratories (VDRL) and fluorescent treponemal antibody absorption test results may be negative. In such cases, biopsy with special stains for spirochetes may be required. Granuloma inguinale is characteristically diagnosed by crush preparations of a friable skin lesion followed by histologic examination. Chancroid is diagnosed by microscopic examination of gram-stained smears of lesions that demonstrate clusters of thin gram-negative rods, the characteristic "schools of fish."

Treatment

Treatment of each of the aforementioned disorders is based on accurate diagnosis and identification of causative microorganisms and their sensitivities to antibiotics. Pyogenic bacterial infections generally respond to treatment with dicloxacillin, cephalexin, or ciprofloxacin. Chlorhexidine gluconate washes of the skin and application of topical antibiotics such as polymyxin B sulfate, bacitracin, or mupirocin ointment preparations into the nostrils may help to eradicate bacterial colonization. Unfortunately, in immunocompromised hosts, recurrence is the rule. Bacillary angiomatosis responds well to treatment with erythromycin ethyl succinate at doses of 500 mg orally four times a day for 4 weeks to 6 months depending on the tendency toward relapse. Doxycycline hydrochloride 100 mg orally twice a day is also effective. Other antibiotics that have been shown to have some efficacy include rifampin, ciprofloxacin, trimethoprim-sulfamethoxazole, and gentamicin. Azithromycin, rozithromycin, and fluoroquinolones such as norfloxacin have also been used with good response. Recent data indicate that trimethoprim-sulfamethoxazole is effective in preventing relapses (Tim Berger, personal communication, 1995).

Cutaneous atypical mycobacterial infections demonstrate variable responses to antibiotics, so it is important to culture the organisms and determine sensitivities. In general, cutaneous tuberculosis responds to antituberculous regimens with isoniazid and ethambutol with or without pyrazinamide. However, multiple drug–resistant tuberculosis has been described that may not respond to any medication currently available, but regimens employing pyrazinamide, amikacin, olfloxacin, and ciprofloxacin have met with some success.[159] Clarithromycin, ansamycin, clofazimine, minocycline, and trimethoprim-sulfamethoxazole all have variable degrees of efficacy in the treatment of atypical mycobacterial infections. One study demonstrated good response of *Mycobacterium chelonae* infection to clarithromycin in a series of non–HIV-infected immunocompromised hosts.[160] *M. haemophilum* is usually sensitive to ciprofloxacin and rifampin, but even in cases when both antibiotics are used, chronic relapse may be noted.

Syphilis responds to penicillin at higher doses that must be continued for longer courses than those in immunocompetent hosts. Recommended treatment of primary syphilis is with penicillin G benzathine 2.4 million units intramuscularly per week for up to three doses. Careful follow-up with repeat serologic testing is recommended. Secondary syphilis should be treated with lumbar puncture and if the test result is positive, high-dose intravenous penicillin G therapy is recommended. In the absence of neurosyphilis, 2.4 million units of penicillin G benzathine intramuscularly per week for three to four doses is required. Tertiary syphilis and neurosyphilis require aqueous penicillin G, 3 million units intravenously every 4 hours for 10 days, followed by penicillin G benzathine, 2.4 million units intramuscularly weekly for three doses. In patients who are allergic to penicillin, desensitization may be attempted, but if this cannot be accomplished, tetracycline or erythromycin at doses of 500 mg orally four times a day for up to 30 days may be substituted. As benzathine penicillin does not cross the blood-brain barrier well, studies using "enhanced" regimens of ampicillin and probenecid are currently ongoing.

Chancroid is treated with erythromycin 500 mg orally four times per day for 7 days, or, alternatively, a single intramuscular injection of ceftriaxone 250 mg may be administered. Lymphogranuloma venereum responds to erythromycin in the same dosage, although doxycycline 100 mg orally twice a day for 7 days and ofloxacin 300 mg orally twice a day for 7 days are also quite effective. Granuloma inguinale responds to treatment with erythromycin or trimethoprim-sulfamethoxazole. Gonorrhea is treated with regimens generally used consisting of penicillin, spectinomycin, or ceftriaxone.

PARASITIC INFECTIONS AND ECTOPARASITIC INFESTATIONS

Definition

In addition to bacterial and fungal infections, a number of parasitic infections and ectoparasitic infestations may be encountered in patients with HIV infection. Some of these include scabies, both classic and crusted types; demodicidosis; *Pneumocystis carinii* infection; acanthamebiasis; leishmaniasis; and toxoplasmosis. As in the case of other infections, these may occur either as localized conditions or as multiorgan visceral disease. Also, as with other infectious disorders in HIV-infected patients, clinical morphologies may be unusual so that skin biopsies and cultures are often necessary to establish an accurate diagnosis.

Epidemiology

Scabies is one of the most frequent skin conditions to develop in patients with HIV infection and is the most common ectoparasitic infestation in these individuals. The causative agent is the mite *Sarcoptes scabiei,* var *humanus.* Although the data regarding the overall incidence of scabies and HIV infection are not well determined, it was reported in one study in 20% of patients.[161]

Papular demodicidosis has also been reported sporadically in patients with HIV infection.[162,163] Approximately five cases of cutaneous *P. carinii* infection have been reported, as have cases of disseminated strongyloidiasis caused by *Strongyloides stercoralis,* acanthamebiasis caused by *Acanthamoeba castellani,* and disseminated toxoplamosis caused by *Toxoplasma gondii.*[164–169] *A. castellani* is part of the normal oral flora and may disseminate to the skin and central nervous system in profoundly immunocompromised patients. One hundred and fifty cases of leishmaniasis in HIV-infected hosts have been diagnosed in India, Southeast Asia, and the Mediterranean coast.[170] The most common infecting organism is *Leishmania donovani,* the protozoan responsible for the visceral form of the disease.

Pathogenesis

Severe infestation with scabies in patients with HIV infection develops as a consequence of the impaired immunity in these individuals. Immunity to scabies is thought to result from the effects of Langerhans' cells and cell-mediated immunity, which destroy mites and inhibit reinfestation. Langerhans' cells are diminished in number and are abnormal in function in patients with HIV disease.[171] Patients with altered neurologic status may fail to scratch away mites, leading to an increase in their number. In immunocompetent hosts, the number of infesting mites ranges from 10 to 20; however, in HIV-infected patients with crusted scabies, they may number in the millions. *P. carinii* infection may affect the skin preferentially in patients who use aerosolized pentamidine for prophylaxis of *P. carinii* pneumonia. By creating a more unfavorable environment in the lung, organisms spread more widely to affect visceral organs as well as the skin. Papular demodicidosis develops as a consequence of excessive proliferation of *Demodex folliculorum* within follicles, leading to inflammation and pruritus. Lowered immunity also predisposes to the development of other opportunistic infections and infestations.

Clinical Manifestations

Scabies may have a number of different clinical manifestations in patients with HIV infection (Figs. 4–45 and 4–46). Hyperkeratotic plaques present on the palms, soles, trunk, or extremities may develop that appear similar to crusted scabies in other settings. In other patients, only scattered pruritic papules accompanied by slight scale of the trunk and extremities may be seen. A widespread papulosquamous eruption that may resemble atopic dermatitis and scalp and facial scaling that may mimic seborrheic dermatitis have also been reported.[167,172–174] Characteristic burrows may be difficult to identify, so virtually any patient with a scaly persistent pruritic eruption should have skin lesions scraped and examined histologically in search of mites of scabies. Severe forms of scabies may be associated with secondary infection, bacteremia, and fatal septicemia, especially in severely immunocompromised patients.[175] Patients usually complain of intractable pruritus that is worse at night. Contacts are almost always infested, especially because of the number of mites present on the skin of index cases.

Demodicidosis generally consists of a persistent pruritic follicular eruption that may be confused with other responses to arthropods, including scabies as well as folliculitis. Lesions may affect the face, trunk, and extremities.

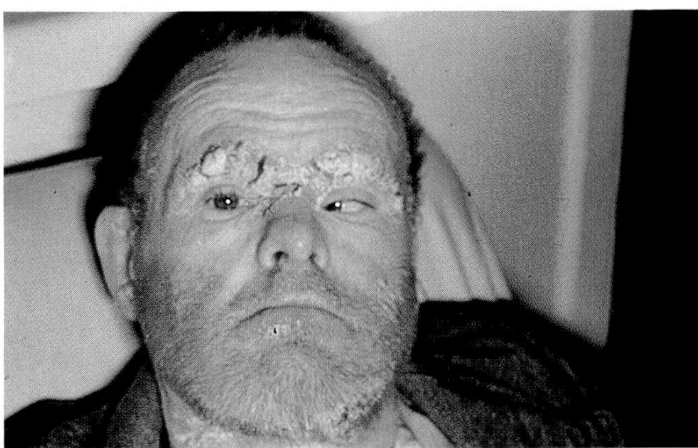

FIGURE 4–45. Norwegian scabies

These markedly hyperkeratotic and crusted plaques were found to have innumerable mites of *Sarcoptes scabei.* This is a florid example of Norwegian scabies.

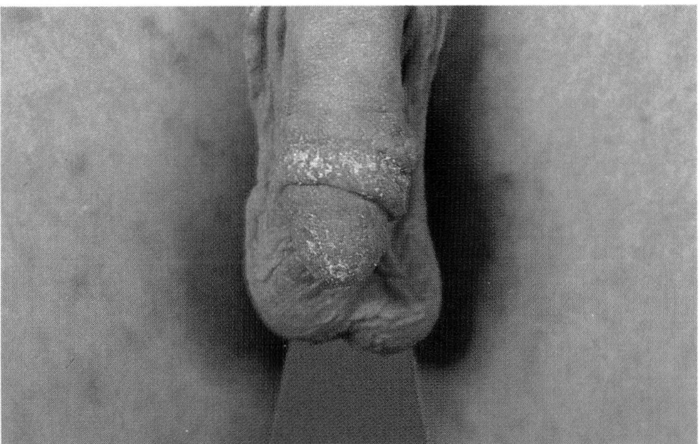

FIGURE 4–46. Norwegian scabies

Papules and slight scaling and crusting were the manifestations of Norwegian scabies in this patient. Notice the marked lack of hyperkeratosis and crusting, as seen in Figure 4–45.

P. carinii may have several different clinical manifestations in the skin (Fig. 4–47). The most commonly reported form is that of friable reddish papules or nodules seen in the ear canal or the nares. Small, translucent, molluscum contagiosum–like papules; bluish, cellulitic, plaque-like lesions; and deep-seated abscesses have also been observed. Leishmaniasis produces skin lesions resembling those of kala-azar, namely, scaly lichenified plaques with dyspigmentation and lichen simplex chronicus. The one case of toxoplasmosis that has been reported had an appearance of a papular dermatitis, and strongyloidiasis gives rise to a rapidly migrating serpiginous urticarial eruption known as larva currens. In some cases, lesions may be reticulate in appearance and have a purpuric quality that mimics livedo reticularis or other forms of vasculitis. Acanthamebiasis consists of painful nodular lesions with ulcerations usually on the trunk or extremities (Fig. 4–48).

Histopathology

Histopathologic findings are generally quite helpful in making accurate diagnoses of these conditions. In crusted scabies there is usually a superficial and mid- to-deep perivascular and interstitial infiltrate of lymphocytes with numerous eosinophils. The epidermis is hyperplastic with prominent crusting and many mites visible in the cornified layer (Fig. 4–49). In patients with postscabetic "id" reactions, a spongiotic dermatitis may be noted, and in nodular scabies, a dense, mixed inflammatory infiltrate with numerous eosinophils in a nodular configuration resembling a pseudolymphoma may be seen. In nodular scabies, the number of mites is few so that it may be difficult to find them.

Demodicidosis characteristically shows abundant *Demodex* mites within follicular infundibula associated with a mixed infiltrate of neutrophils and eosinophils within and around the infundibula of hair follicles. Leishmaniasis usually shows an infiltrate of histiocytes with plasma cells and numerous intracellular and extracellular *Leishmania* organisms with polar densities that represent kinetoplasts.

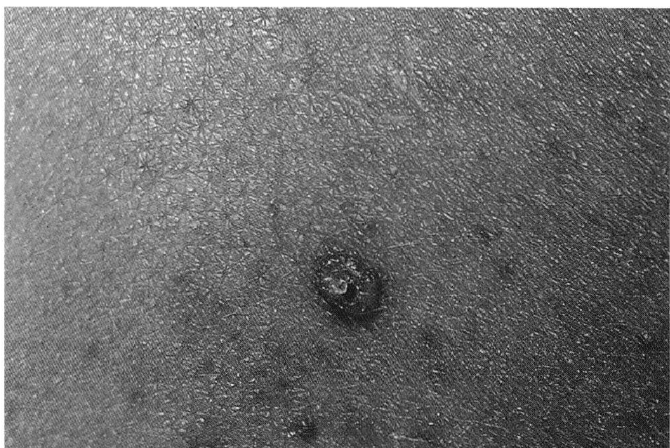

FIGURE 4–47. *Pneumocystis carinii* infection
Cutaneous *P. carinii* infection. There are scattered translucent papules present on the trunk and extremities.

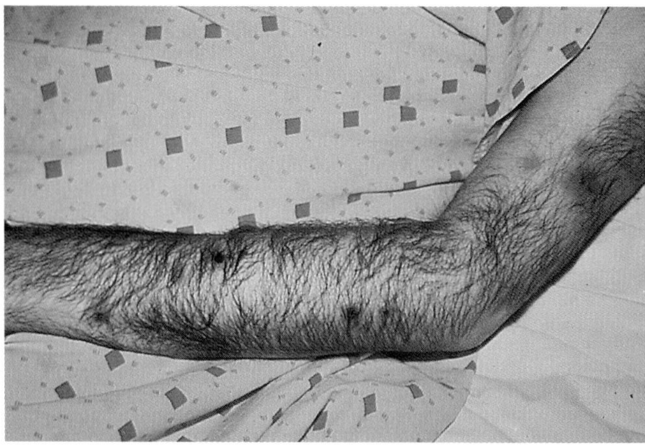

FIGURE 4–48. *Acanthamoeba* infection
Cutaneous *Acanthamoeba* infection. There are numerous painful necrotic nodules present on the extremities of this severely immunocompromised patient. (Photograph courtesy of Deborah Kalter, MD.)

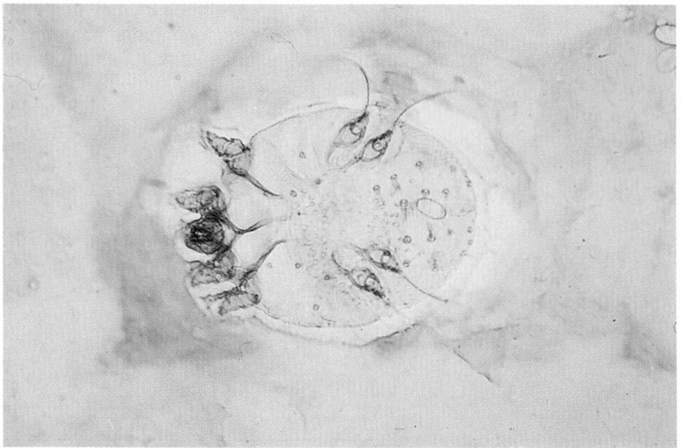

FIGURE 4–49. *Sarcoptes scabiei*
S. scabiei, the mite that causes scabies, seen histologically. Note the small egg within the body near the posterior portion of the organism.

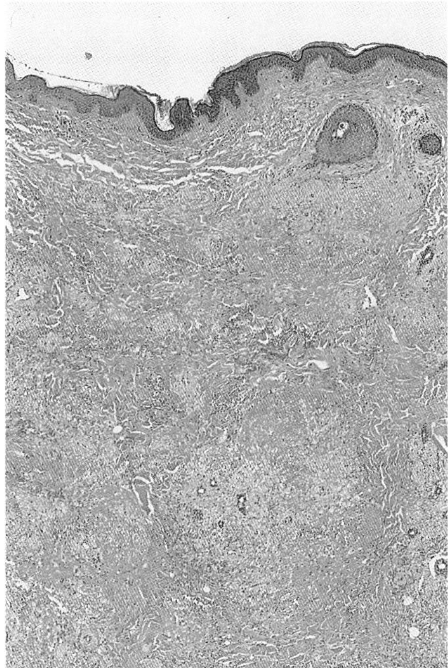

FIGURE 4–50. *Pneumocystis carinii* infection

Histopathologic findings in *P. carinii* infection of the skin. There is a diffuse infiltrate of foamy appearing cells throughout the dermis. Hematoxylin and eosin stain (original magnification ×40).

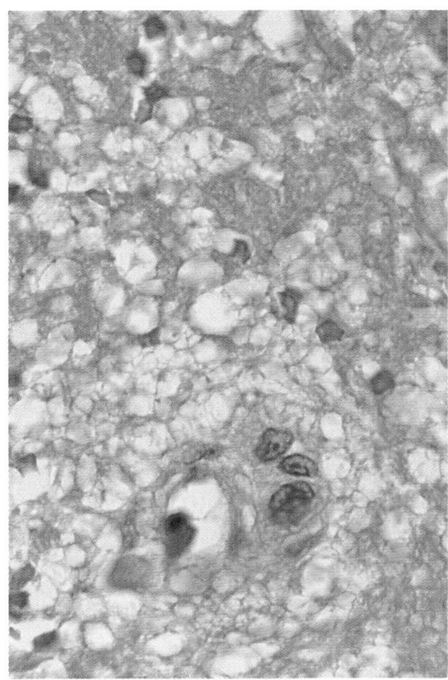

FIGURE 4–51. *Pneumocystis carinii* infection

Higher magnification demonstrates the foamy "bubbly" appearance of the infiltrate. Hematoxylin and eosin stain (original magnification ×600).

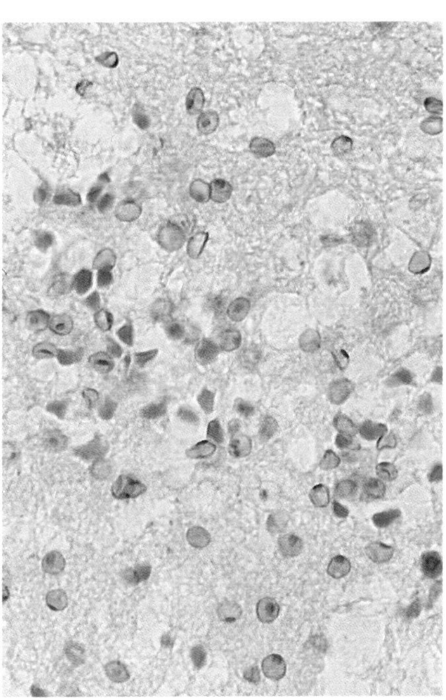

FIGURE 4–52. *Pneumocystis carinii* infection

Gomori's methenamine silver stain highlights the characteristic "teacup and saucer" appearance of the organisms. Gomori's methenamine silver stain (original magnification ×400).

P. carinii in the skin has an appearance similar to that in the lung, with a diffuse infiltrate of foamy-appearing cells, which, when stained with Gomori's methenamine silver or Steiner stains, highlight the microorganisms, resulting in the "teacup and saucer" appearance (Figs. 4–50 through 4–52). Strongyloidiasis generally shows a diffuse infiltrate of lymphocytes and eosinophils scattered throughout the dermis. If an organism itself is contained within the biopsy specimen, it is located in the upper papillary dermis. Acanthamebiasis shows a diffuse infiltrate composed of amebic cysts and trophozoites, especially around blood vessels and in the subcutaneous fat (Figs. 4–53 and 4–54). Careful inspection is required, as these may appear similar to histiocytes or other normal-appearing structures in the skin. Erythrophagocytosis may be noted.

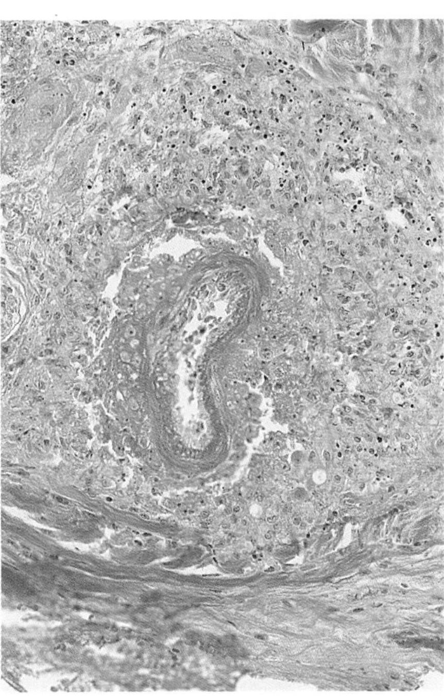

FIGURE 4–53. *Acanthamoeba* infection

Histopathology of cutaneous *Acanthamoeba* infection. Note the abundant pale-staining cells surrounding the large blood vessel in the deep portion of the skin. Hematoxylin and eosin stain (original magnification ×100).

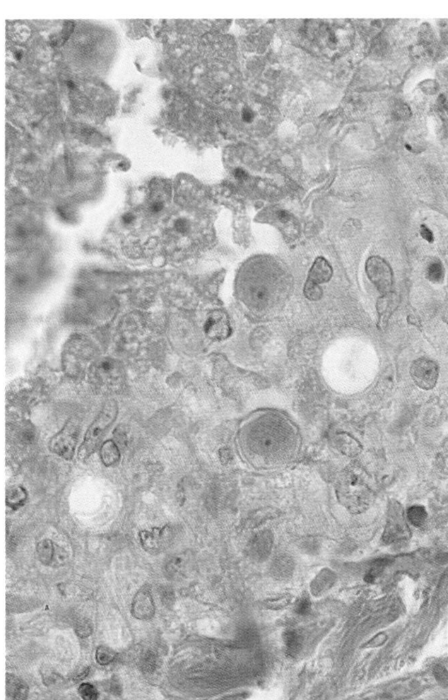

FIGURE 4–54. *Acanthamoeba* infection

Higher magnification demonstrates the numerous amebic trophozoites in the skin. Some have engulfed erythrocytes. Hematoxylin and eosin stain (original magnification ×600).

Laboratory Findings

No specific laboratory findings are seen with any of these infestations, although elevated eosinophil counts are commonly noted. Most patients with these disorders are immunocompromised, having $CD4^+$ cell counts of less than 250 cells/mm^3.

Differential Diagnosis

Scabies in patients with HIV infection must be distinguished from a wide variety of different disorders. Norwegian (crusted) scabies may appear similar to palmoplantar hyperkeratotic disorders such as psoriasis. Diffuse scabies may mimic atopic dermatitis as well as other spongiotic dermatitides such as nummular dermatitis. Occasionally, scabies may affect the scalp with scaling and may simulate seborrheic dermatitis. Nodular scabies may mimic lymphomatoid papulosis as well as other insect bite reactions. Demodicidosis usually appears similar to folliculitis, both eosinophilic pustular folliculitis and bacterial folliculitis. Acne and rosacea may also have similar features and must be excluded on the basis of biopsies and scrapings.

Cutaneous pneumocystosis may mimic molluscum contagiosum and nonspecific bruises of the skin as well as pyogenic granulomas. Strongyloidiasis may simulate urticaria as well as figurate erythema, livedo reticularis, and other causes of cutaneous livedo. Acanthamebiasis is generally nondescript clinically and must be distinguished from other causes of ulcerated nodules in the skin.

Diagnosis

As mentioned previously, the diagnosis of scabies and demodicidosis depends primarily on the clinical appearance of skin lesions and eruptions and the demonstration of mites on microscopic examination of scrapings. Skin biopsies evaluated in the context of clinical history and appearance are important in diagnosing the other conditions discussed earlier. Special serologic and complement fixation tests may be helpful in confirming diagnoses.

Treatment

Scabies generally responds to treatment with lindane cream or lotion or 5% permethrin cream applied from head to toe and left in place for 8 to 12 hours and then washed off. The treatment is repeated in 1 week. In some patients, recurrences develop as a consequence of failure to treat under the fingernails and the intertriginous zones, although resistance to scabicidal medications may develop. Some have recommended alternating treatment with lindane and permethrin. Multiple treatments may be required. Five percent precipitated sulfur in petrolatum applied from the neck down nightly for 3 nights may also be effective. Recent evidence has shown ivermectin at a single oral dose of 150 to 200 micrograms to be highly effective at eradicating scabies; it is hoped that it will be available for this indication soon.[175a]

Postscabetic id reactions must be treated with antihistamines such as doxepin 10 to 25 mg orally two to four times daily with a topical application of corticosteroid preparations to diminish inflammation. In cases of nodules, injection of triamcinolone acetonide may be required. Careful laundering of linen and clothing is necessary, and household and other contacts should be treated. In cases of crusted scabies, entire wards of patients may require therapy.[176] Demodicidosis usually resolves after treatment with an application of metronidazole gel two to three times daily with or without the addition of topical benzoyl benzoate. Systemic metronidazole at doses of 250 mg to 750 mg orally twice a day may be required in cases not responsive to topical measures.

Pneumocystosis responds to the usual treatment for *P. carinii* pneumonia, namely, intravenous pentamidine. Strongyloidiasis requires treatment with thiabendazole 25 mg/kg twice a day for 4 to 5 days to several weeks depending on the immune status of the host. Amebiasis responds to metronidazole at a dosage of 750 mg orally twice a day for 10 days, but as these patients are often quite immunocompromised, response to therapy may be poor. Leishmaniasis may respond to ketoconazole or other new imidazole antifungal medications, but stibogluconate sodium at a dosage of 20 mg/kg per day for 3 to 4 weeks is generally used in immunocompromised patients.

Adjunctive therapies are also important, as pruritus is often severe. Topical application of corticosteroid preparations as well as antipruritic agents containing menthol and phenol, pramoxine, and antihistamines may be required. Four percent doxepin cream (Zonalon) is a valuable antipruritic agent that may be used in patients with refractory pruritus. Exposure to ultraviolet B irradiation and psoralen plus ultraviolet A are also helpful.

SYSTEMIC FUNGAL INFECTIONS

Definition

Blastomycosis, candidiasis, coccidioidomycosis, cryptococcosis, histoplasmosis, paracoccidioidomycosis, and sporotrichosis are some of the systemic fungal infections that occur in HIV-infected individuals. These infections may occur in localized fashion and affect a single tissue or as disseminated multiorgan disease. Mucosal and cutaneous lesions may have a number of different clinical morphologies in HIV-seropositive patients, many of which may be unusual and defy accurate clinical diagnosis.

Epidemiology

The most common opportunistic fungal infections to affect the skin in HIV-seropositive patients are histoplasmosis and cryptococcosis. Nearly 20% of HIV-seropositive individuals with disseminated histoplasmosis and up to 10% of those with disseminated cryptococcosis develop mucocutaneous lesions. Systemic and cutaneous coccidioidomycosis are both being recognized more frequently in HIV-infected patients, although they are still seen only sporadically. Patients infected with HIV who have blastomycosis, paracoccidioidomycosis, or sporotrichosis have also been observed, albeit rarely. Similarly, although mucocutaneous candidiasis occurs commonly in HIV-seropositive individuals, disseminated candidiasis is seldom reported.

Clinical Manifestations

Mucocutaneous lesions associated with systemic fungal infections may assume a number of different features. The most common lesions are pustules and ulcers, although papules and nodules are also frequently observed. Less often, patches, plaques, and mucosal ulcerations are seen.

Blastomycosis. Progressive disseminated blastomycosis has been described in a 30-year-old homosexual HIV-seropositive man who had *Blastomyces dermatitidis*–related pustules, nodules, and cutaneous ulcers.[177] Amphotericin B initially was used to treat the primary pulmonary infection, although when the regimen was changed to fluconazole, multiple pustules that grew *B. dermatitidis* developed. The condition failed to respond well to treatment and eventually proved fatal.

Candidiasis. Oral thrush that affects the tongue or the buccal mucosa or both, with or without esophageal infection, is the most common manifestation of candidiasis in HIV-seropositive patients (Fig. 4–55). Oral candidiasis may be the initial sign of HIV infection in many individuals.

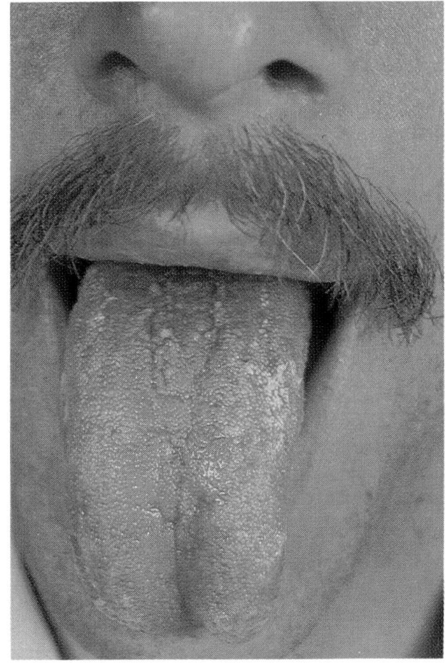

FIGURE 4–55. Candidiasis

A whitish, curd-like exudate present on the tongue or buccal mucosa that can easily be scraped away is characteristic of this condition. This may be an indication that a patient will later develop AIDS.

Other manifestations that may develop include chronic paronychia and onychodystrophy; chronic refractory vaginal candidiasis; distal urethritis; and persistent monilial infection of the axilla, glans penis, groin, or inframammary area, or a combination of these (Fig. 4–56).

Disseminated candidiasis in HIV-infected individuals has been reported in a small number of patients. Administration of broad spectrum antibiotics and total parenteral nutrition, extended placement of central intravenous catheters during prolonged hospitalizations, and, in children, previous oral candidiasis are predisposing factors for systemic infection in these individuals. In one study, only one of 11 patients who had an episode of disseminated candidiasis had cutaneous involvement. The patient had been HIV seropositive since the age of 11 months and developed a culture-positive right infraclavicular *C. albicans* skin abscess. A 28-day course of amphotericin B resulted in complete recovery.[179]

Coccidioidomycosis. Although an increasing number of HIV-infected patients with coccidioidomycosis are being described, only a few of these individuals have been reported with associated skin lesions.[180–182] The first was a 36-year-old man with primary pulmonary coccidioidomycosis who developed lower extremity purpura that proved to be leukocytoclastic vasculitis. Subsequently, cutaneous disease developed that manifested as painful erythema overlying an abscess of the buttock. The infection resolved with amphotericin B and ketoconazole.

A second patient was a 28-year-old man who developed asymptomatic papulopustules on the extremities, chest, back, and palm, from which *Coccidioides immitis* was cultured. The skin lesions involuted after systemic treatment with amphotericin B and ketoconazole. Other skin manifestations that may be seen in coccidioidomycosis include ulcers, abscesses, and nodules.

Cryptococcosis. Cryptococcosis is a not uncommon infection to develop in HIV-infected individuals.[183–185] The incidence of cutaneous involvement was found to be approximately 6 to 7% when a large series of HIV-infected patients with cryptococcosis were evaluated. Mucocutaneous lesions of cryptococcosis are polymorphous and may appear as erythematous papules, nodules, pustules, or ulcers of the skin and mucosa (Figs. 4–57 through 4–59).[186] Cutaneous cryptococcosis, like other opportunistic infections that develop in these patients, may mimic the cutaneous morphology of other disorders such as herpes simplex virus, cellulitis, or molluscum contagiosum infection, as well as soft tissue hypertrophic lesions such as rhinophyma and Kaposi's sarcoma.[187,188] In addition to simulating it, *Cryptococcus neoformans* has been demonstrated within lesions of cutaneous Kaposi's sarcoma.

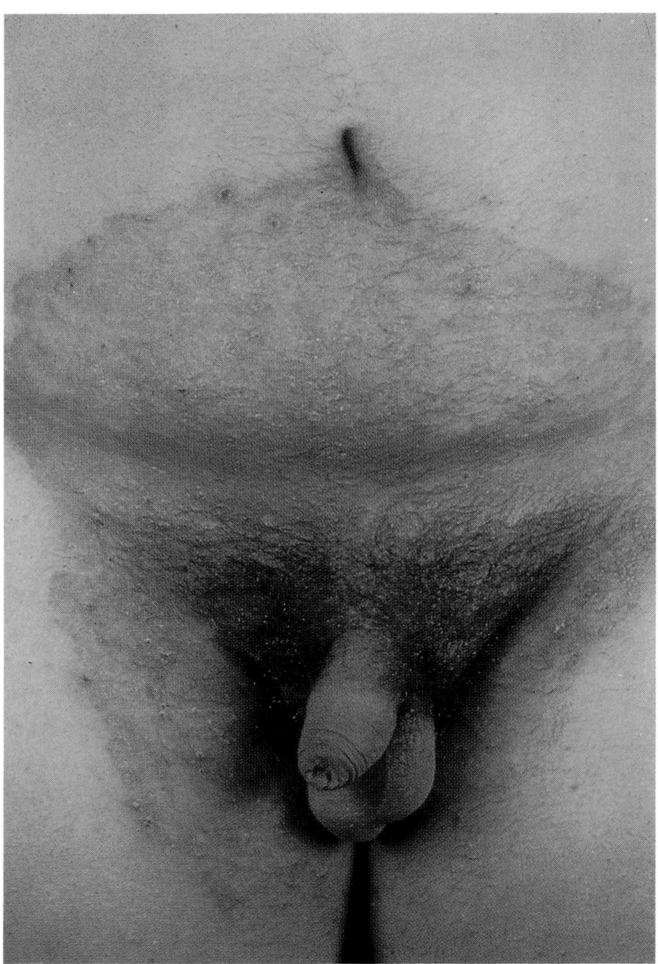

FIGURE 4–56. Mucocutaneous candidiasis

Chronic mucocutaneous candidiasis seen in patient with HIV infection. Note the extensive crusting and scaling as well as the subungual hyperkeratosis.

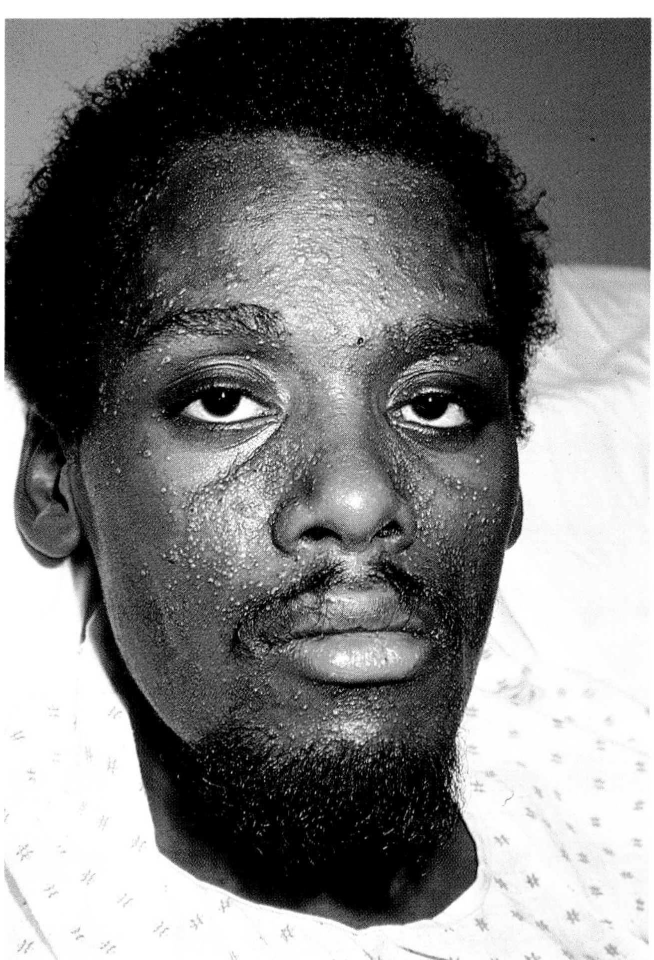

FIGURE 4–57. Cryptococcosis

Crusted umbilicated follicular and perifollicular papules may mimic lesions of molluscum contagiosum infection. They are often multiple and may tend to confluence in both conditions.

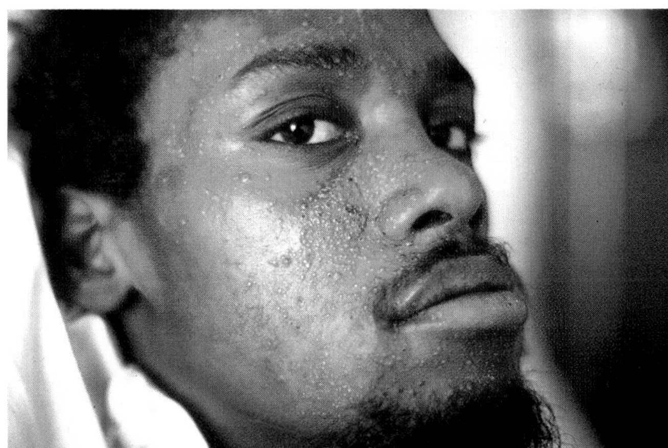

FIGURE 4–58. Cryptococcosis

Close-up view revealing the umbilicated nature of the papules. A biopsy is essential to distinguish this condition from molluscum contagiosum infection.

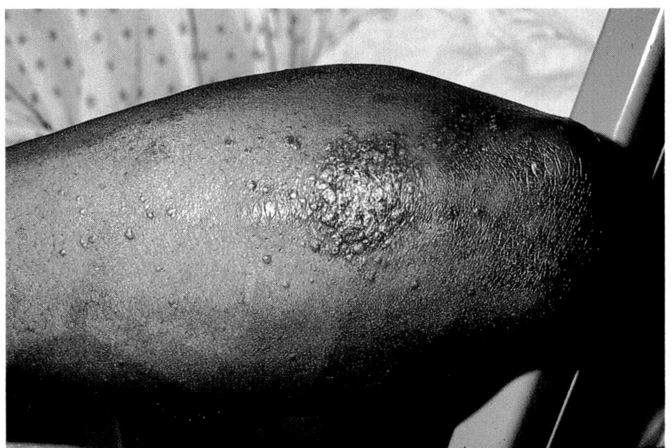

FIGURE 4–59. Cryptococcosis

The lesions have coalesced to form a plaque on the arm.

Histoplasmosis. Cohen and colleagues reviewed cases of 280 HIV-infected individuals with disseminated histoplasmosis and found 48 patients (17%) with histologically or culture-proven mucocutaneous lesions of *Histoplasma capsulatum.*[189] Clinically, the lesions appeared as cutaneous and mucosal ulcers, erythematous macules and patches, fistulae, papules and nodules, pustules, and verrucous plaques (Fig. 4–60).[190–193] Patients with AIDS have been described in whom *H. capsulatum* and Kaposi's sarcoma were found to be coexisting in a single skin lesion, and cases of concomitant psoriasis and histoplasmosis have been described.[193,194] The possibility of human-to-human transmission of histoplasmosis between two HIV-seropositive individuals via close skin contact has been postulated but not proved.[195]

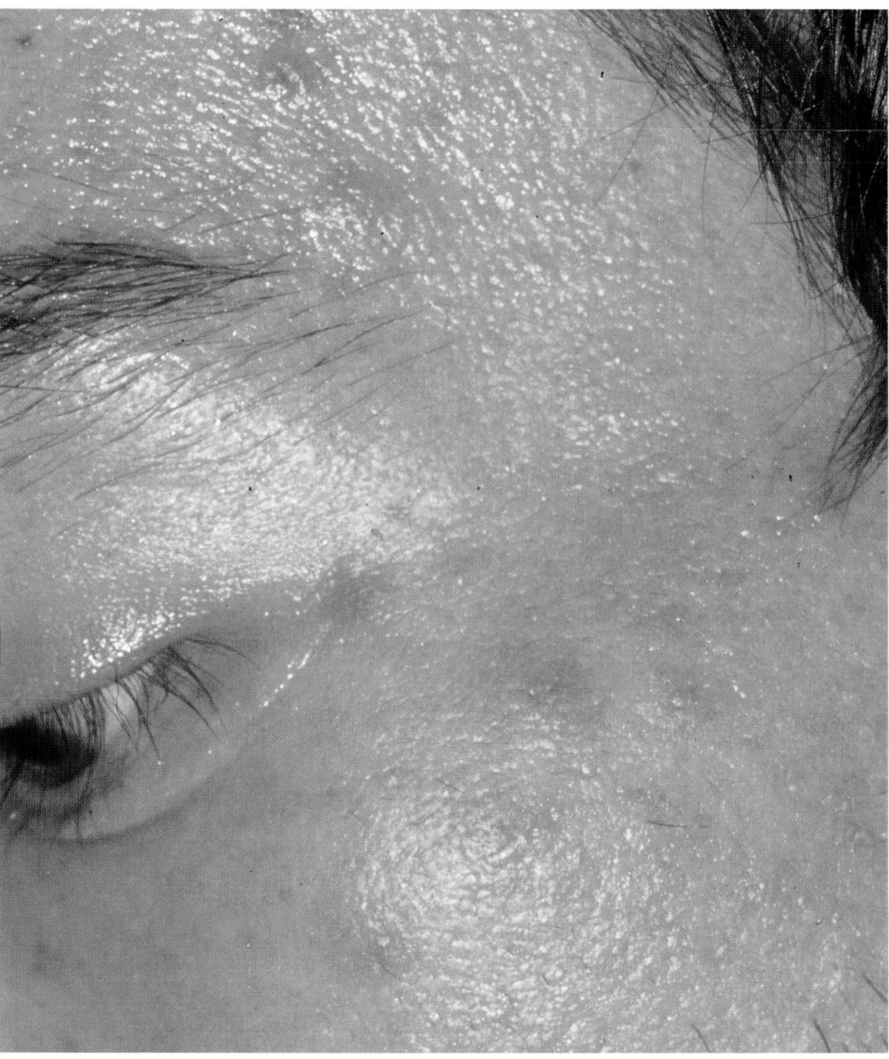

FIGURE 4–60. *Histoplasma capsulatum* infection

Scattered and sometimes widespread acneiform papules or nodules may be caused by a number of different systemic infectious organisms. In this case the cause was *H. capsulatum;* however, cutaneous cryptococcosis and cutaneous *Mycobacterium avium-intracellulare* infection may appear identical.

Paracoccidioidomycosis. Descriptions of disseminated paracoccidioidosis in HIV-infected individuals are rare. One Brazilian AIDS patient with cutaneous lesions of disseminated paracoccidioidomycosis has been described.[196] The man was a 31-year-old homosexual who presented with an abnormal chest roentgenogram, headache, fever, and small, painful ulcers on the face and thigh. *Paracoccidioides brasiliensis* organisms were observed on hematoxylin and eosin–stained sections prepared from a biopsy of the cutaneous ulcers. Both pulmonary and cutaneous lesions healed completely after treatment with amphotericin B.

Sporotrichosis. Clinical forms of sporotrichosis include lymphocutaneous, fixed cutaneous, disseminated cutaneous, and systemic. The last mentioned may manifest either as localized pulmonary disease or as widespread involvement of numerous organs. In patients with HIV infection, skin lesions may be ulcers, papules, nodules, plaques, or pustules, or a combination of these.[197–199] These lesions may be widespread, and internal organ involvement may develop that often proves fatal.

Histopathology

The histopathologic features of the mucocutaneous lesions of systemic fungal infections in HIV-infected patients are generally similar to those seen in immunocompetent hosts with some exceptions. The epidermis usually exhibits pseudocarcinomatous hyperplasia, and there is almost always a suppurative and granulomatous inflammatory infiltrate in the dermis in blastomycosis, coccidioidomycosis, paracoccidioidomycosis, and sporotrichosis. There may be transepidermal elimination of fungal spores. His-

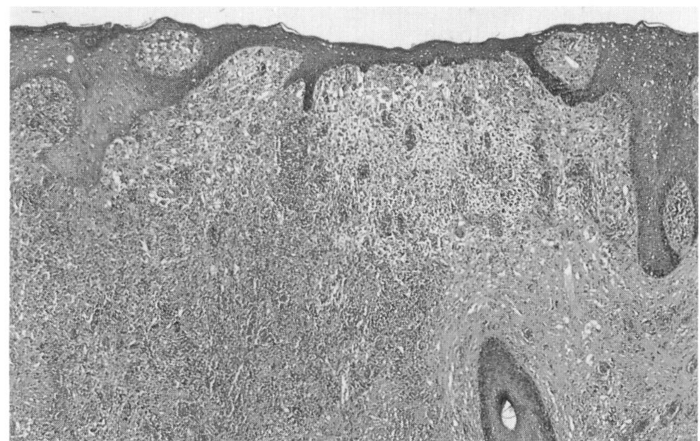

FIGURE 4–61. Histoplasmosis
Note the epidermal hyperplasia and the infiltrate of pale-staining cells in the dermis.

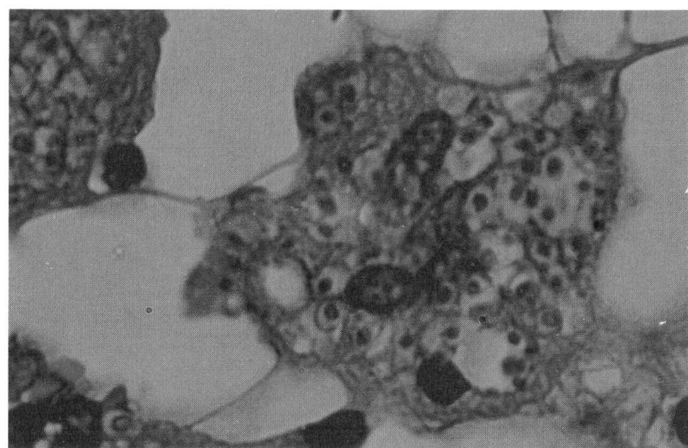

FIGURE 4–62. Histoplasmosis
This histiocyte is virtually filled with *Histoplasma capsulatum* organisms.

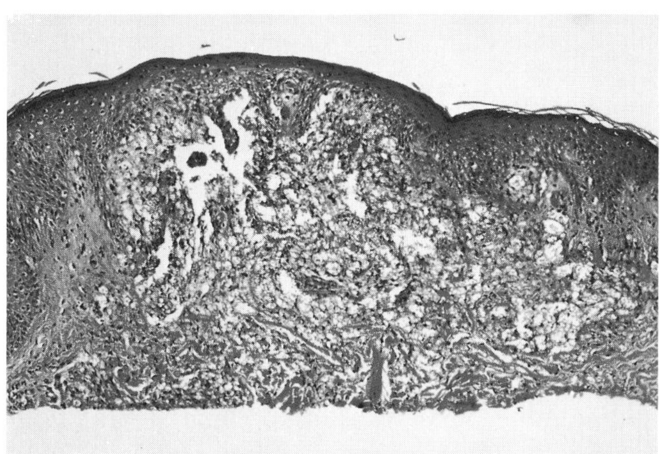

FIGURE 4–63. Cryptococcosis
Shave biopsy of a lesion of cryptococcosis. Note the clear-staining cells present in the dermis.

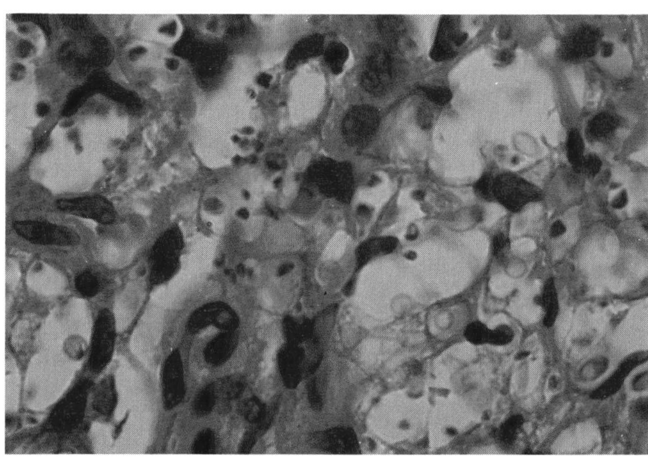

FIGURE 4–64. Cryptococcosis
Higher magnification of the same specimen as in Figure 4–60 reveals numerous organisms of *Cryptococcus neoformans.* The whitish areas represent the abundant mucinous capsular material.

toplasmosis may exhibit a diffuse dermal infiltrate of histiocytes, neutrophils, and leukocytoclasis (Figs. 4–61 and 4–62). Some cases have been histologically confused with leukocytoclastic vasculitis. Cryptococcosis has a characteristic histopathologic appearance in most cases. There is diffuse pallor of the dermis that correlates with the mucoid capsular material of the organisms, which are usually present in abundance (Figs. 4–63 and 4–64). With the exception of disseminated candidiasis and sporotrichosis, fungal spores or hyphae are usually present in number either free in the dermis or within histiocytes, multinucleated giant cells, or abscesses. The organisms can often be identified on hematoxylin and eosin–stained sections, although special stains such as periodic acid–Schiff and Gomori's methenamine silver can be used to facilitate their detection. Examination of multiple sections taken from the biopsy specimen may be necessary to find organisms in disseminated candidiasis and sporotrichosis. Nevertheless, both of these organisms grow readily and rapidly when cultured on Sabouraud's medium. In some immunocompromised hosts infected with HIV, but not in immunocompetent patients, abundant organisms of sporotrichosis may be present and may be visualized microscopically.[200]

Diagnosis

When the possibility that a mucocutaneous lesion in an HIV-infected patient is secondary to dissemination of a systemic fungal infection, a tissue biopsy of that lesion should be performed for histologic evaluation and microbiologic cultures. The growth of a fungal organism in culture is definitive evidence that the lesion is caused by an opportunistic fungus. Unfortunately, several of these organisms require several days to weeks to grow in culture so that more rapid methods to establish a definitive diagnosis are often required. Fungal organisms can be identified readily when the contents from cutaneous lesions are smeared onto a glass slide, treated with 10% potassium hydroxide solution, and examined microscopically. Alternatively, a crushed tissue preparation taken from a lesion immediately after skin biopsy is a simple and expedient technique for detecting fungal organisms. Light microscopic examination after routine staining with hematoxylin and eosin or after special staining for fungi with either periodic acid–Schiff or Gomori's methenamine silver, or both, is also helpful in establishing the existence of a systemic fungal infection. When the number of microorganisms is small, the sensitivity of diagnosis can be increased by immunoperoxidase staining using antibodies directed to fungi or mycobacteria that cross-react with them. Amplification of fungal DNA from small tissue samples using the polymerase chain reaction technique has expedited the diagnosis of some of these infections, but currently, diagnostic molecular microbiology is still a research methodology that is not routinely available. Finally, because fungal infection–associated lesions in HIV-seropositive individuals have been reported to harbor more than one pathogen, a diligent search for concurrent infectious organisms is warranted.

Treatment

The treatment of disseminated fungal infections in HIV-infected patients is currently in flux as new, powerful antifungal medications have been released and are in the process of evaluation.[201] Nevertheless, until these agents have been used to treat significant numbers of HIV-infected patients, amphotericin B remains the drug of choice for many. Thus, for blastomycosis, intravenous amphotericin B is the first-line agent. In disseminated candidiasis, amphotericin B is also the drug of choice, although fluconazole or itraconazole may be effective for initial and maintenance therapy. Localized superficial mucocutaneous candidiasis usually is adequately treated with topical antifungal preparations, although systemic therapy with imidazoles may be required in refractory cases. The treatment of coccidioidomycosis is intravenous amphotericin B, and in some cases, concomitant intrathecal amphotericin B may be required. Cryptococcosis is usually treated with amphotericin B and flucytosine, although imidazoles have shown promise. The treatment of disseminated histoplasmosis and paracoccidioidomycosis is also amphotericin B, although as with *Cryptococcus,* imidazoles have been shown to be effective in both prophylaxis and therapy. Although amphotericin B is the drug of choice for systemic sporotrichosis, ketoconazole, fluconazole, or intraconazole may be effectively used. Lymphocutaneous sporotrichosis can be treated successfully with potassium iodide, although careful monitoring is necessary to avoid recurrences as the drug is not fungicidal.

Other Fungal Infections in Patients with HIV Infection. In addition to the fungal infections described earlier, a number of other fungal infections have been reported in patients with HIV infection. Disseminated *Scedosporium inflatum, Pseudallescheria boydii,* and *Microsporum canis* have been observed in these patients, as have infections with other saprophytic fungi.[202–204] Disseminated *Aspergillus* infection was the cause of facial palsy in one patient as a consequence of involvement of the mastoid sinus.[205] Zygomycosis infection of the head and neck may develop and may manifest as local pain, cutaneous necrosis, and necrotizing ulcerations.[206,207] Deep soft tissue muscular aspergillosis has also been noted. These infections are being encountered more frequently as a consequence of better prophylaxis against other opportunistic infections and because of abnormal neutrophil function that has been demonstrated in these patients.

Penicillium marneffei, a fungus that is endemic in Asia, causes an infection that has been reported with increasing frequency in patients with AIDS in Thailand.[208] Seventy-six percent of affected individuals develop skin disease. Some of the cutaneous manifestations include umbilicated papules that could be confused with molluscum contagiosum, ecthyma-like lesions, folliculitis, subcutaneous nodules, and morbilliform eruptions. The diagnosis is established by histologic evaluation of skin biopsies and by the performance of cultures.

Infection by dermatophytes in HIV-infected individuals may occur on any cornified epithelial surface (Fig. 4–65). HIV-infected homosexual men have been shown to have a 37.3% rate of colonization of the feet compared with a rate of 8.6% in heterosexual men.[209] Dermatophyte infection of the toenails or fingernails also occurs commonly in HIV infection (Fig. 4–66). Proximal white subungual onychomycosis of the toenails has been described as occurring more commonly in patients with HIV infection (Fig. 4–67).[210] In contrast to the classical form of distal subungual onychomycosis in which the fungus infects the nail distally and spreads proximally, proximal white subungual onychomycosis is characterized by involvement of the proximal nail plate beginning under the posterior nail groove and extending distally. Fifty-eight percent of these infections were shown on one study to be caused by *Trichophyton rubrum.* Tinea corporis may manifest as extensive widespread involvement of the trunk and extremities. In any individual with extensive tinea corporis, the possibility of underlying HIV should be entertained.

Pityrosporum ovale and *Pityrosporum orbiculare* are normal residents of the hair follicles of the

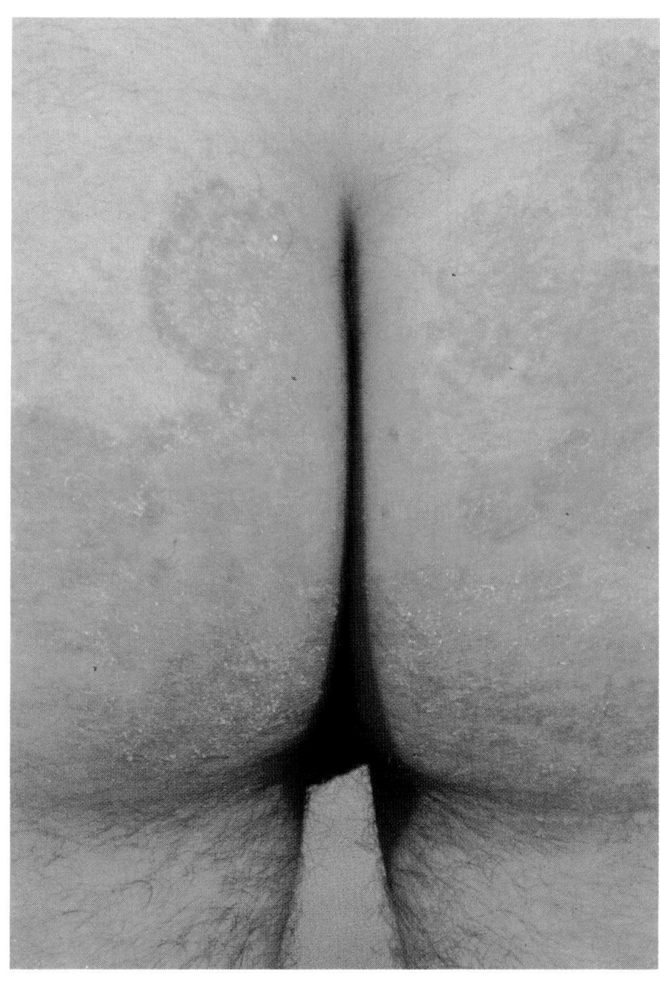

FIGURE 4–65. Dermatophyte infection

Common dermatophyte infections in patients with HIV infection or AIDS on occasion may become rampant because of immunosuppression. Scrapings for microscopic examination and culture should be obtained when such lesions are encountered.

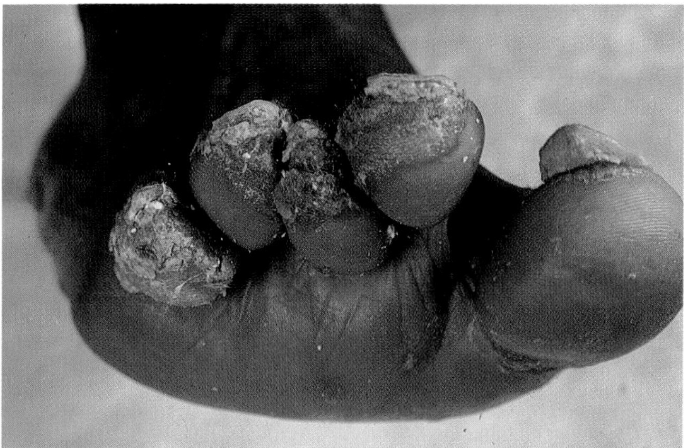

FIGURE 4–66. Onychomycosis

Severe onychomycosis with marked subungual hyperkeratosis and nail dystrophy may also be seen in patients with AIDS. This is usually a chronic condition seen in elderly patients.

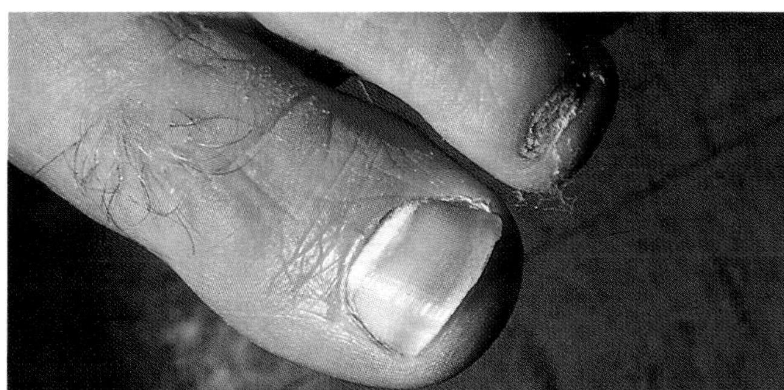

FIGURE 4–67. Proximal subungual onychomycosis

Proximal "white" subungual onychomycosis. In this condition, which is relatively specific for immunocompromised patients, there is penetration of the nail plate by fungus extending from the proximal nailfold distally. This is in contrast to what is seen in immunocompetent hosts in whom fungi first affect the nail plate distally.

scalp and have been suggested to cause or exacerbate seborrheic dermatitis in patients with HIV infection. In one study, the density of *P. ovale* of the affected skin was found to correlate with the severity of seborrheic dermatitis.[211] *Pityrosporum* folliculitis characterized by pruritic papules and pustules on the trunk and extremities also may develop in HIV-infected hosts. Histologic evaluation of potassium hydroxide preparations of scrapings from lesions shows yeasts and pseudohyphal forms of the organisms, and histopathology of skin biopsy specimens also demonstrates numerous organisms within hair follicles. An overgrowth of *P. ovale* of the glabrous skin leads to tinea versicolor that manifests as scaling patches and plaques of the trunk. In patients with HIV infection, it may be very extensive. Treatment with oral imidazole antifungal medications such as fluconazole, itraconazole, or ketoconazole for 14 days is effective, although the condition tends to recur following its discontinuation.

Trichosporonosis, due to infection with *Trichosporon beigelii,* generally causes white piedra, a superficial infection of the hair endemic to tropical and subtropical regions and areas of the southeastern United States. Carriage of this organism has been shown to be increased in homosexual men, and several cases of invasive disease with positive blood and urine cultures have been reported.[212] *Cladosporium cladosporioides* has been reported to cause pustular nodules in an HIV-infected patient.[213] Surgical excision was curative. Cutaneous *Alternaria* infection presenting as an eschar on the leg and *Curvularia* phaeohyphomycosis causing a keratotic lesion on the scrotum have both been observed in HIV-infected individuals.[214,215]

NONINFECTIOUS SKIN DISORDERS

In addition to infectious disorders, a number of noninfectious cutaneous signs and symptoms have been described in patients who are infected with HIV. The development of one or more of these conditions should alert the physician to consider HIV infection as a possible underlying cause of the conditions.

SEBORRHEIC DERMATITIS, PSORIASIS, AND REITER'S SYNDROME

Definition

Seborrheic dermatitis and psoriasis are papulosquamous disorders associated with epidermal hyperplasia, increased epidermal turnover, and scaling. Reiter's syndrome is a condition consisting of urethritis, conjunctivitis, arthritis, and psoriasiform lesions of the glans penis and other parts of the body. Seborrheic dermatitis has a characteristic distribution involving the scalp, nasolabial fold, and presternal areas as well as occasionally intertriginous sites. Psoriasis occurs in a number of different forms, most commonly as scaly plaques of extensor surfaces. All three of these conditions are increased in incidence in patients with HIV infection.

Epidemiology

Seborrheic dermatitis is one of the most common skin conditions that affects patients with HIV infection, seen in up to 85% of all HIV-infected individuals at some point during the course of the disease.[216] Psoriasis develops in 5% of patients with HIV infection, which is much more frequent than the 1 to 2% incidence reported for the general population.[217,218] Up to 10% of the patients with HIV-associated psoriasis may develop arthritis, a figure that is also significantly higher than the 1% of patients with psoriatic arthritis who are immunocompetent. Reiter's syndrome has been reported in 6 to 10% of HIV-infected patients in contrast to an incidence of 0.06% in healthy men.[219,220] As in HIV seronegative immunocompetent hosts, human leukocyte antigen (HLA) B27 is frequently found in HIV-associated Reiter's syndrome patients. In one study, 71% of patients were documented to have HLA-B27. No correlation between the presence of HLA-B27 and psoriatic arthritis has been found, however.[221]

Pathogenesis

The pathogenesis of seborrheic dermatitis remains unknown, although as mentioned earlier, it has been postulated to be caused by a reaction to *P. ovale.* Dysregulation of the immune system may cause the skin of HIV-infected hosts to become acanthotic and psoriasiform possibly as a consequence of cytokine release or an exaggerated inflammatory reaction. Why psoriasis develops in patients with HIV infection remains unknown, although several studies have postulated that the pathogenesis of psoriasis may be related to underlying vascular proliferation. Patients with HIV infection are prone to develop vasoproliferative lesions such as Kaposi's sarcoma so that the same factor that leads to vasoproliferation could be responsible for the increased epidermal turnover associated with psoriasis. Infections may also cause psoriasis to flare in patients with HIV infection, especially those caused by *Candida, Staphylococcus,* and *Streptococcus.* Reiter's syndrome in immunocompetent hosts is commonly triggered by infections with *Shigella flexneri, Campylobacter fetus,* and *Ureaplasma urealyticum.* These organisms are rarely found in HIV-infected patients with Reiter's syndrome, although some patients do have a culture-negative diarrheal illness or culture-negative urethritis at the time of the onset of the disorder.[222] In that HLA-B27 is significantly associated with HIV-associated Reiter's disease, autoimmunity associated with this allele may be important. Recent studies have suggested a small vessel (capillary) vasculitis associated with Reiter's syndrome in which chlamydial arteries were determined.[222a]

Clinical Manifestations

Seborrheic dermatitis most commonly is manifested as slightly indurated, diffuse or confluent, pinkish-red, scaly plaques that affect the face and scalp (Fig. 4–68). These may be large, thickened, and heavily crusted and may be present on other areas such as the upper anterior chest, back, groin, and extremities. In some patients, the condition may affect large areas of the skin, leading to erythroderma. Still other cases may be associated with alopecia. The disease may be more difficult to control with routine therapy in HIV-infected individuals, a finding that should serve as a clue that a patient might be infected with HIV.

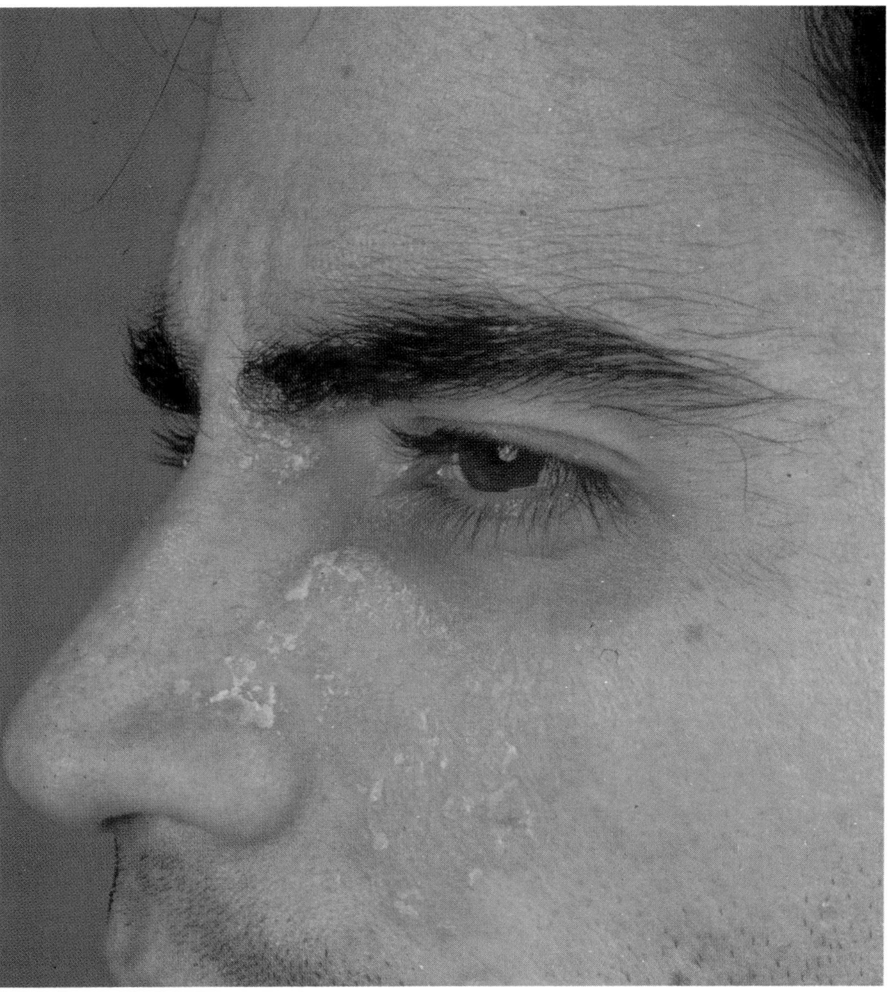

FIGURE 4–68. Seborrheic dermatitis

This eruption is seen in a patient with AIDS. Pinkish red scaly and crusted plaques seen in the malar areas but also in other locations are characteristic of this condition. It is refractory to treatment in most cases.

Psoriasis may have a number of different manifestations (Figs. 4–69 and 4–70). It may resemble classic psoriasis found in immunocompetent hosts consisting of reddish plaques with superficial micaceous scale on the extensor surfaces and nail changes of onycholysis, pitting, and subungual hyperkeratosis. In other patients, severe psoriatic arthritis may be seen. Different forms of psoriasis may be found in the same patient, such as guttate psoriasis associated with classic psoriasis vulgaris. Severe exfoliative erythroderma may develop within several days, and acral pustular lesions of keratoderma blenorrhagicum coexisting with psoriasis or sebopsoriasis have been noted. Concomitant seborrheic dermatitis of the scalp is almost always seen. In addition, HIV-related psoriasis may develop in patients with mild preexisting psoriasis that suddenly undergoes severe exacerbation once AIDS develops, or it may develop spontaneously at some point after HIV seroconversion in an individual who has never before had clinical disease.

Reiter's syndrome is characterized clinically by arthritis (especially sacroiliitis), urethritis, conjunctivitis, and pustular scaling lesions of the glabrous skin, glans penis, and scalp. Debilitating palmoplantar pustular disease is common, and there is generally striking nail dystrophy associated with periungual erythema, inflammation, and hyperkeratosis with prominent crusting (Figs. 4–71 through 4–73).

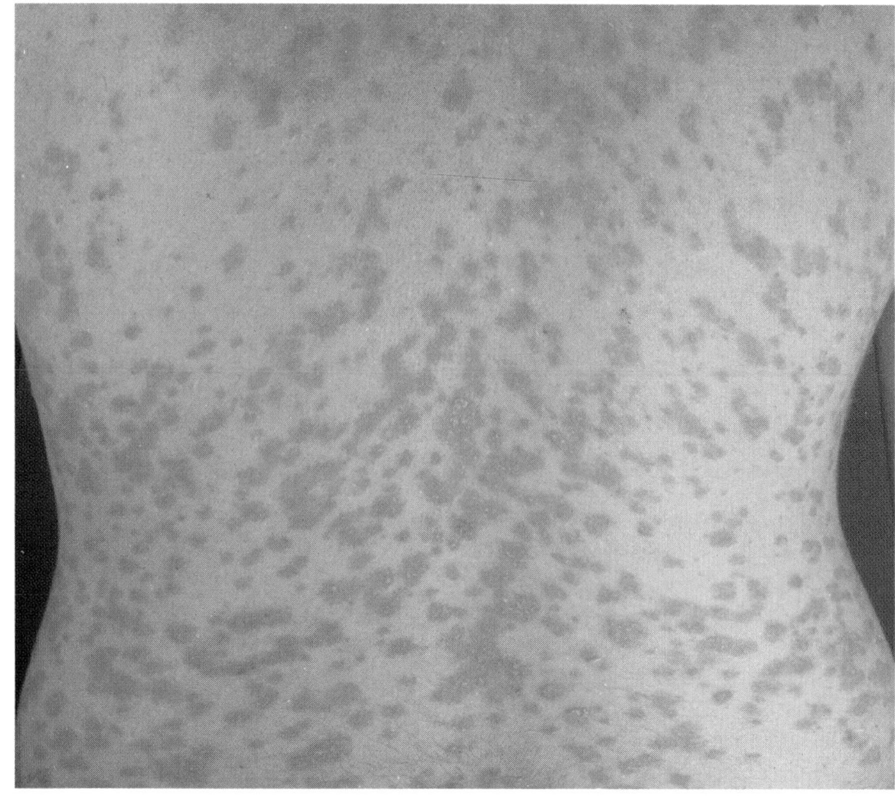

FIGURE 4–69. Psoriasis

Psoriasis in a patient with AIDS. Common psoriasis may be markedly exacerbated in this patient population, and erythroderma may result.

FIGURE 4–70. Eruptive psoriasis

Close-up view of eruptive psoriasis in a patient with AIDS.

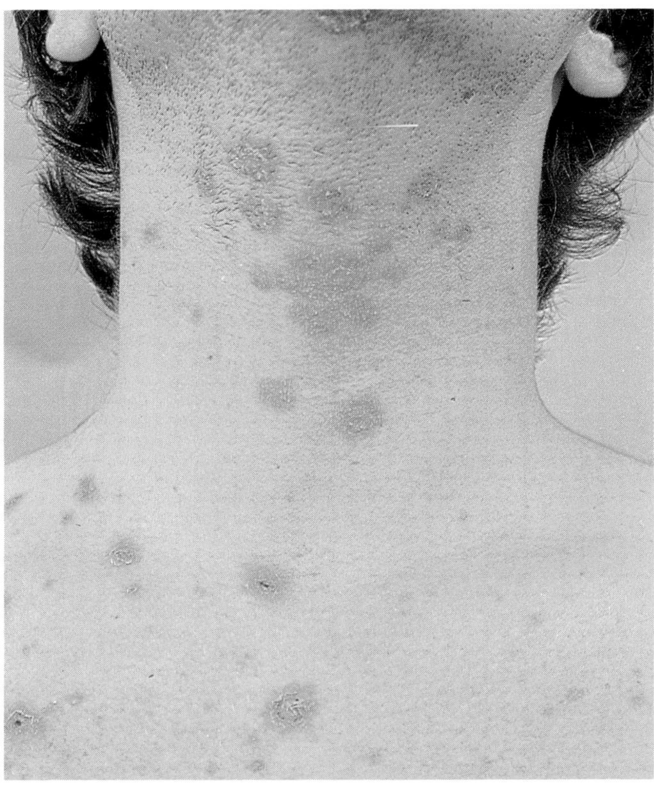

FIGURE 4–71. Reiter's syndrome

Thick, scaly, and crusted plaques present on the trunk, extremities, and acral surfaces are characteristic of Reiter's syndrome.

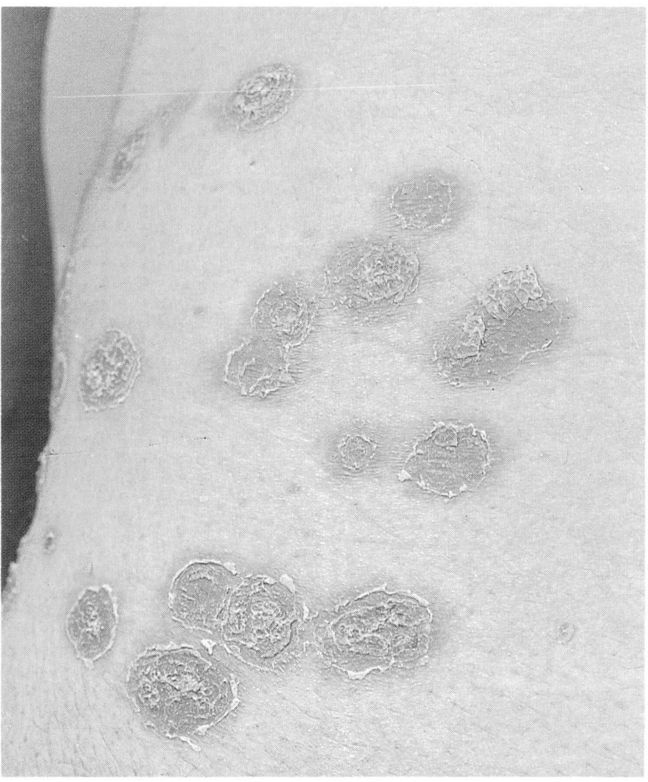

FIGURE 4–72. Reiter's syndrome

Close-up view of individual crusted plaques of Reiter's syndrome. This may represent an unusual, florid manifestation of psoriasis, often exacerbated by underlying infection.

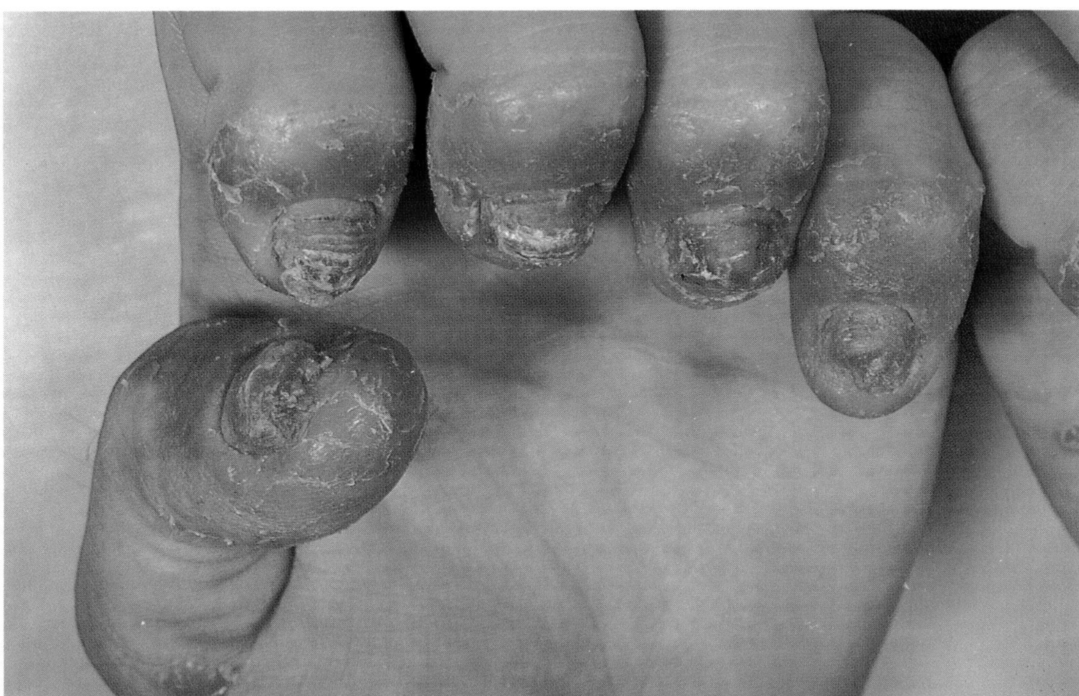

FIGURE 4–73. Reiter's syndrome

Erythema, crusting, and subungual hyperkeratosis are characteristic of the acral lesions of Reiter's syndrome.

Histopathology

The histopathologic findings of seborrheic dermatitis are similar to those seen in patients with non–HIV-associated disease, namely, psoriasiform hyperplasia of the epidermis with mounds of parakeratosis containing neutrophils near ostia of hair follicular infundibula (Figs. 4–74 and 4–75). There is an infiltrate of lymphocytes and scattered plasma cells in the dermis. One finding that is characteristically seen in seborrheic dermatitis in patients with HIV infection and AIDS that is not seen generally in patients with non–HIV-associated seborrheic dermatitis is the presence of scattered individually necrotic keratinocytes.[223] Some have likened this to cutaneous graft versus host disease.[224,225]

Psoriasis, too, has histologic features quite similar to those seen in non–HIV-infected patients. The pattern is generally that of marked acanthosis with regular elongation of epidermal retia associated with dilated tortuous blood vessels in the papillary dermis, thin suprapapillary plates, and mounds of parakeratosis that contain neutrophils. In pustular cases, spongiform areas in the epidermis that contain collections of neutrophils are noted. Reiter's disease has a histologic picture similar to that of pustular psoriasis.

Laboratory Findings

No specific laboratory findings associated with these diseases have been reported other than the presence of HLA-B27 in patients with Reiter's syndrome, as previously mentioned. $CD4^+$ cell numbers may be at any level when seborrheic dermatitis develops, but when it becomes persistent and refractory to therapy, it is generally lower than 250 cells/mm^3. Psoriasis, too, may develop at any point during the course of HIV infection but has been reported to be worse when $CD4^+$ cell numbers are between 500 cells/mm^3 and 50 cells/mm^3. In spite of this, a number of cases have been reported in which severe psoriasis has been seen in patients with profoundly depressed $CD4^+$ cell numbers.

Differential Diagnosis

The differential diagnosis of seborrheic dermatitis includes other papulosquamous dermatoses such as psoriasis, dermatophytosis, and even scabies, as mentioned previously. Psoriasis may have histologic features of other psoriasiform processes including psoriasiform drug eruptions and psoriasiform manifestations of infectious diseases such as histoplasmosis.[193] Other skin disorders that may progress to widespread erythroderma, including cutaneous T-cell lymphoma, drug eruptions, and atopic dermatitis, must also be excluded. Reiter's syndrome must be distinguished from other forms of arthritis such as lupus erythematosus and infectious disorders such as disseminated gonococcal infection.

Diagnosis

The diagnosis of a psoriasiform dermatosis in HIV-infected hosts is generally based on evaluation of clinical and histologic features of the disease in question. In most cases, diagnoses are not difficult to render. Scrapings for microscopic examination should be done to exclude the possibility of fungi and scabies if any question in the diagnosis persists.

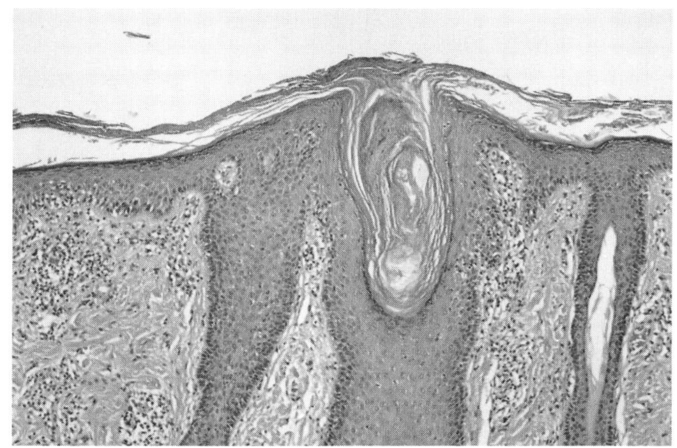

FIGURE 4–74. Seborrheic dermatitis

Photomicrograph. The parakeratosis is present over most of the epidermis as opposed to being located at the side of the follicular ostia.

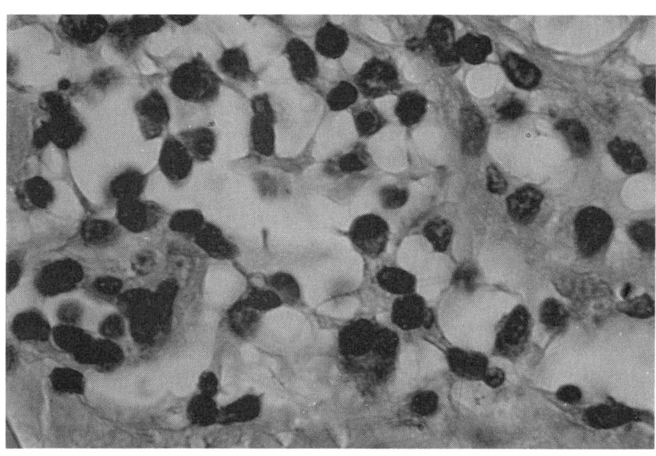

FIGURE 4–75. Seborrheic dermatitis

The inflammatory cell infiltrate in the eruption often consists of many plasma cells.

Treatment

Seborrheic dermatitis is generally treated with topical application of corticosteroid preparations and antifungal creams. In our experience, topical antifungals do not cause significant improvement over what is accomplished by the use of topical corticosteroids. Systemic antifungal treatment with imidazoles such as ketoconazole, itraconazole, and fluconazole have been reported to be of benefit, although patients receiving these medications may develop or present with florid seborrheic dermatitis. Exposure to ultraviolet B phototherapy is also often effective as an adjunct.

Psoriasis may undergo partial remission in response to zidovudine therapy, although recurrence is common.[218] Both spontaneous remission and complete unresponsiveness to all forms of treatment have been observed in HIV-infected patients. Emollients such as hydrophilic petrolatum applied several times daily, 3 to 5% salicylic acid ointment applied once to twice per day for keratolytic effect, and triamcinolone acetonide ointment 0.025 to 0.1% or its equivalent applied for localized short-term therapy are often partially effective. Two percent crude coal tar and petrolatum followed by ultraviolet B phototherapy may also be beneficial. Anthralin 0.1 to 1% cream or ointment applied either overnight or for short duration may have some benefit, but it is not often highly efficacious or well tolerated in HIV-infected patients. In many cases, systemic drugs such as etretinate at a dosage of 1 mg/kg of body weight daily, with or without the addition of dapsone 100 to 200 mg/day, may be required, as may systemic psoralen and ultraviolet A therapy. Methotrexate may be used with extreme caution, beginning at a dosage of 2.5 to 7.5 mg per week, gradually increasing the dose by 2.5 mg per week as needed. More than 20 patients in our institution have been treated without adverse consequences.[226] Patients must be monitored very carefully, however, as this drug may cause worsened immunodepression. Concomitant administration of trimethoprim-containing compounds is contraindicated as the folate reductase–inhibiting effect is synergistic with that induced by methotrexate.[227]

There has been concern that exposure to ultraviolet radiation may cause worsening of immunocompromise in patients with HIV infection, as in vitro exposure of HIV-infected cell lines has been shown to lead to increased production of HIV from latently infected cells.[228] In spite of this, in clinical practice, no evidence of increased immunosuppression or worsening of HIV infection has been observed.[229]

OTHER PAPULOSQUAMOUS DISORDERS

Pityriasis rubra pilaris is a papulosquamous dermatosis characterized by widespread scaly plaques that affect the scalp, trunk, extremities, palms and soles with characteristic follicular involvement and islands of skin that are spared by the disease. Several HIV-infected patients with this disorder have been reported, some of whom developed explosive cystic acne vulgaris in association with the follicular abnormality.[230] Elongated cutaneous follicular spines have been observed, and in one case, histopathologic evidence of mucin deposition was noted.[231] Therapy with 13-cis-retinoic acid (Accutane) or etretinate (Tegison) may be effective, and improvement following the administration of zidovudine may be noted.

Exfoliative erythroderma in patients with HIV infection is most commonly caused by psoriasis although it may be caused by cutaneous T-cell lymphoma, atopic dermatitis, drug eruptions, and severe seborrheic dermatitis.[232–233] A hyperpigmented erythroderma associated with elevated immunoglobulin E levels has also been observed. Staphylococcal scalded skin syndrome as well as toxic streptococcal syndrome are infectious causes of erythroderma and should be considered, as these may be treated with antibiotics.

The psoriasiform dermatitis of AIDS described by Kaplan and associates is a papulosquamous condition that may represent a number of diverse conditions.[234] Histologically, patients with this condition have been shown to have findings similar to those of seborrheic dermatitis or spongiotic dermatitis. Severe xerosis and acquired ichthyosis may develop as a consequence of abnormal nutrition or as secondary to diminished autonomic nervous system function with decreased sweating and diminished sebaceous gland secretion. The problems may develop in 20 to 30% of HIV-infected patients.[235] Patients may bathe frequently using harsh soaps, which also leads to worsening of asteatosis. Treatment consists of the avoidance of soap and water and the application of emollients such as hydrophilic petrolatum or lotions containing 12% lactic acid. Pityriasis rosea may also occur in widespread fashion in patients with HIV infection.

NONINFECTIOUS PAPULAR PRURITIC DISORDERS

Definition

Aside from infestations, a number of cutaneous disorders in patients with HIV infection may be severely pruritic and lead to extreme discomfort. Some of the conditions associated with itchy papular and pustular dermatoses in these individuals include eosinophilic pustular folliculitis, papular dermatitis of AIDS, papular urticaria, severe xerotic dermatitis, and atopic dermatitis. Eosinophilic pustular folliculitis is a condition of widespread follicular papules and pustules that is characterized by an influx of eosinophils in the infundibula of hair follicles. The papular dermatitis of AIDS is a condition of nondescript papules on the trunk and extremities in patients with HIV infection, the etiology of which cannot be determined. Papular urticaria generally refers to reactions to insect bites or possibly to hypersensitivity "recall" reactions to insect bites suffered previously. Xerotic dermatitis refers to severe dryness of the skin, and atopic dermatitis is a condition of heightened sensitivity of the skin to irritating factors that is associated with asthma and elevated circulating levels of immunoglobulin E.

Epidemiology

Pruritic conditions in patients with HIV infection are quite common, although the precise incidence and prevalence are unknown. In a study by Goodman and others, eosinophilic folliculitis was seen in approximately 5% of a series of patients in an HIV-infected population.[235] This number correlates well with figures evaluated in the patient population at our institution. Other studies have shown prevalences of 20 to 30%.[236–238] Other pruritic dermatoses such as papular dermatitis of AIDS, papular urticaria, and atopic dermatitis are seen in variable percentages, probably ranging between 1 and 2% or less. Atopic dermatitis may be seen more commonly in children with HIV infection, having been reported to be present in up to 20% in one study.[239] Xerotic dermatitis is commonly found in patients with advanced HIV infection and AIDS and may be seen to some degree in up to 85% of patients.

Pathogenesis

The pathogenesis of pruritic dermatoses in patients with HIV infection is not entirely clear although several theories may be germane. All patients should be evaluated for the presence of ectoparasites and other pathogens such as scabies and fungi as these may lead to itching. Systemic parasites, too, may lead to itching by inducing urticarial reactions or as a consequence of migrating through the skin. Other causes of hypersensitivity such as drug eruptions and underlying atopic dermatitis may be the cause of itching and should be excluded on clinical grounds. Patients with HIV infection commonly have circulating IgE antibodies to HIV, the levels of which increase as $CD4^+$ cell numbers fall.[240,241] This may correlate with the increased frequency of IgE-mediated disorders in HIV-infected patients such as worsened atopic dermatitis and other hypersensitivity disorders. Basophils have been shown to be hyperreleasable in patients with HIV infection, and it is presumed that mast cells are similarly hyperreleasable.[242] Enhanced degranulation of basophils and mast cells results in increased release of mast cell mediators with attendant inflammatory reactions and pruritus. Patients with HIV infection may also have direct neural infection with HIV which leads to neural irritation and enhanced sensations of itching.[243] This may result in chronic excoriation, lichen simplex chronicus, and prurigo nodularis. Sometimes autonomic dysfunction is associated with diminished sweating and sebaceous gland secretion, both of which lead to worsened xerosis. In addition, patients infected with HIV are under severe stress for a number of reasons, and it is well known that stress may lead to urticaria and itching. Finally, patients with HIV infection may develop pruritus secondary to underlying circulating pruritogens associated with systemic disorders. Liver disease, renal disease, and systemic lymphoma all may be associated with pruritus. All of these factors should be considered when dealing with an itchy HIV-infected patient. In our experience, most patients develop pruritus as a consequence of a primary cutaneous disease rather than secondary to an underlying systemic illness.

Prurigo nodularis is a reaction pattern that may be associated with many of the aforementioned underlying causes of itching. Patients chronically rub and scratch lesions, which results in thickening of the skin.

The pathogenesis of eosinophilic pustular folliculitis is unknown but has been postulated to be a consequence of an exaggerated reaction to *Pityrosporum* yeasts or pseudomonads normally present within follicular infundibula.

Clinical Manifestations

Eosinophilic pustular folliculitis is one of the most characteristic and common pruritic dermatoses to develop in patients with HIV infection. Patients generally present with widespread excoriated follicular papules that commonly affect the trunk, extremities, and head and neck areas (Figs. 4–76 through 4–78).[237] It is important to exclude the diagnosis of scabies, which may look quite similar, by performing scrapings and biopsies if necessary. Although the condition is called eosinophilic pustular folliculitis, it is rare to find intact pustules, as patients are usually so uncomfortable that lesions have been excoriated vigorously by the time they present to the dermatologist. Many patients have clinical appearances that manifest mostly as lichen simplex chronicus and prurigo nodularis.

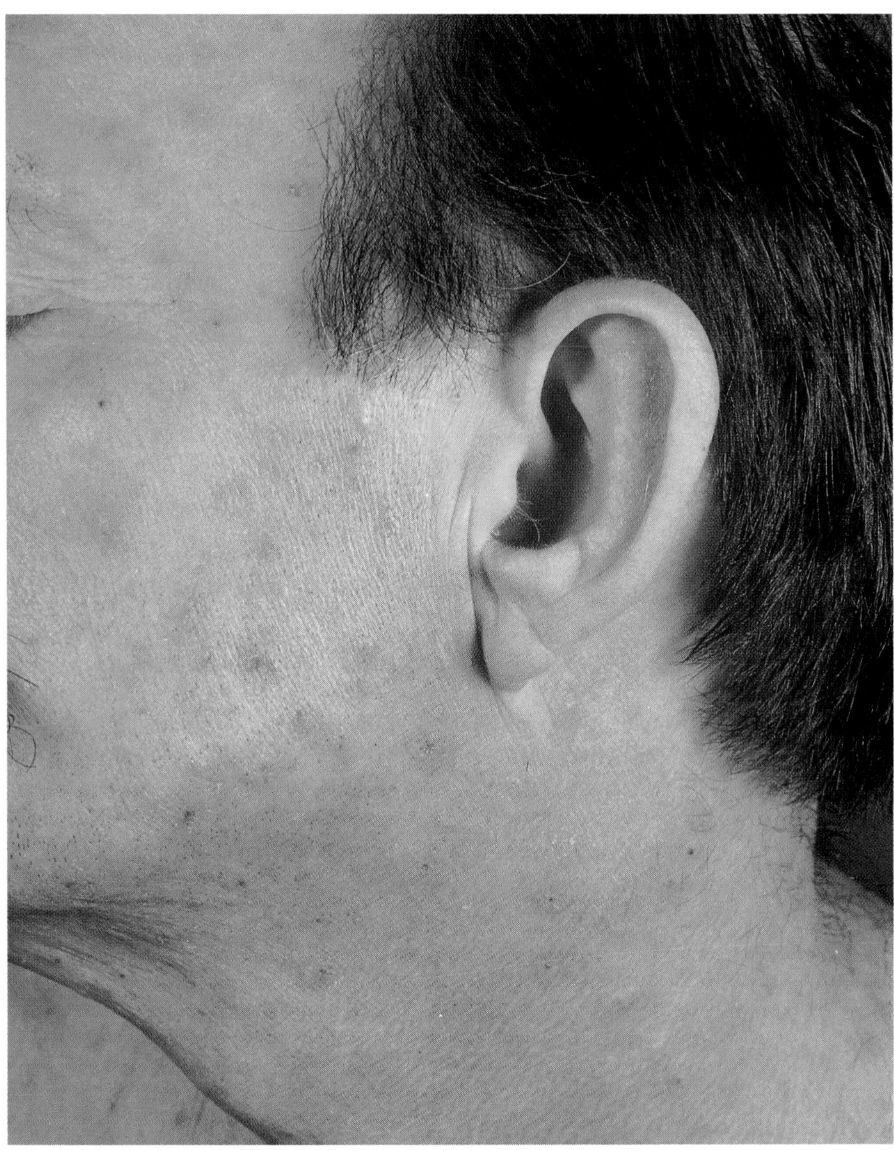

FIGURE 4–76. Eosinophilic pustular folliculitis
This severely pruritic eruption is characterized by generalized perifollicular pustules often involving the head, neck, chest, and back. It usually develops late in the course of HIV infection.

The papular dermatitis of AIDS is a diagnosis that refers to a nondescript papular eruption in patients with HIV infection that cannot be subclassified into any specific category.[241] The original description was that of an eruption of urticarial papules present on the trunk and extremities that were associated with excoriation and rubbing. Many believe that it may represent a reaction to insect bites or eosinophilic pustular folliculitis.

Atopic dermatitis characteristically manifests as erythematous patches and plaques, with fine papulovesicles associated with scaling, crusting, and lichen simplex chronicus. Patients often have associated hyperlinear palms, allergic rhinitis, and asthma. HIV-infected individuals who develop atopic dermatitis may present with severe forms of the disorder with erythroderma.

Xerotic dermatitis generally is characterized by diffuse dryness of the skin with hyperpigmented scales and focal crusting. Many lesions may be fissured, and in some cases, *eczema craquele* develops. This latter complication may lead to localized infection, as the skin is broken and can serve as a portal of entry for bacteria and fungi.

Prurigo nodularis appears as hyperpigmented, dome-shaped, verrucous, often crusted papules and nodules that are usually associated with lichen simplex chronicus. Lesions are induced by chronic rubbing and scratching.

Papular urticaria and chronic urticaria are characterized by pinkish-red erythematous papules and plaques initially with little surface change (Fig. 4–79). Edema and a peau d'orange appearance of the skin are noted. Angioedema may be seen. Although papular urticaria may be excoriated, primary urticaria generally is not.

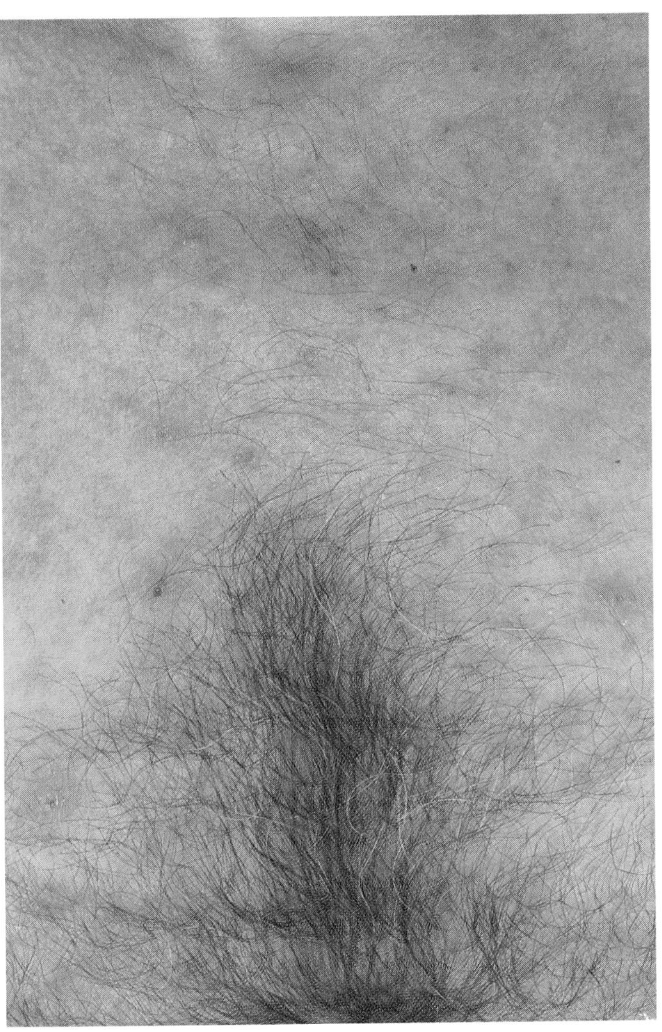

FIGURE 4–77. Eosinophilic pustular folliculitis
Widespread follicular papules, often crusted and excoriated, are seen in this unusual manifestation of AIDS. It is clinically indistinguishable from the appearance of banal folliculitis.

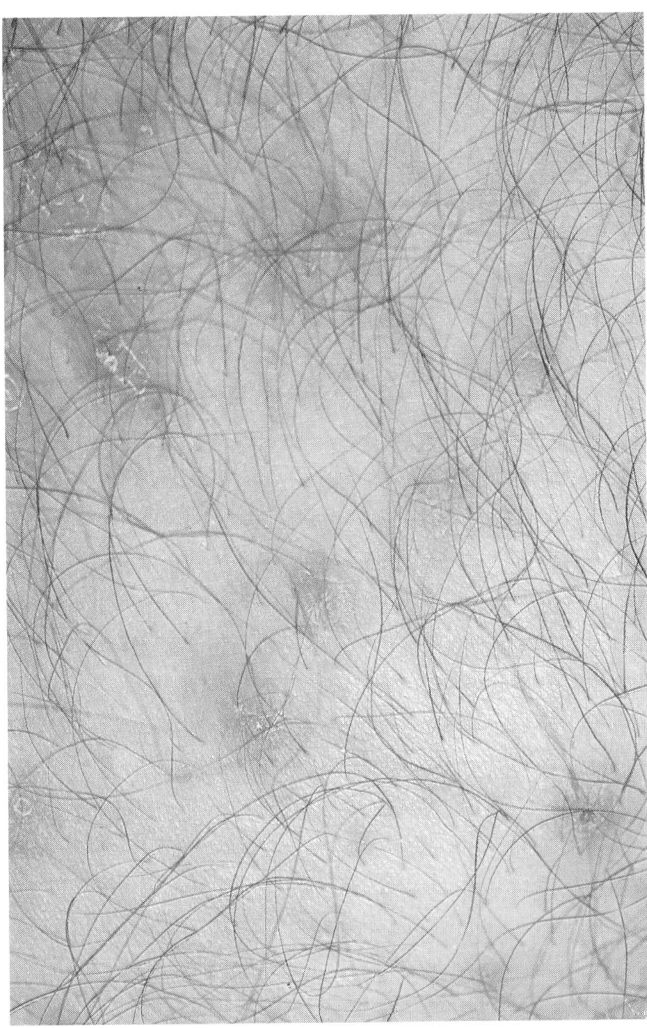

FIGURE 4–78. Eosinophilic pustular folliculitis
Close-up view.

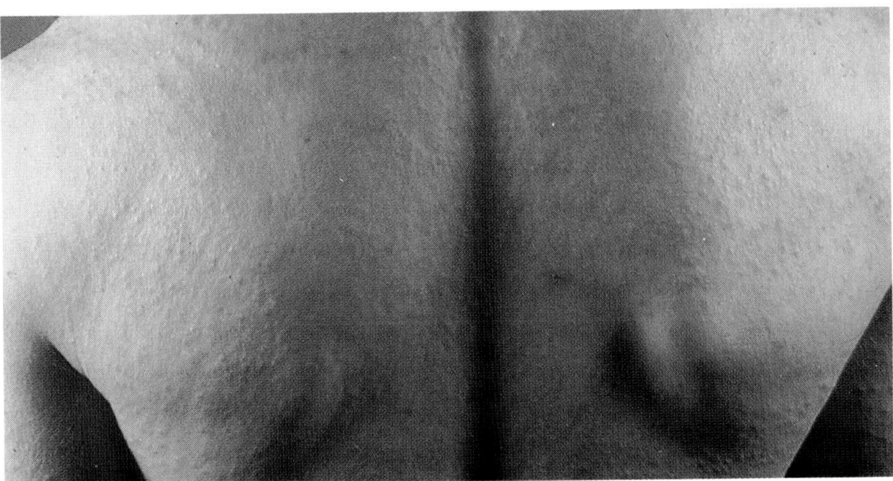

FIGURE 4–79. Papular urticaria
This widespread eruption consists of pinkish red, dome-shaped urticarial papules that are often excoriated. Individual lesions have morphologic appearances similar to those of insect bites.

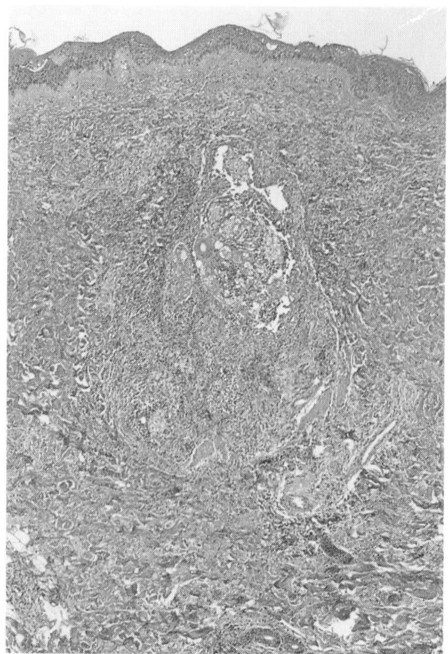

FIGURE 4–80. Eosinophilic pustular folliculitis

Photomicrograph. The inflammatory cell infiltrate is centered within the lumen of the hair follicle, and some is present around it.

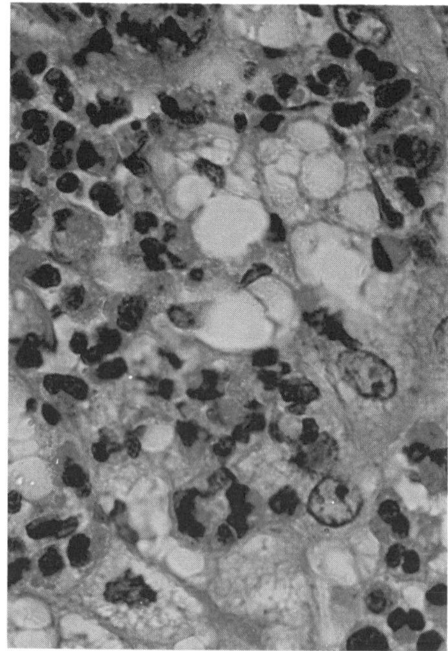

FIGURE 4–81. Eosinophilic pustular folliculitis

Myriad eosinophils in a collection within the affected follicle.

Histopathology

Eosinophilic pustular folliculitis has a characteristic histopathologic appearance that allows the diagnosis to be made in most cases. Within the infundibula of hair follicles are clusters of eosinophils that may be numerous (Figs. 4–80 and 4–81). There is often a perifollicular inflammatory infiltrate of lymphocytes, neutrophils, and some eosinophils, especially in cases in which follicles have ruptured. In some cases, the number of eosinophils may be relatively small in which case the differentiation from bacterial folliculitis may be difficult. When biopsies are performed on long-standing lesions, the primary finding may be that of lichen simplex chronicus or prurigo nodularis, which is manifested by marked acanthosis and hyperkeratosis with coarse, thickened collagen bundles in the papillary dermis.

The papular dermatitis of AIDS has no specific histologic finding but usually has a pattern similar to that seen in insect bite reactions (Figs. 4–82 and 4–83). This pattern most commonly consists of a superficial and deep perivascular and interstitial infiltrate of lymphocytes, some histiocytes, and eosinophils.

Atopic dermatitis has microscopic features of a superficial perivascular infiltrate of lymphocytes and eosinophils with epidermal hyperplasia and foci of spongiosis. Late lesions have a morphology that is primarily that of lichen simplex chronicus. Asteatotic dermatitis or xerotic dermatitis shows very little inflammation in the dermis, with slight epidermal hyperplasia, tiny amounts of spongiosis, and small zones of parakeratosis.

Laboratory Findings

Most patients with eosinophilic pustular folliculitis have $CD4^+$ cell counts of less than 250 cells/mm^3. No other specific findings have been determined in individuals with this condition. Eosinophilia may be found in patients with atopic dermatitis or papular urticaria. Although IgE levels are often elevated, no laboratory test is specific for any of these disorders. If underlying liver or renal impairment is present, characteristic findings of the underlying disorder are usually seen.

Differential Diagnosis

The differential diagnosis of eosinophilic pustular folliculitis includes a number of other pruritic dermatoses that may be found in both HIV-infected individuals and immunocompetent patients. Bacterial folliculitis may be associated with pruritus and has clinical features similar to those of eosinophilic folliculitis. Insect bite reactions, scabies, and dermatitis herpetiformis must all be excluded. In the setting of a pruritic dermatosis in an HIV-seropositive patient with skin scrapings that show no evidence of scabies, the diagnosis can generally be assumed to be eosinophilic pustular folliculitis and treated accordingly without a biopsy in most cases.

Papular urticaria is thought to be a manifestation of insect bite reactions, so it is important to exclude scabies and pediculosis by microscopic examination of skin scrapings. In some cases, careful histories reveal no evidence of insect bite reactions.

Atopic dermatitis must be differentiated from other psoriasiform dermatitides such as psoriasis, cutaneous T-cell lymphoma, and psoriasiform drug eruptions. In general, the presence of severe pruritus and a history of atopy will aid in this diagnosis. Xerotic dermatitis is generally characteristic but should probably be excluded from other forms of dry, scaly dermatoses such as the characteristic "flaky paint" dermatitis seen with kwashiorkor. As both conditions occur in individuals with advanced AIDS, evaluation of nutritional status is essential.

Diagnosis

The diagnosis of these conditions is based on history, physical examination, and performance of biopsies and scrapings when appropriate. As mentioned previously, many of these diagnoses are based on exclusion of other entities, especially scabies, demodicidosis, and pediculosis. Evaluation for causes of chronic urticaria is similar to that undertaken in immunocompetent hosts, although searches for underlying parasitic and protozoal infestations and drug hypersensitivity should be undertaken in all cases because these problems are seen more commonly in HIV-infected patients.

Treatment

Therapy of eosinophilic pustular folliculitis has been the subject of a number of studies because of the frequency of the disorder and the morbidity it induces in HIV-infected individuals. Ultraviolet B exposure has been shown to be quite effective in relieving the pruritus associated with this condition.[238] Patients are generally treated with gradually increasing exposure to ultraviolet B, which is usually administered by phototherapy units. Irradiances beginning at one third of the minimal erythmogenic dose with gradual increase by one third to one half of the previous dose are instituted and continued until remission is experienced. Because exposure to ultraviolet irradiation may be associated with complications of both photosensitivity and activation of HIV-1, indiscriminate use of ultraviolet B or sunlight exposure should be avoided.[228,231] Nevertheless, several studies have demonstrated that moderate exposure to ultraviolet B is safe in the treatment of HIV-related dermatoses if it is administered appropriately.[229] Our experience is similar to that of others, namely, that no worsened immunodeficiency has been noted on clinical ground following exposure to ultraviolet light therapy and that, in fact, the sense of well-being that accompanies this therapy far outweighs the theoretic risk of activation of latent HIV infection. Furthermore, many other agents are administered to patients with HIV infection and AIDS that are known to be associated with activation of HIV, such as granulocyte-macrophage colony-stimulating factor, without adverse consequences. If patients are unable to undergo treatment with ultraviolet B for financial or other reasons, excellent relief may be obtained by exposure to natural sunlight. Use of tanning booths, which provide ultraviolet A, also may be of benefit. In addition to ultraviolet light, administration of itraconazole in doses of 200 mg orally twice a day has been shown to diminish the pruritus of eosinophilic pustular folliculitis.[244] The mechanism of action is unknown, but the drug may act by diminishing the concentration of *Pityrosporum* yeasts within follicular infundibula. Metronidazole, 500 mg orally three times a day,

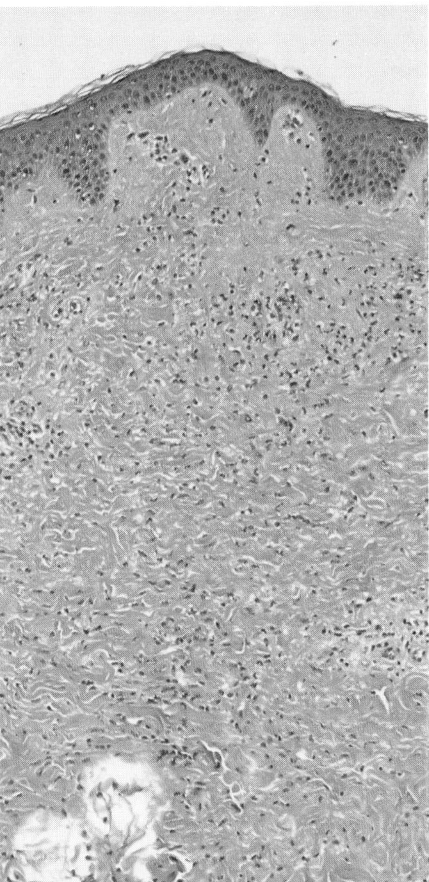

FIGURE 4–82. Papular urticaria
Punch biopsy demonstrates a sparse but diffuse infiltrate in the dermis.

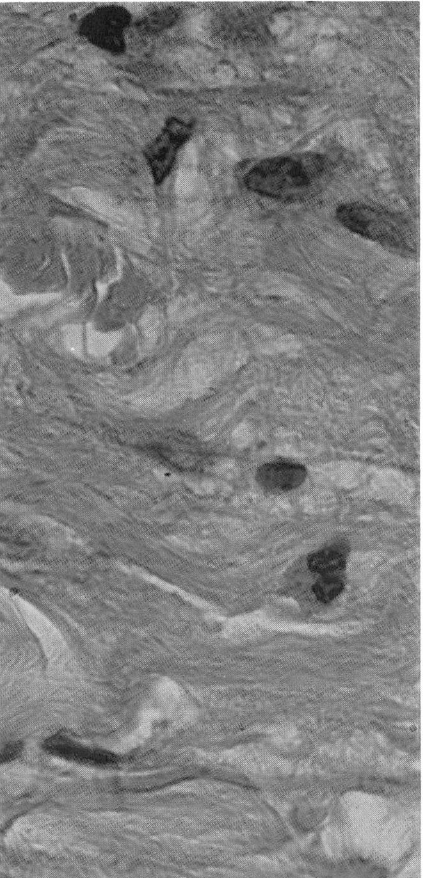

FIGURE 4–83. Papular urticaria
The infiltrate consists of lymphocytes, scattered histiocytes, and numerous eosinophils. The histiologic differential diagnosis includes an insect bite reaction.

also may be beneficial, and in some cases, orally administered tetracycline or erythromycin is effective. Administration of antihistamines such as doxepin at doses of 10 to 20 mg orally every 6 hours as well as topical application of antipruritic agents such as pramoxine and menthol and phenol-containing lotions may also be beneficial in diminishing sensations of itching.

For papular urticaria, systemic antihistamines are generally used. In general, nonsedating antihistamines are not as effective as classic H_1 receptor antagonists that induce somnolence, as this may aid in lessening the perceived sensation of itching. Topical corticosteroid preparations such as triamcinolone acetonide 0.1% ointment or more potent corticosteroid preparations are often beneficial in lessening inflammation. Four percent doxepin cream (Zonalon) is also effective, although no specific effect on the underlying cause is attained with the use of any of these agents. It is important to search for underlying causes of pruritus, such as ingestants that may be causing an allergic reaction. Chronic urticaria is often difficult to control in immunocompetent patients and may be especially problematic in HIV-infected persons. It is usually difficult to establish an etiology.

Xerotic dermatitis generally responds to avoidance of excessive exposure to soap and water and other irritating factors accompanied by the application of potent emollients such as hydrophilic petrolatum and alpha-hydroxy acid–containing preparations. Twelve percent lactic acid lotions such as Lac-Hydrin are quite effective in lessening the severe dryness that may develop in these patients.

Finally, atopic dermatitis usually responds to measures used to treat atopic dermatitis in immunocompetent hosts. These consist of avoidance of irritants and application of emollients and topical corticosteroid preparations.

VASCULITIS AND OTHER VASCULAR-RELATED ABNORMALITIES

Definition

Patients with HIV infection and AIDS develop a number of conditions that either primarily affect the blood vessels with inflammation or are associated with vascular proliferation. Kaposi's sarcoma is discussed under the section on neoplastic disorders. Some of the conditions associated with vascular abnormalities include vasculitis, idiopathic thrombocytopenic purpura, hyperalgesic pseudothrombophlebitis, diffuse facial and truncal telangiectasia, and erythema elevatum diutinum.

Epidemiology

All of these conditions have been reported only sporadically in patients with HIV infection, and thus, no record of a large series of any is available. Approximately 15 cases of erythema elevatum diutinum have been reported in the literature to date.

Pathogenesis

Vasculitis and erythema elevatum diutinum represent manifestations of immune complex–mediated disease. Antigen-antibody complexes collect within blood vessels, leading to deposition of fibrin in walls of blood vessels and attendant signs of inflammation. As the $CD4^+$ cell count falls, the B-cell arm of the immune response may become hyperactive, leading to a relative overabundance of antibody secretion. The altered concentration of antigen to antibody in the circulation leads to precipitation and abnormal clearance of immune complexes.[245] This may be related to the development of idiopathic thrombocytopenic purpura as well. Extravasated erythrocytes result in the characteristic clinical picture of palpable purpura and petechiae. Erythema elevatum diutinum has been associated with chronic infectious diseases such as streptococcal infection, hyperimmunoglobulinemic states, and neoplastic disorders.

Hyperalgesic pseudothrombophlebitis is thought to be related to deeply seated Kaposi's sarcoma with associated secretion of cytokines and inflammatory mediators.[246] Widespread telangiectasias may be associated with a circulating vascular proliferation factor that may be related to fibroblast growth factor or other vasoproliferative agents.

Clinical Manifestations

Leukocytoclastic vasculitis may progress clinically through several stages, beginning as urticarial papules or small petechiae. In most cases, characteristic palpable purpuric papules develop. Lesions are most commonly situated on the extremities, although any body site may be affected. In patients with HIV infection, lesions may be more numerous and more florid than those in immunocompetent hosts. In addition to palpable purpuric papules, pustules, ulcers, and bullae may be seen.[246,247] Erythema elevatum diutinum is a manifestation of chronic leukocytoclastic vasculitis which generally begins as palpable purpuric papules and plaques that in time evolve into indurated reddish plaques often over the joints. The dorsal surfaces of the hands, especially over the knuckles and around the ankles and knees, are common sites of involvement. Plaques may assume a somewhat yellowish color as a consequence of the influx of numerous neutrophils and their degradation, which correlates with the clinical name of extracellular cholesterolosis that was previously applied to this condition. In time, plaques give way to firm, thick, fibrotic nodules that may extend to affect volar skin surfaces. Generally, lesions are asymptomatic, but if they are located on sites of weight bearing, they may be painful.[248,249] Idiopathic thrombocytopenic purpura usually manifests as petechiae or palpable purpura and may simulate leukocytoclastic vasculitis.

Hyperalgesic pseudothrombophlebitis is associated with diffuse swelling of an extremity with extreme tenderness.[250] Patients note marked sensitivity to even the lightest touch. No thrombophlebitic cords can be palpated. Diffuse telangiectasia has a clinical appearance somewhat similar to that of Civatte's poikiloderma.[251] Reddish telangiectatic areas on the cheeks, neck, chest, and trunk are characteristically seen, often in areas that are not significantly associated with sun exposure.

Histopathology

Leukocytoclastic vasculitis has a characteristic histopathologic appearance that is usually diagnostic. Very early urticarial or petechial lesions are characterized by a perivascular and interstitial infiltrate that contains lymphocytes, neutrophils, and eosinophils with abundant nuclear dust. Minimal involvement of blood vessels themselves may be noted so that no fibrin within the walls of vessels is appreciated. In time, inflammatory cells are noted within the walls of small and medium-sized blood vessels with abundant deposition of fibrin. In fully developed lesions, there may be significant thrombi within vascular lumina. Erythema elevatum diutinum also manifests similar histologic findings initially, but in due course, abundant fibrosis is noted around blood vessels and in the stroma. An increase in the number of MAC-387–positive histiocytes and fibroblasts can be demonstrated with immunoperoxidase stains.[248] Only minimal granulomatous inflammation is seen although in some lesions, cholesterol clefts are observed in the interstitium. Collections of neutrophils and eosinophils are seen in late fibrotic lesions even though vasculitis may have abated.

No specific histologic findings have been described for either hyperalgesic pseudothrombophlebitis or diffuse telangiectasias. Some studies have noted a suggestion of diffuse vascular proliferation in random biopsies of normal-appearing skin in patients with Kaposi's sarcoma, although that finding has not been repeatably verified.

Laboratory Findings

Elevated erythrocyte sedimentation rates may be found in patients with leukocytoclastic vasculitis and erythema elevatum diutinum. If an underlying cause of vasculitis is present such as a connective tissue disease, characteristic laboratory findings of the underlying disease are found in most cases. $CD4^+$ cell counts are variable and have ranged from higher than 500 cells/mm^3 to lower than 10 cells/mm^3. Hypocomplementemia may be noted, and if vasculitis affects the kidneys, findings of renal dysfunction such as elevated serum creatinine levels may be present. Prolonged bleeding times will be noted in idiopathic thrombocytopenic purpura. Elevated antistreptolysin O titers or elevated immunoglobulin levels may be found in patients with erythema elevatum diutinum. No known abnormalities are found in patients with either hyperalgesic pseudothrombophlebitis or diffuse telangiectasia.

Differential Diagnosis

The differential diagnosis of leukocytoclastic vasculitis includes other causes of palpable purpura, which are relatively few in number. Schamberg's pigmented purpuric dermatosis or Gougerot-Blum syndrome (pigmented purpuric lichenoid dermatitis) may have clinical features of petechiae and palpable purpuric papules. Urticarial vasculitis must be distinguished from true urticaria. Purpura secondary to abnormal clotting parameters and disseminated intravascular coagulation must be distinguished from leukocytoclastic vasculitis as well, both of which may develop in patients with HIV infection. Generally, biopsies aid in the distinction between these entities. Erythema elevatum diutinum, especially in the nodular stage, must be distinguished from other causes of periarticular nodules, including rheumatoid nodules, nodules associated with rheumatic fever, and juxta-articular nodes of syphilis. Gout and multicentric reticulohistiocytosis may also cause periarticular nodules.

True thrombophlebitis must be excluded in cases of suspected hyperalgesic pseudothrombophlebitis as must diffuse lymphangitic spread of Kaposi's sarcoma. Plethysmography and venography may be required to establish this diagnosis. Diffuse telangiectasia must be distinguished from other causes of poikiloderma, such as poikiloderma vasculare atrophicans, dermatomyositis, and Civatte's poikiloderma, which is a manifestation of chronic sun exposure.

Diagnosis

Diagnosis of each of these conditions is based on characteristic clinical findings and exclusion of other diseases in combination with histopathologic findings. In most cases, the diagnosis is relatively straightforward. Appropriate evaluation for underlying disorders must be taken in the proper clinical context, such as in searching for possible underlying causes of vasculitis.

Treatment

Treatment of vasculitis consists primarily of identifying the underlying cause and correcting the associated abnormalities. In some cases, administration of nonsteroidal anti-inflammatory agents may be beneficial. Colchicine, dapsone, or systemic corticosteroids such as prednisone may be required in severe cases. Before cyclophosphamide, methotrexate, or other potentially immunosuppressive immunomodulators are administered, careful assessment of the immune status of the patient must be undertaken. All patients who are to be treated with agents such as these must be monitored carefully. Idiopathic thrombocytopenic purpura responds to splenectomy.

Erythema elevatum diutinum in immunocompetent patients often responds to treatment with dapsone. In HIV-infected patients, the response to dapsone may be blunted, or there may be no response at all. Surgical excision has been effective in some cases.

Hyperalgesic pseudothrombophlebitis is treated primarily with analgesics. Narcotic analgesics may be required, as the condition is extremely painful. Bed rest, warm compresses, leg elevation, and administration of nonsteroidal anti-inflammatory agents may be useful.

Diffuse telangiectasia may be treated by selective laser destruction using argon or tunable dye laser. Electrocoagulation may also be beneficial. Cosmetic camouflage using green-tinted makeup is helpful in masking the red appearance.

PHOTOINDUCED AND PHOTOAGGRAVATED CONDITIONS

Definition

Several skin disorders that are worsened with light exposure may be associated with HIV infection. These include chronic actinic dermatitis, porphyria cutanea tarda, photoexacerbated drug eruptions, and photoexacerbated rosacea. Granuloma annulare may also be widely disseminated in patients with HIV infections, and this, too, may be exacerbated following ultraviolet light exposure.

Epidemiology

No specific figures exist regarding the prevalence of these conditions, in that most have been reported only sporadically. Porphyria cutanea tarda, however, is being reported with some frequency, although the overall prevalence of this condition remains low. We have observed five HIV-infected patients with porphyria cutanea tarda in the patient population within the last 3 years.

Pathogenesis

Chronic actinic dermatitis may be associated with HIV infection because of the exaggerated B-cell immunity that may be present in these individuals. Patients may develop allergies to drugs and other substances, and, with alteration of the immune system, underlying allergic phenomena may be recalled. Patients with HIV infection are known to produce greater concentrations of porphyrins, possibly as a consequence of abnormal liver function secondary to hepatitis, such as hepatitis C, or other factors. Hepatitis C is of prime importance as more than 50% of all patients with porphyria cutanea tarda have been found to be coinfected with this virus.

Clinical Manifestations

Chronic actinic dermatitis of HIV infection characteristically manifests as psoriasiform lichenified plaques, which are often hyperpigmented, scaly, and pruritic, in the sun-exposed areas of the body.[252,253] Lesions are generally located on the dorsal surfaces of the hands, forearms, face, upper anterior chest, and posterior neck. Extensive lichenification is often seen, and patients may have an appearance similar to what has been described with actinic reticuloid. The appearance of porphyria cutanea tarda is virtually identical to that seen in immunocompetent hosts with blisters on the dorsal surfaces of the hands and other sun-exposed areas that are associated with crusting, milia formation, dyspigmentation, and scarring (Fig. 4–84).[254–256] There is also often hyperpigmentation and hypertrichosis of the malar areas of the face. Patients may describe the excretion of dark urine. Actinically aggravated rosacea looks similar to acne rosacea in immunocompetent hosts with an eruption of follicular papules and pustules on the face. Extrafacial lesions may be seen. Dermal waxy papules may represent granulomatous rosacea that may also be worsened by sunlight exposure. Widespread granuloma annulare manifests as small pinkish dermal papules distributed on sun-exposed areas.[257] Photoexacerbated drug eruptions often appear lichenoid or erythematous distributed on photoexposed sites.

Histopathology

Chronic actinic dermatitis generally is manifested as a superficial and often deep psoriasiform dermatitis with an infiltrate of lymphocytes and abundant eosinophils. Some cases may be associated with a band-like infiltrate and epidermotropism of lymphocytes, many of which may be atypical in appearance. Spongiosis is generally seen and necrotic keratinocytes may be noted. Porphyria cutanea tarda has histologic findings that are similar to those seen in immunocompetent individuals and manifests as a subepidermal blister with minimal inflammation in the dermis. Preservation of dermal papillae, so-called festooning, is seen, as are thick hyaline periodic acid-Schiff–positive rims surrounding blood vessels in the upper dermis. Elongated aggregations of necrotic keratinocytes are often present in the epidermis overlying the blister that have been referred to as "caterpillar bodies."[256] Granuloma annulare also has a histologic pattern similar to that seen in immunocompetent hosts, namely, a diffuse infiltrate of histiocytes arranged in palisaded fashion in the dermis with mucin in the center of the palisade. Eruptive forms of granuloma annulare may be associated only with an interstitial infiltrate without significant palisading. Rosacea histologically has a perifollicular infiltrate of lymphocytes, some neutrophils, and follicular pustules. Often, scattered demodectic mites may be found within the infundibula of follicles.

Laboratory Findings

The only significant laboratory findings are those associated with porphyria in which elevated circulating and urinary uroporphyrins and coproporphyrins are characteristically found. Uroporphyrin levels up to 9000 IU/ml have been reported.[258] Patients with porphyria cutanea tarda have $CD4^+$ cell numbers that range from 3 to more than 500 cells/mm^3, indicating that the disorder may develop at any stage of HIV infection. As porphyria may be associated with liver abnormalities, there is often an elevation of serum glutamic-oxaloacetic transaminase and serum glutamate pyruvate transaminase enzyme levels and, occasionally, hyperbilirubinemia. Of interest, many patients with HIV infection and porphyria are anemic rather than polycythemic. This is important because treatment with phlebotomy cannot be undertaken in such patients.

No specific findings have been reported for patients with any of the other photoaggravated disorders, although most have occurred in patients with $CD4^+$ cell counts below 200 cells/mm^3.

Differential Diagnosis

The differential diagnosis of chronic actinic dermatitis includes true actinic reticuloid as well as persistent light reactivity. Other photodermatoses such as pellagra must also be excluded. Porphyria cutanea tarda must be differentiated from other primary blistering disorders of the skin that may rarely be seen in patients with HIV infection. These include epidermolysis bullosa acquisita, bullous pemphigoid, and bullae associated with ischemia. Drug-induced pseudoporphyria and porphyria associated with renal disease may have virtually identical clinical features and must also be excluded. The differential diagnosis of eruptive granuloma annulare and HIV-associated rosacea include other papular, pustular, and follicular disorders, as well as other forms of granulomatous dermatitis. The possibility of miliary acid-fast bacillary infections and fungal infections must be entertained and appropriate biopsies with special stains and cultures should be performed to exclude those more serious diagnoses.

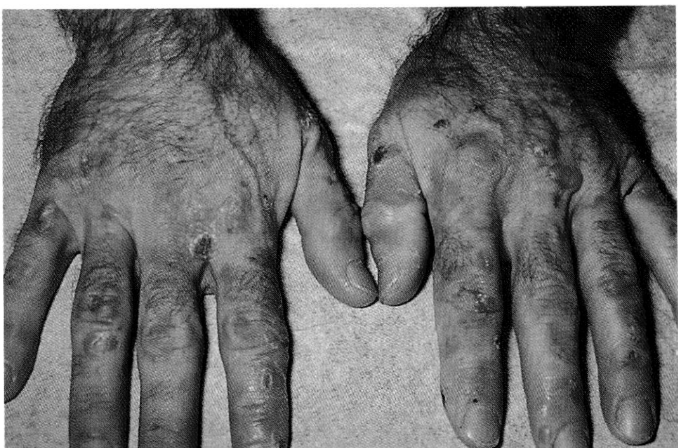

FIGURE 4–84. Porphyria cutanea tarda

There are subepidermal bullae on the dorsal surfaces of the hands that are associated with cutaneous fragility and milia.

Histopathologically, the interstitial form of granuloma annulare may appear similar to Kaposi's sarcoma. Stains to demonstrate the presence of mucin or to define the cells as representing histiocytes or endothelial cells can be used to distinguish the two in difficult cases.

Diagnosis

The diagnosis of chronic actinic dermatitis may be corroborated by the performance of phototesting. Thorough questioning is important to elicit a history of recent exposure to potential photoallergens or phototoxins as well as past histories of exposure to such that may have been reactivated. Porphyria is diagnosed on the basis of clinical and histologic findings as well as demonstration of elevated urinary uroporphyrins and coproporphyrins. Actinically exacerbated granulomatous disorders are diagnosed on the basis of exclusion of infectious diseases and, as mentioned earlier, in the context of characteristic clinical findings.

Treatment

Treatment of chronic actinic dermatitis consists of the avoidance of photoallergens and phototoxins and the application of topical corticosteroid preparations. Avoidance of ultraviolet light is also important. In some cases, even visible light may precipitate a flare of the condition; in these cases, complete light avoidance is essential, because even light emitted from television monitors may be sufficient to worsen the condition. Paradoxically, the use of psoralen and ultraviolet A therapy may "harden" the skin and lead to remission. Administration of hydroxychloroquine sulfate (Plaquenil Sulfate) at doses of 200 mg orally once to twice a day may also be beneficial. Fortunately, the incidence of this often difficult-to-manage condition remains low.

The classic treatment for porphyria is repeated phlebotomy. In patients with HIV infection, who are often anemic, this treatment cannot be used. Low doses of hydroxychloroquine beginning at 25 mg weekly and increasing to 200 mg weekly may be effective in mobilizing accumulated porphyrin in the liver.[259] Erythropoietin has been shown to be effective in treatment of porphyria cutanea tarda by enhancing heme biosynthesis.[260] This results in mobilization of porphyrins. Thus, although expensive, this might be the most beneficial form of treatment, as it tends to correct the hematologic deficit as well as the metabolic one.

Rosacea is treated with the usual antirosacea regimen of tetracycline and topical benzoyl peroxide preparations. Topical metronidazole gel (MetroGel) or systemic metronidazole at doses of 250 to 750 mg orally three times a day may also be beneficial, as *Demodex* mites are thought to play a role in the pathogenesis in some cases. Widespread granuloma annulare may respond to treatment with nicotinamide or the application of topical corticosteroid preparations. As these two disorders may be exacerbated by exposure to light, avoidance of ultraviolet light is necessary in such cases.

CUTANEOUS DRUG ERUPTIONS

Definition

Drug eruptions are cutaneous disorders caused by the oral or parenteral administration of therapeutic drugs. Most are hypersensitive in nature, although others are a consequence of direct toxicity or unusual idiosyncratic reactions.

Epidemiology

Cutaneous drug reactions are the most common manifestation of drug hypersensitivity. A study of 684 HIV-infected patients in Boston revealed that 79% had one or more dermatologic diagnoses, 188 of which included cutaneous reactions to drugs.[261] The incidence of many of these reactions is higher in HIV-infected patients than in the general population, including hypersensitivity to multiple drugs. The best known example of a drug that causes hypersensitivity reactions in HIV-infected persons is trimethoprim-sulfamethoxazole. In some studies, 50 to 60% of HIV-positive patients have been shown to develop a cutaneous eruption that is due to this agent.[262] Up to 45% of patients develop morbilliform eruptions, with variable numbers of other reactions being reported. Black patients seem to have a lower risk of cutaneous trimethoprim-sulfamethoxazole reactions as manifested by a lowered incidence of this eruption in HIV-positive patients treated in Zaire, Haiti, and the United States. Stevens-Johnson syndrome and toxic epidermal necrolysis occur sporadically, with fewer than 50 cases in the literature having been reported.[263] Other antibiotics are common offenders. Morbilliform eruptions may be seen in 10% of patients on antituberculous regimens and in 40% of patients treated with amoxicillin-clavulanic acid.[264–266] In one series, 52% of patients taking a combination of clindamycin and primaquine developed morbilliform eruptions, and in another study, 33% of patients receiving intravenous clindamycin for *Toxoplasma* encephalitis developed an exanthem.[267] Fusidate sodium caused an eruption in 100% of patients with AIDS and 70% of individuals with AIDS-related complex in one study.[268] Thalidomide used for treatment of aphthous ulcers may cause a widespread maculopapular exanthem in 38% of HIV-positive patients treated with this agent.[269] Zidovudine, too, may cause an exanthematous eruption in 1% of patients that may warrant its discontinuation.[270] Other eruptions and toxic drug effects have been reported to occur sporadically.

Pathogenesis

Drug eruptions develop as a consequence of any of the classic hypersensitivity reactions described by Coombs and Gel. Immediate hypersensitivity mediated by immunoglobulin E may lead to anaphylactoid and urticarial reactions. Type 2 reactions involving IgG and IgM antibody may induce hemolytic anemia and thrombocytopenia. Immune complex mediated–reactions may produce serum sickness–like eruptions, drug-induced lupus erythematosus, or morbilliform eruptions, although morbilliform eruptions may also be the result of cell-mediated (type 4) immune reactions. Although the pathogenesis of some of these eruptions is unknown, underlying infection with CMV or Epstein-Barr virus may predispose to adverse drug reactions in an analogous fashion to what is seen with Epstein-Barr virus–induced infectious mononucleosis and ampicillin.[271]

Clinical Manifestations

Trimethoprim-sulfamethoxazole is the best known and most common allergic drug eruption to develop in patients with HIV infection. In most cases, a widespread eruption of fine pink to red macules and papules that affect the trunk and extremities develops 8 to 12 days after initiating therapy and reaches maximal intensity 1 to 2 days later (Figs. 4–85 and 4–86). In some cases, desquamation may supervene. The eruption may disappear within 3 to 5 days even though therapy is continued, although in some cases, the eruption may persist for days to weeks after discontinuation of the medication. Cutaneous eruptions due to trimethoprim-sulfamethoxazole do not always recur with drug rechallenge in HIV-infected patients; however, if the agent is to be reinstituted, it should be done under controlled circumstances to monitor for possible anaphylactoid reactions. Stevens-Johnson syndrome and toxic epidermal necrolysis may also develop as a consequence of trimethoprim-sulfamethoxazole administration. Stevens-Johnson syndrome is characterized by fever and widespread blistering of the skin and mucous membranes of the eye, mouth, or genitals. Toxic epidermal necrolysis is a more serious manifestation of the same process that involves widespread areas of the skin with confluent bullae that can lead to loss of skin in massive sheets. Thirty-five cases of toxic epidermal necrolysis have been reported in HIV-infected individuals.

Anaphylactoid reactions are characterized by fever, urticarial papules, and plaques associated with angioedema, shortness of breath, and bronchospasm. Many patients may have a history of having suffered a maculopapular eruption before the development of the reaction. These eruptions are less common than morbilliform ones but are usually caused by antibiotics.

Zidovudine may induce several different cutaneous complications. The most common reaction is hyperpigmentation of the nails. Blue to brown-black nail discoloration has been reported to occur in more than 40% of patients.[272,273]

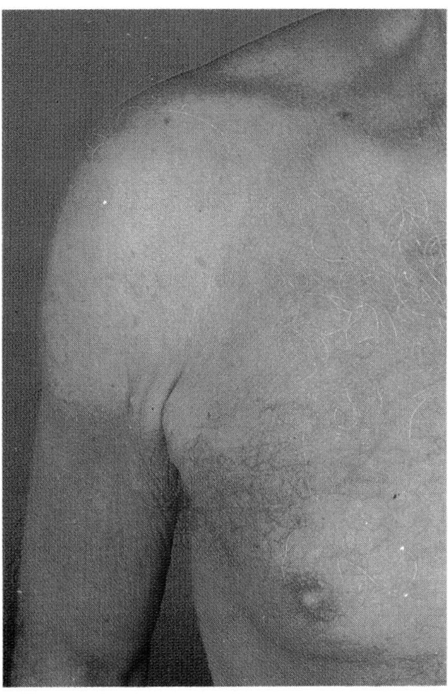

FIGURE 4–85. Morbilliform drug eruption A widespread eruption consisting of pruritic, pinkish red macules and papules is commonly seen following administration of trimethoprim-sulfamethoxazole for *Pneumocystis carinii* pneumonia. The morphologic appearance of this eruption is quite similar to that seen in patients with infectious mononucleosis who have received ampicillin.

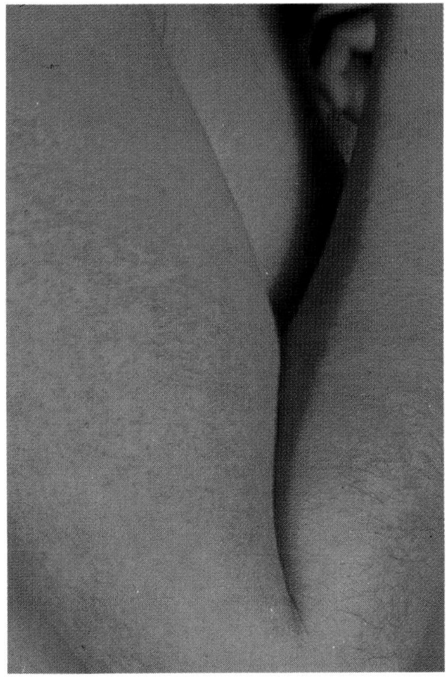

FIGURE 4–86. Morbilliform drug eruption Close-up view shows fine, morbilliform macules and papules.

It is more common in blacks and usually begins 4 to 8 weeks after initiating treatment or may occur as late as 1 year. Longitudinal streaks are most common, but diffuse pigmentation and transverse bands may occur. The thumbnails are affected most frequently. Zidovudine may also induce hyperpigmentation of the mucous membranes and the skin that may mimic that seen with adrenal insufficiency.[274,275] In addition to pigmentary abnormalities, severe exanthematous eruptions may develop within 1 to 2 weeks following the initiation of zidovudine therapy. Lichenoid reactions may appear almost identical to lichen planus, with whitish, lacy plaques of the mucous membranes as well as polygonal pink papules on flexural surfaces of glabrous skin.[276] Other manifestations include acral and periarticular reticulate erythema that may simulate dermatomyositis.[277]

Penile ulcerations due to foscarnet develop following a mean of 11 to 16 days after initiation of therapy. Lesions range in number from two to five, are usually 1 to 5 cm in diameter, and consist of erosive, bullous, tender ulcerations.[278] They usually occur at sites of high urine concentration such as the urethral meatus and scrotum where the tip of the penis rests. Oral and esophageal ulcers may also develop. In addition to ulcerations, a generalized cutaneous eruption has been reported.[279] Widespread erythroderma has been reported in association with rifampin administration.

Parenteral pentamidine may cause severe adverse reactions in 20% of AIDS patients, ranging from morbilliform to urticarial eruptions.[280] Sulfadoxine-pyrimethamine (Fansidar) may cause erythema multiforme and toxic epidermal necrolysis, and aerosolized pentamidine may cause a widespread erythematous maculopapular pruritic eruption.[281,282] Other causes of toxic epidermal necrolysis include chlormezanone, fluoxetine, and thiacetazone.[264,283] Unfortunately, patients sensitive to trimethoprim-sulfamethoxazole also often react to dapsone, so these two agents may not be able to be substituted successfully in every case.[284] In addition to causing an eruption that is similar to that caused by trimethoprim-sulfamethoxazole, the sulfone syndrome has been observed in patients taking dapsone for prophylaxis against *P. carinii* infection.[285] Finally, systemic treatment with methotrexate for psoriasis and with corticosteroids for vasculitis, non-Hodgkin's lymphoma, and opportunistic infections has precipitated both the rapid proliferation and the sudden appearance of Kaposi's sarcoma.[286]

Histopathology

The histopathology of morbilliform drug eruptions typically consists of a superficial perivascular inflammatory infiltrate of lymphocytes with scattered eosinophils associated with vacuolar alteration of the dermoepidermal junction and individually necrotic keratinocytes. In some cases, spongiosis is prominent. Slight parakeratosis may be noted, and scattered plasma cells may be seen. Erythema multiforme, Stevens-Johnson syndrome, and toxic epidermal necrolysis are all characterized by prominent vacuolar interface changes with extensive keratinocytic necrosis of the epidermis. In toxic epidermal necrolysis, the number of inflammatory cells in the dermis may be minimal, although there is confluent epidermal necrosis with no parakeratosis, a consequence of the rapidity of progression of the eruption. Urticarial allergic eruptions are usually characterized by mixed infiltrates of inflammatory cells interstitially in the dermis with minimal epidermal change. Ulcerations due to foscarnet generally show a mixed perivascular and interstitial infiltrate in the dermis with ulceration and epidermal necrosis, although inflammation may be minimal. The changes are relatively nonspecific, and no evidence of vasculitis or thrombosis of vessels is noted. Zidovudine-induced lichenoid eruptions may appear histologically identical to lichen planus, whereas zidovudine-induced nail pigmentation generally consists of an increase in the amount of melanin within melanocytes associated with scattered melanophages in the dermis.

Laboratory Findings

In most cases, laboratory findings are nonspecific, although patients with cutaneous drug eruptions tend to have $CD4^+$ cell numbers below 250 cells/mm^3. Eosinophilia may be noted as a general sign of hypersensitivity. As drugs may induce a number of other systemic problems, it is not uncommon to see accompanying changes such as neutropenia, thrombocytopenia, elevation of transaminases, and anemia. Anemia has been reported to occur in up to 40% of patients receiving trimethoprim-sulfamethoxazole. Neutropenia developed in 35% of patients receiving pentamidine, and anemia developed in 24%. Hypoglycemia may also develop. Transaminase elevations have been observed in HIV-infected patients treated with trimethoprim-sulfamethoxazole, trimethoprim-dapsone, fusidate, and antituberculous drugs. As mentioned previously, IgE levels are also routinely elevated and rise with diminishing $CD4^+$ cell numbers.

Differential Diagnosis

The differential diagnosis of morbilliform drug eruptions includes other morbilliform eruptions such as those caused by viruses. Ulcerations caused by foscarnet may mimic fixed drug eruptions or ulcers of a number of other causes, including those due to infectious agents such as herpesvirus, CMV and opportunistic bacteria and fungi. Lichenoid eruptions due to zidovudine must be distinguished from true lichen planus. Zidovudine-induced nail pigmentation must be differentiated from other causes of pigmented bands in the nail plate such as junctional nevi and acrolentiginous melanoma. Acral and periarticular reticulate erythema induced by zidovudine may mimic dermatomyositis or other connective tissue diseases. Toxic epidermal necrolysis is generally characteristic but must be distinguished from staphylococcal scalded skin syndrome and toxic strep syndrome. Skin biopsy or frozen section evaluation of the roof of the blister will demonstrate confluent epithelial necrosis in erythema multiforme and sloughing of the stratum corneum in staphylococcal scalded skin syndrome.

Phototoxic drug eruptions are reported uncommonly in patients with HIV infection but must be distinguished from chronic actinic dermatitis and subacute cutaneous lupus erythematosus.

Diagnosis

Diagnosis is usually made on the basis of the clinical appearance of the eruption correlated with the history of drug intake. Generally, diagnosis of drug hypersensitivity can be rendered with ease, although because many of the eruptions that develop in patients with HIV infection are unusual and nondescript, the diagnosis occasionally is difficult. Furthermore, identification of the specific offending agent is often challenging, as patients are often treated with many drugs that may not be able to be discontinued and reinstituted sequentially. As a general rule, antibiotics are the most common offenders, followed by anticonvulsants, nonsteroidal anti-inflammatory agents, and zidovudine.[261] Furthermore, patients may be sensitive to multiple drugs. Biopsies may be required, and, in some cases, rechallenge with the suspected offending allergen may be necessary to prove the diagnosis.

Treatment

The most important aspect of the treatment of a cutaneous drug eruption relates to the avoidance of serious complications that may arise if the diagnosis is not made in a timely fashion and the offending agent is not withdrawn. The most serious cutaneous complication is the development of toxic epidermal necrolysis. Other complications include systemic toxicity such as hepatotoxicity or renal damage associated with the sulfone syndrome. Toxic epidermal necrolysis may lead to secondary infection, sepsis, volume depletion, and high output cardiac failure as a consequence of widespread denudation of the skin. Patients who develop this must be treated aggressively in intensive care settings. Whether systemic corticosteroids should be used remains controversial.

Hypersensitivity to trimethoprim-sulfamethoxazole has been treated successfully with desensitization. Desensitization may also be attempted with other antibiotics when necessary.[287]

HAIR AND NAIL ABNORMALITIES

A number of abnormalities of hair and nails may be encountered in patients with HIV infection. Chronic inflammatory and noninflammatory alopecia has been observed (Figs. 4–87 and 4–88).

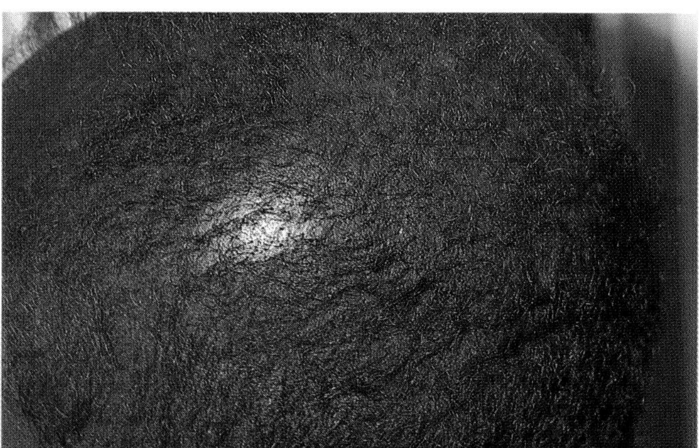

FIGURE 4–87. Alopecia of AIDS

There is a fine, downy quality to the hair, which is increased in density. Notice the relative lack of inflammation seen clinically.

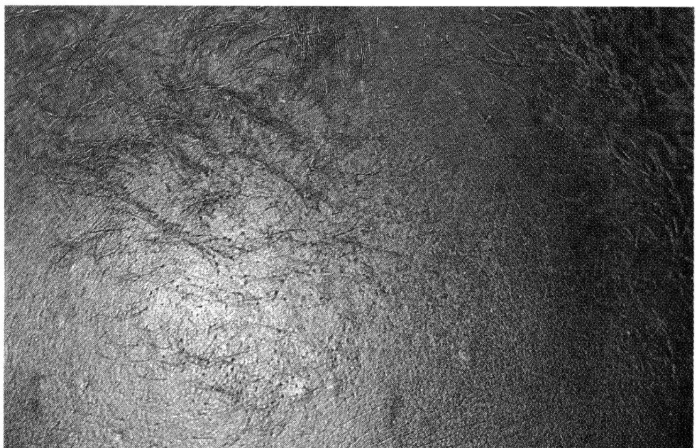

FIGURE 4–88. Alopecia of AIDS

Close-up view. Occasionally scattered follicular papules may be seen that probably represent slight folliculitis.

The hair may become lusterless and dull, and straightening is often noted in patients with curly hair.[288] Although these hair changes may be related to HIV infection of the follicular epithelium as well as concomitant nutritional abnormalities, diffuse alopecia may also be associated with underlying connective tissue diseases or syphilis; these should be excluded on clinical and histologic grounds. Biopsies of the scalp have shown histologic features both of noninflammatory telogen effluvium–like alopecia as well as dense inflammatory cell infiltrates containing lymphocytes, histiocytes, and plasma cells with destruction of follicles.[289] Diffuse, fine, downy alopecia that may or may not be associated with scaling has also been observed, usually in patients with end-stage AIDS. Finally, patients with HIV infection may develop serious infections with fever leading to true telogen effluvium.

In addition to loss of scalp hair, there may be elongation of the eyelashes, a sign of a prolonged anagen phase. This condition has been termed *trichomegaly of the eyelashes* (Fig. 4–89).[290–292] The cause of this phenomenon is unknown, but in some cases it is associated with the administration of drugs such as recombinant interferon A. The frequency with which this problem develops is unclear, but it has been reported in as many as 20% of HIV-infected patients in one study.[290] Other changes of the hair seen in HIV-infected patients include premature canities and alopecia areata.[293,294]

Nail disorders, too, commonly develop in patients with HIV infection. Patients receiving zidovudine may develop elongated pigmented grayish streaks on multiple nail plates, as mentioned previously. Nail plate thickening with subungual hyperkeratosis and dystrophy may be associated with fungal infections due to dermatophytes, *Candida,* and *Hendersonula toruloidea, Scytalidium* spp. and other nondermatophyte fungi. The yellow nail syndrome secondary to metabolic abnormalities, lymphedema, and hypoxia has been reported to develop in HIV-infected patients, as has transverse and longitudinal ridging.[295,296] Diminished thickness of the nail plate may also be seen. Increased nail plate opacity as well as both Muehrcke's and Terry's nails have been seen. Ridging and nail thickness changes are most likely a consequence of diminished matrix growth with decreased nail plate turnover. Just as in immunocompetent patients, Beau's lines may be seen 2 to 3 months after an episode of a serious infection. Involvement of the periungual tissues by infectious agents, psoriasis, and erythema with features similar to those of Gottron's papules may also be seen.

MISCELLANEOUS INFLAMMATORY AND METABOLIC SKIN DISORDERS ASSOCIATED WITH HIV INFECTION

Calciphylaxis is a disorder that represents a manifestation of hyperparathyroidism that develops in association with renal failure.[297] Patients become "sensitized" to elevated circulating levels of parathyroid hormone, following which an insult such as an infection or another metabolic alteration leads to widespread calcification of the skin, soft tissues, blood vessels, and viscera. Diminished levels of protein C may be important in the pathogenesis of the disorder. Histopathologically, there is extensive calcification of small and medium-sized blood vessels throughout the dermis and subcutaneous fat with secondary cutaneous necrosis and prominent thrombosis. Calcification of soft tissues may also be seen. Clinically, skin lesions may appear as livedo reticularis–like areas of the skin with hemor-

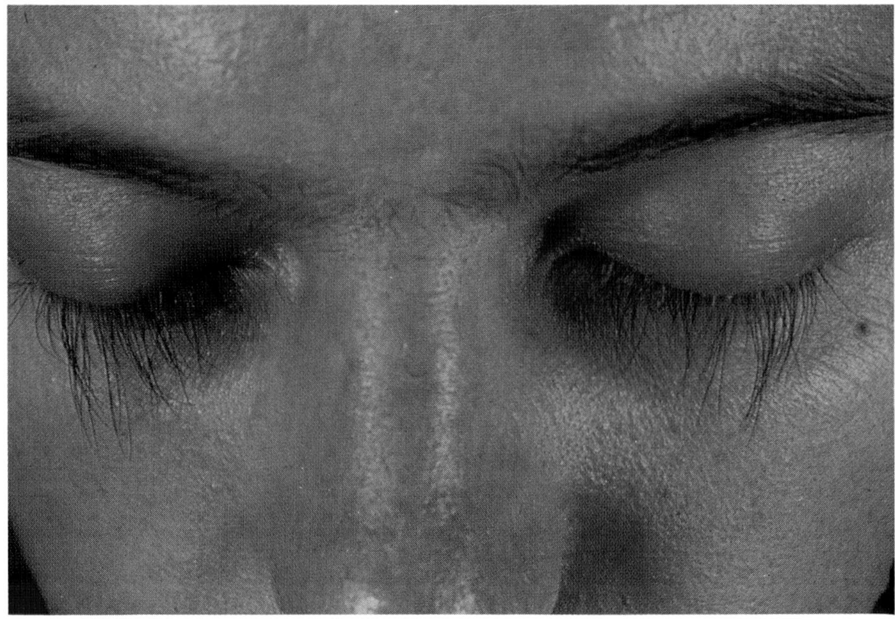

FIGURE 4–89. Trichomegaly of the eyelashes
This phenomenon has been observed in patients who received recombinant leukocyte A interferon, although it is commonly seen in patients with HIV infection or AIDS.

rhage, purplish discoloration, and erythema. They may become extremely painful and progress to necrosis and gangrene over the course of a few days. Treatment consists of correction of serum calcium and phosphorous abnormalities as well as emergency parathyroidectomy. Some patients may have no detectable abnormalities in either parathormone, calcium, or phosphorous levels.

In addition to the diseases described previously, a host of poorly defined inflammatory skin disorders have been noted in patients with HIV infection. These are thought to occur as a consequence of cutaneous eruptions developing in the setting of an abnormal immune state that includes diminished neutrophil function, elevated serum levels of IgE, abnormal T-cell, B-cell, and macrophage function; and the presence of circulating antiepidermal antibodies that have been identified. Widespread scaly dermatoses, serum sickness–like eruptions, diffuse noninfectious granulomatous dermatitis, and gyrate erythema-like eruptions have all been observed, many of which correlate poorly, if at all, with classic descriptions of clinical disorders. In addition to unusual clinical pictures, histopathologic findings correlate with clinical findings in only 30% of cases.[222] Other unusual cutaneous conditions in HIV-infected individuals include lichenoid granulomatous dermatitis, exaggerated responses to insect bites, and nonspecific cellulitis.[298,299]

Adult Kawasaki's disease has been described in four patients with AIDS. Unusual features include the age of onset, pneumonia, arthritis, aseptic meningitis, and the absence of cardiac involvement or thrombocytosis.[300] Clinically, all patients had fever of more than 5 days' duration that was unresponsive to antibiotics and was associated with bilateral conjunctivitis, a generalized confluent macular eruption with edema of the hands that underwent desquamation, oral mucous membrane changes, and cervical adenopathy. The differential diagnosis includes infectious processes such as Rocky Mountain spotted fever and connective tissue diseases.

Acute allergic contact dermatitis and acute anaphylactic reactions as a consequence of latex sensitivity have also been reported in HIV-infected patients.[301] With the increased use of gloves and condoms that contain latex to prevent the spread of HIV disease, the incidence of these conditions is likely to increase.

As patients live longer with HIV infection, it has become increasingly recognized that malnutrition is a common problem that may develop in these individuals. Cutaneous manifestations of protein and vitamin deficiencies may be encountered. An eruption of multiple spiny follicular papules known as phrynoderma may be a manifestation of vitamin A deficiency.[302] Vitamin C deficiency results in scurvy which is manifested as bleeding gums and perifollicular petechiae. Pellagra is manifest as a blistering photosensitive eruption with hyperpigmentation that is associated with diarrhea and dementia. The condition arises as a consequence of pyridoxine deficiency. Kwashiorkor manifests as dry, scaly areas of the skin, which tend to desquamate, giving rise to the so-called flaky paint dermatitis. Diminished luster to the hair with assumption of a reddish-orange color may also be noted. Periorificial erythema with crusting and blistering may be a manifestation of acrodermatitis enteropathica, a sign of zinc deficiency.[303] Once the disorder is recognized, treatment consists of nutritional zinc replacement.

NEOPLASTIC DISORDERS

A number of different neoplastic disorders may develop in patients with HIV infection. These may be classified as epithelial, lymphoreticular, vascular, smooth muscle, and melanocytic. Only the first two are discussed in this chapter.

EPITHELIAL CUTANEOUS NEOPLASMS

Definition

Epithelial neoplasms are either benign or malignant proliferations that exhibit differentiation toward cells of epithelial structures. Some of those that have been described in HIV-seropositive patients include neoplasms of the anorectal area including anal intraepithelial neoplasia, squamous cell carcinoma in situ, fully developed squamous cell carcinoma, and cloacogenic carcinoma; both cervical intraepithelial neoplasia and fully developed cervical carcinoma in HIV-infected women; Bowenoid papulosis; basal cell carcinoma, both primary and metastatic; multiple cutaneous squamous cell carcinomas associated with epidermodysplasia verruciformis; and multiple sebaceous gland tumors. Other noncutaneous epithelial neoplasms that have been observed in patients with HIV infection include small cell carcinoma of the lung, anaplastic carcinoma, testicular germ cell tumors, seminoma, and transitional cell carcinoma of the bladder.

Epidemiology

The incidence of epithelial neoplasms in patients infected with HIV is markedly increased, most commonly in oral, cervical, and anorectal locations. Women with AIDS have been found to have a twofold increased risk for the development of cervical cancer compared with the risk for the general population.[304,305] American patients with AIDS have been shown to have a greater than fortyfold increased risk for the development of anal cancer, and anal intraepithelial neoplasia has been found in a high percentage of patients with AIDS.[306] In one study, cytologic specimens from the anorectal mucosa of homosexual men with AIDS demonstrated abnormalities ranging from atypia in 19% to fully developed anal intraepithelial neoplasia in 15%. Bowenoid papulosis, cloacogenic carcinoma, and transitional cell carcinoma are also increased in incidence in these patients. These neoplasms as well as carcinoma of the cervix are thought to be related to repeated trauma and HPV infection. Human papillomavirus DNA has been detected from the lower gastrointestinal tract and perianal mucosa in up to 54% of HIV-infected male homosexuals.[307] Cytologic techniques used in cervical Papanicolaou smears applied to smears obtained from the anorectal junction in these individuals indicate an HPV infection rate of greater than 50%. The likelihood for the development of anal intraepithelial neoplasia and carcinoma rise as $CD4^+$ cell numbers fall. Up to 11% of homosexual men develop anal intraepithelial neoplasia when $CD4^+$ counts are lower than 50 cells/mm^3.

Women infected with HIV have been shown to have cervical dysplasia rates five to 10 times higher than those of non–HIV-infected women, that is, up to 33% in one study.[308] Furthermore, HPV infection is highly prevalent in these individuals as was demonstrated in one study of HIV-infected women in which 74% had vulvar HPV infection, 47% had condyloma acuminata, and 26% had vulvar intraepithelial neoplasia.[305] It is anticipated that invasive squamous cell carcinoma arising in HPV-induced anal intraepithelial neoplasia or cervical intraepithelial neoplasia may become a major clinical problem as patients survive longer with HIV infection.[309]

Cutaneous epithelial malignancies, although reported in association with HIV infection, have not been shown to be present in significant numbers. In a study of HIV-infected individuals in a military setting, it was found that basal cell and squamous cell carcinoma developed in less than 5% of patients.[310] However, epidermodysplasia verruciformis, a condition of widespread HPV infection with multiple carcinomas, has been reported in several patients with HIV infection.[79,80]

Pathogenesis

Infection with HPV is thought to play an important role in the development of epithelial neoplasia in patients with HIV infection. The HIV *tat* protein upregulates the expression of HPV in tissue, a finding that would be expected to lead to an exaggerated expression of HPV-induced lesions, especially in the context of immunocompromise.[72] Furthermore, the E6 protein derived from HPV-16 interacts with p53 tumor suppressor gene product, causing its inactivation, which may promote the development of neoplasms.[311]

Although HPV infection is prevalent in these patients, only certain types are oncogenic. Thus, HPV-16, 18, 31, and 33 are associated with malignant potential on mucosal sites, whereas HPV-5 and 8 are found in association with epidermodysplasia verruciformis. However, HPV types not usually associated with intraepithelial neoplasia or squamous cell carcinoma have been detected in invasive squamous cell carcinoma in some cases.

Clinical Manifestations

Anal intraepithelial neoplasia and cervical intraepithelial neoplasia are asymptomatic clinically and may have no visible findings. Evidence that these conditions exist are found only by microscopic evaluation of biopsy specimens or exfoliative cytology. Cervical carcinoma initially appears as a red friable area that mimics chronic cervicitis and can only be detected by colposcopically directed biopsy or exfoliative cytology. Similar findings are noted in anal squamous cell carcinoma in situ. Over the course of time, invasive verrucous squamous cell carcinoma may occur either in the cervix or in the anorectal area. These lesions are manifested as indurated cauliflower-like areas that may be deeply infiltrating. Lesions may ulcerate, undergo necrosis, and become painful if nerves are involved. Cloacogenic carcinoma has a similar clinical appearance. Bowenoid papulosis generally manifests as brownish flat-topped papules on the labia or penile skin. Lesions are often hyperpigmented, but in some cases, they appear identical to condylomata acuminata. Rarely, brownish macules may be the only manifestation of the disease. Epidermodysplasia verruciformis has a clinical appearance of widespread warty papules that are either pink or red. In some cases, diffuse erythematous pruritic areas of the skin may be seen.[312] Biopsies are necessary to establish this diagnosis. Basal cell carcinoma reported in HIV-seropositive patients has had clinical appearances similar to those seen in immunocompetent hosts, although multiple primary nodular and superficial basal cell carcinomas may develop (Figs. 4–90 and 4–91). In some cases, metastases of basal cell carcinoma occur, probably as a consequence of immunocompromise.[313] Most metastases have been to draining lymph nodes and the lung.

Histopathology

The histopathologic findings of these conditions range from subtle atypical intraepithelial prolif-

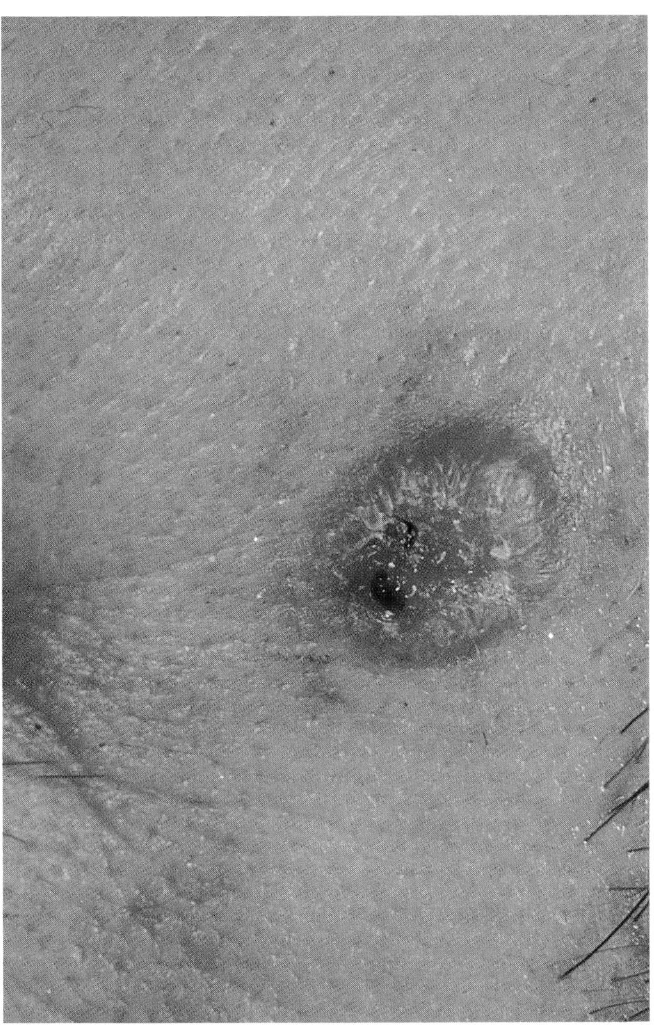

FIGURE 4–90. Basal cell carcinoma

A characteristic reddish, ulcerated, pearly nodule seen on the side of the face of a patient with AIDS. Basal cell carcinomas often behave more aggressively in this patient population.

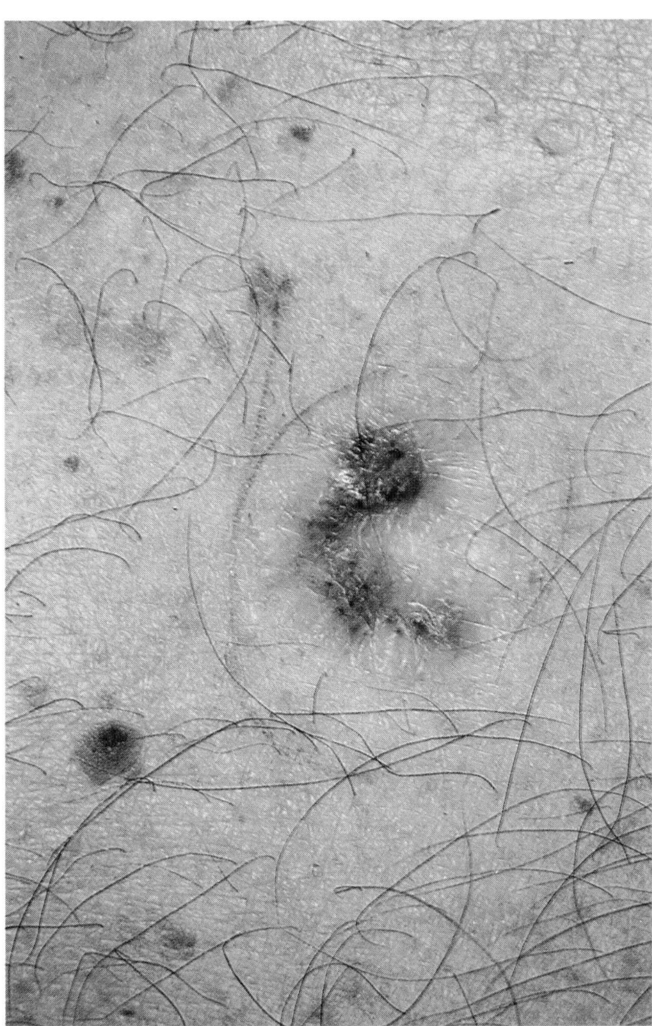

FIGURE 4–91. Basal cell carcinoma

This multifocal pigmented basal cell carcinoma is another example of the types of lesions that may be seen in patients with HIV infection. It should be remembered that these may be multiple and have been reported to metastasize.

erations within stratified squamous epithelial cells that begin at the basal cell layer to full-thickness involvement of the epithelium by atypical neoplastic keratinocytes. Rete ridges are expanded and replaced by atypical cells, many of which are strikingly pleomorphic and in mitosis. In time, bulbous aggregations of neoplastic cells extend from the epithelium into the underlying lamina propria and reticular dermis. Involvement of deeper soft tissues, nerves, and blood vessels may develop in due course. Lesions are often digitated, verrucous, and associated with prominent necrosis.

Bowenoid papulosis manifests histologically by similar cytologic features except that lesions have a histologic architectural pattern similar to that of condyloma acuminatum. Epidermodysplasia verruciformis is characterized by a diffuse infiltrate of pale-appearing cells in the epidermis that represent koilocytes.[79] There is also dyskeratosis and characteristic "corps rond–like" structures in the stratum corneum. Basal cell carcinoma has a histologic appearance that is identical to that seen in immunocompetent hosts.

Laboratory Findings

No specific abnormalities are found in the blood that relate directly to these neoplasms except for the fact that $CD4^+$ cell counts are often well below 500 cells/mm^3 at the time of diagnosis. Immunoperoxidase staining for HPV is usually strongly positive, and HPV genomic DNA can be identified with neoplastic cells by the polymerase chain reaction in many cases.

Differential Diagnosis

Bowenoid papulosis clinically may appear similar or identical to condyloma acuminata so that biopsies are necessary to establish the diagnosis. Squamous cell carcinoma may have clinical and histologic features similar to those of pseudocarcinomatous hyperplasia, including that induced by infectious agents. Giant HPV-induced verrucous carcinoma may have histologic features similar to those of giant condylomata. These lesions are similar clinically to those of the Buschke-Löwenstein variant of verrucous carcinoma. Clinically, epidermodysplasia verruciformis may simulate widespread warts or, in some cases, other forms of erythroderma or widespread erythematous scaly dermatoses. Basal cell carcinoma may mimic molluscum contagiosum as well as nondescript papular lesions of opportunistic infections.

Diagnosis

Diagnosis is established primarily on the basis of clinical appearance and skin biopsy. Of interest, recent studies have evaluated the efficacy of exfoliative cytology in determining the presence of intraepithelial neoplasia of the cervix and anal areas and have found a high rate of false-negative results compared with those from colposcopically or sigmoidoscopically directed tissue biopsies.[314]

Treatment

Treatment of squamous cell carcinoma usually requires excision or aggressive destructive measures. Cryotherapy, generally used for the management of cervical intraepithelial neoplasia, has been shown in one study to have an overall efficacy of 25%, significantly below that observed in HIV-seronegative patients.[315] Carbon dioxide laser destruction may be more effective in this setting. Bowenoid papulosis, although generally treated with simple cryosurgical destruction or topical application of 5-fluorouracil, should be treated with either electrodesiccation and curettage or other destructive surgical measures, with biopsy confirmation of removal, rather than with conservative topical measures. Basal cell carcinoma also should be treated aggressively with destructive measures such as cryosurgery or excision, as there is the potential for metastasis in HIV-infected immunocompromised hosts. Epidermodysplasia verruciformis may be refractory to all forms of therapy. Any neoplasms that develop should be destroyed or excised. Systemic administration of retinoids such as etretinate or isotretinoin at doses of 1 to 2 mg/kg may be effective in preventing development of carcinomas.

LYMPHORETICULAR MALIGNANCIES

Definition

A number of different lymphoreticular malignancies of both B- and T-cell lineage may develop in patients with HIV infection. The majority of these affect the lymph nodes and the reticuloendothelial system although the skin may be involved primarily or secondarily. Non-Hodgkin's lymphoma and mostly high grade (small, noncleaved cell and large cell immunoblastic) and intermediate grade (diffuse large cell) B-cell lymphomas are seen most commonly, although cutaneous T-cell lymphomas, Hodgkin's disease, lymphomatoid granulomatous (angiocentric peripheral T-cell) lymphoma, and adult T-cell leukemia-lymphoma caused by human T-cell leukemia-lymphoma virus–1 have been reported.

Incidence

The greatest proportion of the increase in incidence of non-Hodgkin's lymphomas has been in patients with HIV infection. The incidence of non-Hodgkin's lymphoma in never-married men in the Los Angeles area is nearly twice that of married men aged

15 to 54.[316] In San Francisco, the rate of non-Hodgkin's lymphoma is five times greater in patients with HIV infection than in non–HIV-infected individuals.[317] Hodgkin's disease that is associated with HIV infection is less well appreciated, but several studies have demonstrated a statistically significant increase in the incidence of this neoplasm as well. Other lymphomas such as cutaneous T-cell lymphoma have been reported sporadically.

Pathogenesis

Approximately 25% of AIDS patients with non-Hodgkin's lymphoma have had a prior history of generalized lymphadenopathy with histologic findings of follicular hyperplasia observed on biopsy. These lymph nodes contain polyclonal proliferations of B lymphocytes, a finding similar to what is seen in African children with endemic Burkitt's lymphoma as well as in iatrogenically immunosuppressed patients.[318] Polyclonal B-cell proliferation is thought to be caused directly by a viral infection or as a consequence of the loss of T-cell immunoregulation. Clonal immunoglobulin heavy chain rearrangements, however, have been found in HIV-associated lymph node hyperplasia, suggesting a premalignant nature of such proliferations. In most cases, lymphomas associated with HIV infection represent monoclonal lymphocytic neoplasia, although on occasion more than one neoplastic clone may be demonstrated. Chromosomal abnormalities are also well documented in patients with HIV-related lymphoma, with translocations between chromosomes 8 and 14 being found in the majority of endemic and nonendemic Burkitt's lymphoma–like tumors.[319] The translocation breakpoint in chromosome 8 is near the c-*myc* proto-oncogene region, which suggests that rearrangements of the c-*myc* oncogene may be related to malignant transformation in these patients. Juxtaposition of this gene to important regulatory regions may cause unregulated transcriptional activation and monoclonal proliferation of tumor cells. Other chromosomal abnormalities that have been documented in patients with AIDS-related lymphoma include duplications and deletions of chromosomes 1, 7, 9, and 12.[319]

Epstein-Barr virus infection is another factor of importance in the pathogenesis of HIV-related lymphoma, as this virus may be found in a high percentage of HIV-associated non-Hodgkin's lymphomas. Activation of the B-cell arm of the immune system develops in HIV-infected patients as a consequence of constant stimulation by foreign antigens. Concomitant infection by Epstein-Barr virus may lead to immortalization of infected lymphocytes, resulting in uncontrolled lymphoproliferation and, eventually, malignancy.

Clinical Manifestations

Most cases of lymphoma in HIV-infected patients involve visceral sites. When the skin is affected by non-Hodgkin's lymphoma, the disease usually manifests as pink to purplish papules or nodules (Fig. 4–92). Any site may be affected, including the head and neck, trunk, or extremities. Deeply seated soft tissue involvement may expand superficially, forming dome-shaped nodules that often ulcerate. Cutaneous Hodgkin's disease appears similar to non-Hodgkin's lymphoma either as diffuse nodular lesions or as a "panniculitis." Cutaneous T-cell lymphoma that is related to HIV may have a clinical appearance similar to that of mycosis fungoides, manifesting as widespread plaques that may progress

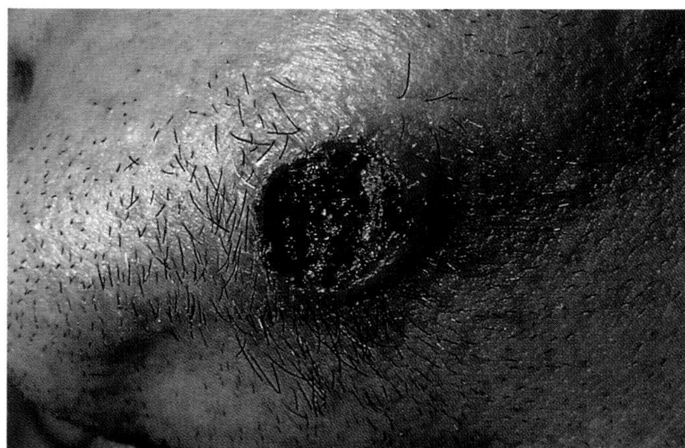

FIGURE 4–92. Cutaneous B-cell lymphoma
In this patient, necrotic nodules were present on the head and neck in association with systemic lymphomatosis.

to erythroderma.[320] Human T-cell lymphotropic virus-1–associated lymphoma may also resemble mycosis fungoides although it may have a clinical picture of an acute viral exanthem with an eruption of morbilliform papules and small, fine vesicles.[321]

Histopathology

When the skin is affected by lymphoma, there is generally a diffuse infiltrate of atypical lymphoid cells that are monomorphous in appearance (Figs. 4–93 and 4–94). Many of the cells are large, pleomorphic, and in mitosis. The infiltrate tends to be deeply situated, affecting the lower portions of the dermis and the subcutaneous fat, and extensive necrosis often occurs along with obliteration of preexisting adnexal structures. Hodgkin's disease may have an appearance similar to that of an inflammatory infiltrate in the skin, although the diffuse nature of the infiltrate and the presence of large, atypical cells having a Reed-Sternberg–like morphology generally aid in making the diagnosis. Cutaneous T-cell lymphoma is usually manifested histologically by psoriasiform hyperplasia of the epidermis with a band-like infiltrate of atypical lymphocytes, many having convoluted nuclei with a cerebriform appearance. These cells are also present in the epidermis, where they often form small collections. In some cases, minimal epidermotropism is noted, but the atypical nature of the cells allows the diagnosis to be made. In cases of lymphoma that are associated with human T-cell lymphotropic virus-1, neoplastic lymphocytes are often extremely large and multilobulated, having a "cloverleaf" appearance. There is also usually prominent exocytosis, and, because there is an associated leukemia, atypical lymphoid cells are often seen in blood vessels and lymphatics.

Laboratory Findings

In patients with systemic lymphoma, no specific laboratory findings are noted although patients generally have $CD4^+$ counts of less than 250 cells/mm^3 when the diagnosis of lymphoma is made. Patients may have abundant circulating atypical lymphocytes that may number up to 600,000 cells/mm^3 in Sézary's syndrome and in adult T-cell lymphoma-leukemia. In contrast, when hemophagocytosis or extensive bone marrow involvement supervenes, there may be profound anemia and pancytopenia.

Differential Diagnosis

The differential diagnosis of malignant lymphomas in the skin includes other lymphoid infiltrates such as inflammatory pseudolymphomas and other malignant neoplasms that may spread to the skin. Cutaneous T-cell lymphoma may mimic inflammatory dermatoses including psoriasis, atopic dermatitis, and other forms of erythroderma. Ulcerated nodules of lymphoma may be nondescript and may simulate any cause of cutaneous ulceration in the skin ranging from infection to trauma.

Diagnosis

The routine diagnosis of these neoplasms is based on the characteristic clinical appearance taken in the context of histopathologic features. In many cases, the use of gene rearrangement studies, flow cytometric immunologic analysis, and DNA probes is necessary to further characterize and subtype the neoplasm. Immunophenotyping of mycosis fungoides–like CTCL in HIV patients may be characterized by an infiltrate of $CD8^+$ lymphocytes in some cases.[321] Human T-cell lymphotropic virus-1–associated leukemia-lymphoma is characterized by an infiltrate of $CD4^+$ cells with absent $CD2^+$ and $CD7^+$ antigens.[322]

Treatment

Treatment consists of the usual therapy for systemic lymphoma. Some of the regimens utilized include methotrexate, prednisone, bleomycin, doxorubicin (Adriamycin), cyclophosphamide, and vincristine. Cutaneous T-cell lymphoma may respond to psoralen and ultraviolet A therapy, total body electron beam, and topical nitrogen mustard. As expected, however, these lymphomas tend to be more aggressive than those in patients who are immunocompetent; survival is generally between 5 and 10 months following diagnosis.[323] As patients are already immunocompromised, administration of many of these agents may cause profound immunocompromise and acceleration of death.

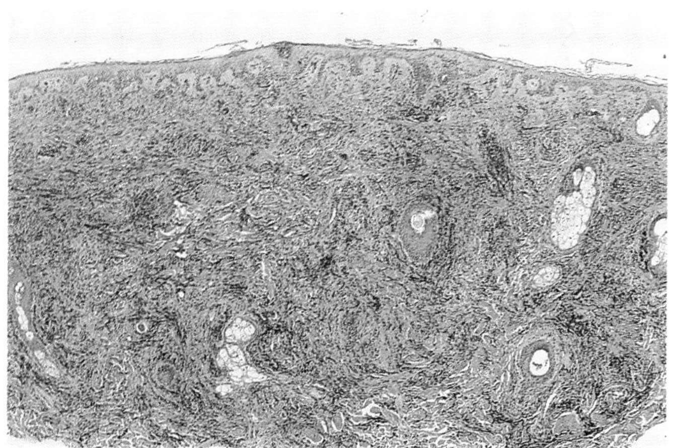

FIGURE 4–93. Histopathology of cutaneous B-cell lymphoma
There is a diffuse infiltrate of darkly staining cells extending throughout the dermis. Hematoxylin and eosin stain (original magnification ×40).

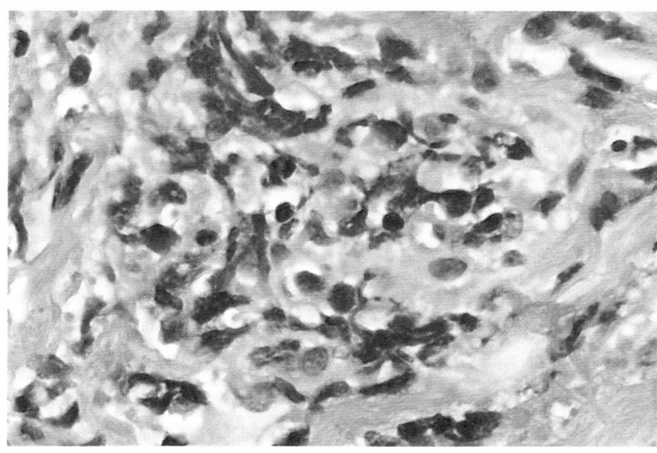

FIGURE 4–94. Cutaneous B-cell lymphoma
Higher magnification demonstrates the pleomorphism and cytologic atypia of neoplastic lymphocytes. In this case, the cells stain positively with antibodies directed to CD20, a B-cell marker.

References

1. Lange JM, Boucher CA, Hollak CE, Wiltink EH, Reiss P, van Royen EA, Roos M, Danner SA, Goldsmit J. Failure of zidovudine prophylaxis after accidental exposure to HIV-1. N Engl J Med 1990;322:1375–1377.
2. Collier AC, Meyers JD, Corey L, Murphy VL, Roberts PL, Handsfield HH. Cytomegalovirus infection in homosexual men. Relationship to sexual practices, antibody to human immunodeficiency virus and cell-mediated immunity. Am J Med 1987;82:593–601.
3. Lin CS, Penha PD, Krishnan MN, Zak FG. Cytomegalic inclusion disease of the skin. Arch Dermatol 1981;117:282–284.
4. Feldman PS, Walker AN, Baker R. Cutaneous lesions heralding disseminated cytomegalovirus infections. J Am Acad Dermatol 1982;7:545–548.
5. Muehler-Stamou A, Sen HJ, Emodi G. Epidermolysis in a case of severe cytomegalovirus infection. BMJ 1974;3:609–611.
6. Minars N, Silverman JF, Escobar MR, Martinez AJ. Fatal cytomegalic inclusion disease: Associated skin manifestations in a renal transplant patient. Arch Dermatol 1977;113:1569–1571.
7. Horn TD, Hood AF. Cytomegalovirus is predictably present in perineal ulcers from immunosuppressed patients. Arch Dermatol 1990;126:642–644.
8. Lee JY, Peel R. Concurrent cytomegalovirus and herpes simplex virus infections in skin biopsy specimens from two AIDS patients with fatal CMV infection. Am J Dermatopathol 1989;11:136–143.
9. Greenspan JS, Greenspan D, Lennette ET, Abrams DI, Conant MA, Petersen V, Freese UK. Replication of Epstein-Barr virus within the epithelial cells of oral "hairy" leukoplakia, an AIDS associated lesion. N Engl J Med 1985;313:1564–1571.
10. Reichart PA, Langford A, Gelderblom HR, Pohle HD, Becker J, Wolf H. Oral hairy leukoplakia: Observations in 95 cases and review of the literature. J Oral Pathol Med 1989;18:410–415.
11. Greenspan D, Greenspan JS, Overby G, Hollander H, Abrams DI, MacPhail L, Borowsky C, Feigal DW Jr. Risk factors for rapid progression from hairy leukoplakia to AIDS: A nested case-control study. J Acquir Immune Defic Syndr 1991;4:652–658.
12. Worrell JT, Cockerell CJ. Histopathologic findings of cutaneous nerves in herpes simplex and varicella zoster virus infection. J Cutan Pathol, in press.
13. Smith KJ, Skelton HG, Angritt P. Histopathologic features of HIV-associated skin disease. Dermatol Clin 1991;9:551–578.
14. Cockerell CJ. Mucocutaneous signs of AIDS other than Kaposi's sarcoma. In: Friedman-Kien AE, ed. Color Atlas of AIDS. Philadelphia: WB Saunders; 1989:96.
15. DeSouza YG, Greenspan D, Felton JR, Hartzog GA, Hammer M, Greenspan JS. Localization of Epstein-Barr virus DNA in the epithelial cells of oral hairy leukoplakia by in situ hybridization of tissue sections (letter). N Engl J Med 1989;320:1559.
16. Tindall B, Barker S, Donovan B, Barnes T, Roberts J, Kronenberg C, Gold J, Penny R, Cooper D. Characterization of the acute clinical illness associated with human immunodeficiency virus infection. Arch Intern Med 1988;148:945–949.
17. Sinicco A, Palestro G, Caramello P, Giacobbi D, Guiliani G, Paggi G, Sciandra M, Gioannini P. Acute HIV-1 infection: Clinical and biologic study of twelve patients. J Acquir Immune Defic Syndr 1990; 3:260–265.
18. Gaines H. Primary HIV infection. Clinical and diagnostic aspects. J Infect Dis (suppl) 1989;61:1–46.
19. Ho DD, Sarngadharan MG, Resnick L, Dimarzoveronese F, Rota TR, Hirsh MS. Primary human T-lymphotropic virus type III infection. Ann Intern Med 1985;103:880–883.
20. Ciesielski C, Metler R, Hammett T, Ward J, Berkelman R. National surveillance for occupationally acquired HIV infections in the United States. Poster presentation, VIII International Conference on AIDS, Amsterdam, July 19–24, 1992.
21. Kinlock S, de Saussure PH, Vanhems PH, Hirshel B, Perrin L. Primary HIV infection: A prospective and retrospective study. Poster presentation, VIII International Conference on AIDS, Amsterdam, July 19–24, 1992.
22. Rabeneck L, Popovic M, Gartner S, McLeod WA, Read E, Wong KK, Boyko WJ. Acute HIV infection presenting with painful swallowing and esophageal ulcers. JAMA 1990;263:2318–2322.
23. Isaksson B, Albert J, Chiodi F, Furucrona A, Krook A, Putkonen P. AIDS two months after primary human immunodeficiency virus infection. J Infect Dis 1988;158:866–868.
24. McMillan A, Bishop PE, Aw D, Peutherer JF. Immunohistology of the skin rash associated with acute HIV infection. AIDS 1989;3:309–312.
25. Henderson DK, Gerberding JL. Prophylactic zidovudine after occupational exposure to the human immunodeficiency virus: An interim analysis: J Infect Dis 1989;160:321–323.
26. Looke DFM, Grove DI. Failed prophylactic zidovudine after needlestick injury (letter): Lancet 1990; 335:1280.
27. Safran S, Ashley R, Houlihan C, Cusick PS, Mills J. Clinical and serologic features of herpes simplex virus infection in patients with AIDS. AIDS 1991;5:1107–1110.
28. Klatt EC, Shibata D. Cytomegalovirus infection in the acquired immunodeficiency syndrome. Arch Pathol Lab Med 1988;112:540–544.
29. Masur H. Clinical implications of herpes virus infections in patients with AIDS. Am J Med 1992; 92(2A):1S–2S.
30. Corey YL, Spear PG. Infections with herpes simplex viruses (part II). N Engl J Med 1986;314:749–756.
31. Simonson JN, Cameron WD, Gakenya MN, et al. Human immunodeficiency virus infection among men with sexually transmitted diseases: Experience from a center in Africa. N Engl J Med 1988;319:274–278.
32. Stamm WE, Hansfield HH, Rompalo AM, Ashley RL, Roberts PL, Corey L. The association between genital ulcer disease and acquisition of HIV infection in homosexual men. JAMA 1988;260:1429–1433.
33. Lawrence J. Perspective. Molecular interactions among herpes viruses and human immunodeficiency viruses. J Infect Dis 1990;162: 338–347.
34. Friedman-Kien AE, LaFleur FL, Gendler EC, Hennessey NP, Montagna R, Halbert S, Rubinstein P, Krasinski K, Zang E, Poiesz B. Herpes zoster: A possible early clinical sign for development of acquired immunodeficiency syndrome in high-risk individuals. J Am Acad Dermatol 1986;14:1023–1028.
35. Rogues AM, Dupon M, Ladner J, Ragnaud JM, Pellegrin JL, Dabis F. Herpes zoster and human immunodeficiency virus infection: A cohort study of 101 co-infected patients (letter). J Infect Dis 1993;168:245.
36. Buchbinder SP, Katz MH, Hessol NA, Liu JY, O'Malley PM, Underwood R, Holmberg SD. Herpes zoster and human immunodeficiency virus infection. J Infect Dis 1992;166:1153–1156.
37. Melbye EM, Grossman RJ, Goedert J, Eyster ME, Biggar RJ. Risk of AIDS after herpes zoster. Lancet 1987;1: 728–731.
38. Siegal FP, Lopez C, Hammer GS, Brown AE, Kornfeld SJ, Gold J, Hassett J, Hirschman SZ, Cunningham-Rundles C, Adelsberg BR, et al. Severe acquired immunodeficiency in male homosexuals, manifested by chronic perianal ulcerative herpes simplex lesions. N Engl J Med 1981;305:1439–1444.
39. Norris SA, Kessler HA, Fife KH. Severe progressive herpetic whitlow caused by an acylovir-resistant virus in a patient with AIDS (letter). J Infect Dis 1988;157:209–210.
40. Zimmerli W, Bianchi L, Goudat F, et al. Disseminated herpes simplex type 2 in systemic *Candida* infection in a patient with previous asymptomatic

human immunodeficiency virus infection (letter). J Infect Dis 1988;157: 597–598.
41. Marks GL, Nolan PE, Erlich KS, Ellis MN. Mucocutaneous dissemination of acylovir-resistant herpes simplex virus in a patient with AIDS. Rev Infect Dis 1989;11:474–476.
42. Jura E, Chadwick EG, Josephs HS, Steinberg SP, Yogev R, Gershon AA, Krasinski KM, Borokowski W. Varicella zoster virus infections in children infected with human immunodeficiency virus. Pediatr Infect Dis J 1989;8:586–590.
43. Pahwa S, Biron K, Lim W, Swenson P, Kaplan MH, Sadick N, Pahwa R. Continuous varicella zoster infection associated with acyclovir resistance in a child with AIDS. JAMA 1988;260:2879–2882.
44. Williamson BC. Disseminated herpes zoster in a human immunodeficiency virus-positive homosexual man without complications. Cutis 1987;40: 45–46.
45. Gilson IH, Barnett JH, Conant MA, Laskin OL, Williams J, Jones PG. Disseminated ecthymatous varicella-zoster virus infection in patients with acquired immunodeficiency syndrome. J Am Acad Dermatol 1989;20:637–642.
46. Janier M, Hillion B, Baccard M, Morinet F, Scieux C, Perol Y, Civatte J. Chronic varicella zoster infection in acquired immunodeficiency syndrome (letter). J Am Acad Dermatol 1988;18:584–585.
47. Cohen PR, Beltranny VP, Grossman ME. Disseminated herpes zoster in patients with immunodeficiency virus infection. Am J Med 1988;84:1076–1080.
48. Jacobson MA, Berger TG, Fikrig S, Becherer P, Moohr JW, Stanat SC, Biron KK. Acyclovir-resistant varicella zoster virus infection after chronic oral acyclovir therapy in patients with the acquired immunodeficiency syndrome (AIDS). Ann Intern Med 1990;112:187–191.
49. Jacobson MA, Mills J. Serious cytomegalovirus disease in the acquired immunodeficiency syndrome (AIDS). Ann Intern Med 1988;108:585–594.
50. Fowler CD, Reed KD, Brannon RB. Intranuclear inclusions correlate with the ultrastructural detection of herpes-type virions in oral hairy leukoplakia. Am J Surg Pathol 1989;13:114–119.
51. Gaglioti D, De Pietro M, Ficarra G, Paci P, Ravina A. Oral hairy leukoplakia: Clinical behavior and treatment results (abstract). V International Conference on AIDS. Montreal, June 4–9, 1989:473.
52. Hardy WD. Foscarnet treatment of acyclovir-resistant herpes simplex virus infection in patients with acquired immunodeficiency syndrome: Preliminary results of a controlled, randomized, regimen-comparative trial. Am J Med 1992;92:30s–35s.
53. Chatis PA, Miller CH, Schrager LE, Crumpacker CS. Successful treatment with foscarnet of an acyclovir-resistant mucocutaneous infection with herpes simplex virus in a patient with acquired immunodeficiency syndrome. N Engl J Med 1989; 320:297–300.
54. Collaborative DHPG Treatment Study Group. Treatment of serious cytomegalovirus infections with 9-(1,3-dihydroxy-2-propoxymethyl) guanine in patients with AIDS and other immunodeficiencies. N Engl J Med 1986;314:801–805.
55. Kessler HA, Benson CA, Urbanski P. Regression of oral hairy leukoplakia during treatment with azidothymidine. Ann Intern Med 1988;148: 2496–2497.
56. Schofer H, Ochsendorf FR, Helm EB, Milbradt R. Treatment of oral hairy leukoplakia in AIDS patients with vitamin A acid (topically) or acyclovir (systemically) (letter). Dermatologica 1987;174:150–151.
57. Bauer HM, Ting Y, Greer CE, Chambers JC, Tashiro CJ, Chimera J, Reingold A, Manos MM. Genital HPV infection in female university students as determined by a PCR-based method. JAMA 1991; 265:472–477.
58. Koutsky LA, Galloway DA, Holmes KK. Epidemiology of genital human papillomavirus infection. Epidemiol Rev 1988;10:122–163.
59. Beutner KR, Becker TM, Stone KM. Epidemiology of HPV infections. Dermatol Clin 1991;9:211–218.
60. Matis WL, Triana A, Shapiro R, Eldred L, Polk BF, Hood AF. Dermatologic findings associated with human immunodeficiency virus infection. J Am Acad Dermatol 1987; 17:746–751.
61. Palefsky JM, Gonzales J, Greenblatt RM, Ahn DK, Hollander H. Anal intraepithelial neoplasia and anal papillomavirus infection among homosexual males with group IV HIV disease. JAMA 1990;263:2911–2916.
62. Oreal JD. Natural history of genital warts. Br J Vener Dis 1971;47:1–13.
63. Stolar JH, Wolensky SM, Whitback A. Differentiation-linked human papillomavirus type VI and XI transcription and genital condylomata revealed by in situ hybridization with message-specific RNA probes. Arch Dermatol 1989;172:331–340.
64. Braun L, Farmer ER, Shah KV. Immunoperoxidase localization of papillomavirus antigen and cutaneous warts in bowenoid papulosis. J Med Virol 1983;12:187–193.
65. McCance DJ, Walker PG, Dyson JL. Presence of human papillomavirus DNA sequences in cervical intraepithelial neoplasia. BMJ 1983;287:784–788.
66. Dyson N, Hoelwy PM, Munger K, Harlow E. The human papillomavirus-16—E7 oncoprotein is able to bind to the retina blastoma gene products. Science 1989;243:934–937.
67. Chardonnet Y, Viac J, Staqnet MJ. Cell mediated immunity to human papillomavirus. Clin Dermatol 1985;3:156–161.
68. Sillman FH, Sedliss A. Anogenital papillomavirus infection and neoplasia in immunodeficient women. Obstet Gynecol Clin North Am 1987;14:537–558.
69. Byrne MA, Taylor-Robinson D, Munday PE, Harris JR. The common occurrence of human papillomavirus in intraepithelial neoplasia in women infected by HIV. AIDS 1989;3:379–382.
70. Frazer JH, Medley G, Cratper RM. Association between anorectal dysplasia, human papillomavirus and immunodeficiency virus infection in homosexual men. Lancet 1986;2:657–660.
71. Doherty R, Tanskanen E, Churchill MJ, Deacon NJ. Interactions between human immunodeficiency virus and human papillomavirus. Poster presentation, VIII International Conference on AIDS, Amsterdam, July 19–24, 1992.
72. Tornesello ML, Buonaguro FM, Galloway DA, Beth-Giraldo E, Giraldo G, McDougall JK. HIV and HPV interaction: Transactivation of HPV long control region by HIV-*tat* protein. Poster presentation, VIII International Conference on AIDS, Amsterdam, July 19–24, 1992.
73. Rüdlinger R, Grob R, Buchmann P, Christen D, Steiner R. Anogenital warts of the condyloma acuminatum type in HIV-positive patients. Dermatologica 1988;176:277–281.
74. Syrjanen SM, von Krogh G, Syrjanen KJ. Anal condylomas in men. 1. Histopathological and virological assessment. Genitourin Med 1989;65:216–224.
75. Rütlinger R, Buchmann P. HPV 16—Positive bowenoid papulosis and squamous cell carcinoma in an HIV-positive man. Dis Colon Rectum 1989;32:1042–1045.
76. Rosemberg SK. Subclinical papilloviral infection of male genitalia. Urology 1985;26:552–557.
77. Campion MJ. Clinical manifestations and natural history of genital human papillomavirus infection. Obstet Gynecol Clin North Am 1987;14:363–388.
78. Ocagaki T, Clark BA, Zachow KR. Presence of human papillomavirus in verrucus carcinoma (Ackerman) of vagina: Immunocytochemical ultrastructural or DNA hybridization studies. Arch Pathol Lab Med 1984;108:567–570.
79. Berger TG, Sawchuk WS, Leonardi C, Langenberg A, Tappero J, Leboit PE. Epidermodysplasia verruciformis–associated papillomavirus infection complicating human immu-

nodeficiency virus disease. Br J Dermatol 1991;124:79–83.

80. Grusendorf-Conen EI. Papillomavirus-induced tumors of the skin: Cutaneous warts in epidermodysplasia verruciformis in papillomaviruses. In: Syrjanen K, Gisman L, Kist LG, eds. Human Disease. Berlin: Springer-Verlag; 1987:158–181.
81. McMillan A, Bishop PE. Clinical course of anogenital warts in man infectd with HIV. Genitourin Med 1989;65:225–228.
82. Oriole JD. Natural history of genital warts. Br J Vener Dis 1971;47:1–13.
83. Beckmann AM, Myerson D, Daling Jr, Kiviat NB, Fenoglio CM, McDougall JK. Detection and localization of human papillomavirus DNA in human genital condylomas by in situ hybridization with biotinylated probes. J Med Virol 1985;16:265–273.
84. Cargen JR, Zur Hausen H. Workshop on the papillomaviruses in cancer. Cancer Res 1979;39:545–546.
85. Shibata KK, Arnheim M, Martin WJ. Detection of human papillomavirus in paraffin-embedded tissue using the polymerase chain reaction. J Exp Med 1988;167:225–230.
86. Cornelissen MT, van den Tweel JG, Struyk AP, Jebbink ME, Briet M, van der Noordaa J, ter Schegget JT. Localization of human papillomavirus type 16 DNA using the polymerase chain reaction in the cervix uteri of women with cervical intraepithelial neoplasia. J Gen Virol 1989;70:2555–2562.
87. Melchers W, Van Den Brule A, Walboomers J, et al. Increased detection rate of human papillomavirus in cervical scrapes by the polymerase chain reaction as compared to modified FISH and southern blot analysis. J Med Virol 1989;27:329–335.
88. Fisher AA. Severe systemic and local reactions to topical podophyllin resin. Cutis 1981;28:233–266.
89. Stoeh GP, Peterson AL, Taylor WJ. Systemic complications of local podophyllin therapy. Ann Intern Med 1978;89:362–363.
90. Slater GE, Rumack BH, Peterson RG. Podophyllin poisoning: Systemic toxicity following cutaneous application. Obstet Gynecol 1978;52:94–96.
91. Beutner KR, Conant MA, Friedman-Kien AE, Illeman M, Artman NN, Thisted RA, King DH. Patient-applied podofilox for treatment of genital warts. Lancet 1989;1:831–834.
92. Godley MJ, Bradbeer CS, Gellan M, Thin RN. Cryotherapy compared with trichloracetic acid in treating genital warts. Genitourin Med 1987;63:390–392.
93. Baggish MS. Improved laser techniques for the elimination of genital and extragenital warts. Am J Obstet Gynecol 1985;153:545–550.
94. Sawchuck WS, Weber PJ, Lowry DR, Dzubow LM. Infectious papillomavirus in the vapor of warts treated with carbon dioxide laser or electrocoagulation: Detection and protection. J Am Acad Dermatol 1989;21:41–49.
95. Friedman-Kien AE, Eron LJ, Conant M, Growdon W, Badiak H, Bradstreet PW, Fedorczyk D, Trout JR, Plasse TF. Natural interferon alfa for treatment of condylomata acuminata. JAMA 1988;259:533–538.
96. Katzman M, Carey JT, Elmets CA, Jacobs GH, Lederman MM. Molluscum contagiosum and AIDS: Clinical and immunologic details of two cases. Br J Dermatol 1987;116:131–138.
97. Redfield RR, Wright DC, James WD, Jones TS, Brown C, Burke DS. Disseminated vaccinia in a military recruit with human immunodeficiency virus (HIV) disease. N Engl J Med 1987;316:673–676.
98. Fivenson DP, Weltman RE, Gibson SH. Giant molluscum contagiosum presenting as basal cell carcinoma in an AIDS patient (letter). J Am Acad Dermatol 1988;19:912–914.
99. Berger TG, Greene I. Bacterial, viral, fungal and parasitic infections in HIV Disease and AIDS. Dermatol Clin 1991;3:465–492.
100. Smith KJ, Skelton HG, Yeager J, James WD, Wagner KF. Molluscum contagiosum. Ultrastructure evidence for its presence in skin adjacent to clinical lesions in patients infected with human immunodeficiency virus type 1. Arch Dermatol 1992;128:223–227.
101. Kerl H. Personal communication, 1993.
102. Torok TJ. Parvovirus and human disease. Adv Intern Med 1992;37:431–455.
103. Coldiron BM, Freeman RG, Beaudoing DL. Isolation of adenovirus from a granuloma annulare-like lesion in the acquired immunodeficiency syndrome-related complex. Arch Dermatol 1988;124:654–655.
104. Markowitz LE, Chandler FW, Roldan EO, Saldana MJ, Roach KC, Hutchins SS, Preblud SR, Mitchell CD, Scott GB. Fatal measles pneumonia without rash in a child with AIDS. J Infect Dis 1988;158:480–483.
105. Ross LA, Kim KS, Comport Z. Successful treatment of disseminated measles in a patient with acquired immune deficiency syndrome: Consideration of anti-viral and passive immunotherapy. Am J Med 1990;88:313–314.
106. Ganesh R, Castle D, Gibbon D, McGibbon D, Phillips I, Bradbeer C. Staphylococcal carriage and HIV infection (letter). Lancet 1989;2:558.
107. Nichols SL, Balog K, Silverman M. Bacterial infection and AIDS. Clinical pathologic correlations in a series of autopsy cases. Am J Clin Pathol 1989;92:787–790.
108. Pitrack DL, Pall AK, Back PA. Serious *Pseudomonas aeruginosa* infection complicating AIDS. Poster presentation, IX International Conference on AIDS, Berlin, June 6–12, 1993.
109. Steinhart R, Reingold AL, Taylor F, Anderson G, Wenger JD. Invasive *Haemophilus influenzae* infections in men with HIV infection. JAMA 1992;268:3350–3352.
110. Barbaro DJ, Orcutt VL, Coldiron BM. *Mycobacterium avium–Mycobacterium intracellulare* infection limited to the skin and lymph nodes in patients with AIDS. Rev Infect Dis 1989;11:625–628.
111. Rogers PL, Walker RE, Lane HC, Witebsky FG, Kovacs JA, Parrillo JE, Masur H. Disseminated *Mycobacterium haemophilum* infection in two patients with AIDS. Am J Med 1988;84:640–642.
112. Rohatgi PK, Palazzolo JV, Saini NB. Acute military tuberculosis of the skin in acquired immunodeficiency syndrome. J Am Acad Dermatol 1992;26:285–287.
113. Boudes P, Sobel A, Deforges L, Leblic E. Disseminated *Mycobacterium bovis* infection from BCG vaccination and HIV infection (letter). JAMA 1989;262:2386.
114. Quinn TC, Cannon RO, Glasser D, Groseclose SL, Brathwaite WS, Fauci AS, Hook EW III. The association of syphilis with risk of human immunodeficiency virus infection in patients attending sexually transmitted disease clinics. Arch Intern Med 1990;150:1297–1302.
115. Kimura S, Goto M, Teramura M, Oka S, Suganoya Y, Mitamura K, Shimada K. Decreased function of granulocytes in patients with HIV infection. Poster presentation, VIII International Conference on AIDS, Amsterdam, July 19–24, 1992.
116. Gendelman HE, Orenstein JM, Baca LM, Weiser B, Burger H, Kalter DC, Meltzer MS. The macrophage in the persistence and pathogenesis of HIV infection. AIDS 1989;3:475–495.
117. Pahwa SG, Quilop MT, Lange M, Pahwa RN, Grieco MH. Defective B-lymphocyte function in homosexual men in relation to acquired immunodeficiency syndrome. Ann Intern Med 1984;101:757–763.
118. Ellis M, Gupta S, Galant S, Hakim S, Vande Ven C, Toy C, Cairo MS. Impaired neutrophil function in patients with AIDS or AIDS-related complex: A comprehensive evaluation. J Infect Dis 1988;158:1268–1276.
119. Raviglione MC, Battan R, Pablos-Mendez A, Aceves-Casillas P, Mullen MP, Taranta A. Infections associated with Hickman catheters in patients with acquired immunodeficiency syndrome. Am J Med 1989;86:780–786.
120. Paganelli R, Scala E, Mezzaroma I, Ansotegui IJ, D'Offizi GP, Pinter E, Aiuti F. sCD23 levels in human immunodeficiency virus (HIV) infection with hyper-IgE and chronic dermatitis. Poster presentation, VIII Interna-

tional Conference on AIDS, Amsterdam, July 19–24, 1992.

121. Adal KA, Cockerell CJ, Petrie WA Jr. Cat scratch disease, bacillary angiomatosis, and other infections due to *Rochalimaea* (review). N Engl J Med, 1994; 330:1509–1515.
122. Patterson JW, Kitces EN, Neafie RC. Cutaneous botryomycosis in a patient with acquired immunodeficiency syndrome. J Am Acad Dermatol 1987;16:238–242.
123. Gaut P, Wong PK, Meyer RD. Pyomyositis in a patient with the acquired immunodeficiency syndrome. Arch Intern Med 1988;148:1608–1610.
124. Janssen F, Zelinsky-Gurung A, Caumes E, and Decazed JM. Group A streptococcal cellulitis-adenitis in a patient with the acquired immunodeficiency syndrome. J Am Acad Dermatol 1991;24:363–365.
125. Weitzner JM, Dhawan SS, Rosen LB, and Reznick L. Successful treatment of botryomycosis in a patient with acquired immune deficiency syndrome. J Am Acad Dermatol 21:1312–1314.
126. Patterson JW, Kitces EN, Neafie RC. Cutaneous botryomycosis in a patient with acquired immune deficiency syndrome. J Am Acad Dermatol 1987;16:238–242.
127. Becker BA, Odom RB, Berger TG: Atypical plaque-like staphylococcal folliculitis in human immunodeficiency virus infected persons. J Am Acad Dermatol 1989;21:1024–1026.
128. Kline MW, Dunkle LM: Toxic shock syndrome in the acquired immunodeficiency syndrome. Pediatr Dis J 1988;7:736–738.
129. Cipriano J, Feranno J, Ferranti E. Acquired immunodeficiency syndrome in non-menstrual toxic shock syndrome (letter). Ann Intern Med 1986;105:300.
130. el Baze P, Thyss A, Vinti H, Deville A, Dellamonica P, Ortonne JP. A study of nineteen immunocompromised patients with extensive skin lesions caused by *Pseudomonas aeruginosa* with and without bacteremia. Acta Dermatol Venereol 1991;71:411–415.
131. Kielhofner M, Atmar RL, Hamill RF, Musher DM. Life-treatening *Pseudomonas aeruginosa* infections in patients with human immunodeficiency virus infection. Clin Infect Dis 1992;14:403–411.
132. Sangeorzan JA, Bradley SF, Kaufman CA. Cutaneous manifestation of *Pseudomonas* infection in the acquired immune deficiency syndrome. Arch Dermatol 1990;126:832–833.
133. Raiteri R, Pippione M, Picciotto L, Martinetto P, Sinicco A. Job's-like syndrome in HIV-1 page infection. Abstract, VIII International Conference on AIDS, Amsterdam, July 19–24, 1992.
134. Cone LA, Woodard DR, Byrd RG, Schulz K, Kopp SM, Schlivert PM. A recalcitrant, erythematous, desquamating disorder associated with toxin-producing staphylococci in patients with AIDS. J Infect Dis 1992;165:638–643.
135. Javaly K, Horowitz HW, Wormser GP. Nocardiosis in patients with human immunodeficiency virus infection. Medicine 1992;71:128–138.
136. Watkins KV, Richmond AS, Langstein IM. Nonhealing extraction site due to *Actinomyces naeslundii* in patients with AIDS. Oral Surg Oral Med Oral Pathol 1991;71:675– 677.
137. Drancourt M, Bonnet E, Gallais H, Paloux Y, Raoult D. *Rhodococcus equi* infection in patients with AIDS. J Infect 1992;24:123–131.
138. Patey O, Halioua B, Casciani D, Emond JP, Dublanchet A, Lafaix C. *Corynebacterium diphtheriae* septicemia in an AIDS patient (abstract). VIII International Conference on AIDS, Amsterdam, July 19–24, 1992.
139. Raffi F, Billaud E, Dutartre H, Milpied B. Thoracic *Salmonella typhimurium* abscess in an AIDS patient (letter). Eur J Clin Microbiol Infect Dis 1990;9:53–54.
140. Cockerell CJ, LeBoit PE. Bacillary angiomatosis: A novel pseudoneoplastic, infectious vascular disorder. J Am Acad Dermatol 1990;22:501–519.
141. Cockerell CJ, Whitlow MA, Webster GF, Friedman-Kien AE. Epithelioid angiomatosis: A distinct vascular disorder in patients with acquired immunodeficiency syndrome or AIDS-related complex. Lancet 1987;2:654–656.
142. LeBoit PE, Berger TG, Egbert BM, Beckstead JH, Yen TS, Stoler MH. Bacillary angiomatosis. The histopathology and differential diagnosis of a pseudoneoplastic infection in patients with human immunodeficiency virus disease. Am J Surg Pathol 1989;13:909–920.
143. Baron AL, Steinbach LS, LeBoit PE, Mills CM, Gee JH, Berger TG. Osteolytic lesions in bacillary angiomatosis in HIV infection: Radiologic differentiation from AIDS-related Kaposi's sarcoma. Radiology 1990;177:77–81.
144. Berger TG, Tappero JW, Kaymen A, LeBoit PE. Bacillary (epithelioid) angiomatosis and concurrent Kaposi's sarcoma in acquired immunodeficiency syndrome. Arch Dermatol 1989;125:1543–1547.
145. Schwartzman WA, Marchevski A, Meyer RD. Epithelioid angiomatosis or cat-scratch disease with splenic and hepatic abnormalities in AIDS: Case report or review of the literature. Scand J Infect Dis 1990;22:121–133.
146. Knobler EH, Silvers DN, Fein KC, Lefkowitch JH, Grossman ME. Unique vascular skin lesions associated with human immunodeficiency virus. JAMA 1988;260:524–527.
147. Roth C, Theodore C, Aitkin C, Shaw E, Forster G, Cerio R. Presumed disseminated *Mycobacterium tuberculosis* infection presenting with cutaneous lesions in a patient with AIDS (abstract). VIII International Conference on AIDS, Amsterdam, July 19–24, 1992.
148. Rogers PL, Walker RE, Lane HC, Witebsky FG, Kovacs JA, Parrillo JE, Masur H. Disseminated *Mycobacterium haemophilum* infection in two patients with AIDS. Am J Med 1988;84:640–642.
149. Piketty C, Lons Danic D, Weiss L, Bu Hoi A, Kazatchkine MD. Atypical sporotrichosis-like infection caused by *Mycobacterium avium* in AIDS (abstract). VIII International Conference on AIDS, Amsterdam, July 1992.
150. Centers for Disease Control. Tuberculosis and human immunodeficiency virus infection: Recommendations of the Advisory Committee for the Elimination of Tuberculosis (ACET). MMWR 1989;38:236–250.
151. Gregory N, Sanchez M, Buchness MR. The spectrum of syphilis in patients with human immunodeficiency virus infection. J Am Acad Dermatol 1990;22:1061–1067.
152. Glover RA, Piaquadio DJ, Kern S, Cockerell CJ. An unusual presentation of secondary syphilis in a patient with human immunodeficiency virus infection. A case report and review of the literature. Arch Dermatol 1992;128:530–534.
153. Ficarra G, Zaragoza AM, Stendardi L, Parri F, Cockerell CJ. Early oral presentation of lues maligna in a patient with HIV infection. A case report. Oral Surg Oral Med Oral Pathol 1993;75:728–732.
154. Johns DR, Tierney M, Felsenstein D. Alteration of the natural history of neurosyphilis by concurrent infection with the human immunodeficiency virus. N Engl J Med 1987;316:1569–1572.
155. Quale J, Tepletts E, Augenbraun F. Atypical presentation of chancroid in a patient infected with the human immunodeficiency virus. Am J Med 1990;88(suppl 5):43–44.
156. Strongin IS, Kale SA, Raymond MK, Luskin RL, Weisberg GW, Jacobs JJ. An unusual presentation of gonococcal arthritis in an HIV-positive patient. Ann Rheum Dis 1991; 50:572–573.
157. Regnery RL, Anderson BE, Clarridge JE III, Rodriguez-Barradas MC, Jones DC, Carr JH. Characterization of a novel *Rochalimaea* species, *R. henselae* sp. nov., isolated from blood of a febrile, human immunodeficiency virus–positive patient. J Clin Microbiol 1992;30:265–274.
158. Koehler JE, Quinn FD, Berger TG, LeBoit PE, Tappero JW. Isolation of *Rochalimaea* species from cutaneous and osseous lesions of bacillary angiomatosis. N Engl J Med 1992;327:1625–1631.
159. Geman MD. Treatment of multidrug

resistant tuberculosis. N Engl J Med 1993;329:784–791.
160. Wallace RJ, Tanner PJ, Brown BA. Clinical trial of clarithromycin for cutaneous (disseminated) infection due to *Mycobacterium chelonae.* Ann Intern Med 1993;119:482–486.
161. Sadick N, Kaplan MH, Pahwa SG, Sarngadharan MG. Unusual features of scabies complicating human T-lymphotrophic virus type III infection. J Am Acad Dermatol 1986;15:482–486.
162. Dominey A, Roen R, Tschen J. Papulonodular demodicidosis associated with acquired immunodeficiency syndrome. J Am Acad Dermatol 1989;20:197–201.
163. Girault C, Borsa-Lebas F, Humbert G. Papulonodular demodicidosis: A new opportunistic infection in AIDS. Poster presentation, VIII International Conference on AIDS, Amsterdam, July 19–24, 1992.
164. Gherman CR, Ward RR, Bassis ML. *Pneumocystis carinii* otitis media and mastoiditis as the initial manifestation of the acquired immunodeficiency syndrome. Am J Med 1991;127:250–252.
165. Hennessey NP, Parro EL, Cockerell CJ. Cutaneous *Pneumocystis carinii* infection in patients with acquired immunodeficiency syndrome. Arch Dermatol 1991;127:1699–1701.
166. Litwin MA, Williams CM. Cutaneous *Pneumocystis carinii* infection mimicking Kaposi's sarcoma. Ann Intern Med 1992;117:48–49.
167. Hirschmann JV, Chu AC. Skin lesions with disseminated toxoplasmosis in a patient with the acquired immunodeficiency syndrome. Arch Dermatol 1988;124:1446–1447.
168. Portnoy BL, Micheletti GA. *Acanthamoeba* infection of skin and sinuses in an AIDS patient: Diagnosis and treatment (abstract). VIII International Conference on AIDS, Amsterdam, July 19–24, 1992.
169. Glezerov V, Masci JR. Disseminated strongyloidiasis and other selected unusual infections in patients with acquired immunodeficiency syndrome. Prog AIDS Pathol 1990;2:137–142.
170. Montelban C, Martinez-Fernandez R, Calleja JL, Garcia-Diaz JD, Rubio R, Dronda F, Moreno S, Yebra M, Barros C, Cobo J. Visceral leishmaniasis (kala-azar) as an opportunistic infection in patients infected with the human immunodeficiency virus in Spain. Rev Infect Dis 1989;11:655–660.
171. Belsito DV, Sanchez MR, Baer RL, Valentine F, Thorbecke GJ. Reduced Langerhans' cell Ia antigen and ATPS activity in patients with the acquired immunodeficiency syndrome. N Engl J Med 1984; 310:1279–1282.
172. Insera DW, Bickley LK. Crusted scabies in acquired immunodeficiency syndrome. Int J Dermatol 1990;29:287–289.
173. Raur C, Baird IM. Crusted scabies in a patient with acquired immunodeficiency syndrome (letter). J Am Acad Dermatol 1986;15:1058–1059.
174. Jucowics P, Ramon ME, Don PC, Stone RK, Bamji M. Norweigan scabies in an infant with acquired immunodeficiency syndrome. Arch Dermatol 1989;125:1670–1671.
175. Skinner SM, DeVillez RL. Sepsis associated with Norwegian scabies in patients with acquired immunodeficiency syndrome. Arch Dermatol 1992;50:213–216.
175a. Meinking TL, Taplin D, Hermida JL, Pardo R, Kerdel FA. The treatment of scabies with ivermectin. N Engl J Med 1995;333(1):26–30.
176. O'Donnell BF, O'Loughlin S, Powell FC. Management of crusted scabies. Int J Dermatol 1990;29:258–266.
177. Fraser VJ, Keath EJ, Powderly WG. Two cases of blastomycosis from a common source: Use of DNA restriction analysis to identify strains. J Infect Dis 1991;163:1378–1381.
178. Klein RS, Harris CA, Small CB, Moll B, Lesser M, Friedland GH. Oral candidiasis in high-risk patients as the initial manifestation of the acquired immunodeficiency syndrome. N Engl J Med 1984;311:354–358.
179. Leibovitz E, Rigaud M, Chandwani S, Kaul A, Greco MA, Pollack H, Lawrence R, Di John D, Hanna B, Krasinski K, Borkowsky W. Disseminated fungal infections in children infected with human immunodeficiency virus. Pediatr Infect Dis J 1991;10:888–894.
180. Wolf JE, Little JR, Pappagianis D, Kobayashi GS. Disseminated coccidioidomycosis in a patient with the acquired immune deficiency syndrome. Diagn Microbiol Infect Dis 1986;5:331–336.
181. Prichard JG, Sorotzkin RA, James RE III. Cutaneous manifestations of disseminated coccidioidomycosis in the acquired immunodeficiency syndrome. Cutis 1987;39:203–205.
182. Fish DG, Ampel NM, Galgiani JN, Dols CL, Kelly PC, Johnson CH, Pappagianis D, Edwards JE, Wasserman RB, Clark RJ, Antoniskis D, Larsen RA, Englender SJ, Petersen EA. Coccidioidomycosis during human immunodeficiency virus infection: A review of 77 patients. Medicine 1990;69:384–391.
183. Manrique P, Mayo J, Alvarez JA, Ganchegui X, Zabalza I, Flores M. Polymorphous cutaneous cryptococcosis: Nodular, herpes-like, and molluscum-like lesions in a patient with the acquired immunodeficiency syndrome. J Am Acad Dermatol 1992;26:122–124.
184. Cusini M, Cagliani P, Grimalt R, Tadini G, Alessi E, Fasan M. Primary cutaneous cryptococcosis in a patient with the acquired immunodeficiency syndrome (letter). Arch Dermatol 1991;127:1848–1849.
185. Jones C, Orengo I, Rosen T, Ellner K. Cutaneous cryptococcosis simulating Kaposi's sarcoma in the acquired immunodeficiency syndrome. Cutis 1990;45:163–167.
186. Lynch DP, Naftolin LZ. Oral *Cryptococcus neoformans* infection in AIDS. Oral Surg Oral Med Oral Pathol 1987;64:449–453.
187. Rico NJ, Penneys NS. Cutaneous cryptococcosis resembling molluscum contagiosum in a patient with AIDS. Arch Dermatol 1985;121:901–902.
188. Mares M, Sartori MT, Carretta M, Bertaggia A, Girolami A. Rhinophyma-like cryptococcal infection as an early manifestation of AIDS in a hemophilia B patient. Acta Haematol 1990;84:101–103.
189. Cohen PR, Grossman ME, Silvers DN. Disseminated histoplasmosis and human immunodeficiency virus infection. Int J Dermatol 1991; 30:614–622.
190. Hazelhurst JA, Vismer JF. Histoplasmosis presenting with unusual skin lesions in acquired immunodeficiency syndrome (AIDS). Br J Dermatol 1985;113:345–348.
191. Kalter DC, Tschen JA, Klima M. Maculopapular rash in a patient with acquired immunodeficiency syndrome. Arch Dermatol 1985;121:1455–1456.
192. Lindgren AM, Fallon JD, Horan RF. Psoriasiform papules in the acquired immunodeficiency syndrome. Disseminated histoplasmosis in AIDS. Arch Dermatol 1991;127:722–723, 725–726.
193. Chaker MB, Cockerell CJ. Concomitant psoriasis, seborrheic dermatitis and disseminated cutaneous histoplasmosis in a patient infected with human immunodeficiency virus. J Am Acad Dermatol 1993;29:311–313.
194. Cole MC, Cohen PR, Satra KH, Grossman ME. The concurrent presence of systemic disease pathogens and cutaneous Kaposi's sarcoma in the same lesion: *Histoplasma capsulatum* and Kaposi's sarcoma coexisting in a single skin lesion in a patient with AIDS. J Am Acad Dermatol 1992;26:285–287.
195. Cohen PR, Held JL, Grossman ME, Ross MJ, Silvers DN. Disseminated histoplasmosis presenting as an ulcerated verrucous plaque in a human immunodeficiency virus-infected man: Report of a case possibly involving human-to-human transmission of histoplasmosis. Int J Dermatol 1991;30:104–108.
196. Bakos L, Kronfeld M, Hampe S, Castro I, Zampese M. Disseminated paracoccidioidomycosis with skin lesions in a patient with acquired immunodeficiency syndrome (letter). J Am Acad Dermatol 1989;20:854–855.
197. Lipstein-Kresch E, Isenberg HD, Singer C, Cooke O, Greenwald RA. Disseminated *Sporothrix schenckii* infection with arthritis in a patient

with acquired immunodeficiency syndrome. J Rheumatol 1985;12:805–808.
198. Shaw JC, Levinson W, Montanara A. Sporotrichosis in the acquired immunodeficiency syndrome. J Am Acad Dermatol 1989;21:1145–1147.
199. Fitzpatrick JE, Eubanks S. Acquired immunodeficiency syndrome presenting as disseminated cutaneous sporotrichosis. Int J Dermatol 1988;27:406–407.
200. Bibler MR, Luber HJ, Glueck HI, Estes SA. Disseminated sporotrichosis in a patient with HIV infection after treatment for acquired factor VIII inhibitor. JAMA 1986;256:3125–3126.
201. Terrell CL, Hughes CE. Antifungal agents used for deep-seated mycotic infections. Mayo Clin Proc 1992;67:69–91.
202. Wood GM, McCormack JG, Muir DB, Ellis DH, Ridley MF, Pritchard R, Harrison M. Clinical features of human infection with *Scedosporium inflatum*. Clin Infect Dis 1992; 14:1027–1033.
203. Scherr GR, Evans SG, Kiyabu MT, Klatt EC. *Pseudallescheria boydii* in the acquired immunodeficiency syndrome. Arch Pathol Lab Med 1992;116:535–536.
204. Hevia O, Kligman D, Penneys NS. Non-scalp hair infection caused by *Microsporum canis* in a patient with acquired immunodeficiency syndrome. J Am Acad Dermatol 1991;24:789–790.
205. Sachot LJ, Hadderingh RJ, Devriese PP. Facial palsy and HIV infection (abstract). VIII International Conference on AIDS, Amsterdam, July 19–24, 1992.
206. Frazier R, Stoole E, Gathe J Jr, Le Blanc M, Nichols M, Flaitz C. Head and neck *Zygomycetes/Aspergillus* infections in patients with AIDS. Poster presentation, IX International Conference, Berlin, Germany, June 6–12, 1993.
207. Sanders M, Panza-Wilson I. Cutaneous zygomycosis. Poster presentation, IX International Conference, Berlin, Germany, June 6–12, 1993.
208. Supparatpinyo K, Chiewchanvit S, Hirunsri P, Uthammachai C, Nelson KE, Sirisanthana T. *Penicillium marneffei* infection in patients infected with HIV. Poster presentation, VIII International Conference on AIDS, Amsterdam, July 19–24, 1992.
209. Torssander J, Karlsson A, Morfeldt-Månson L, Putkonen PO, Wasserman J. Dermatophytosis and HIV infection. A study in homosexual men. Acta Derm Venereol (Stockh) 1988;68:53–56.
210. Noppakun N, Head ES. Proximal white subungual onychomycosis in a patient with acquired immunodeficiency syndrome. Int J Dermatol 1986;25:586–587.
211. Heng MC, Henderson CL, Barker DC, Haberfelde G.: Correlation of *Pityrosporum ovale* density with clinical severity of seborrheic dermatitis as assessed by simplified technique. J Am Acad Dermatol 1990;23:82–86.
212. Lief HL, Semperkopf MS. Invasive trichosporosis in a patient with AIDS. J Infect Dis 1989;160:356–357.
213. Drabick JJ, Gomatos PJ, Solis JB. Cutaneous cladosporiosis as a complication of skin testing in a man positive for HIV. J Am Acad Dermatol 1990;22:135–136.
214. Lévy-Klotz B, Badillet G, Cavelier-Balloy, Chemaly P, Leverger G, Civatte J. Alternariose cutanée au cours d'un SIDA. Acta Dermatol Venereol 1985;112:739–740.
215. Duvic M, Lowe L, Rios A, MacDonald E, Vance P. Superficial phaeohyphomycosis of the scrotum in a patient with AIDS (letter). Arch Dermatol 1987;123:1597–1599.
216. Mathes BM, Douglass MC. Seborrheic dermatitis in patients with acquired immunodeficiency syndrome. J Am Acad Dermatol 1985;13:947–951.
217. Duvic M, Johnson TM, Rapini RP, Freese T, Brewton G, Rios A. Acquired immunodeficiency syndrome–associated psoriasis and Reiter's syndrome. Arch Dermatol 1987;123: 1622–1632.
218. Kaplan MH, Sadick NS, Wieder J, Farber BF, Neidt GW. Antipsoriatic effects of zidovudine in human immunodeficiency virus–associated psoriasis. J Am Acad Dermatol 1989;20:76–82.
219. Kaye BR: Rheumatologic manifestations of infection with human immunodeficiency virus (HIV). Ann Intern Med 1989;111:158–167.
220. Solomon G, Brancato LJ, Itescu S, Skovorn ML, Mildvan D, Winchester RJ. Arthritis, psoriasis and related syndromes associated with HIV infection (abstract). Arthritis Rheum 1988;31(suppl 2):S12.
221. Lin RY. Reiter's syndrome in human immunodeficiency virus infection. Dermatologica 1988;176:39–42.
222. Winchester R, Bernstein DH, Fischer HD, Enlow R, Solomon G. The co-occurrence of Reiter's syndrome and acquired immunodeficiency. Ann Intern Med 1987;106:19–26.
222a. Magro CM, Crowson AN, Peeling R. Vasculitis as the basis of cutaneous lesions in Reiter's disease. Hum Pathol 1995;26(6):633–638.
223. Rao BK, Cockerell CJ. Histologic findings in inflammatory dermatoses in a patient with HIV infection. Poster presentation, VII International Conference on AIDS, Florence, Italy, 1991.
224. Smith J, Skelton HG. Pathogenesis of inflammatory dermatoses in patients with HIV infection. Poster presentation, American Society of Dermatopathology, San Francisco, California, December 1, 1992.
225. Habeshaw J, Hounsell E, Dalgleish A. Does the HIV envelope induce a chronic graft-versus-host–like disease? Immunol Today 1992;13:207–210.
226. Cockerell CJ. Personal observation, 1993.
227. Auerbach R. Personal communication, 1993.
228. Valerie K, Delers A, Bruck C, Thiriart C, Rosenberg H, Debouck C, Rosenberg M. Activation of human immunodeficiency virus type 1 by DNA damage in human cells. Nature 1988;333:78–81.
229. Meola T, Soter NA, Ostrecher R, Sanchez M, Moy JA. The safety of UVB phototherapy in patients with HIV infection. J Am Acad Dermatol 1993;29(2 pt 1):216–220.
230. Martin AG, Weaver CC, Cockerell CJ, Berger TG. Pityriasis rubra pilaris in the setting of HIV infection: Clinical behaviour and association with explosive cystic acne. Br J Dermatol 1992;126:617–620.
231. Le Bozec P, Janier M, Reygagnee P, Pinquier L, Blanchet-Bardon C, Dubertret L. Pityriasis rubra pilaris in a patient with AIDS. Acta Dermatol Venereol 1991;118(11):862–864.
232. Herman LE, Curbin AK. Eryrthroderma as a manifestation of the AIDS-related complex. J Am Acad Dermatol 1987;17:507–508.
233. Janier M, Katlama C, Flageul B, Valensi F, Moulonguet I, Sigaux F, Dompmartin D, Civatte J. Pseudo-Sézary's syndrome with CD-8 phenotype in a patient with AIDS. Ann Intern Med 1989;110:738–740.
234. Kaplan MH, Sadick N, McNutt NS, Meltzer M, Sarngadharan MG, Pahwa S. Dermatologic findings and manifestations of acquired immunodeficiency syndrome. J Am Acad Dermatol 1987;16:485–506.
235. Goodman DS, Teplitz ED, Wishner A, Klein RS, Burk PG, Hershenbaum E. The prevalence of cutaneous disease in patients with AIDS or ARC. J Am Acad Dermatol 1987;17:210–220.
236. Soeprono FF, Schinella RA. Eosinophilic pustular folliculitis in patients with acquired immunodeficiency syndrome. J Am Acad Dermatol 1986;14:1020–1022.
237. Rosenthal D, LeBoit PE, Klumpp L, Berger TG. Human immunodeficiency virus–associated eosinophilic folliculitis: A unique dermatitis associated with advanced human immunodeficiency virus infection. Arch Dermatol 1991;127:206–209.
238. Buchness MR, Lim HW, Hatcher VA, Sanchez M, Soter NA. Eosinophilic pustular folliculitis in the acquired immunodeficiency syndrome. Treatment with ultraviolet B phototherapy. N Engl J Med 1988;318:1183–1186.
239. Ball LM, Harper JI. Atopic eczema in HIV-seropositive hemophiliacs. Lancet 1987;2:627–628.

240. Dikeacou T, Lowenstein W, Romana C, Carabinis A, Renieri N, Balamotis A, Petrides A, Chatzivassiliou M, Fragouli E, Katsambas A, Stragios J. Relation of allergy to HIV infection. J Eur Acad Dermatol Venereol 1993;2:180–187.
241. Sadik NS, McNutt NS. Cutaneous hypersensitivity reactions in patients with AIDS. Int J Dermatol 1993;32:621–627.
242. Miadonna A, Leggieri E, Tedeschi A, Lazzarin A, Chianura L, Froldi M, Zanussi C. Enchanced basophil releasability in subjects infected with human immunodeficiency virus. Clin Immunol Immunopathol 1990;54: 237–246.
243. Tateno M, Gonzales-Scarano F, Levy JA. Human immunodeficiency virus type 1 can infect CD-4 negative human fibroblastoid cells. Proc Natl Acad Sci USA 1989;11:4287–4290.
244. King DA, Ion D, Berger TG, Conant M. Itraconazole for treatment of HIV-associated eosinophilic folliculitis. Poster presentation, IX International Conference on AIDS, Berlin, Germany, June 6–12, 1993.
245. Pantaleo G, Graziosi C, Fauci AS. Immunopathogenesis of human immunodeficiency virus infection. N Engl J Med 1993;328:327–335.
246. Raffi F, Testa A, Magadur G, Barrier JH. Schönlein-Henoch purpura and glomerulonephritis as the initial manifestation of HIV infection. VII International Conference on AIDS, Florence, Italy, June 16–21, 1991.
247. Chren MM, Silverman RA, Sorensen RU, Elmets CA. Leukocytoclastic vasculitis in a patient infected with HIV. J Am Acad Dermatol 1989;21:1161–1164.
248. LeBoit PE, Cockerell CJ. Nodular lesions of erythema elevatum diutinum in patients with human immunodeficiency infection. J Am Acad Dermatol 1993;28:919–922.
249. de Cunha Bang F, Weismann K, Ralfkiaer E, Pallesen G, Lange Wantzin G. Erythema elevatum diutinum and pre-AIDS. Acta Derm Venereol (Stockh) 1986;66:272–274.
250. Abramson SB, Odajnyk CM, Grieco AJ, Weissmann G, Rosenstein E. Hyperalgesic pseudothrombophlebitis: New syndrome in male homosexuals. Am J Med 1985;78:317–320.
251. Fallon T, Abell E, Kingsley L, et al. Telangiectasis of the anterior chest in homosexual men. Ann Intern Med 1986;105:679–682.
252. Toback AC, Longley J, Cardello AC, et al. Severe chronic photosensitivity in association with acquired immunodeficiency syndrome. Arch Dermatol 1986;15:2056–2057.
253. Tojo N, Yoshimura N, Yoshizawa M, Ichioka M, et al. Vitiligo and chronic photosensitivity in human immunodeficiency virus infection. Jpn J Med 1991;30:255–259.
254. Lobato MN, Berger TG. Porphyria cutanea tarda associated with the acquired immunodeficiency syndrome. Arch Dermatol 1988;124:1009–1010.
255. Herranz MT, el Amrani A, Aranegui P, Jimenez-Alonse JF, et al. Porphyria cutanea tarda and acquired immunodeficiency syndrome: Pathogenetic mechanisms. Arch Dermatol 1991;12:1585–1586.
256. Egbert BM, LeBoit PE, McCalmont T, Hu CH, Austin C. Caterpillar bodies: Distinctive, basement membrane–containing structures in blisters of porphyria. Am J Dermatopathol 1993;15(3):199–202.
257. Ghadially R, Sibbald RG, Walter JB, Haberman HF. Granuloma annulare in patients with human immunodeficiency virus infections. J Am Acad Dermatol 1989;20:232–235.
258. Picard C, Crickx B, Fegueux S, Carbon C, Margent P, Belaich S. Porphyria cutanea tarda in HIV infection. Poster presentation, VII International Conference on AIDS, Florence, Italy, June 16–21, 1991.
259. Cockerell CJ. Successful treatment of HIV-related porphyria cutanea tarda with low-dose oral hydroxychloroquine. Submitted for publication.
260. Anderson KE, Goeger DE, Carson RW, Lee SM, Stead RB. Erythropoietin for the treatment of porphyria cutanea tarda in a patient on long-term hemodialysis. N Engl J Med 1990;322:315–317.
261. Coopman SA, Johnson RA, Platt R, Stern RS. Cutaneous disease and drug reactions in HIV infection. N Engl J Med 1993;328:1670–1674.
262. Gordin FM, Simon GL, Wofsy CD, Mills J. Adverse reactions to trimethoprim-sulfamethoxazole in patients with the acquired immunodeficiency syndrome. Ann Intern Med 1984;100:495–499.
263. Raviglione MC, Dinan WA, Pablo-Mendez A, Palagiano A, Sabatini MT. Fatal toxic epidermal necrolysis during prophylaxis with pyrimethamine and sulfadoxine in a human immunodeficiency virus–infected person. Arch Intern Med 1988;148:2683–2685.
264. Nunn P, Wasunna K, Kwanyah G, Gathua S, Imalingat A, Lucas S, Gilks C, Brindle R, Omwega M, Were J, et al. Cutaneous hypersensitivity reactions to thiacetazone among HIV-1 seropositive tuberculosis patients in Nairobi. Poster presentation, VII International Conference on AIDS, Florence, Italy, June 16–21, 1992.
265. Snider DE, Graczyk J, Bek E, Rogowski J. Supervised six-month treatment of newly diagnosed pulmonary tuberculosis using isoniazid, rifampin and pyrazinamide with and without streptomycin. Am Rev Respir Dis 1984;130:1091–1094.
266. Battegay M, Opravil M, Wuthrich B, Luthy R. Rash with amoxicillin-clavulanate therapy in HIV-infected patients (letter). Lancet 1989;2:1100.
267. Toma E, Fournier S, Poisson M, Morisset R, Phaneuf D, Vega C. Clindamycin with primaquine for *Pneumocystis carinii* pneumonia. Lancet 1989;1:1046–1048.
268. Youle MS, Hawkins DA, Lawence AG, Tenant-Howers M, Shanson DC, Gazzard BG. Clinical, immunological, and virological effects of sodium fusidate in patients with AIDS or AIDS-related complex (ARC): An open study. J Acquir Immune Defic Syndr 1989;2:59–62.
269. Williams I, Weller IV, Malni A, Anderson J, Waters MF. Thalidomide hypersensitivity in AIDS (letter). Lancet 1991;337:436–437.
270. Bayard PJ, Berger TG, Jacobsen MA. Drug hypersensitivity reactions in human immunodeficiency virus disease. J Acquir Immune Defic Syndr 1992;5:1237–1257.
271. Greenberger RG, Patterson R. Management of drug allergy in patients with acquired immunodeficiency syndrome. J Allergy Clin Immunol 1987;79:484–488.
272. Don PC, Fusco F, Fried P, Batterman A, Duncanson FP, Lenox TH, Klein NC. Nail dyschromia associated with zidovudine. Ann Intern Med 1990; 112:145–146.
273. Furth PA, Kazakis AM. Nail pigmentation changes associated with azidothymidine (zidovudine). Ann Intern Med 1987;107:350.
274. Greenberg RG, Berger TG. Nail and mucocutaneous hyperpigmentation with azidothymidine therapy. J Am Acad Dermatol 1990;327:330.
275. Merenich JA, Hannen RN, Gentry RH, Harrison SM. Azidothymidine-induced hyperpigmentation mimicking primary adrenal insufficiency. Am J Med 1989;86:469–470.
276. Gaglioti D, Ficarra G, Adler-Storthz K, Pimpinelli N, Piluso S, Meli M. Zidovudine-related oral lichenoid reactions. Poster presentation, VII International Conference on AIDS, Florence, Italy, June 16–21, 1991.
277. Bessen LJ, Greene JB, Louie E, Setizman P, Weinberg H. Severe polymyositis-like syndrome associated with zidovudine therapy of AIDS and ARC (letter). N Engl J Med 1988;318:708.
278. Van Der Pijl JW, Frissen PH, Reiss P, Hulsebosch HJ, Van Den Tweel JG, Lange JM, Danner SA. Foscarnet and penile ulceration. (letter) Lancet 1990;335:286.
279. Blanshard C. Generalized cutaneous rash associated with foscarnet usage in AIDS. J Infect Dis 1991;23:336–337.
280. Greenberger RG, Patterson R. Management of drug allergy in patients with acquired immunodeficiency syndrome. J Allergy Clin Immunol 1987;79:484–488.
281. Raviglione MC, Dinan WA, Pablos-

Mendez A, Palagiano A, Sabatini MT. Fatal toxic epidermal necrolysis during prophylaxis with pryimethamine and sulfadoxine in a human immunodeficiency virus–infected person. Arch Intern Med 1988;148:2683–2685.

282. Berger TG, Tappero JW, Leoung GS, Jacobson MA. Aerosolized pentamadine and cutaneous eruptions (letter). Ann Intern Med 1989;110:1035–1036.
283. Rosenthal E, Pesce A, Vinti H, Chichmanian RM, Bodokh I, Vitetta A, Dubois D, Cassuto JP. Two original observations of chlormezanone and fluoxetine induced toxic epidermal necrolysis in HIV-infected patients. Poster presentation, VII International Conference on AIDS, Florence, Italy, June 16–24, 1991.
284. Jorde UP, Horowitz HW, Wormser GP. Limitations of dapsone as PCP prophylaxis in HIV-infected patients intolerant of trimethoprim/sulfamethoxazole. Poster presentation, VIII International Conference on AIDS, Amsterdam, July 19–24, 1991.
285. Mohle-Boetani J, Akula S, Holodny M, Katzenstein D, Garcia G. The sulfone syndrome during dapsone treatment for *Pneumocystis carinii* pneumonia prophylaxis. Poster presentation, VII International Conference on AIDS, Florence, Italy, June 16–21, 1991.
286. Gill PS, Loureiro C, Bernstein-Singer M, Rarick MU, Sattler F, Levine AM. Clinical effects of glucocorticoids on Kaposi's sarcoma related to the acquired immunodeficiency syndrome. Ann Intern Med 1989;110:937–940.
287. Feingold I. Oral desensitization of trimethoprim-sulfamethoxasole in a patient with acquired immunodeficiency syndrome. J Allergy Clin Immunol (leter). 1986;78:905.
288. Leonidas JR. Hair alteration in black patients with acquired immunodeficiency syndrome. Cutis 1987;39:537–538.
289. Cockerell CJ. Personal observation, 1993.
290. Casanova JM, Puig T, Rubio M. Hypertrichosis of the eyelashes in acquired immunodeficiency syndrome. Arch Dermatol 1987;123:1599–1601.
291. Foon KA, Dougher G. Increased growth of eyelashes in a patient given leukocyte A interferon (letter). N Engl J Med 1984;311:1259.
292. Kaplan MH, Sadik NS, Talmor M. Acquired trichomegaly of the eyelashes. A cutaneous marker of acquired immunodeficiency syndrome. J Am Acad Dermatol 1991;25:801–804.
293. Schonwetter RS, Nelson EB. Alopecia areata and the acquired immunodeficiency syndrome related complex. Ann Intern Med (letter). 1986;104:287.
294. Sadick NS. Clinical and laboratory evaluation of AIDS trichopathy. Int J Dermatol 1993;32:33–38.
295. Chernosky ME, Findley VK. Yellow-nail syndrome in patients with AIDS. J Am Acad Dermatol 1985;13:731–737.
296. Scher RK. Acquired immunodeficiency syndrome and yellow nails. J Am Acad Dermatol 1988;18:758–759.
297. Cockerell CJ, Dolan ET. Widespread cutaneous and systemic calcification (calciphylaxis) in patients with the acquired immunodeficiency syndrome and renal disease. J Am Acad Dermatol 1992;26:559–562.
298. Cockerell CJ. Noninfectious inflammatory skin diseases in HIV infected individuals. Dermatol Clin 1991;9:531–541.
299. Viraben R, Dupre A. Lichenoid granulomatous papular dermatosis associated with human AIDS. J Am Acad Dermatol 1988;18:1140–1141.
300. Porwancher RB, Sajjad S. Adult Kawasaki disease in HIV infected patients. Poster presentation, VIII International Conference on AIDS, Amsterdam, July 19–24, 1992.
301. Fisher AA. Condom conundrums. Cutis 1991; 48:359–360.
302. Karter DL, Karter AJ, Yarrish R, Patterson C, Nord J, Sepulveda J, Kislak J. Vitamin A deficiency in patients with AIDS. Poster presentation, VIII International Conference on AIDS, Amsterdam, July 19–24, 1992.
303. Reichel M, Mauro TM, Ziboh VA, Huntley AC, Fletcher MP. Acrodermatitis enteropathica in a patient with the acquired immunodeficiency syndrome. Arch Dermatol 1992;128:415–417.
304. Nelson AM, Mvula M, St. Louis M, Brown C, Lebughe I, Jingu M, Laga M, Kaseka N, Goeman J, O'Leary T. Increased rates of cervical dysplasia associated with clinical and immunological evidence of immunodeficiency. Poster presentation, VIII International Conference on AIDS, Amsterdam, July 19–24, 1992.
305. Galfetti M, Irion O, Beguin F. Vulvar and cervical pathologies in HIV-seropositive (HIV+) women followed in a colposcopy outpatient clinic (abstract, vol II). VI International Conference on AIDS, San Francisco, California, June 20–24, 1990:337.
306. Palefsky JM, Gonzales J, Greenblatt RM, Ahn DK, Hollander K. Anal intraepithelial neoplasia and anal papillomavirus infection among homosexual males with group IV HIV disease. JAMA 1990;263:2911–2916.
307. Beck DE, Jaso RF, Zajac RA. Surgical management of anal condylomata in the HIV-positive patient. Dis Colon Rectum 1990;33:180–183.
308. Marte C, Cohen M, Fruchter R, Kelly P. Pap test and STD findings in HIV positive women at ambulatory care sites (abstract, vol I). VI International Conference on AIDS, San Francisco, California, June 20–24, 1990:211.
309. Goedert JJ, Caussy D, Palefsky J, Gonzales J, Grossman RJ, DiGioia RJ, Sanchez WC. Interaction of HIV and papillomaviruses: Association with anal intraepithelial abnormality in homosexual men (abstract, vol I). VI International Conference on AIDS, San Francisco, California, June 20–24, 1990:201.
310. Smith KJ, Skelton HG, Yeager J, Angritt P, Wagner KF. Cutaneous neoplasms in a military population of HIV-1–positive patients. J Am Acad Dermatol 1993;29:400–406.
311. Yabe Y, Tanimura Y, Sakai A, Hitsumoto T, Nohara N. Molecular characteristics and physical state of human papillomavirus DNA change with progressing malignancy: Studies in a patient with epidermodysplasia verruciformis. Int J Cancer 1989;43:1022–1028.
312. Pandya AG, Cockerell CJ. Personal observation, 1993.
313. Sitz KV, Keppen M. Metastatic basal cell carcinoma in acquired immunodeficiency syndrome–related complex. JAMA 1987;257:340–343.
314. Fink MJ, Fruchter R, Maiman M, Webber CA, Chen P, Kelly P. Cytology, colposcopy and histology in HIV-positive women. Poster presentation, IX International Conference on AIDS, Berlin, Germany, June 6–12, 1993.
315. Guinness K, LaGuardia K. Cryotherapy in the management of cervical dysplasia in HIV-infected women. Poster presentation, IX International Conference on AIDS, Berlin, Germany, June 6–12, 1993.
316. Bernstein L, Levin D, Menck H, Ross RK. AIDS-related secular trends in cancer in Los Angeles County men: A comparison by marital status. Cancer Res 1989;49:466–470.
317. Harnly ME, Swan SH, Holly EA, Kelter A, Padian N. Temporal trends in the incidence of non-Hodgkin's lymphoma and selected malignancies in a population with a high incidence of acquired immunodeficiency syndrome (AIDS). Am J Epidemiol 1988;128:261–267.
318. Chadbourne A, Metroka C, Nmuradian J. Progressive lymph node histology and its prognostic value in patients with acquired immunodeficiency syndrome and AIDS-related complex. Hum Pathol 1989;20:579–587.
319. Bernheim A, Berger R. Cytogenic studies of Burkitt's lymphoma/leukemia in patients with acquired immunodeficiency syndrome. Cancer Genet Cytogenet 1988;32:67–74.
320. Parker SC, Fenton DA, McGibbon DH. L'homme rouge and the acquired immunodeficiency syndrome. N Engl J Med 1989;321:906–907.
321. Kobayashi M, Yoshimoto S, Fujishita M, Yano S, Niiya K, Kubonishi I, Taguchi H, Miyoshi I. HTLV-positive T-cell lymphoma/leukemia in an AIDS

patient (letter). Lancet 1984;1:1361–1362.

322. Nagatani T, Miyazawa M, Matsuzaki T, Iemoto G, Ishii H, Kim ST, Baba N, Miyamoto H, Minato K, Motomura S, et al. Adult T-cell leukemia/lymphoma (ATL)—Clinical, histopathological, immunological and immunohistochemical characteristics. Exp Dermatol 1992;1:248–252.
323. Knowles DM, Chamulak G, Subar M, Pelicci PG, Dugan M, Burke JS, Raphael B, Dalla-Favera R. Clinicopathologic immunophenotypic and molecular genetic analysis of AIDS-associated lymphoid neoplasia: Clinical and biologic implications (rewiew). Pathol Annu 1988;23:33–67.

Additional Relevant References

Beral V, Peterman TA, Berkelman RL, Jaffe HW. Kaposi's sarcoma among persons with AIDS: A sexually transmitted infection? Lancet 1990;335:123–128.

Cohen PR, Bank DE, Silvers DN, Grossman ME. Cutaneous lesions of disseminated histoplasmosis in human immunodeficiency virus–infected patients. J Am Acad Dermatol 1990;23:422–428.

Duvic M, Lowe L, Rapini RP, Rodriguez S, Levy ML. Eruptive dysplastic nevi associated with the human immunodeficiency virus infection. Arch Dermatol 1989;125:397–401.

Friedman-Kien AE, Saltzman BR. Clinical manifestations of classical endemic African, and epidemic AIDS-associated Kaposi's sarcoma. J Am Acad Dermatol 1990;22:1237–1250.

Friedman-Kien AE, Saltzman RR, Cao YZ, Nestor MS, Mirabile M, Li JJ, Peterman TA. Kaposi's sarcoma in HIV-negative homosexual men (letter). Lancet 1990;335:168–169.

Haverkos HW. Factors associated with the pathogenesis of AIDS. J Infect Dis 1987;156:251–257.

Hennessey NP, Armington KG. Multiple tumors of sebaceous gland origin in an AIDS patient. Poster presentation, IX International Conference on AIDS, Berlin, Germany, June 6–12, 1993.

Hicks CB, Benson PM, Lupton GP, Tramont EC. Seronegative secondary syphilis in a patient infected with the human immunodeficiency virus (HIV) with Kaposi's sarcoma. Ann Intern Med 1987;107:492–495.

Huang YQ, Li JJ, Rush MG, Poiesz BJ, Nicolaides A, Jacobson M, Zhang WG, Coutavas E, Abbott MA, Friedman-Kien AE. HPV-16–related DNA sequences in Kaposi's sarcoma. Lancet 1992;339:515–518.

Janier M, Moral P, Civatte J. The Koebner phenomenon in AIDS-related Kaposi's sarcoma. J Am Acad Dermatol 1990;22:125–126.

Krigel RL, Friedman-Kien AE. Epidemic Kaposi's sarcoma. Semin Oncol 1990;17:350–360.

Krown SF, Golft JWM, Niedzwicki D. Interferon and zidovudine—Safety tolerance and clinical and virological effects in patients with Kaposi's sarcoma associated with the acquired immunodeficiency syndrome (AIDS). Ann Intern Med 1990;112:812–821.

Martinez-Maza O, Dourado I, Kishimoto T, Fahey JL, Detels R. Elevated serum IL-6 levels are associated with the development of AIDS-related Kaposi's sarcoma. Poster presentation, IX International Conference on AIDS, Berlin, Germany, June 6–12, 1993.

Massarelli G, Scott CA, Ibba M, Tanda F, Cossu A. Immunocytochemical profile of Kaposi's sarcoma cells: Their reactivity to a panel of antibodies directed against different tissue cell markers. Appl Pathol 1989;7(1):34–41.

Nickoloff BJ, Wood GS, Chu M, Beckstead JH, Griffiths CE. Disseminated dermal dendrocytomas. A new fibrohistiotic proliferative disorder? Am J Surg Pathol 1990;14(9):867–871.

Nodal myofibroblastoma in an AIDS patient with disseminated Kaposi's sarcoma. Poster presentation, IX International Conference on AIDS, Berlin, Germany, June 6–12, 1993.

Orlow SJ, Kamino H, Lawrence RL. Multiple subcutaneous leiomyosarcomas in an adolescent with AIDS. Am J Pediatr Hematol Oncol 1992;14:265–268.

Rendon MI, Roberts LJ, Tharp MD. Linear cutaneous lesions of Kaposi's sarcoma: A clinical clue to the diagnosis of AIDS. J Am Acad Dermatol 1988;19:327–329.

Rutherford GW, Payne SF, Lemp GF. The epidemiology of AIDS-related Kaposi's sarcoma in San Francisco. J Acquir Immune Defic Syndr 1990;3(suppl 1):S4–S7.

Safai B, Johnson KG, Myskowski PL, Koziner B, Yang SY, Cunningham-Rundles S, Godbold JH, Dupont B. The natural history of Kaposi's sarcoma in the acquired immunodeficiency syndrome (review). Ann Intern Med 1985;103:744–750.

Salahuddin SZ, Nakamura S, Biberfeld P, Kaplan MH, Markham PD, Larsson L, Gallo RC. Angiogenic properties of Kaposi's sarcoma-derived cells after long term culture in vitro. Science 1988;242:430–433.

Simpson JK, Cottrell CP, Miller RF, Spitel MF. Liposomal doxorubicin: Initial experience of a major London center. Poster presentation, IX International Conference on AIDS, Berlin, Germany, June 6–12, 1993.

Tikjb G, Russel M, Petersen CS, Gerstoft J, Kobayasi T. Seronegative secondary syphilis in a patient with AIDS: Identification of *Treponema pallidum* in biopsy specimen. J Am Acad Dermatol 1991;24:506–508.

Tindall B, Finlayson R, Mutimer K, Billson FA, Munro VF, Cooper DA. Malignant melanoma associated with human immunodeficiency virus infection in three homosexual men. J Am Acad Dermatol 1989;20:587–591.

ORAL MANIFESTATIONS OF HIV INFECTION

Deborah Greenspan
John S. Greenspan

5

The oral mucosa is perhaps the earliest and most frequent location of the opportunistic infections, neoplasms, and other lesions found in patients infected with human immunodeficiency virus (HIV).[1–3] Cross-sectional studies of HIV-infected men show a prevalence of oral lesions of approximately 30%, with the two commonest lesions being oral candidiasis (about 20%) and oral hairy leukoplakia (about 10%).[4] We have found HIV-positive women to have similar levels of oral disease, with prevalences of 22% of any oral lesion, 15% of oral candidiasis, and 10% of oral hairy leukoplakia.[5] The presence of oral lesions determines the patient's category in several widely used classifications of HIV disease and acquired immunodeficiency syndrome (AIDS).[6] The presence of oral lesions is an important factor in the staging of HIV infection, in the assessment of progression of disease, and in the assessment of response to antiretroviral therapy.[7,8] The presence of oral candidiasis and oral hairy leukoplakia has been used as an entry criterion or an end point in the treatment of HIV infection and AIDS.[9]

This chapter is a modification of Greenspan D, Greenspan JS. The mouth in human immunodeficiency virus infection. Semin Dermatol 1994;13:144–150.

ORAL CANDIDIASIS

Oral candidiasis was included in the first descriptions of AIDS, has been described as a feature of primary HIV infection, and is, of course, widely found in later-stage disease.[10,11] *Candida albicans* is the commonest species found, although numerous other species have been described in some cases.[12] It must be emphasized that *C. albicans* is a not uncommon commensal in the oral cavity, even in healthy persons, although the number of fungal organisms rises in many disease states, including HIV infection, particularly as the CD4 count drops.[13] We recognize three clinical manifestations of oral candidiasis in HIV-infected patients: pseudomembranous candidiasis, erythematous candidiasis, and angular cheilitis. Pseudomembranous candidiasis (Fig. 5–1), sometimes called thrush, is characterized by the presence on the oral mucosa of white or yellowish removable plaques. When the plaques are wiped off, a red surface is revealed. The erythematous form appears as a flat red lesion, and the most common locations include the palate (Fig. 5–2) and the dorsal surface of the tongue, where there may be patchy depapillated areas (Fig. 5–3). Angular cheilitis takes the form of cracks, fissures, or ulcers at the corners of the mouth (Fig. 5–4) and can occur alone or in conjunction with either of the other forms. Erythematous candidiasis is easily missed on clinical examination, but its detection is important, for we have found that erythematous candidiasis and pseudomembranous candidiasis are both equally predictive of the subsequent development of AIDS.[14]

The clinician should remember that oral candidiasis may be associated with other conditions in addition to HIV infection, such as xerostomia, diabetes, antibiotic use, and a wide range of immunosuppressive conditions, including those induced by steroids and other drugs. The diagnosis of oral

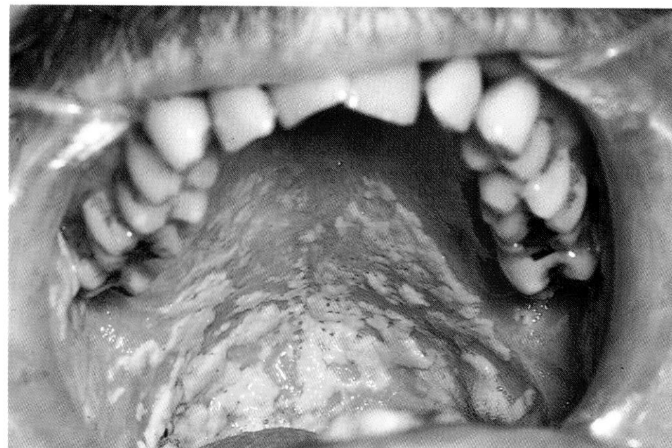

FIGURE 5–1. Candidiasis

One of the commonest clinical features of human immunodeficiency virus infection, the pseudomembranous form of oral candidiasis, also known as thrush, consists of white or creamy removable plaques and can be seen anywhere in the oropharynx. They are often asymptomatic, but sometimes they are associated with pain or changes in taste.

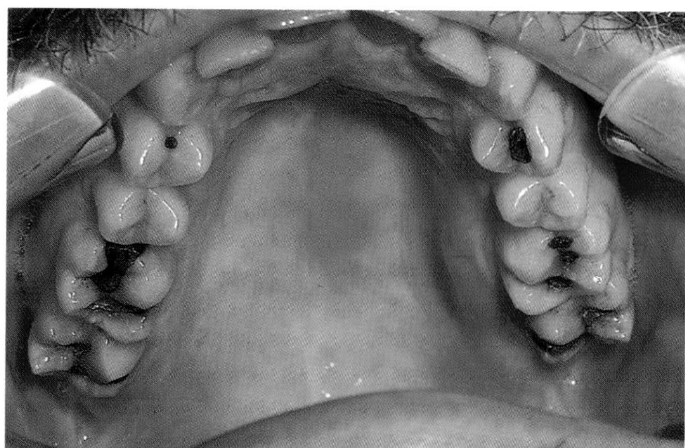

FIGURE 5–2. Erythematous candidiasis

Equally common and equally significant in the progression of human immunodeficiency virus infection but subtle in its clinical presentation, erythematous candidiasis is here seen as a red patch on the palate.

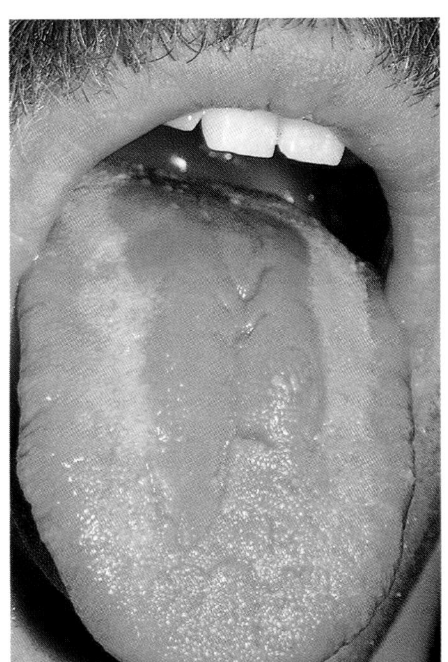

FIGURE 5–3. Erythematous candidiasis
Erythematous candidiasis seen as a red, smooth, depapillated area on the dorsal tongue.

candidiasis is usually straightforward, for the clinical appearances are fairly distinctive. The patient may complain of a burning mouth, a metallic taste, or a change in taste. We have found potassium hydroxide suspension of smears from the lesions to be helpful in revealing hyphae and blastospores. Culture results can be disappointing unless quantified, for the carrier state is extremely common.

Treatment of oral candidiasis requires the use of topical or systemic antifungal drugs.[15] Oral topical medications include clotrimazole (Mycelex) oral troche 10-mg tablets, one tablet dissolved slowly in the mouth five times a day; and nystatin (Mycostatin) oral pastille 200,000 units, one or two pastilles dissolved slowly in the mouth five times a day. Mycolog cream, clotrimazole cream, or ketoconazole cream are useful in the treatment of angular cheilitis. Systemic medications include fluconazole (Diflucan), 100-mg tablet taken daily for 7 to 14 days, and ketoconazole (Nizoral) 200-mg tablets, one or two tablets daily with food for 7 to 14 days.[16] Ketoconazole may not be well absorbed in those with low gastric pH and therefore sometimes may not be effective. Itraconazole (Sporanox) has been reported to be effective in the treatment of oral candidiasis.[17] Several cases have been reported of strains of *Candida* that are resistant to fluconazole.[18,19] Although oral candidiasis is by far the commonest fungal disease seen in the mouth in HIV infection, occasional cases are seen of histoplasmosis, cryptococcosis, geotrichosis, and penicillosis.[20,21]

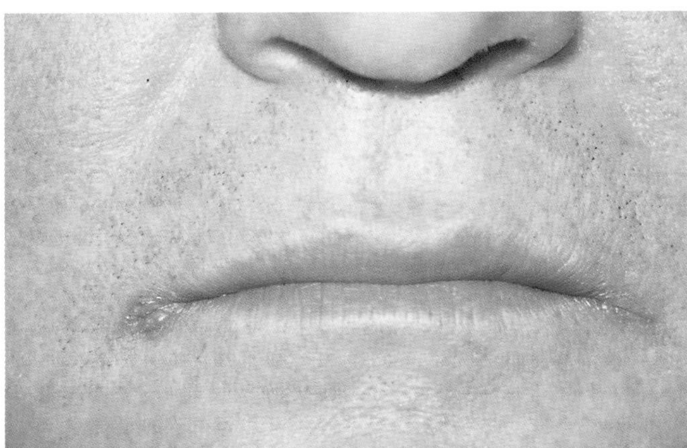

FIGURE 5–4. Angular cheilitis
Angular cheilitis is less common than the other two forms of oral candidiasis and here is seen as redness and cracking at the corners of the mouth.

HIV-ASSOCIATED PERIODONTAL DISEASE

Unusual and severe forms of periodontal disease can affect persons who are infected with HIV.[22,23] The lesions include gingivitis; a severe often localized periodontitis; and a severe spreading destructive infection of gingiva, soft tissue, and associated bone called *necrotizing stomatitis,* resembling noma, or cancrum oris[24] (Fig. 5–5). The gingivitis, currently called *linear gingival erythema,* manifests as a bright red line along the gingival margin, with minimal plaque. The periodontitis may be of rapid onset with significant bone and soft tissue loss and sometimes may result in loosening or loss of teeth. Patients usually experience considerable "deep" pain. This condition may become more widespread, affecting larger areas of the oral mucosa and leading to necrotizing stomatitis, with destruction of large areas of soft tissue and exposure of the underlying bone and subsequent necrosis and sequestration. Treatment by the dentist involves thorough débridement of the affected areas, using scaling, root planing, and currettage.[25] These local approaches are accompanied by the use of antibiotics; additional antibacterial measures that are helpful include local irrigation with povidone-iodine and daily mouth rinses with chlorhexidine gluconate.

WARTS

Oral lesions associated with human papillomavirus include pilliferous warts and flat warts (focal epithelial hyperplasia) (Fig. 5–6). Treatment of the warts is by excision, either surgically or with the carbon dioxide laser. Cryosurgery and electrosurgery may be useful in some locations, but these techniques can sometimes cause edema and pain when used intraorally. The warts tend to recur, however, no matter which approach is adopted.

HERPES SIMPLEX

Oral herpes simplex lesions include ulcers and vesicles on the keratinized mucosa of the palate or gingiva and occasionally on the dorsal surface of the tongue[26] (Figs. 5–7 and 5–8). Diagnosis can be made from culture or cytologic smears showing characteristic viral giant cells. Confirmation can also be made through the use of monoclonal antibody tests.[27] These lesions may sometimes persist for several weeks, and treatment with oral acyclovir may be indicated. Topical acyclovir has not been shown to be effective in the treatment of intraoral herpes simplex virus infection. Rare cases of acyclovir-resistant oral and perioral lesions have been described.[28]

HERPES ZOSTER

Varicella-zoster virus causes oral and facial herpes zoster. The intraoral lesions appear as vesicles and ulcers and may occur on any mucosal surface. The distribution of the ulcers is usually unilateral, following the distribution of the trigeminal nerve, with a characteristic change from affected mucosa to normal mucosa at the midline. Occasionally, the lesions may be preceded by complaints of pain from the teeth in the absence of dental problems. Acyclovir, 3 to 4 grams per day, should be started as soon as possible and continued until the lesions disappear.

ORAL HAIRY LEUKOPLAKIA

Oral hairy leukoplakia is a white lesion found predominantly on the lateral margins of the tongue.[29] It is seen mostly in people with HIV infection and has been noted in all the risk groups for AIDS. It has also been seen, in very rare instances, in other immunosuppressed individuals, including recipients of cardiac, renal, or bone marrow transplants.[30] The lesion is white, does not rub off, and occurs on the tongue and occasionally elsewhere in the mouth and oropharynx (Fig. 5–9). The surface may be smooth, corrugated, or markedly folded (see Fig. 5–4). Microscopically, there are surface folds or corrugations, hyperparakeratosis, acanthosis, vacuolation of bands or clumps of prickle cells, and little, if any, subepithelial inflammation.

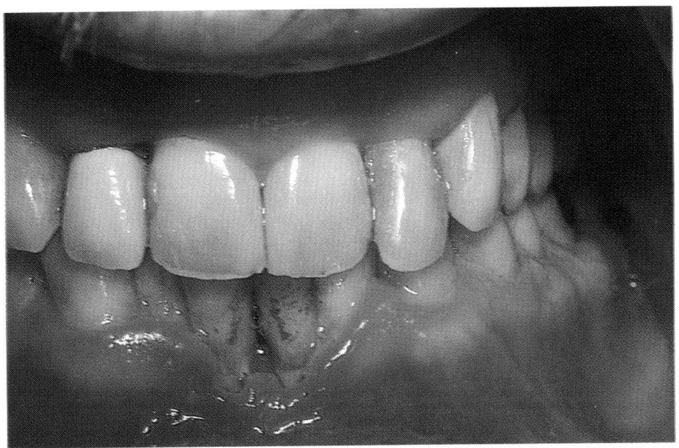

FIGURE 5–5. Necrotizing periodontitis

Rapid onset of pain and bleeding preceded diagnosis of this necrotizing periodontitis of the anterior mandible.

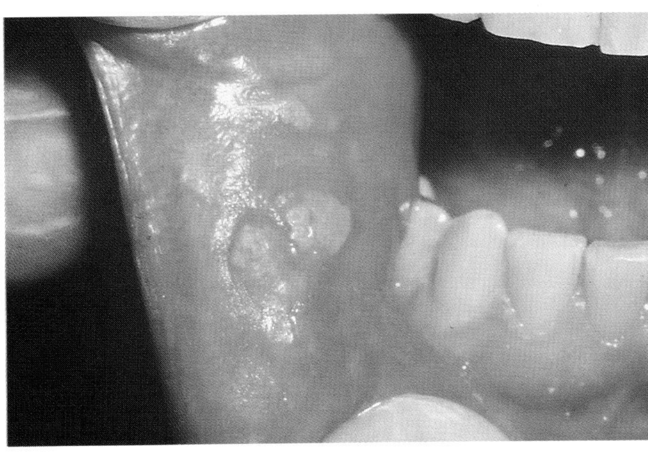

FIGURE 5–6. Flat wart

A flat wart (focal epithelial hyperplasia due to herpesvirus type 13) on the labial mucosa.

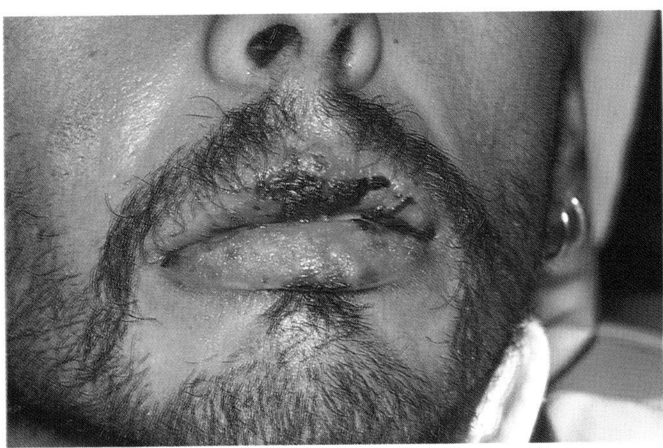

FIGURE 5–7. Herpes simplex virus 2 lesions

Crusted lesions appearing on the lip in this HIV-positive individual caused by reactivation of herpes simplex virus 2.

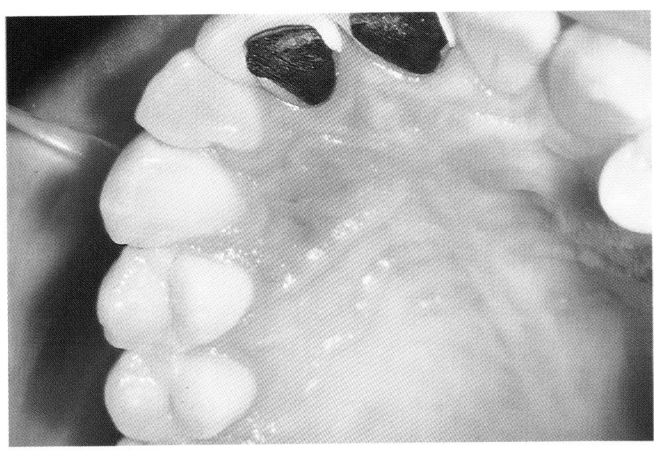

FIGURE 5–8. Herpes simplex virus ulcers

These small ulcers on the hard palate represent recurrent intraoral herpes simplex virus. Note the location on keratinized mucosa.

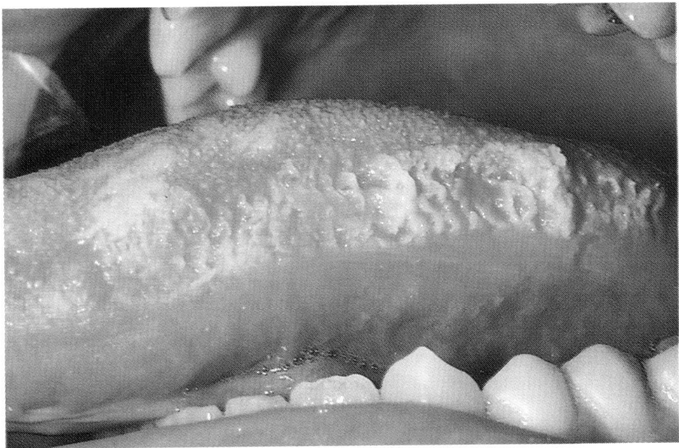

FIGURE 5–9. Oral hairy leukoplakia

Oral hairy leukoplakia manifesting as white corrugations on the lateral margin of the tongue.

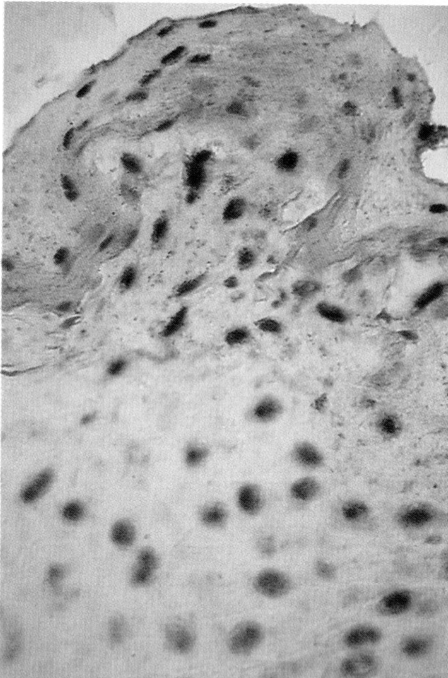

FIGURE 5–10. Epstein-Barr virus
Epstein-Barr virus DNA demonstrated by in situ hybridization in oral hairy leukoplakia.

The epithelial cells of oral hairy leukoplakia are heavily infected with Epstein-Barr virus[31] (Fig. 5–10). Oral hairy leukoplakia lesions should be distinguished from other white oral lesions, such as lichen planus, frictional keratosis, leukoplakia, and geographic tongue. They are usually asymptomatic but sometimes may produce problems because of their appearance or discomfort in the mouth. In such cases treatment may be indicated. Acyclovir at high doses, 3 to 4 grams per day for 2 weeks, may result in resolution, but when treatment is stopped oral hairy leukoplakia usually recurs within 3 to 4 months[31] (Figs. 5–11 and 5–12). Some case reports suggest that oral hairy leukoplakia may disappear in patients who are taking such drugs as ganciclovir or who are using topical tretinoin (Retin-A), applied daily for 1 to 2 weeks.[32] Oral hairy leukoplakia may disappear and reappear in people taking zidovudine.[18,33,34]

KAPOSI'S SARCOMA

The first lesions of Kaposi's sarcoma are often seen in the mouth, and most are seen in men, although a small number of cases have been described in women.[35,36] The lesions may be red, blue, or purple and may be flat or raised, solitary or multiple[31] (Figs. 5–13 and 5–14). The hard palate is the most common location, although lesions may be found on any part of the oral mucosa, including the gingiva, soft palate, tongue, and buccal mucosa (see Fig. 5–5). The lesions may become so large that patients experience difficulty maintaining good oral hygiene, and the lesions may become infected. Treatment for oral Kaposi's sarcoma is similar to that used to treat other manifestations of this disease and includes intralesional chemotherapy, systemic chemotherapy, and radiation therapy.[37,38] In the mouth, however, surgical debulking or application of sclerosing agents may be a very useful adjunct to therapy, improving both function and aesthetic appearance. Good oral hygiene and a clean mouth are essential to reduce morbidity. This can be achieved by frequent professional scaling and polishing of the teeth and the use of chlorhexidine mouth rinse.

NON-HODGKIN'S LYMPHOMA

In some cases of non-Hodgkin's lymphoma, the oral lesions are the presenting feature. The lesions can manifest as painful or painless swellings or ulcers and can occur anywhere in the oral cavity.[39,40]

ORAL ULCERS

Although recurrent aphthous ulcers are fairly common in the general population, there may be a recurrence of this condition in HIV-positive individuals who have been free of ulcers for many years, and in some cases they occur when there has never been a history of ulcers at all.[41] The lesions have the typical appearance of aphthous ulcers, being well-circumscribed ulcers with an erythematous halo. They may be solitary or multiple and may range in size from 1 to 2 mm (herpetiform recurrent aphthous ulcers [RAU]), to 4 to 6 mm (minor RAU)[31] (Fig 5–15), to large 1 to 4 cm (major RAU)[31] (Fig 5–16). The ulcers appear on nonkeratinized mucosa such as the buccal mucosa, the soft palate, the lateral and ventral tongue, and the tonsillar pillar. Similar ulcers have been described in other parts of the gastrointestinal tract. Large and long-standing ulcers can mimic malignant disease, such as lymphoma, and should undergo biopsy. The ulcers usually respond to treatment with topical steroids such as fluocinonide or clobetasol ointment 0.05% mixed half and half with Orabase and applied to the lesions several times a day.[42] Occasionally, systemic steroids may be indicated. Sometimes the lesions may become secondarily infected, and the additional use of antibiotics may be indicated. Thalidomide has been used with some success in some studies.[43,44] Similar ulcers are a complication of zalcitabine (ddC) use.[45] These too respond to steroid therapy.

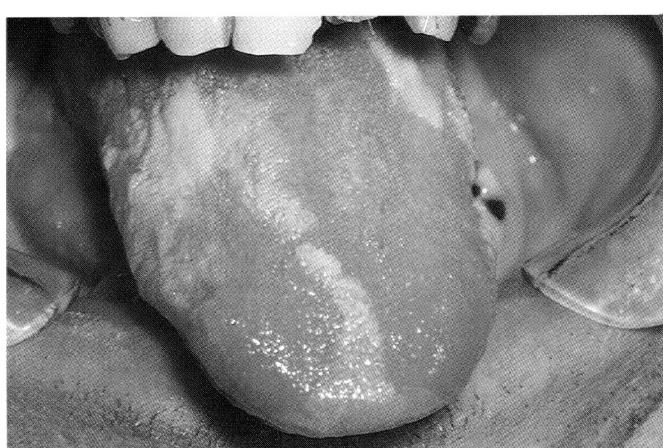

FIGURE 5–11. Oral hairy leukoplakia (before treatment)
Oral hairy leukoplakia on the dorsal surface of the tongue before treatment.

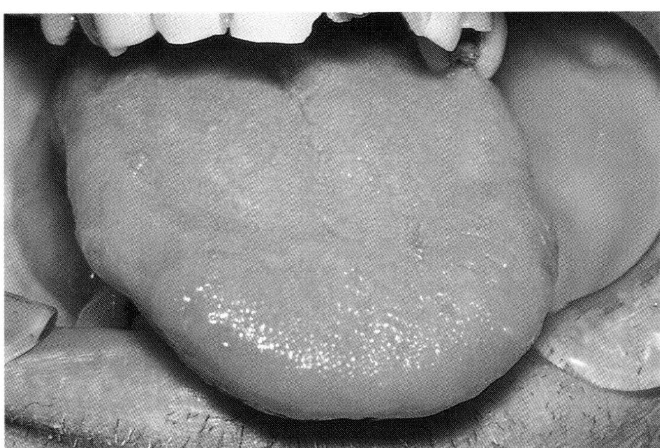

FIGURE 5–12. Oral hairy leukoplakia (after treatment)
After treatment with acyclovir, the oral hairy leukoplakia has disappeared.

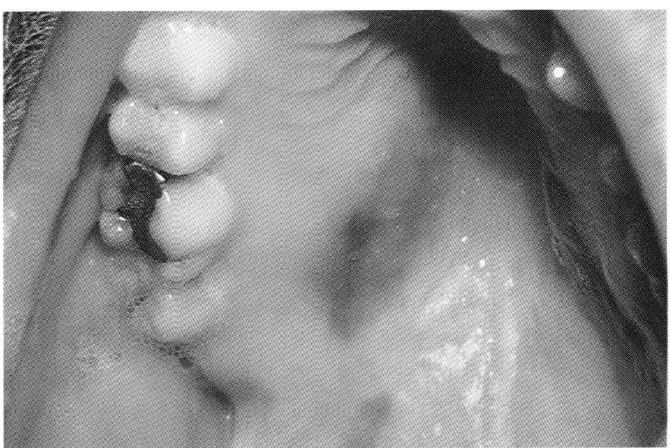

FIGURE 5–13. Flat Kaposi's sarcoma
Flat Kaposi's sarcoma lesion on the palate.

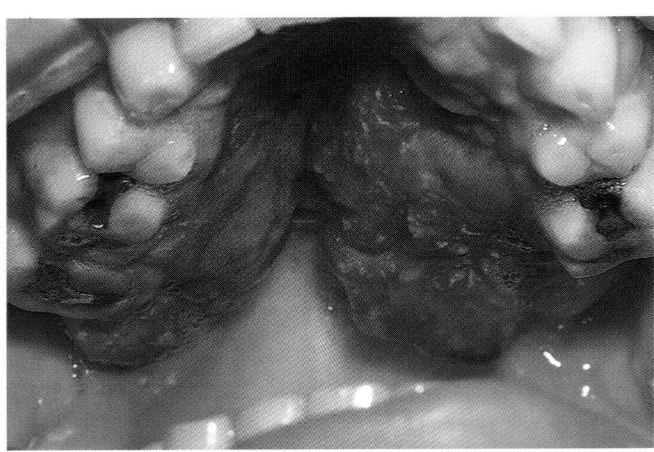

FIGURE 5–14. Nodular Kaposi's sarcoma
Advanced nodular Kaposi's sarcoma of the palate.

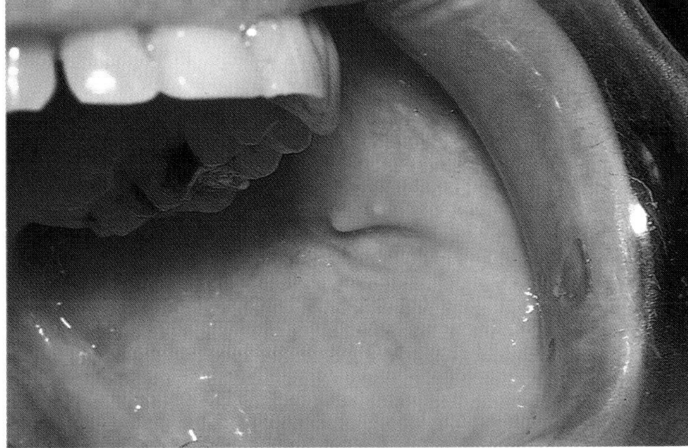

FIGURE 5–15. Minor aphthous ulcer
Minor aphthous ulcer (<5 mm in diameter) on the labial mucosa.

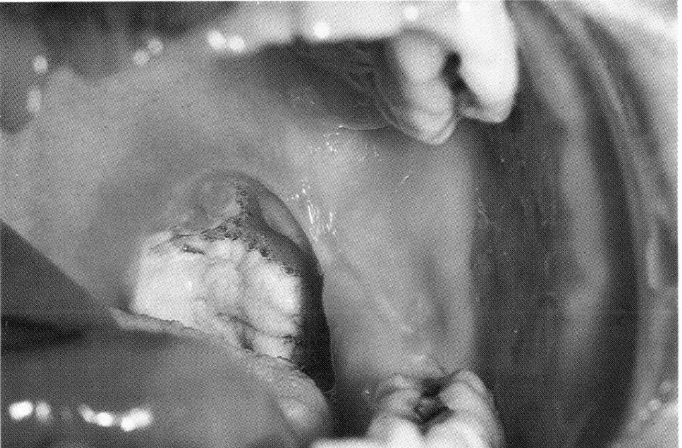

FIGURE 5–16. Major aphthous ulcers
Major aphthous ulcers (>5 mm in diameter) occurring on the tonsillar pillar. Biopsy is indicated for diagnosis to rule out other lesions such as non-Hodgkin's lymphoma or opportunistic infections.

SALIVARY GLAND DISEASE

Salivary gland enlargement, most commonly affecting one or both parotid glands and less frequently the other salivary glands, is sometimes seen in association with HIV infection.[46,47] The enlarged glands are soft and painless and may have a cystic component[31] (Fig 5–17). The glands enlarge slowly but can increase so significantly that patients request removal of the affected gland for aesthetic reasons. Xerostomia may sometimes be present. Xerostomia has also been reported as a complication of therapy with dideoxyinosine (ddI).[48] Treatment of hyposalivation should include local measures to relieve the symptoms of xerostomia, such as the use of saliva substitutes, and topical fluoride applications to reduce the risk of dental caries.

References

1. Melnick SL, Engel D, Truelove E, et al. Oral mucosal lesions: Association with the presence of antibodies to the human immunodeficiency virus. Oral Surg Oral Med Oral Pathol 1989; 68:37–43.
2. Katz MH, Greenspan D, Westenhouse J, Hessol NA, Buchbinder SP, Lifson AR, Shiboski S, Ormond D, Moss A, Samuel M, Lang W, Feigal DW, Greenspan JS. Progression to AIDS in HIV-infected homosexual and bisexual men with hairy leukoplakia and oral candidiasis. AIDS 1992;6:95–100.
3. Katz MH, Mastrucci MT, Leggott PJ, Westenhouse J, Greenspan JS, Scott GB. Prognostic significance of oral lesions in children with perinatally acquired human immunodeficiency virus infection. Am J Dis Child 1993; 147(1):45–48.
4. Feigal DW, Katz MH, Greenspan D, Westenhouse J, Winkelstein W Jr, Lang W, Samuel M, Buchbinder SP, Hessol NA, Lifson AR, Rutherford GW, Moss A, Osmond D, Shiboski S, Greenspan JS. The prevalence of oral lesions in HIV-infected homosexual and bisexual men: Three San Francisco epidemiological cohorts. AIDS 1991;5:519–525.
5. Shiboski CH, Hilton JF, Greenspan D, Westonhouse JL, Devish P, Vranizan K, Lifson AR, Canchola A, Katz MH, Cohen JB, Moss AR, Greenspan JS. HIV-related oral manifestations in two cohorts of women in San Francisco. J Acquir Immune Defic Syndr 1994; 7:964–971.
6. Royce RA, Luckmann RS, Fusaro RE,

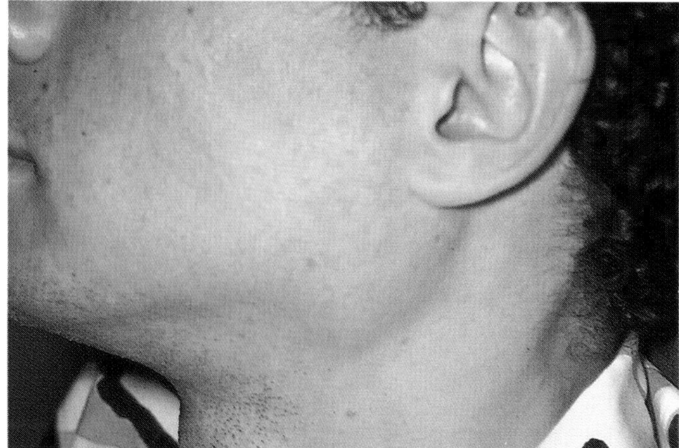

FIGURE 5–17. Salivary gland disease
Enlargement of the left parotid gland in a patient with salivary gland disease caused by human immunodeficiency virus. The lesions were soft, painless, and bilateral.

Winkelstein WJ. The natural history of HIV-1 infection: Staging classifications of disease. AIDS 1991;5(4):355–364.
7. Aylward RB, Vlahov D, Munoz A, Rapititi E. Validation of the proposed World Health Organization staging system for HIV disease and infection in a cohort of intravenous drug users. AIDS 1994;8:1129–1133.
8. Lamster IB, Begg MD, Mitchell-Lewis D, Fine JB, Grbie JT, Todak GG, El-Sadr W, Gorman JM, Zambon JJ, Phelan JA. Oral manifestations of HIV infection in homosexual men and intravenous drug users. Oral Surg Oral Med Oral Pathol 1994;78:163–174.
9. Fischl MA, Richmann DD. Hansen N, et al. The safety and efficacy of zidovudine (AZT) in the treatment of subjects with mildly symptomatic human immunodeficiency virus type 1 (HIV) infection. Ann Intern Med 1990; 112:727–737.
10. Klein RS, Harris CA, Small CR, et al. Oral candidiasis in high-risk patients as the initial manifestation of the acquired immunodeficiency syndrome. N Engl J Med 1984;311:354–358.
11. Dull JS, Sen P, Raffanti S, Middleton JR. Oral candidiasis as a marker of acute retroviral illness. S Med J 1991;84:733–739.
12. Samaranayake LP, Holmstrup P. Oral candidiasis and human immunodeficiency virus infection. J Oral Pathol Med 1989;18(10):554–564.
13. Tylenda CA, Larsen J, Yeh CK, Lane HC, Fox PC. High levels of oral yeasts in early HIV-1 infection. J Oral Pathol Med 1989;18(9):520–524.
14. Dodd CL, Greenspan D, Katz MH, Westenhouse JL, Feigal DW, Greenspan JS. Oral candidiasis in HIV infection: Pseudomembranous and erythematous candidiasis show similar rates of progression to AIDS. AIDS 1991;5:1339–1343.
15. Greenspan D. Treatment of oral candidiasis in HIV infection. Oral Surg Oral Med Oral Pathol 1994;78:211–215.
16. Just-Nubling G, Gentschew G, Meisner K, et al. Fluconazole prophylaxis of recurrent oral candidiasis in HIV-positive patients. Eur J Clin Infect Dis 1991;10:917–921.
17. Smith DE, Midgley J, Allan M, Connolly GM, Gazzard BG. Itraconazole versus ketoconazole in the treatment of oral and oesophageal candidosis in patients infected with HIV. AIDS 1988;5(11):1367–1371.
18. Warnock DW, Burke J, Cope NJ, Johnson EM, von Fraunhofer NA, Williams EW. Fluconazole resistance in *Candida glabrata* (letter). Lancet 1988;2(8623):1310.
19. Baily GG, Perry FM, Denning DW, Mandal BK. Fluconazole-resistant candidosis in an HIV cohort. AIDS 1994; 8:787–792.
20. Heinic G, Greenspan D, MacPhail LA, Schiødt M, Miyasaki SH, Kaufman L, Greenspan JS. Oral *Histoplasma capsulatum* in association with HIV infection: A case report. J Oral Pathol Med 1992;21:85–89.
21. Vithayasai P, Vithayasai V. Clinical manifestations of 174 AIDS cases in Maharaj Nakorn Chiang Mai Hospital. J Dermatol 1993;20(7):389–393.
22. Winkler JR, Herrera C, Westenhouse J, Robinson P, Hessol N, Buchbinder S, Greenspan JS, Katz MH. Periodontal disease in HIV-infected and uninfected homosexual and bisexual men (letter). AIDS 1992;6:1041–1043.
23. Masouredis CM, Katz MH, Greenspan D, et al. Prevalence of HIV-associated periodontitis and gingivitis in HIV-infected patients attending an AIDS clinic. J Acquir Immune Defic Syndr 1992;5:479–483.
24. Barr C, Lopez MR, Rua DA. Periodontal changes by HIV serostatus in a cohort of homosexual and bisexual men. J Clin Periodontol 1992;10:794–801.
25. Winkler JR, Murray PA, Grassi M, Hammerle C. Diagnosis and management of HIV-associated periodontal lesions. J Am Dent Assoc 1989; 119(suppl):S25–S34.
26. Greenspan D, Greenspan JS, Pindborg JJ, Schiodt M. AIDS and the Mouth. Copenhagen: Munksgaard; 1990.
27. MacPhail LA, Hilton JF, Heinic GS, Greenspan D. Direct immunofluorescence vs. culture for detecting HSV in oral ulcers: A comparison. J Am Dent Assoc 1995;126:74–78.
28. MacPhail LA, Greenspan D, Schiodt M, et al. Acyclovir-resistant, foscarnet-sensitive oral herpes simplex type 2 lesion in a patient with AIDS. Oral Surg Oral Med Oral Pathol 1989; 67:427–432.
29. Greenspan D, Greenspan JS, Conant M, Petersen V, Silverman S Jr, DeSouza Y. Oral "hairy" leucoplakia in male homosexuals: Evidence of association with both papillomavirus and a herpes-group virus. Lancet 1984;2:831–834.
30. Epstein JB, Sherlock CH, Greenspan JS. Hairy leukoplakia-like lesions following bone marrow transplantation (letter). AIDS 1991;5:101–102.
31. Greenspan JS, Greenspan D, Lennette ET, et al. Replication of Epstein-Barr virus within the epithelial cells of "hairy" leukoplakia, an AIDS-associated lesion. N Engl J Med 1985; 313:1564–1571.
32. Schofer H, Ochsendorf FR, Helm EB, Milbracht R. Treatment of oral hairy leukoplakia in AIDS patients with vitamin A acid (typically) or acyclovir (systemically) (letter). Dermatologica 1987;74:150–151.
33. DeSouza YG, Freese UK, Greenspan D, Greenspan JS. Diagnosis of Epstein-Barr virus infection in hairy leukoplakia by using nucleic acid hybridization and noninvasive techniques. J Clin Microbiol 1990;28: 2775–2778.
34. Katz MH, Greenspan D, Heinic GS, Chan AK, Hollander H, Chernoff D, Greenspan JS. Resolution of hairy leukoplakia: An observational trial of zidovudine versus no treatment (letter). J Infect Dis 1991;164:1240–1241.
35. Dodd CL, Greenspan D, Greenspan JS. Oral Kaposi's sarcoma in a woman as a first indication of infection with the human immunodeficiency virus. J Am Dent Assoc 1991;122:61–63.
36. Ficarra G, Person AM, Silverman S, et al. Kaposi's sarcoma of the oral cavity: A study of 134 patients with a review of the pathogenesis, epidemiology, clinical aspects, and treatment. Oral Surg Oral Med Oral Pathol 1988;66: 543–550.
37. Lucatorto FM, Sapp JP. Treatment of oral Kaposi's sarcoma with a sclerosing agent in AIDS patients. Oral Surg Oral Med Oral Pathol 1993;75:192–198.
38. Epstein JB, Scully C. Intralesional vinblastine for oral Kaposi's sarcoma in HIV infection. Lancet 1989;2:1100–1101.
39. Dodd CA, Greenspan D, Schiødt M, Daniels TE, Beckstead JH, MacPhail LA, Miyasaki S, Greenspan JS. Unusual oral presentation of non-Hodgkin's lymphoma in association with HIV infection. Oral Surg Oral Med Oral Pathol 1992;73:603–608.
40. Zeigler JL, Beckstead JA, Volberding PA, et al. Non-Hodgkins lymphoma in 90 homosexual men: Relation to generalized lymphadenopathy and the acquired immunodeficiency syndrome. N Engl J Med 1984;311:565–570.
41. Muzyka BC, Glick M. Major aphthous ulcers in patients with HIV disease. Oral Surg Oral Med Oral Pathol 1994;77:116–120.
42. MacPhail LA, Greenspan D, Greenspan JS. Recurrent aphthous ulcers in association with HIV infection: Diagnosis and treatment. Oral Surg Oral Med Oral Pathol 1992;73:283–288.
43. Revuz J, Guillaume JC, Janier M, et al. Crossover study of thalidomide vs placebo in severe recurrent aphthous stomatitis. Arch Dermatol 1990;126: 923–927.
44. Ryan J, Colman J, Pedersen J, Benson E. Thalidomide to treat esophageal ulcer in AIDS (letter). N Engl J Med 1992;327:208–209.
45. Greenspan D, Hilton J, Canchola AJ, MacPhail LM. Association between oral ulcers and zalcitabine. X International Conference on Acquired Immunodeficiency Syndrome. Yokohama, Japan, 1994.
46. Schiødt M, Dodd CL, Greenspan D, et al. Natural history of HIV-associated salivary gland disease. Oral Surg Oral Med Oral Pathol 1992;74:326–331.
47. Itescu S, Brancato LJ, Buxbaum J, et al. A diffuse infiltrative CD8 lymphocytosis syndrome in human immunodeficiency virus (HIV) infection: A host immune response associated with HLA-DR5. Ann Intern Med 1990;112: 3–10.
48. Dodd CL, Greenspan D, Westenhouse JL, Katz M. Xerostomia associated with didanosine. Lancet 1992;340:790.

MUCOCUTANEOUS MANIFESTATIONS OF PEDIATRIC HIV INFECTION

Ross E. McKinney, Jr.
Neil S. Prose

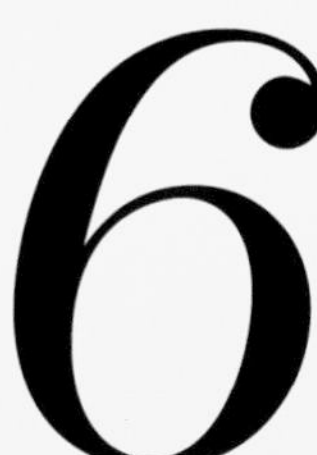

The basic pathogenesis of human immunodeficiency virus (HIV) infection in children is no different from that in adults, but the clinical manifestations of HIV infection are quite different. These variations probably reflect a combination of the age of the child at the time of the infection and the limited ability of a young child to respond immunologically to the infection. Pediatric HIV infection is more aggressive than the same infection in adults, particularly in regard to central nervous system involvement.

A SHORT HISTORY OF PEDIATRIC HIV INFECTION

The initial recognition that children suffered from a unique form of acquired immunodeficiency syndrome (AIDS) was made by Oleske and Rubinstein during 1981 and 1982.[1,2] They began to encounter children who seemed to be suffering from a new form of immunodeficiency that was very similar to one that had been recently described in adults. Like adults, the children had T-cell depletion and unusual opportunistic infections, particularly candidiasis and *Pneumocystis carinii* pneumonia. Oleske and Rubinstein reported their findings and were greeted by a surprising amount of skepticism. The absence of a diagnostic test made their reports somewhat conjectural, but they eventually were confirmed as correct once the retrovirus causing AIDS was recognized and a diagnostic assay developed.

TRANSMISSION OF HIV INFECTION TO CHILDREN

Most HIV-infected children acquire their infection from their mother either in utero or in the peripartum (birth) process. The exact timing of most infection is unknown, although the relatively small number of HIV-infected children who test positive for the virus on culture shortly after birth makes it seem likely that the majority of children are infected during the birth process.[3,4] However, interventions such as caesarean sections, which might be expected to affect a peripartum route of transmission, have been of no benefit. Goedert and colleagues published a study of twin deliveries in which there was a clearly higher rate of HIV transmission to the first-born twin, increasing the likelihood that the critical events for transmission occur around the time of delivery.[5]

The other risk factors for HIV transmission are increasingly less significant in children before adolescence. The majority of hemophiliacs treated with factor replacement before 1985 are infected with HIV, and a substantial number of children were infected by HIV-contaminated transfusions. Breast-feeding by HIV-infected women, particularly if the mother acquires her HIV infection during the period in which she is nursing, can lead to transmission through breast milk. The sexual route of transmission has also been documented, both in adolescents and in sexually abused young children.[6]

THE DIAGNOSIS OF HIV INFECTION IN CHILDREN

The fact that HIV-infected mothers transport anti-HIV antibody across the placenta to their fetus virtually 100% of the time but transmit HIV to only 15 to 40% of children has led to a great deal of clinical confusion. If a mother is infected with HIV, she has synthesized anti-HIV antibodies against the virus in her blood and cells. The term *HIV positive* when applied to adults means that an individual is positive for both the virus and the antibodies against it. However, for children the term *HIV positive* has no clear meaning, and its use brings confusion. Early in life, children who were exposed to HIV in utero are *HIV antibody positive*. If they subsequently turn out to be infected, they will be *HIV culture* (or *PCR*) *positive*, or simply *HIV infected*. Many families and clinicians have been confused by calling a child HIV positive because it does not spell out whether the child is infected. During the period in which a child is known to be antibody positive but before it can be determined whether the child is HIV infected, the indeterminate status is referred to as *CDC Class P-0*. A child who is HIV infected but asymptomatic is *CDC Class P-1*, and children with symptoms are referred to as *CDC Class P-2* (Table 6–1).

The median age for the disappearance of maternal antibodies from an uninfected child is roughly 10 months.[7] Some children may lose their maternal antibodies sooner, and some uninfected toddlers may be antibody positive as late as 15 to 18 months old. Because of the rapid progression of pediatric HIV and the need to start antiretroviral therapy early in the infected children, waiting for the maternal antibodies to be metabolized as a means to diagnose HIV infection is not acceptable. Further testing is necessary.

The major function of antibody testing in a child younger than 15 months old is to establish which children are at risk for HIV infection. This risk can be ascertained by testing either the mother or the child. To then identify which children are among the 15 to 40% who are infected requires further evaluation using three major elements: (1) attempts to isolate HIV

TABLE 6–1. SUMMARY OF THE CLASSIFICATION OF HIV INFECTION IN CHILDREN UNDER 13 YEARS OF AGE

Class P-0. Indeterminate infection

Class P-1. Asymptomatic infection

Subclass A. Normal immune function
Subclass B. Abnormal immune function
Subclass C. Immune function not tested

Class P-2. Symptomatic infection

Subclass A. Nonspecific findings
Subclass B. Progressive neurologic disease
Subclass C. Lymphoid interstitial pneumonitis
Subclass D. Secondary infectious diseases
- Category D-1. Specified secondary infectious diseases listed in the Centers for Disease Control and Prevention (CDC) surveillance definition for AIDS
- Category D-2. Recurrent serious bacterial infections
- Category D-3. Other specified secondary infectious diseases

Subclass E. Secondary cancers
- Category E-1. Specified secondary cancers listed in the CDC surveillance definition for AIDS
- Category E-2. Other cancers possibly secondary to HIV infection

Subclass F. Other diseases possibly due to HIV infection

or its components; (2) demonstration of immunologic changes; and (3) observation for clinical abnormalities.

The gold standard for the identification of HIV is culture. Unfortunately, HIV culture is expensive and slow and requires specialized laboratory personnel, equipment, and supplies. Also, HIV culture is not widely available. An alternative is to look for the genes of HIV using a technique called *polymerase chain reaction*, or PCR. This tool amplifies specific genetic sequences and can identify small quantities of HIV genome. Studies to date have demonstrated that PCR and HIV culture have comparable sensitivity, but PCR is cheaper, faster, and likely to be more widely available. The difficulty with PCR is the risk of a false-positive result as a result of low-level contamination, a risk that is made greater by the extreme sensitivity of the PCR assay. Consequently, most physicians who rely on PCR for diagnosis repeat a positive assay result before informing the family or beginning therapy. In addition, neither PCR nor HIV culture identifies all infected children, particularly during the first few months of life, and negative assay results should be repeated several times to be certain a child is not infected.

P24 antigen assays measure the amount of one of the core virus proteins in the blood stream. The sensitivity of P24 detection is less than that for culture and PCR, but it quantifies the amount of virus present when the assay result is positive. When P24 assays are available, they are generally inexpensive and can be performed relatively quickly. However, a negative P24 antigen result provides little reassurance, because the majority of HIV-infected children are P24 assay negative during most of their course. An advancement in P24 technology has been the inclusion of an acid dissociation step.[8] By lowering the pH of the serum, P24 and anti-P24 antibodies are split apart and the P24 can then be detected. Although this step improves the sensitivity of P24 detection, the reproducibility of the assay results for quantitative purposes is somewhat diminished.

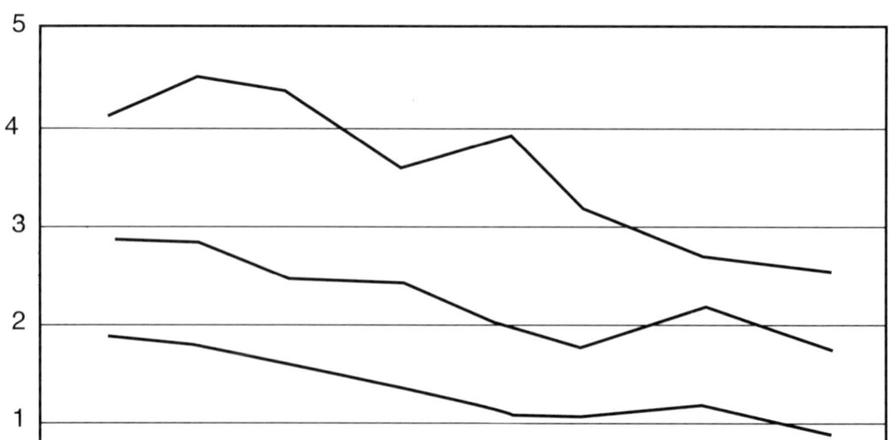

FIGURE 6–1. Normal CD4+ lymphocyte counts

The ninetieth, fiftieth, and tenth percentiles for $CD4^+$ lymphocyte counts (cells/mm^3) in children who are not infected with HIV. (Adapted from McKinney RE Jr, Wilfert CM. Lymphocyte subsets in children younger than 2 years old: Normal values in a population at risk for HIV infection and diagnostic and prognostic application to infected children. Pediatr Infect Dis J 1992;11:641. Copyright Williams & Wilkins.)

Using PCR or culture, the HIV infection status of most children can be determined by 6 months of age. A single PCR or culture result in the first 8 weeks of life is positive in roughly 50% of HIV-infected children. By the time the patient is 8 to 12 weeks old, the sensitivity increases to more than 95%, probably reflecting an increase in viral burden over time.

Children infected with HIV experience progressive losses in their $CD4^+$ lymphocyte counts. The degree of this loss can be difficult to sort out during the first 2 years of life because all children, whether HIV-infected or not, begin with very high $CD4^+$ counts that decrease over time. Consequently, tables of normal counts (Fig. 6–1) should be used to determine the child's status relative to age-appropriate expectations.[9]

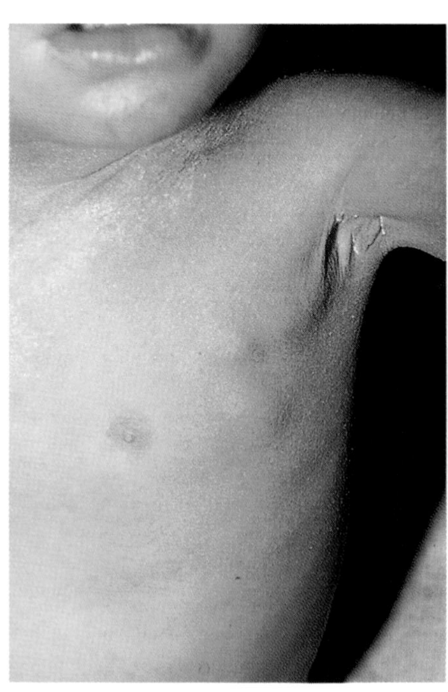

FIGURE 6–2. Lymphadenopathy

Generalized lymphadenopathy is often an early physical finding in children with perinatally acquired HIV infection.

Regulation of immunoglobulin synthesis is disrupted by HIV infection, leading to an increased synthesis of nonspecific IgG, IgA, and IgM antibodies. At birth, many children born to HIV-infected women have high IgG concentrations because of the transport of IgG across the placenta from their mothers, who also have high IgG levels. In contrast, IgA and IgM are not transported transplacentally, and so the child's levels should be normal at birth. If the amount of any of the immunoglobulin classes increases to substantially above normal, the child may be infected.

Physical examination and clinical history are the other important pieces of information in sorting out whether a child is infected with HIV. On examination, infected children may have several findings: generalized lymphadenopathy (Fig. 6–2), hepatomegaly, splenomegaly, oral candidiasis, enlarged parotid glands, developmental delay, or hyperreflexia. Their history may indicate an unusual number of infections, particularly with bacteremia, or an opportunistic infection. The high incidence and mortality of *P. carinii* pneumonia in the first few months of life is, in fact, one of the major factors creating an urgency about the need for an early diagnosis of HIV infection.

The evaluation of an infant for HIV infection is most effective if the mother is seen before the child is born. Studies are ongoing since 1992 to determine whether treating a pregnant woman with antiretroviral therapy during pregnancy can decrease the rate of HIV transmission from mother to child (vertical transmission). Screening for HIV is important because not all women with HIV infection have identified risk factors for the disease. The most common risk factors are a history of intravenous drug use, a sexual partner who is an intravenous drug user or is bisexual, or a history of multiple sex partners. However, many HIV-infected women have no identified risk factors. Consequently, screening of women during pregnancy is probably the best way to identify at-risk children early. An alternative is to screen all newborns for HIV antibodies, which can be done either on phlebotomized samples or on filter papers such as those obtained by heelstick in the newborn nursery. There are some who recommend that routine screening for HIV should be initiated once the maternal seroprevalance rate exceeds one infected delivery per 1000. The United States seroprevalence rate between 1989 and 1993 was that 1.6 to 1.7 deliveries per 1000 were to an HIV-infected woman.[10]

CLINICAL MANAGEMENT OF THE HIV-INFECTED CHILD

The management of pediatric HIV infection is a complex endeavor. Certain broad areas warrant discussion. Children infected with HIV require attention to *P. carinii* pneumonia prophylaxis, their neurodevelopmental function, and antiretroviral therapy.

P. carinii pneumonia prophylaxis is somewhat controversial.[11] The factor that seems to determine the degree of risk for *P. carinii* pneumonia is the $CD4^+$ count. Some clinicians wait until the $CD4^+$ count is below a critical threshold before they start prophylaxis. The standard starting points are a $CD4^+$ count of less than 1500/mm^3 during the first year of life, less than 750 during the second year, less than 500 until 5 years of age, and less than 250 thereafter. Some clinicians are more conservative and start all HIV seropositive children on *P. carinii* pneumonia prophylaxis when they are 3 weeks old and continue the medication until the child is clearly going to maintain a $CD4^+$ count higher than 1500/mm^3. The primary option for *P. carinii* pneumonia prophylaxis is trimethoprim-sulfamethoxazole, and alternatives are dapsone and pentamidine (either intravenous in young children or aerosolized in older, cooperative children). All HIV-infected children deserve close follow-up of their central nervous system functioning, because abnormalities in this realm are very common. Typical manifestations include lower extremity hyperreflexia, failure to attain the usual cognitive or motor developmental milestones, or loss of previously acquired skills. Some children can advance to a spastic diplegia, which is distinguishable from cerebral palsy by the fact that AIDS encephalopathy is progressive and cerebral palsy is static.

CUTANEOUS MANIFESTATIONS OF PEDIATRIC HIV INFECTION

Human immunodeficiency virus infection in children has a wide range of cutaneous manifestations. The majority of these disorders, such as oral candidiasis and seborrheic dermatitis, are common pediatric dermatoses. These tend to be more severe and less responsive to treatment in the child with HIV infection than in the otherwise healthy child.[12] A number of adult mucocutaneous manifestations of HIV infection, including Kaposi's sarcoma and oral hairy leukoplakia, are extremely unusual in children.

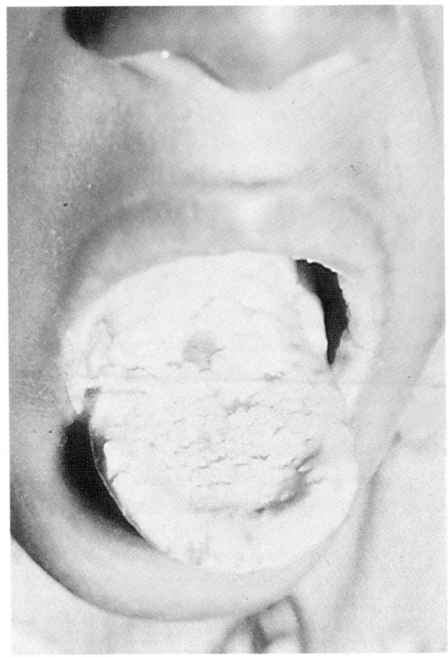

FIGURE 6–3. Oral candidiasis
A 6-year-old girl with AIDS and severe oral thrush. In this patient, the involvement of the tongue and buccal mucosa was accompanied by the presence of esophageal candidiasis. (From Rico MJ, Prose NS. Cutaneous diseases associated with HIV infection. In: Sauer GC. Manual of Skin Diseases. Philadelphia: JB Lippincott; 1991.)

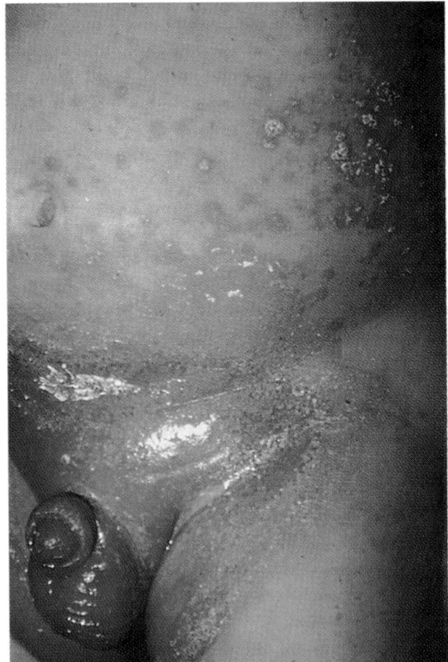

FIGURE 6–4. Candidal diaper dermatitis
Confluent erythema in the diaper area is associated with satellite papules and pustules. In the HIV-infected child, lesions of this type may tend to recur after successful topical therapy with an imidazole cream.

CANDIDIASIS

Oral and cutaneous candidiasis are the most common mucocutaneous manifestations of HIV infection in children. Oral thrush, associated with *Candida albicans*, is usually characterized by creamy white or yellowish plaques on the oral mucosa[13] (Fig. 6–3). The plaques can be removed with scraping, and the underlying surface may bleed. Children may have simultaneous angular cheilitis.

Oral thrush is an extremely common disorder in healthy children under the age of 6 months but is relatively uncommon beyond that age. Persistence of oral thrush beyond 6 months of age, poor response to treatment, and development of recurrent episodes are sometimes seen in children with HIV infection. Dysphagia or loss of appetite in a child with thrush may signal the development of candidal esophagitis. Treatment with nystatin drops or with nystatin or clotrimazole troches is effective in controlling oral candidiasis in most children with early HIV infection. Many children go on to require treatment with ketoconazole (5–10 mg/kg/day).

Infants with HIV infection may also develop persistent candidal diaper dermatitis[14] (Fig. 6–4). Involvement of other intertriginal areas, including the neck folds and axilla, has been noted. Chronic candidal paronychiae (Fig. 6–5) and severe nail dystrophy are additional complications and occur especially in older children.

HERPES SIMPLEX INFECTION

Herpetic gingivostomatitis is a particularly common manifestation of pediatric HIV infection.[15] Children with this form of infection develop painful ulcerations of the lips, tongue, and oral mucosa. Skin lesions due to herpes simplex may also occur on the hands (Fig. 6–6), buttocks, and other locations. The persistence of lesions despite therapy with intravenous acyclovir may signal the development of a strain of virus resistant to that drug.[16] Intravenous foscarnet has been used successfully in some adult patients.[17]

DERMATOPHYTE INFECTIONS

A number of dermatophytes may also cause cutaneous disease in children with HIV infection. Severe tinea capitis, onychomycosis, and widespread tinea corporis have all been observed. Tinea capitis requires treatment with griseofulvin (10–15 mg/kg/day) for 4 to 6 weeks. Infections of the skin in areas other than the scalp may be treated with a topical imidazole cream. In some HIV-infected children, dermatophyte infection tends to recur after the discontinuation of either topical or oral therapy.

VARICELLA-ZOSTER INFECTION

Primary Varicella-Zoster (Chickenpox)

Chickenpox in a child with HIV infection may be a prolonged and severe disease.[18,19] Pneumonia, hepatitis, or both were observed in seven of eight HIV-infected children during the course of their chickenpox.[18] Other complications include pancreatic and central nervous system involvement and a profuse, hemorrhagic exanthem. Treatment with intravenous acyclovir is indicated for most children who develop chickenpox during the course of HIV infection; oral therapy is useful only in children with mild immunosuppression.

Herpes Zoster (Shingles)

Herpes zoster is a relatively rare disorder in healthy children, with

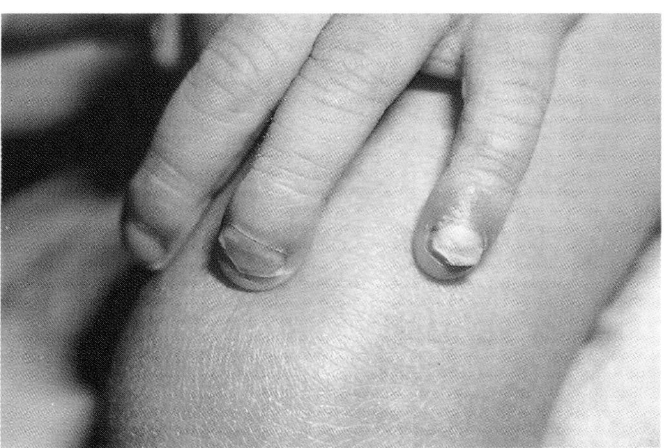

FIGURE 6–5. Proximal candidal paronychia
Chronic candidal infection of the nail fold may lead to nail dystrophy in the child with HIV infection. (From Prose NS. HIV infection in childhood, the disease and its cutaneous manifestations. Adv Dermatol 1990;5:113–130. Copyright 1990, Year Book Medical Publishers, Inc.)

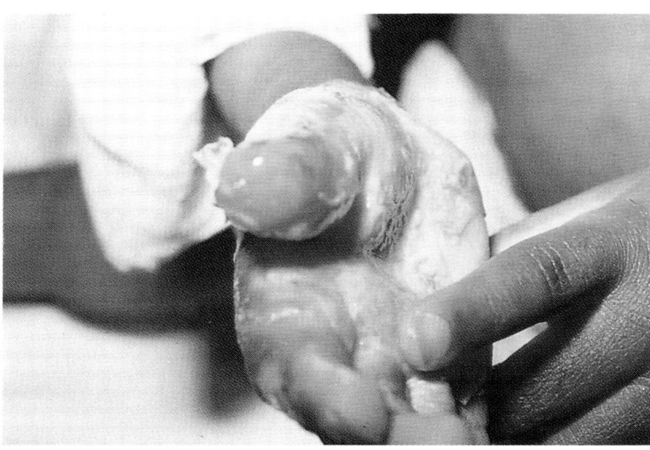

FIGURE 6–6. Herpes simplex
Severe herpetic infection of the hand in a child with simultaneous gingivostomatitis. This infection responded well to treatment with intravenous acyclovir. (From Prose N. Cutaneous manifestations of HIV infection in children. Dermatol Clin 1991; 9:543–550.)

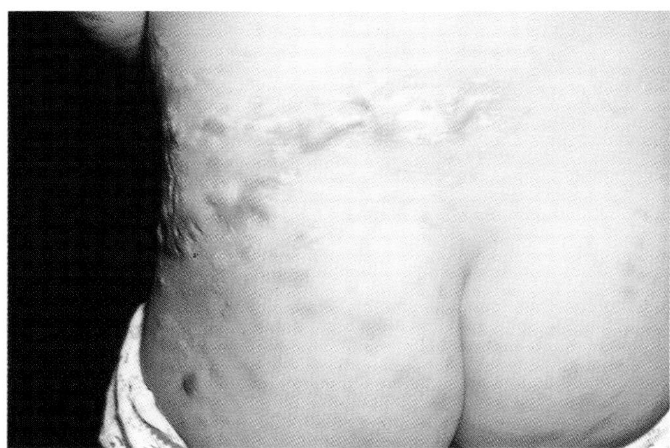

FIGURE 6–7. Scarring secondary to varicella-zoster infection
This 3-year-old girl with HIV infection developed severe scarring despite therapy with intravenous acyclovir. (From Weinberg S, Prose NS. Color Atlas of Pediatric Dermatology. 2nd ed. New York: McGraw-Hill; 1990:162.)

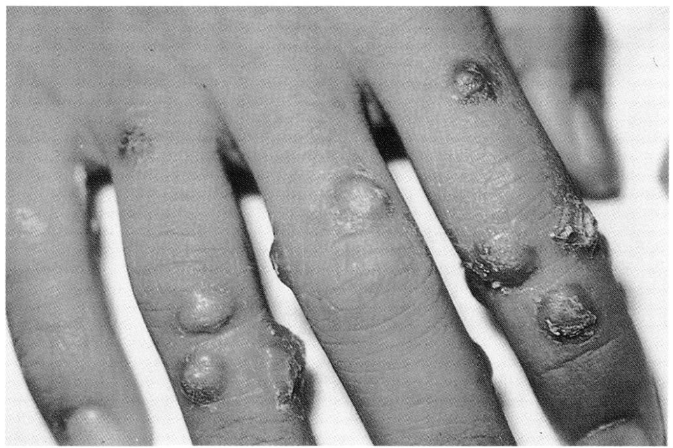

FIGURE 6–8. Chronic varicella-zoster infection
Patients with chronic infection with varicella-zoster may develop widespread keratotic nodules.

a frequency of 0.15 per 1000 person-months.[20] The incidence of this disorder appears to be considerably higher in the context of pediatric HIV infection. The disease tends to be more severe and painful than in the healthy child, with a higher incidence of recurrent episodes and of scarring (Fig. 6–7).

Treatment of herpes zoster consists of intravenous acyclovir (500 mg/m^2/dose, every 8 hours). Lesions near the eye or at the tip of the nose may signal the involvement of intraocular structures; prompt evaluation by an ophthalmologist is mandatory.

Chronic Varicella-Zoster Infection

Chronic varicella-zoster infection has been observed in a number of children and adults with AIDS.[21,22] This cutaneous eruption may develop after episodes of either chickenpox or herpes zoster. The lesions are widespread keratotic or ulcerated nodules and plaques (Fig. 6–8).

Repeated culture of lesions may be required to establish this diagnosis. Treatment consists of intravenous acyclovir. The occurrence of new lesions despite this therapy suggests the presence of a strain resistant to this drug. Central nervous system involvement and death from dissemination has been reported.[23]

MOLLUSCUM CONTAGIOSUM

In children with HIV infection, the umbilicated papules typical of molluscum contagiosum may be particularly widespread and resistant to treatment. Giant lesions of molluscum contagiosum have also been observed in these patients.

CYTOMEGALOVIRUS INFECTION

A single case of cutaneous cytomegalovirus infection in an infant with AIDS has been reported.[24] This 6-month-old child developed a pustular and vesicular diaper dermatitis.

ORAL HAIRY LEUKOPLAKIA

Oral hairy leukoplakia is characterized by the presence of white, corrugated plaques on the lateral surface of the tongue. This disorder appears to be extremely unusual in children, but it has been reported to occur.[25]

HUMAN PAPILLOMAVIRUS INFECTION

Children with HIV infection may develop widespread verrucae. A more unusual manifestation of human papillomavirus infection in these patients is the occurrence of widespread flat warts[26] (Fig. 6–9). Rarely, confluent plaques on the face and upper back and chest may mimic the appearance of epidermodysplasia verruciformis. Extensive lesions of condyloma acuminatum have also been noted in children with AIDS[27] (Fig. 6–10). In one such case, the warts recurred after cryotherapy under general anesthesia.[28]

BACTERIAL INFECTIONS

Infection with HIV in children has a significant effect on humoral immunity; patients are at risk for meningitis and bacterial sepsis.[29,30] Cutaneous infections in HIV-infected children include wound infections, cellulitis, and impetigo. Recurrent staphylococcal folliculitis and toxic shock syndrome have also been noted.[31,32]

SCABIES

Crusted scabies, with widespread areas of erythema and scaling, is usually accompanied by severe pruritus. This unusual form of infestation with *Sarcoptes scabiei* has been described in an infant with AIDS.[33] Patients with this form of scabies are extremely contagious to family members and health care providers. The preferred treatment of scabies in infants with HIV infection is the single overnight application of 6% permethrin cream. In severe cases, repeat applications may be required.

SEBORRHEIC DERMATITIS

Seborrheic dermatitis may be a significant symptom, especially in children who develop severe immunosuppression during the first year of life. Scaling and erythema tend to affect the scalp, face, axillae, and diaper area (Fig. 6–11). A generalized erythroderma may occur. In children older than 5 years, involvement of the nasolabial folds, eyebrows, and skin behind the ears is particularly characteristic.

HYPERREACTIVITY TO INSECT BITES

Children with HIV infection have been noted to develop severe local reactions to common insect bites (e.g., mosquitoes and fleas). Increased antibody titers to mosquito salivary gland antigens have been documented in some patients with HIV infection.[34]

DRUG ERUPTIONS

Drug eruptions are a significant problem in children with HIV infection. The most common cause is trimethoprim-sulfamethoxazole, which is used for both treatment and prophylaxis of *P. carinii* pneumonia. In one study, 16% of children with HIV infection developed a hypersensitivity-like rash after treatment with this drug.[31]

The majority of drug eruptions are morbilliform or papular and rapidly resolve after discontinuing the causative medication. However, cases of Stevens-Johnson syndrome and toxic epidermal necrolysis have been reported in children with HIV infection.[35,36]

VASCULITIS

Chronic leukocytoclastic vasculitis, mimicking Schönlein-Henoch purpura, may occur in children with HIV infection. In one such patient, palpable purpuric lesions were the sole manifestation of HIV infection for more than 6 months.[37]

PYODERMA GANGRENOSUM

An association between pyoderma gangrenosum and pediatric HIV infection has been reported.[38] In one patient, treatment with dapsone resulted in resolution of the skin lesions. Lesions of pyoderma gangrenosum must be differentiated from the chronic ulcers that may be caused by either herpes simplex or varicella-zoster virus.

KAPOSI'S SARCOMA

The occurrence of Kaposi's sarcoma of the skin is extremely rare in children with AIDS. In one case, cutaneous lesions were present in the 6-day-old infant of a seropositive mother.[39] The appearance of skin lesions is identical to that seen in adult patients.[40]

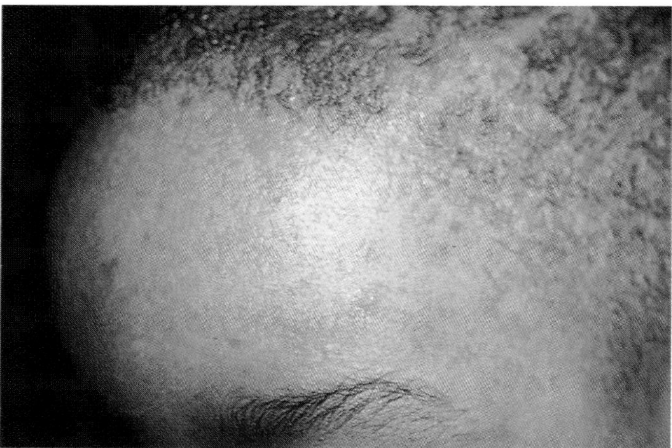

FIGURE 6–9. Widespread flat warts

Older children with HIV infection may develop numerous flat warts on the face and upper trunk. In this 8-year-old boy, the lesions had become confluent on the forehead. (From Prose NS, von Knebel Doeberitz C, Miller S, Milburn P, Heilman E. Widespread flat warts associated with human papillomavirus type 5: A cutaneous manifestation of human immunodeficiency virus infection. J Am Acad Dermatol 1990;23:978–981.)

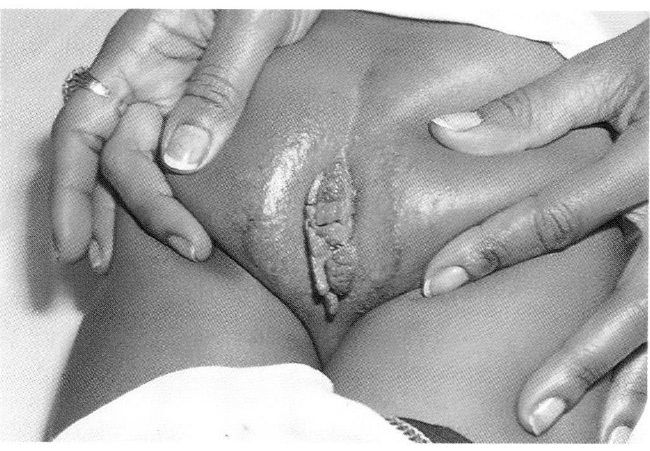

FIGURE 6–10. Severe condyloma acuminatum

Children with HIV infection are at risk for developing large lesions of condyloma acuminatum that are resistant to conventional therapies. Warts of this type may sometimes be an indicator of sexual abuse. (Reprinted by permission of the publisher from Prose NS. Skin manifestations of HIV-1 infection in children. Clin Dermatol 1991;9:59–64. Copyright 1991 by Elsevier Science Inc.)

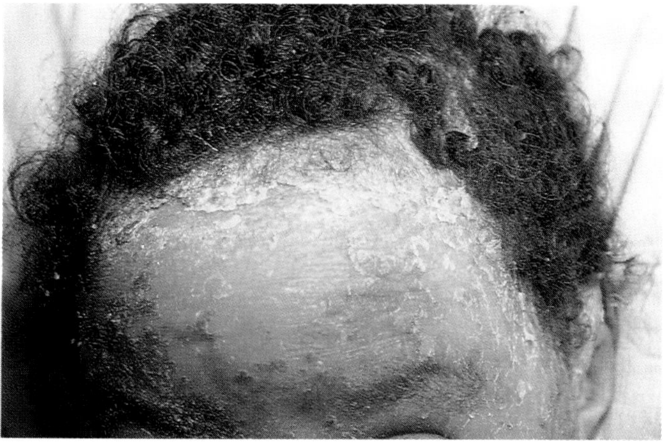

FIGURE 6–11. Seborrheic dermatitis

Severe seborrheic dermatitis may be a marker for the presence of HIV infection during infancy. (Reprinted by permission of the publisher from Prose NS. Skin manifestations of HIV-1 infection in children. Clin Dermatol 1991;9:59–64. Copyright 1991 by Elsevier Science Inc.)

ANTIRETROVIRAL THERAPY

The goal of antiretroviral therapy is to limit HIV replication and by so doing slow the progression of HIV disease. To date, the major target of successful antiretroviral drugs has been the viral reverse transcriptase enzyme. Human immunodeficiency virus includes a reverse transcriptase used to copy its RNA molecule into DNA, which is subsequently processed by cellular enzymes. Uninfected human cells do not transcribe RNA into DNA and so do not normally possess reverse transcriptase. Molecules such as zidovudine (also called AZT or azidothymidine) and didanosine (ddI, or dideoxyinosine) are modifications of normal nucleosides, which lack the ability to link into growing DNA chains. As a result, when they are incorporated into a DNA molecule, they terminate its growth. There are many nucleosides with this property, but zidovudine and didanosine are used by the reverse transcriptase in preference to the unmodified thymidine and adenosine to which they are related. In contrast, human transcriptases recognize zidovudine and ddI as defective and preferentially reject them. The result is that these modified nucleosides can inhibit HIV replication while having less effect on human cellular replication.

Zidovudine has been documented to have many benefits for HIV-infected children, including improved central nervous system function, weight growth, immunoglobulin concentrations, and probably survival.[41] The usual dose is 120 mg/m^2/dose given every 8 hours. Didanosine has been less tested in children but appears to have similar benefits. It may have less central nervous system penetration but is at least as effective as zidovudine. Combination didanosine and zidovudine also appears to be an effective regimen. Zalcitabine (ddC or dideoxycytidine) has been approved for adults in combination with zidovudine, but its pediatric utility is uncertain. Lamivudine (3TC) in combination with zidovudine is another promising antiretroviral therapy.

Other therapeutic approaches to HIV infection have been tested in vitro but not yet in children. Examples include the HIV-specific protease inhibitors. These drugs will probably be undergoing clinical trials over the next several years.

SUPPORTIVE CARE

As noted before, the management of HIV-infected children is complicated. As part of supportive care, many clinicians advocate the inclusion of routine intravenous immunoglobulin infusions on a monthly basis to decrease the number of bacterial infections in those children with high enough CD4$^+$ counts to benefit.[42]

Vaccination is another care issue for HIV-infected children. Essentially, these patients should receive routine childhood immunizations, except that inactivated polio vaccine should be substituted for the attenuated oral polio vaccine. Strong consideration should be given to administering pneumococcal and meningococcal vaccine after the child's second birthday.

Perhaps the most difficult aspect of care is the need to provide intense support to the families of HIV-infected children. In most cases, one or both parents are also HIV infected and may be more ill than the child. A high proportion of children with HIV infection come from families whose problems include intravenous drug use, poverty, abuse and neglect, and a tradition of avoiding authority figures (including physicians). The result is often a very difficult situation that requires the close cooperation of social workers, nurses, physicians, and community resource groups.

References

1. Oleske J, Minnefor A, Cooper R, Thomas K, dela Cruz A, Ahdiel H, Guerrero I, Joshi W, Desposito F. Immune deficiency in children. JAMA 1983;249:2345–2349.
2. Rubinstein A, Sicklick M, Gupta A, Bernstein L, Klein N, Rubinstein E, Spigland I, Fruchter L, Litman N, Lee H, Hollander M. Acquired immunodeficiency with reversed T4/T8 ratios in infants born to promiscuous and drug addicted mothers. JAMA 1983;249: 2350–2356.
3. Alimenti A, Luzuriaga K, Stechenberg B, Sullivan JL. Quantitation of human immunodeficiency virus in vertically infected infants and children. J Pediatr 1991;119:225–229.
4. Krivine A, Firtion G, Cao L, Francoual C, Henrion R, Lebon P. HIV replication during the first weeks of life. Lancet 1992;339:1187–1189.
5. Goedert JJ, Duliege A-M, Amos CI, Felton S, Biggar RJ, International Registry of HIV Exposed Twins. High risk of HIV-1 transmission for first-born twins. Lancet 1991;338:1471–1475.
6. Gutman LT, St. Claire KK, Weedy C, Herman-Giddens M, McKinney RE Jr. Human immunodeficiency virus transmission by child sexual abuse. Am J Dis Child 1991;145:137–141.
7. European Collaborative Study. Children born to women with HIV-1 infection: Natural history and risk of transmission. Lancet 1991;337:253–260.
8. Walter EB, Weinhold KJ, Wilfert CM. Enhanced p24 antigen detection in sera from HIV infected children. Pediatr Infect Dis J 1993;12:94–96.
9. McKinney RE, Wilfert CM. Lymphocyte subsets in children younger than 2 years old: Normal values in a population at risk for human immunodeficiency virus infection and diagnostic and prognostic application to infected children. Pediatr Infect Dis J 1992; 11:639–644.
10. Centers for Disease Control and Prevention. Update: AIDS among women —United States, 1994. MMWR 1995; 44:81–84.
11. Centers for Disease Control. Guidelines for prophylaxis against *Pneumocystis carinii* pneumonia for children infected with human immunodeficiency virus. MMWR 1991;40(RR-2):1–13.
12. Prose N. Pediatric human immunodeficiency virus infection in childhood; the disease and its cutaneous manifestations. Adv Dermatol 1990;5:113–130.
13. Leggott PJ, Robertson P, Greenspan D, Wara DW, Greenspan JS. Oral manifestations of primary and acquired immunodeficiency diseases in children. Pediatr Dent 1987;9:98–194.
14. Prose N, Mendez H, Menikoff H, Miller HJ. Pediatric human immunodeficiency virus infection and its cutaneous manifestations. Pediatr Dermatol 1987;4:67–74.
15. Scott GB, Buck BE, Leterman JG, Bloom FL, Parks WP. Acquired immunodeficiency syndrome in infants. N Engl J Med 1984;310:76–81.
16. Erlich KS, Mills J, Chatis P, Mertz GJ, Busch DF, Follansbee S. Acyclovir-resistant herpes simplex virus infections in patients with the acquired immunodeficiency syndrome. N Engl J Med 1989;320:293–296.
17. Sall RK, Kauffman CL, Levy CS. Successful treatment of progressive acyclovir-resistant herpes simplex virus using intravenous foscarnet in a patient with acquired immunodeficiency syndrome. Arch Dermatol 1989;125: 1548–1550.
18. Perronne C, Lazanas M, Leport C, Simon F, Salmon D, Dallot A, Vilde J-L. Varicella in patients infected with the human immunodeficiency virus. Arch Dermatol 1990;126:1033–1036.
19. Jura E, Chadwick EG, Josephs SH, Steinberg SP, Yogev R, Gershon AA, Krasinski KM, Borkowsky W. Varicella-zoster virus infections in children infected with human immunodeficiency virus. Pediatric Infect Dis J 1989;8:586–590.
20. Baba K, Yabuuchi H, Takahashi M, Ogra PL. Increased incidence of herpes zoster in normal children infected with varicella zoster virus during infancy: Community-based follow-up study. J Pediatr 1986;108:372–377.
21. Pahwa S, Biron K, Lim W, et al. Continuous varicella-zoster infection associated with acyclovir resistance in a child with AIDS. JAMA 1988;260: 2879–2882.
22. Gilson IH, Barnett JH, Conant MA, Laskin OL, Williams J, Jones PG. Disseminated ecthymatous herpes varicella-zoster infection in patients with acquired immunodeficiency syndrome. J Am Acad Dermatol 1989; 20:637–642.
23. Pahwa S, Biron K, Lim W, Swanson P, Kaplan MH, Sadick N, Pahwa R. Continuous varicella-zoster infection associated with acyclovir resistance in a child with AIDS. JAMA 1988;260: 2879–2882.
24. Thiboutot DM, Beckford A, Mart CR, Sexton M, Maloney ME. Cytomegalovirus diaper dermatitis. Arch Dermatol 1991;127:396–398.
25. Greenspan JS, Mastrucci MT, Leggott PJ, Freese UK, De Souza YG, Scott GB, Greenspan D. Hairy leukoplakia in a child. AIDS 1988;2:143.
26. Prose NS, von Knebel Doeberitz C, Miller S, Milburn P, Heilman E. Widespread flat warts associated with human papillomavirus type 5: A cutaneous manifestation of human immunodeficiency virus infection. J Am Acad Dermatol 1990;23:978–981.
27. Laraque D. Severe anogenital warts in a child with HIV infection (letter). N Engl J Med 1989;320:1220–1221.
28. Forman A, Prendiville J. Association of human immunodeficiency virus seropositivity and extensive perineal condylomata acuminata in a child. Arch Dermatol 1988;124:1010–1011.
29. Bernstein LJ, Ochs HD, Wedgwood RJ, Rubinstein A. Defective humoral immunity in pediatric acquired immunodeficiency syndrome. J Pediatr 1985; 107:352–357.
30. Bernstein LJ, Krieger BZ, Novick B, Sicklick MJ, Rubinstein A. Bacterial infection in the acquired immunodeficiency syndrome in children. Pediatr Infect Dis J 1985;4:472–475.
31. Straka BF, Whitaker DL, Morrison SH, Oleske JM, Grant-Kels JM. Cutaneous manifestations of the acquired immunodeficiency syndrome in children. J Am Acad Dermatol 1988;18: 1089–1102.
32. Kline MW, Dunkle LM. Toxic shock syndrome and the acquired immunodeficiency syndrome. Pediatr Infect Dis J 1988;7:736–737.
33. Jucowics P, Ramon ME, Don PC, Stone RK, Bamji M. Norwegian scabies in an infant with acquired immunodeficiency syndrome. Arch Dermatol 1989;125:1670–1672.
34. Penneys NS, Nayar JK, Bernstein H, Knight JW. Chronic pruritic eruption in patients with acquired immunodeficiency syndrome associated with increased antibody titers to mosquito salivary gland antigens. J Am Acad Dermatol 1989;21:421–425.
35. Revuz J. Nécrolyse épidermique toxique par les sulfamides au cours du SIDA; à propos de 3 cas (abstract). J Dermatol Paris 1986;153.
36. Hira SK, Wadhawan D, Kamanga J, Kavindele D, Macuacua R, Patil PS, Ansary MA, Macher AM, Perine PL. Cutaneous manifestations of human immunodeficiency virus in Lusaka, Zambia. J Am Acad Dermatol 1988; 19:451–457.
37. Chren MM, Silverman RA, Sorensen RU, Elmets CA. Leukocytoclastic vasculitis in a patient infected with human immunodeficiency virus. J Am Acad Dermatol 1989;21:1161–1164.
38. Paller AS, Sahn EE, Garen PD, Dobson RL, Chadwick EG. Pyoderma gangrenosum in pediatric acquired immunodeficiency syndrome. J Pediatr 1990;117:63–66.
39. Gutierrez-Ortega P, Hierro-Orozoco S, Sanchez-Cisneros R, Montaño LF. Kaposi's sarcoma in a 6 day-old infant with human immunodeficiency virus. (letter). Arch Dermatol 1989;125:432–433.
40. Connor E, Boccon-Gibod L, Joshi V, Just J, Grimfeld A, Morrison S, McSherry G, Oleske J. Cutaneous acquired immunodeficiency syndrome–associated Kaposi's sarcoma in pediatric patients. Arch Dermatol 1990;126: 791–793.
41. McKinney RE Jr, Maha M, Connor EM, Feinberg J, Scott GB, Wulfsohn M, McIntosh K, Borkowsky W, Modlin JF, Weintrub P, et al. A multicenter trial of oral zidovudine in children with advanced human immunodeficiency virus disease. N Engl J Med 1991;324:1018–1025.
42. The National Institute of Child Health and Human Development Intravenous Immunoglobulin Study Group. Intravenous immune globulin for the prevention of bacterial infections in children with symptomatic human immunodeficiency virus infection. N Engl J Med 1991;325:73–80.

OCULAR COMPLICATIONS OF HIV INFECTION

Dorothy Nahm Friedberg

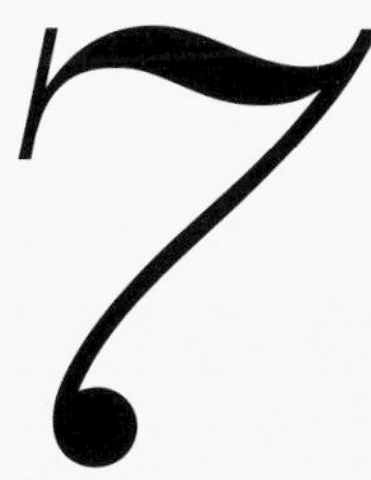

The acquired immunodeficiency syndrome (AIDS) can affect the visual system at all levels from the lids and ocular adnexa to the retina and choroid to the occipital cortex. The manifestations are as diverse as those in other organ systems and include opportunistic infections and malignancies as well as unusual manifestations of diseases seen in immunocompetent patients. This chapter reviews a selection of these conditions, concentrating on those in which photographs can enhance the clinician's ability to diagnose and treat the condition.

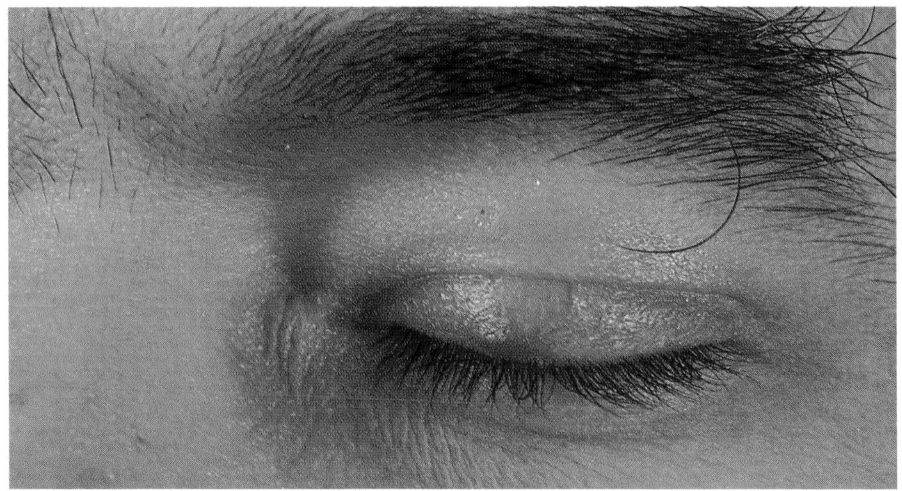

FIGURE 7–1. Kaposi's sarcoma of the eyelid, plaque stage

Lesion was initially thought to be a stye, but a biopsy was performed when it did not respond to therapy.

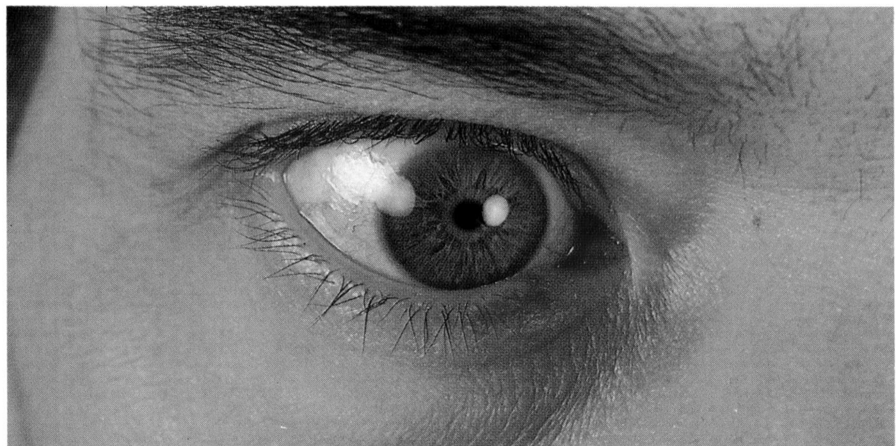

FIGURE 7–2. Kaposi's sarcoma of the eyelid, patch stage

One of many skin lesions in a bisexual male, this developed into a nodule that responded to local radiotherapy.

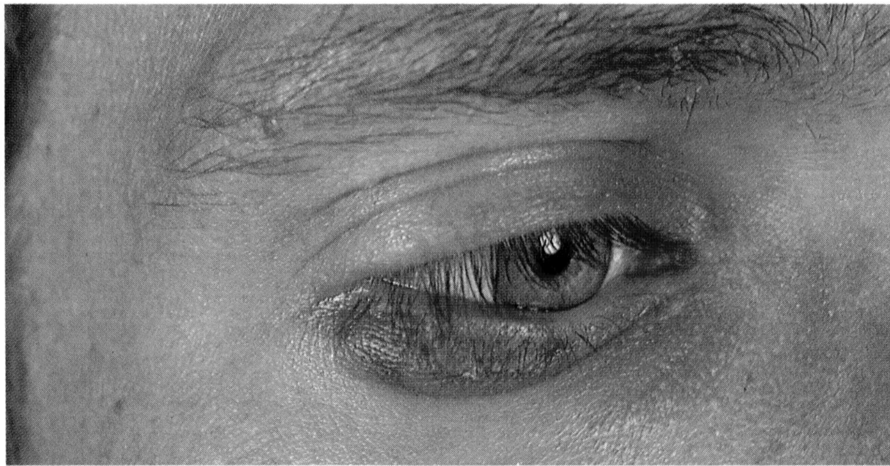

FIGURE 7–3. Kaposi's sarcoma of the eyelid, plaque stage

Indurated violaceous lesion of the left lower eyelid.

LIDS AND ADNEXA

The most common ocular manifestation of AIDS affecting the lids is lesions of Kaposi's sarcoma. These lesions do not differ significantly from the manifestation of Kaposi's sarcoma on other areas of the skin; however, treatment of lid lesions requires careful attention to the effects on the globe itself of the various therapeutic methods, including surgery, radiation, cryotherapy, and chemotherapy, both local and systemic.[1,2] Appearance on the lid margin may be subtle and in early lesions may be misdiagnosed as a chalazion or blepharitis (Fig. 7–1). Lesions of Kaposi's sarcoma on the eyelid rarely affect vision, and decisions concerning treatment are usually based on cosmesis (Figs. 7–2 and 7–3). Patients with AIDS may develop a dry eye syndrome secondary to a diffuse interstitial lymphocytic infiltration of the lacrimal gland.[3] Others have described symptoms of keratoconjunctivitis sicca in 20% of men who tested positive for the human immunodeficiency virus (HIV) who had abnormal results on Schirmer's tests.[4]

Herpes zoster ophthalmicus (Fig. 7–4), a disease that was a harbinger of the AIDS epidemic, does not usually differ in appearance or course in HIV-infected patients from the disease in persons who are not infected with HIV.[5–7] It is most significant when seen in patients who do not know their HIV status; these patients should be counseled to have a medical evaluation to explore the possibility of immunodeficiency. Patients who have had an episode of cutaneous zoster are at risk for the development of acute retinal necrosis.[8]

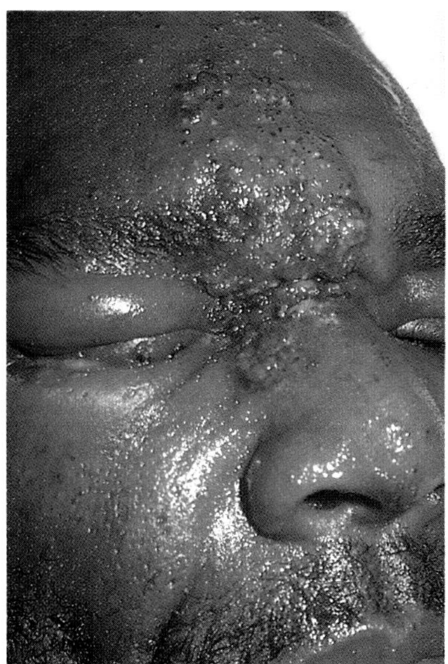

FIGURE 7–4. Herpes zoster

Herpes zoster ophthalmicus. (Courtesy of AE Friedman-Kien, New York University Medical Center, Department of Dermatology.)

Molluscum contagiosum can affect the eyelids.[9,10] This disease illustrates the difference in response between immunocompromised and immunocompetent patients. In immunocompetent patients, a tiny single molluscum lesion produces a virulent conjunctivitis that often resolves only after removal of the lid lesion. Patients with AIDS may have multiple molluscum lesions on the eyelid without any associated conjunctivitis (Fig. 7–5). A case of perilimbal molluscum was without significant conjunctival reaction (Figs. 7–6 through 7–8).

CONJUNCTIVA AND CORNEA

Kaposi's sarcoma can affect the tarsal or the bulbar conjunctiva. When the lesion is small and underneath the lids the patient may complain of recurrent or nonresolving subconjunctival hemorrhage. On careful examination, the cause of this can be identified as conjunctival Kaposi's sarcoma lesion (Fig. 7–9). Lesions rarely affect vision, and the decision about therapy is often based on cosmesis, as it is with lid lesions (Fig. 7–10). A series of different proposals have been made for local treatment of conjunctival Kaposi's sarcoma, and the decision about whether therapy is necessary depends on lesion size, interference with lid function, cosmesis, and whether the patient will be receiving chemotherapy for more widespread disease.[1,11,12] It is unusual for conjunctival lesions to be so large that they interfere with lid function; however, if necessary, the lesions can be debulked, and they do respond well to radiotherapy (Fig. 7–11).

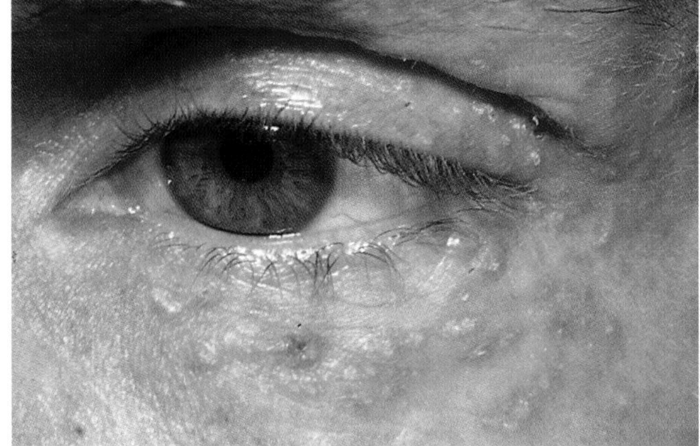

FIGURE 7–5. Molluscum contagiosum
Molluscum contagiosum of the eyelids. Multiple, papular, umbilicated lesions affect the upper and lower lids. Note the lack of conjunctival reaction.

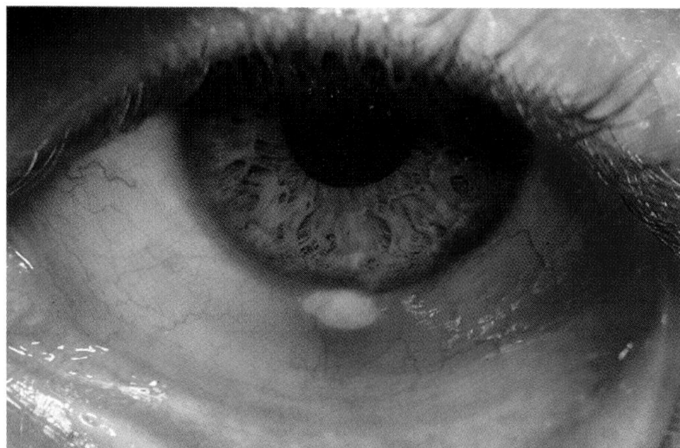

FIGURE 7–6. Molluscum contagiosum
Molluscum contagiosum of the conjunctiva. Note the white perilimbal nodule without conjunctival injection. (From Charles NC, Friedberg DN: Epibulbar molluscum contagiosum in acquired immune deficiency syndrome. Case report and review of the literature. Published courtesy of Ophthalmology 1992;99:1123–1126.)

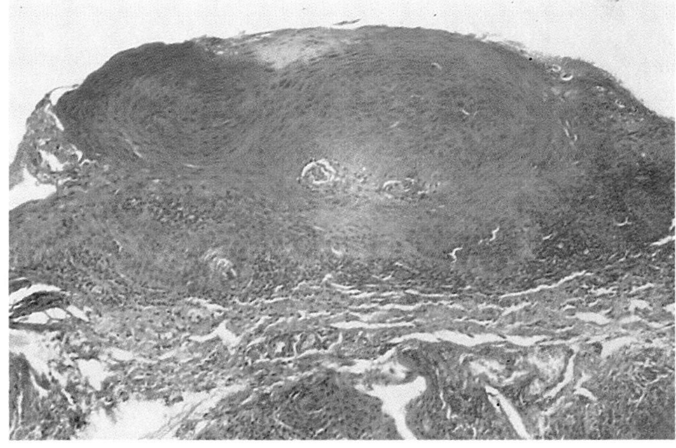

FIGURE 7–7. Molluscum contagiosum

Photomicrograph of molluscum lesion of the conjunctiva, showing an umbilicated, acanthotic lesion with hyperkeratosis and chronic nongranulomatous inflammation. Hematoxylin and eosin (original magnification, ×64). (From Charles NC, Friedberg DN: Epibulbar molluscum contagiosum in acquired immune deficiency syndrome. Case report and review of the literature. Published courtesy of Ophthalmology 1992;99:1123–1126.)

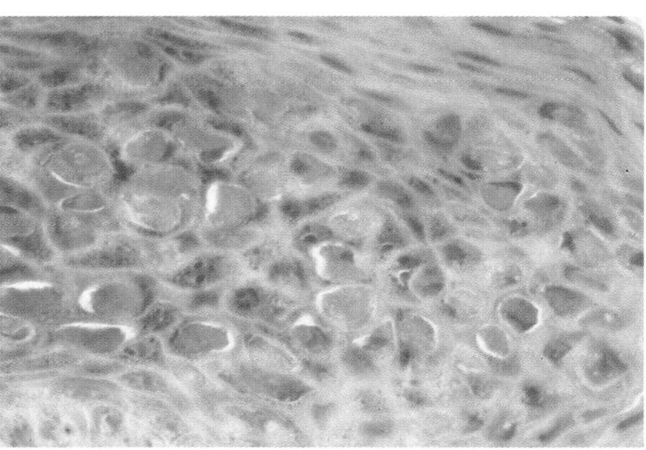

FIGURE 7–8. Molluscum contagiosum

Molluscum of the conjunctiva. Photomicrograph of granular and prickle cell layers showing cells with intracytoplasmic eosinophilic inclusions that push the nuclei peripherally. Hematoxylin and eosin (original magnification, ×512). (From Charles NC, Friedberg DN: Epibulbar molluscum contagiosum in acquired immune deficiency syndrome. Case report and review of the literature. Published courtesy of Ophthalmology 1992;99:1123–1126.)

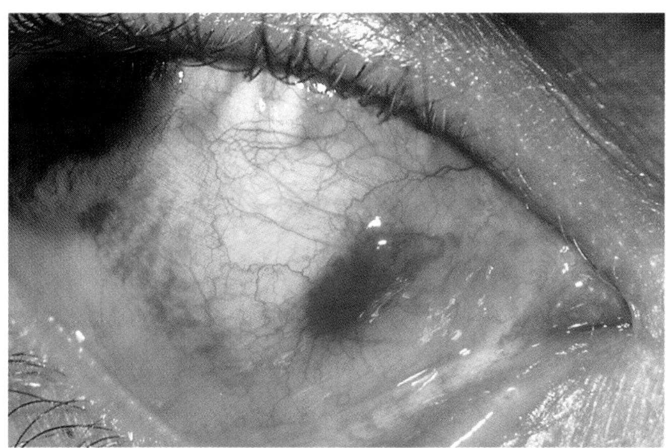

FIGURE 7–9. Kaposi's sarcoma

Kaposi's sarcoma of the conjunctiva with adjacent subconjunctival hemorrhage.

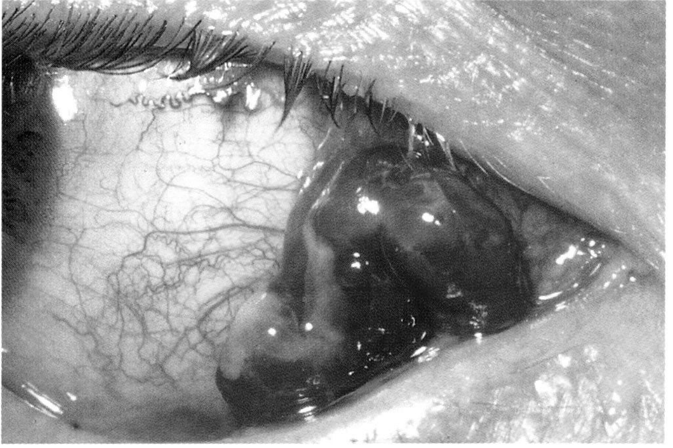

FIGURE 7–10. Kaposi's sarcoma

Large Kaposi's sarcoma lesion of the plica, which was the presenting tumor in this patient.

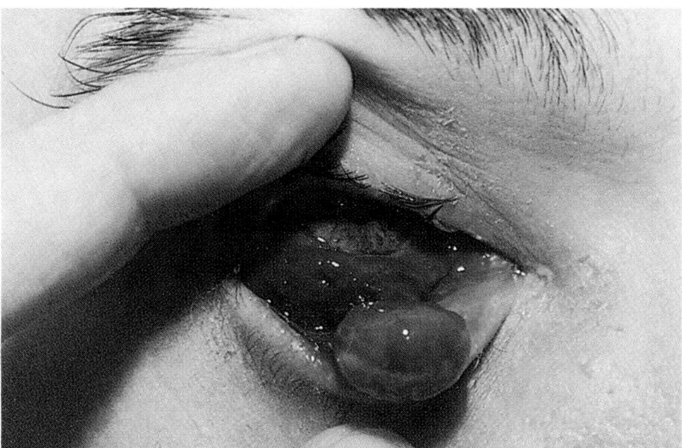

FIGURE 7–11. Kaposi's sarcoma

Pedunculated recurrence of Kaposi's sarcoma of the conjunctiva, preventing proper lid closure. The lesion responded to a combination of surgical debulking and radiotherapy.

Local excision is possible, but if lesions are large and multicentric, too much conjunctival tissue may be destroyed. When lesions are relatively flat, they respond well to cryotherapy.[12] There have been reports of resolution of lesions with injection of interferon-α.[13] When conjunctival Kaposi's sarcoma lesions are part of significant systemic disease, patients should be reassured that the conjunctival lesions respond well to systemic therapy.

Microsporidian keratoconjunctivitis was first described in patients with AIDS in 1990.[14,15] Prior ocular infection with Microsporida occurring in immunocompetent patients affected the deeper as well as the superficial layers of the cornea.[16,17] In AIDS patients microsporidian infection is seen only in the corneal epithelium and in the superficial layers of the conjunctiva and can be identified both from corneal and conjunctival scrapings (Fig. 7–12). Initially the organisms were identified by electron microscopy as members of the *Encephalitozoon* species, most likely *Encephalitozoon cuniculi* (Figs. 7–13 and 7–14). Further study, which included growing the organisms in tissue culture and immunologic studies, revealed that they were a new species, *Encephalitozoon hellum*.[18] Although originally thought to be a purely ocular organism, it has been identified in the urinary tract and tracheobronchial tree.[19] Patients with ocular microsporidiosis may be completely asymptomatic, but they often complain of a foreign body sensation and have minimal conjunctival injection (Fig. 7–15). The cornea may be covered with punctate grayish spots, some of which stain with fluorescein; there is no accompanying uveitis (Figs. 7–16 and 7–17). Treatment has been difficult; success has been reported with topical fumagillin, a water-insoluble antibiotic isolated from *Aspergillus fumigatus*, which has been used extensively by veterinarians in treating nosematosis, a microsporidian infection in honeybees.[21]

ANTERIOR CHAMBER

Uveitis has been described in HIV-infected patients; it can be solely an anterior uveitis or may include a vitritis.[22] The uveitis is thought to be a result of HIV infection, and response to zidovudine has been reported in these cases. Before making a diagnosis of HIV-associated uveitis, other treatable causes of uveitis should be excluded, particularly syphilis and toxoplasmosis. A newly reported syndrome of severe uveitis sometimes accompanied by hypopyon has been described in patients treated with rifabutin.[23] This responds to aggressive treatment with topical steroids and cycloplegics. There have been reports of infectious entities in the anterior chamber, including a filtering bleb infected with *Mycobacterium avium*[24] and a cryptococcal iris nodule (Fig. 7–18).[25]

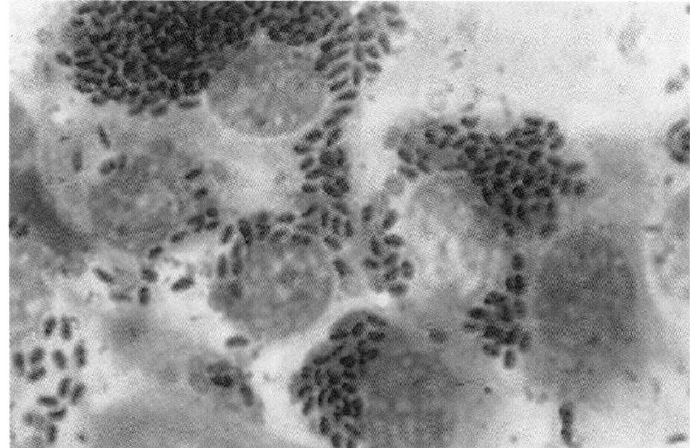

FIGURE 7–12. Microsporidial keratoconjunctivitis
Photomicrograph of conjunctival scraping showing multiple gram-positive ovoid organisms within conjunctival epithelial cells Gram's stain (original magnification, ×500). (From Friedberg DN, Stenson SM, Orenstein JM, et al: Microsporidial keratoconjunctivitis in acquired immunodeficiency syndrome. Arch Ophthalmol 1990;108:504–508. Copyright 1990, American Medical Association.)

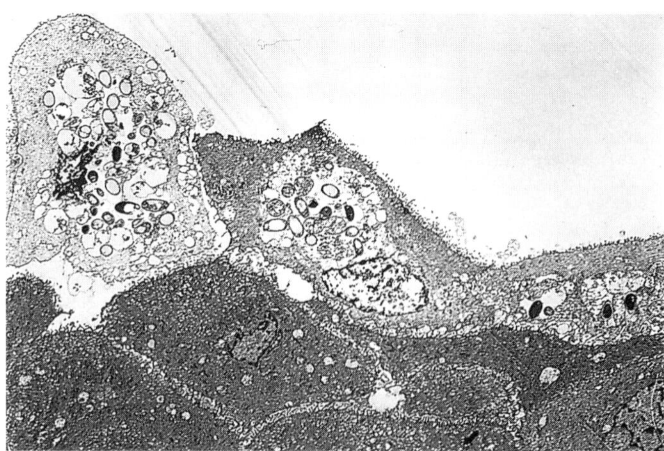

FIGURE 7–13. Microsporidial keratoconjunctivitis
Electron micrograph from conjunctival biopsy, demonstrating three superficial cells with clear parasitophorous vacuoles containing parasites at various developmental stages (original magnification, ×2700). (From Friedberg DN, Stenson SM, Orenstein JM, et al: Microsporidial keratoconjunctivitis in acquired immunodeficiency syndrome. Arch Ophthalmol 1990;108:504–508. Copyright 1990, American Medical Association.)

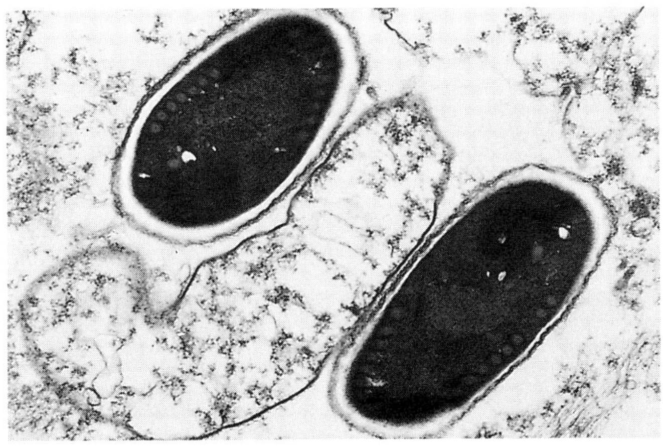

FIGURE 7–14. Microsporidial keratoconjunctivitis

Electron micrograph from conjunctival biopsy of mature electron-dense spore with seven turns of the polar tubule (original magnification, ×45,000). (From Friedberg DN, Stenson SM, Orenstein JM, et al: Microsporidial keratoconjunctivitis in acquired immunodeficiency syndrome. Arch Ophthalmol 1990;108:504–508. Copyright 1990, American Medical Association.)

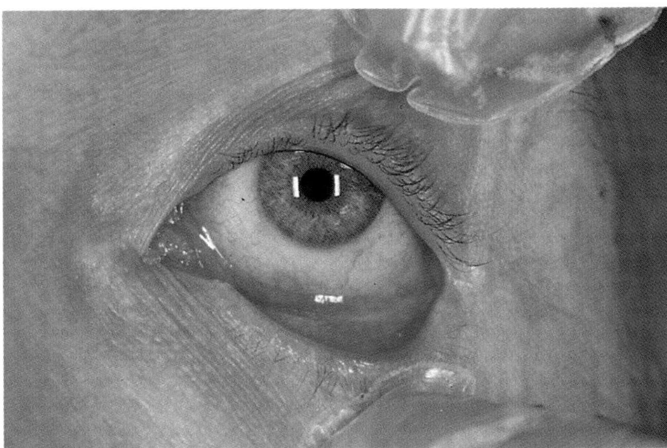

FIGURE 7–15. Microsporidial keratoconjunctivitis

Minimal conjunctival hyperemia in a patient with microsporidial keratoconjunctivitis. (From Friedberg DN, Stenson SM, Orenstein JM, et al: Microsporidial keratoconjunctivitis in acquired immunodeficiency syndrome. Arch Ophthalmol 1990;108:504–508. Copyright 1990, American Medical Association.)

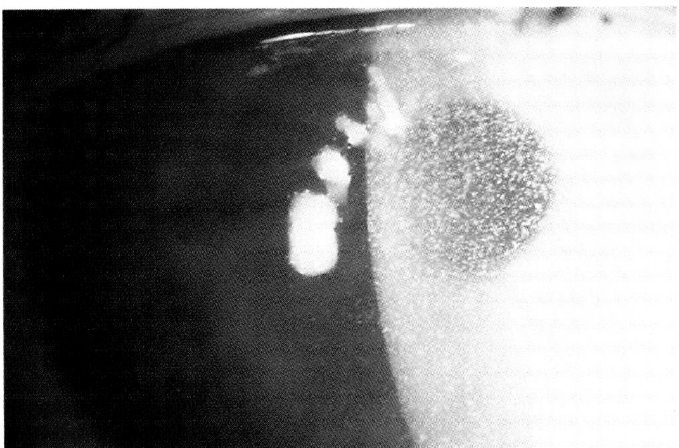

FIGURE 7–16. Microsporidial keratoconjunctivitis

Cornea with diffuse, coarse, superficial, epithelial keratitis. (From Friedberg DN, Stenson SM, Orenstein JM, et al: Microsporidial keratoconjunctivitis in acquired immunodeficiency syndrome. Arch Ophthalmol 1990; 108:504–508. Copyright 1990, American Medical Association.)

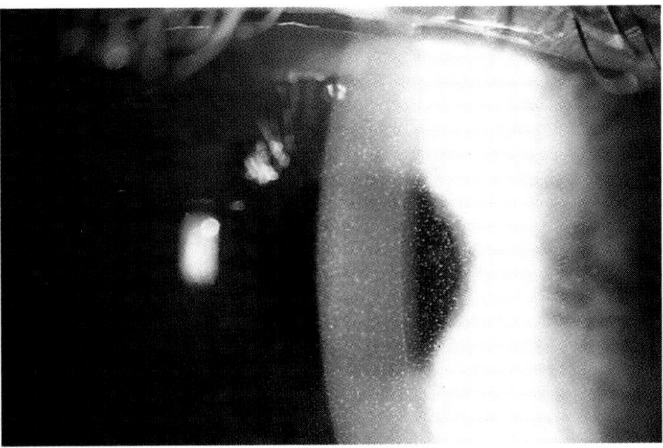

FIGURE 7–17. Microsporidial keratoconjunctivitis

Cornea with superficial epithelial keratitis, finer than that shown in Figure 7–16. (From Friedberg DN, Stenson SM, Orenstein JM, et al: Microsporidial keratoconjunctivitis in acquired immunodeficiency syndrome. Arch Ophthalmol 1990;108:504–508. Copyright 1990, American Medical Association.)

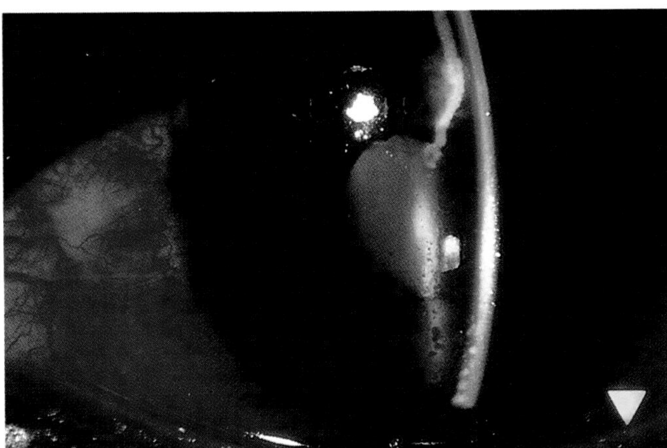

FIGURE 7–18. Cryptococcal iris nodule

Cryptococcal nodule of the iris; slit lamp photograph. (From Charles NC, Boxrud CA, Small EA: Cryptococcosis of the anterior segment in acquired immune deficiency syndrome. Published courtesy of Ophthalmology 1992;99:813–816).

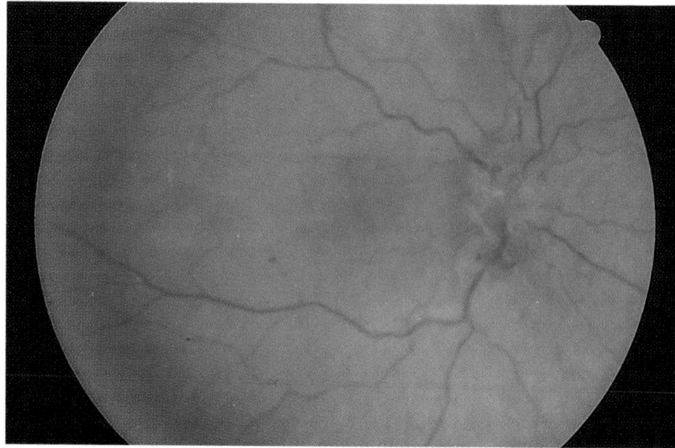

FIGURE 7–19. Papilledema
Papilledema in a patient with cryptococcal meningitis.

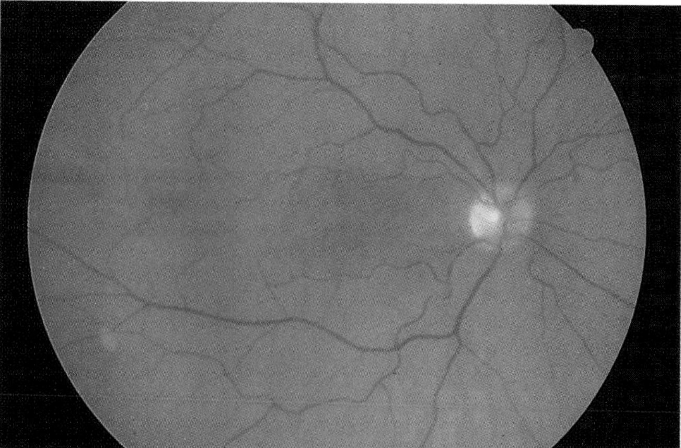

FIGURE 7–20. Papilledema
Disk of patient in Figure 7–19 returned to normal after treatment for cryptococcal infection.

ORBIT AND CENTRAL NERVOUS SYSTEM

Many of the central nervous system conditions seen in AIDS patients can have neuro-ophthalmic manifestations. These include central nervous system toxoplasmosis, central nervous system and orbital lymphoma, cryptococcal meningitis, and progressive multifocal leukoencephalopathy.[26–28] The most common findings include papilledema (Figs. 7–19 and 7–20), diplopia, and visual field abnormalities. Orbital aspergillosis has become an increasing problem in AIDS patients, and even aggressive management may not control it adequately (Fig. 7–21*A* and *B*).[29] Orbital lymphoma may manifest with minimal proptosis, and diagnosis may be missed on early imaging studies.[30–32] A persistent complaint of orbital pain with or without diplopia and proptosis requires aggressive evaluation.

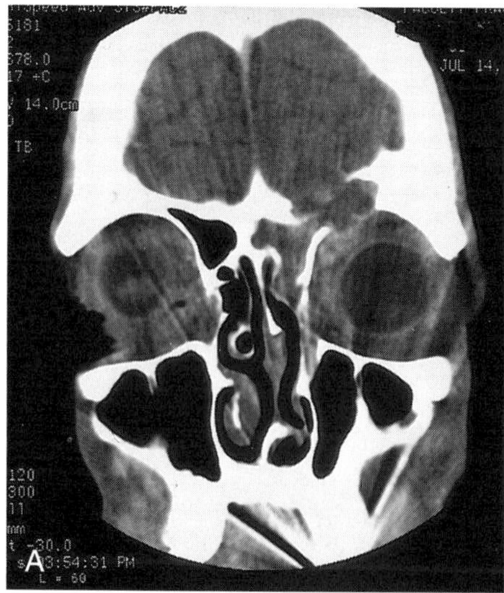

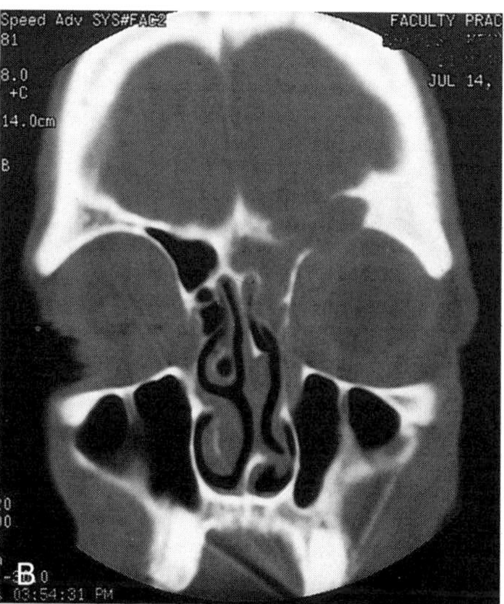

FIGURE 7–21. Orbital aspergillosis
Orbital aspergillosis. Coronal computed tomography scan, normal *(A)* and soft tissue window *(B)*, showing left frontoethmoid sinusitis, subdural empyema with possible intraparenchymal abscess in the left frontal lobe, and a subperiosteal abscess supermedially.

Some patients may demonstrate a more fulminant course with rapidly progressive proptosis (Figs. 7–22 and 7–23).

RETINA AND CHOROID

MICROANGIOPATHY

Retinal vascular abnormalities including hemorrhages (Fig. 7–24), microaneurysms, and cotton-wool spots (Figs. 7–25 and 7–26) similar to those seen in diabetes, hypertension, and collagen vascular diseases have been described in HIV-infected patients.[33] These rarely have any effect on vision and usually wax and wane. Although microvascular changes are not associated with any particular opportunistic infection, they occur more frequently as immunosuppression progresses.[34] It is important to recognize HIV-associated microangiopathy and to reassure patients that their vision will not be affected and that no treatment is required. Branch and central retinal vein occlusions can also be seen in HIV-infected patients (Fig. 7–27). Patients with AIDS who have a coexisting disease that affects the retinal microvasculature, such as diabetes, may have a worsening of their disease.[35]

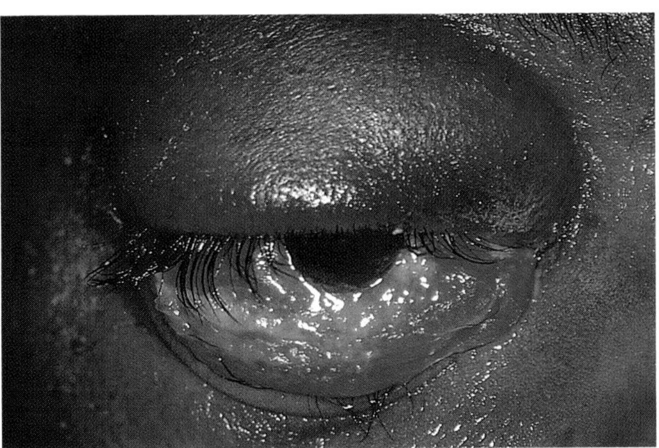

FIGURE 7–22. Orbital lymphoma
Orbital lymphoma with marked chemosis and proptosis.

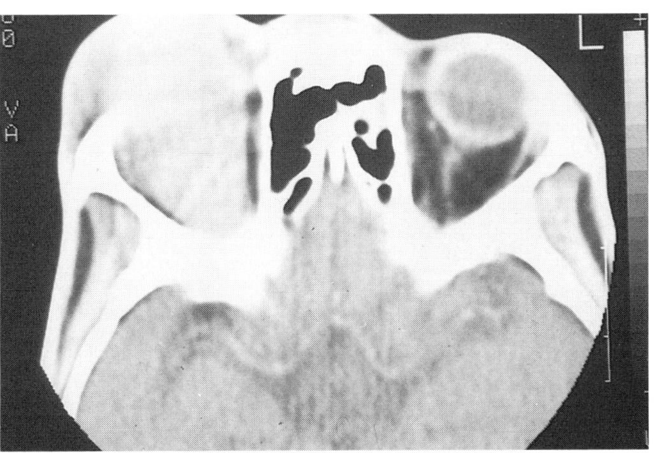

FIGURE 7–23. Orbital lymphoma
Orbital lymphoma; computed tomography scan of the patient in Figure 7–22.

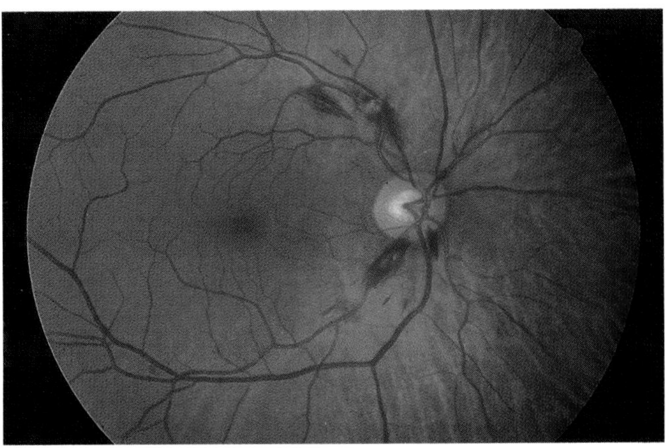

FIGURE 7–24. Microangiopathy
Retinal microangiopathy. Multiple retinal hemorrhages, some white-centered, in a severely anemic HIV-positive patient.

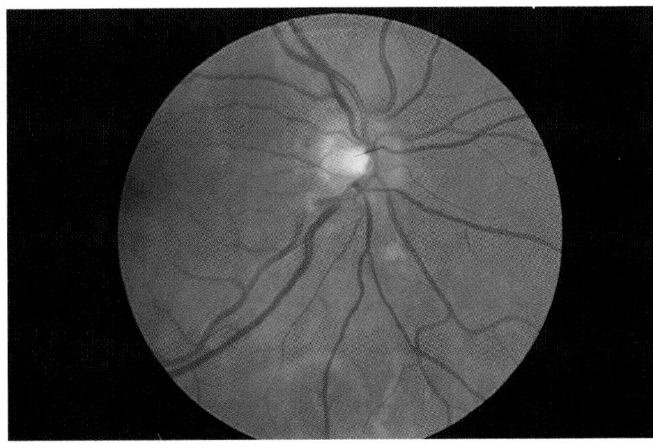

FIGURE 7–25. Microangiopathy
Retinal microangiopathy, two cotton-wool spots. Note feathery edges and superficial position.

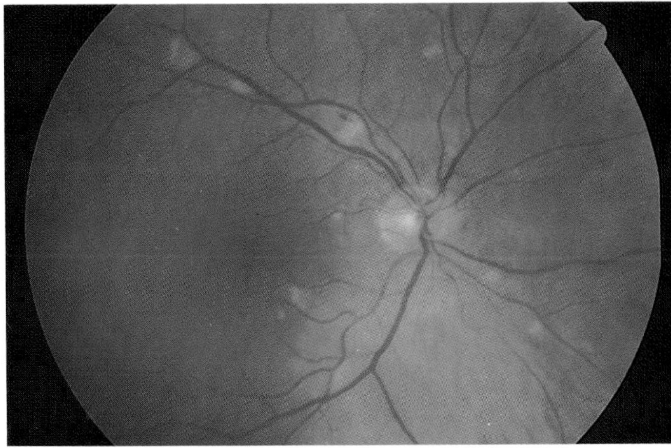

FIGURE 7–26. Microangiopathy
Retinal microangiopathy. Multiple cotton-wool spots, one of which is superotemporal to the disk with an adjacent superficial hemorrhage.

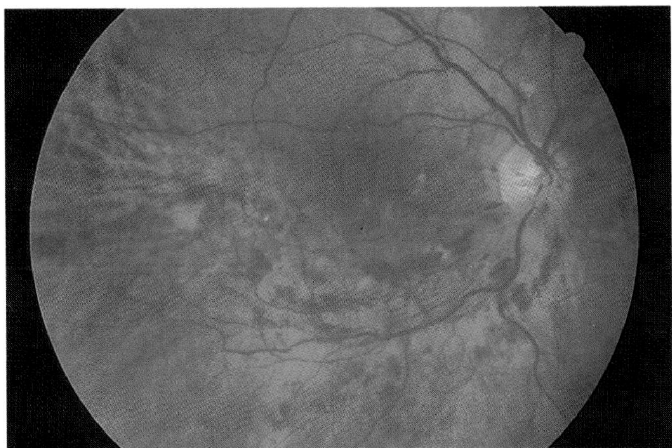

FIGURE 7–27. Microangiopathy
Retinal microangiopathy. Inferior temporal branch vein occlusion in an HIV-positive patient with elevated anticardiolipin antibodies.

PNEUMOCYSTIS CARINII *INFECTION*

Choroidal lesions due to disseminated *Pneumocystis carinii* infection were first described in 1989.[36,37] For several years they were seen with increasing frequency, probably owing to the use of aerosolized pentamidine for *P. carinii* pneumonia prophylaxis. Current prophylaxis for *P. carinii* pneumonia using systemic medication has resulted in a decrease in pneumocystic choroidopathy.

Pneumocystic choroidopathy is usually an asymptomatic condition (Fig. 7–28).[38] It is remarkable that even patients with parafoveal lesions can have perfect visual acuity, although threshold perimetry demonstrates some subtle changes over the lesions. Lesions can be single or multiple and are in the choroid, deep to the retinal vessels. They are yellow to orange and usually rounded. There is no overlying vitreous inflammation except when other infectious processes, such as cytomegalovirus (CMV) retinitis, are present (Fig. 7–29).[39] Pneumocystic choroidopathy establishes the diagnosis of disseminated infection and necessitates vigorous systemic therapy. Choroidal lesions clear slowly after treatment and should not be used as a marker for therapeutic success (Fig. 7–30*A*, *B*, and *C*).

TOXOPLASMOSIS

Retinochoroiditis secondary to toxoplasmosis manifests with the same symptoms as CMV retinitis: light flashes, floaters, and obscured vision. There is frequently an associated anterior uveitis, and the accompanying vitritis may be severe enough to make visualization of the fundus difficult (Figs. 7–31 and 7–32). Lesions may be single or multiple and are white to whitish-yellow in color; hemorrhage is rare. In contrast to ocular toxoplasmosis in immunocompetent patients, the lesions in AIDS patients are often free of the pigmentary scarring that indicates prior infection (Figs. 7–33 and 7–34). Central nervous system toxoplasmosis is more common in AIDS patients than is ocular toxoplasmosis, and careful evaluation for central nervous system involvement is indicated in AIDS patients with retinal lesions from toxoplasmosis. Treatment for ocular toxoplasmosis is systemic and required close cooperation between the primary AIDS-treating physician and the ophthalmologist. After the acute infection subsides, some continued treatment is necessary to prevent reactivation.[40]

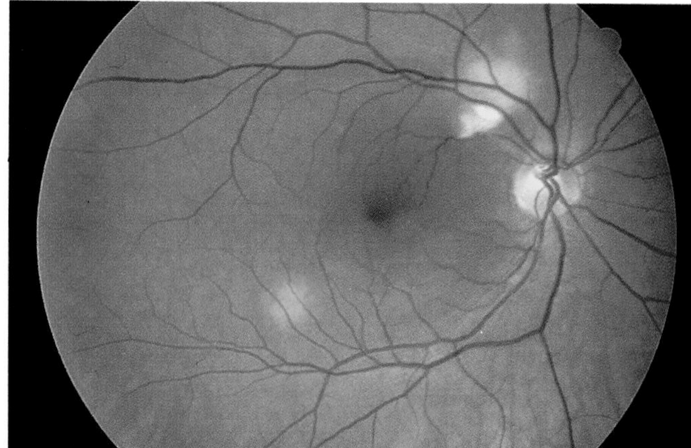

FIGURE 7–28. Pneumocystic choroidopathy
Pneumocystis carinii choroidopathy. Two deep yellowish lesions, one with an adjacent cotton-wool spot, in a patient who had no pulmonary symptoms but had abnormal findings on chest radiograph.

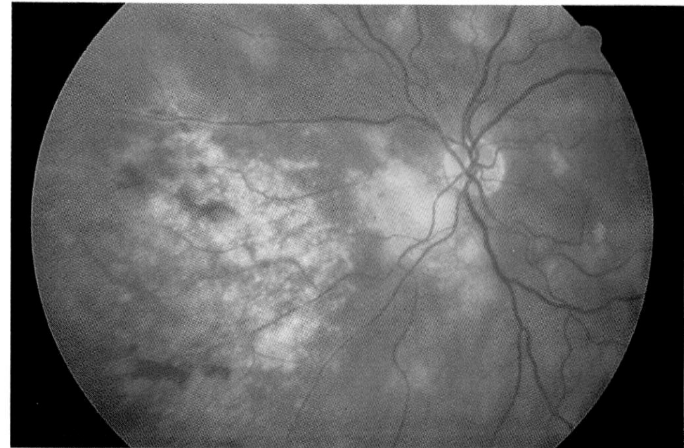

FIGURE 7–29. Pneumocystic choroidopathy
Pneumocystis carinii choroidopathy. Multiple yellow lesions and concurrent cytomegalovirus retinitis (white hemorrhagic lesion nasal to the optic disk).

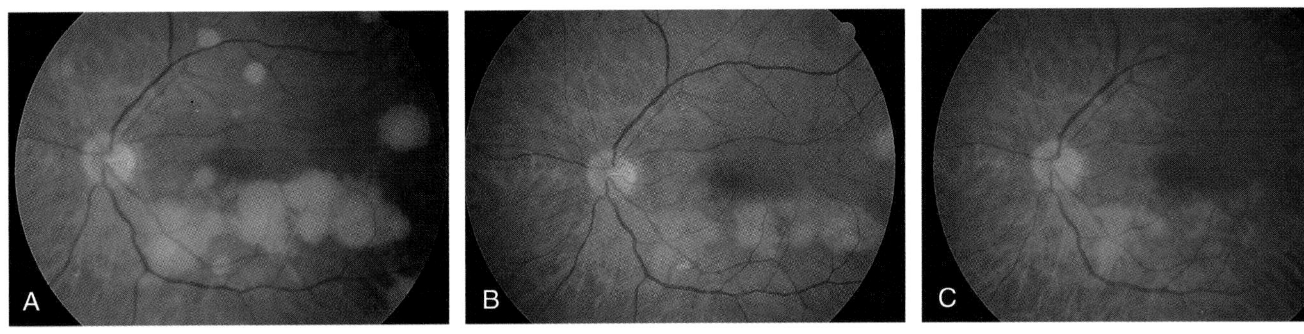

FIGURE 7–30. Pneumocystic choroidopathy

Pneumocystis carinii choroidopathy. *A,* Acute lesions (10/92); *B,* after treatment (12/92); *C,* further fading (8/93).

FIGURE 7–31. Toxoplasmosis

Ocular toxoplasmosis. Acute lesion with intense vitritis that limits the view of the fundus.

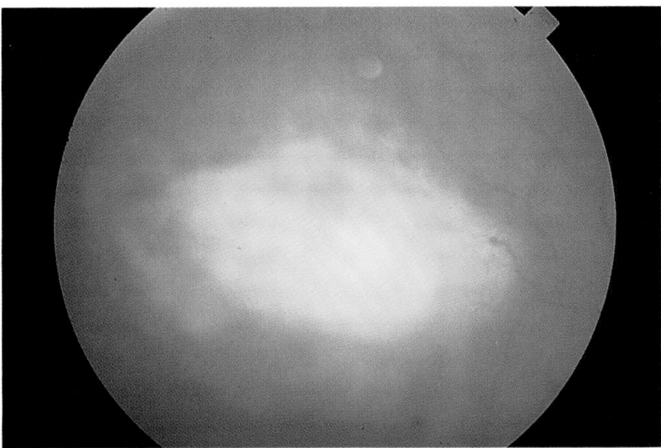

FIGURE 7–32. Toxoplasmosis

Ocular toxoplasmosis. A view of the lesion in Figure 7–31 after 3 months of treatment. The borders of the lesion can now be seen because of decreased vitreous inflammation.

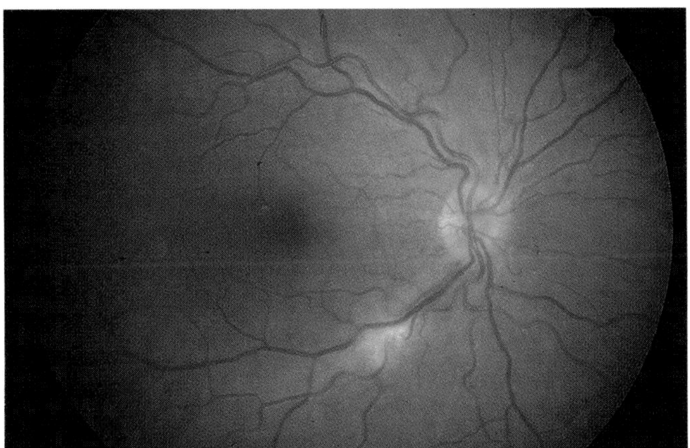

FIGURE 7–33. Toxoplasmosis

Ocular toxoplasmosis. Small early lesion along inferotemporal arcade with minimal vitritis.

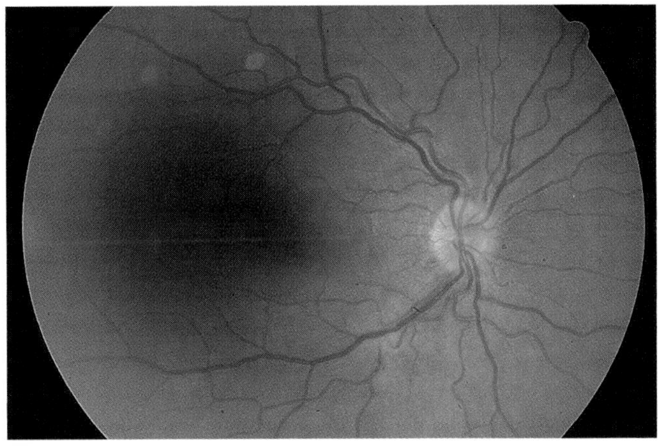

FIGURE 7–34. Toxoplasmosis

Ocular toxoplasmosis. The scar after treatment of the lesion shown in Figure 7–33.

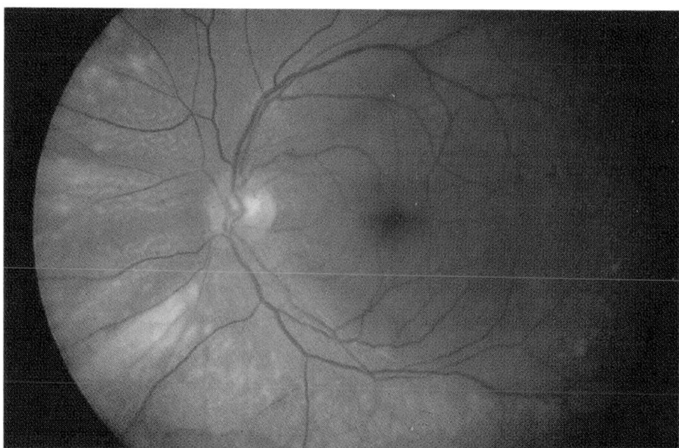

FIGURE 7–35. Progressive outer retinal necrosis
Note the lack of retinal hemorrhage and accompanying retinal detachment.

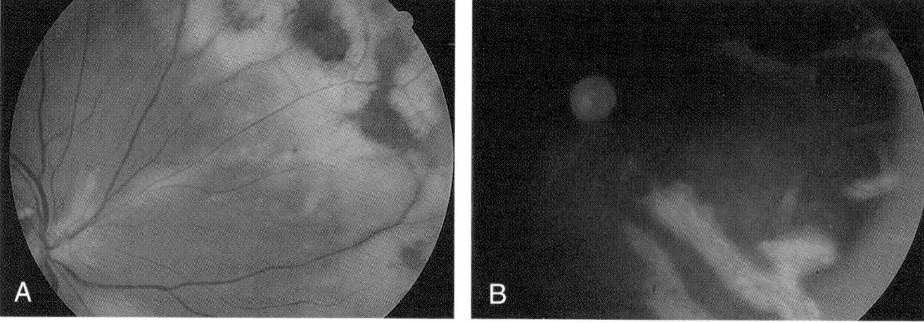

FIGURE 7–36. Progressive outer retinal necrosis
Progressive outer retinal necrosis at presentation *(A)* and after treatment *(B)* with a combination of foscarnet and ganciclovir. This patient retained functional vision in one of his two affected eyes.

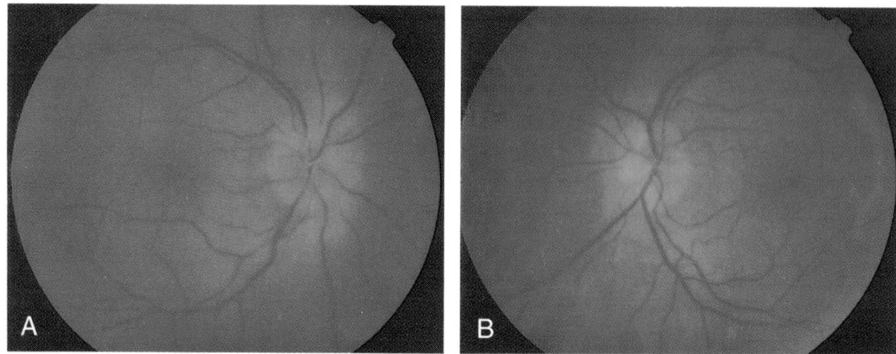

FIGURE 7–37. Syphilitic papillitis
Right and left optic nerves of a patient with syphilis who responded to treatment with penicillin.

HERPES ZOSTER

Herpes zoster can cause a devastating, rapidly progressive retinal necrosis that often results in blindness regardless of vigorous therapy. Manifestation of this infection is varied, which has led to the somewhat confusing nomenclature.[41] Acute retinal necrosis was initially described in immunocompetent patients and, although often causing severe visual loss, in some cases responded well to treatment with acyclovir. The retinal necrosis, which is accompanied by an intense vitritis, manifests initially in the retinal periphery, can become confluent rapidly, and often results in retinal detachment. Studies of pathologic specimens of eyes from patients with acute retinal necrosis have shown herpesvirus particles.

A new and even more aggressive form of retinal necrosis from herpes zoster infection has been described in the last few years in AIDS patients. Progressive outer retinal necrosis is an acute outer retinal necrosis that may begin either peripherally or centrally.[42,43] It spreads rapidly to affect the entire retina. In contrast to acute retinal necrosis, there is little accompanying intraocular inflammation in progressive outer retinal necrosis. Patients often complain of a loss of peripheral vision when they seek care. Retinal detachment is common (Fig. 7–35). Therapy with a variety of antiviral compounds has met with limited success. High-dose intravenous acyclovir, alone or in combination with ganciclovir or foscarnet, and ganciclovir or foscarnet, alone or in combination, have all been used.[44,45] The most encouraging results to date seem to be with combination of high doses of ganciclovir and foscarnet (Fig. 7–36*A* and *B*).

SYPHILIS

As in other organs, the manifestations of syphilis in the eye are protean. Uveitis and syphilitic papillitis (Fig. 7–37*A* and *B*) can be seen as well as placoid chorioretinitis and a widespread retinitis (Fig. 7–38).[46] In AIDS patients, ocular syphilis must be treated as vigorously as neurosyphilis; less aggressive therapy has resulted in relapses.[47–49]

TUBERCULOSIS

Most reports of ocular tuberculosis have come from pathologic studies of autopsy specimens; both infection with *Mycobacterium tuberculosis* and *M. avium* have been described.[50,51] There have been some clinical reports of miliary tuberculous nodules in AIDS patients that responded to antituberculous therapy.[52] With the increased incidence of tuberculosis in the AIDS population, more ocular infections should be expected (Fig. 7–39).[53]

Intraocular lymphoma,[31,32,54] bacterial[55] and cryptococcal infection, (Fig. 7–40) and histoplasmosis[56] have been described in patients with AIDS.

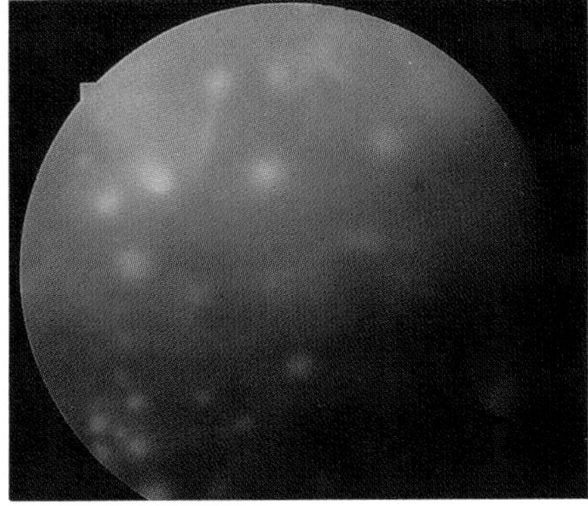

FIGURE 7–38. Syphilitic retinitis
Syphilitic retinitis, with multiple punctate lesions throughout the retina.

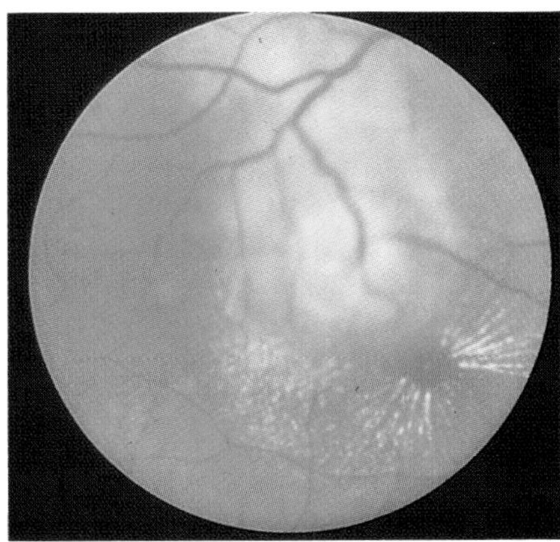

FIGURE 7–39. Tuberculous choroiditis
Tuberculous choroiditis in a patient with miliary tuberculosis. Note the inferior macular exudates. (Photograph courtesy of Alan H. Friedman, MD.)

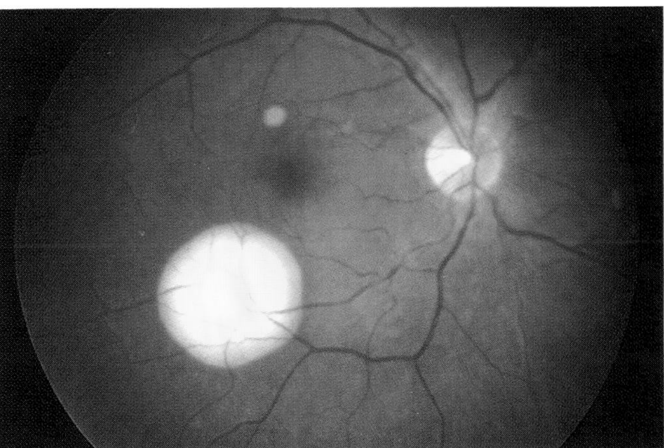

FIGURE 7–40. Cryptococcal choroiditis
Cryptococcal choroiditis, showing a single white lesion along the inferotemporal arcade in a patient with cryptococcal meningitis. The small white dot above the fovea is an artifact.

CYTOMEGALOVIRUS RETINITIS

Cytomegalovirus retinitis is the most common ocular opportunistic infection in AIDS patients.[57] In early case reports, the infection was relentless progressive, and frequently preterminal.[58,59] Most patients who develop CMV retinitis are severely immunosuppressed, with mean CD4 counts under 50/mm^3.[60,61] Patients frequently complain of flashes of light in their vision, multiple floating spots, cloudy vision, or loss of peripheral or central vision. If the infection is in the retinal periphery, there may be no symptoms.

Diagnosis of Cytomegalovirus Retinitis

As with other retinal and choroidal manifestations of AIDS, CMV retinitis is diagnosed clinically. The appearance of the retinal lesions is varied, and familiarity with different manifestations allows differentiation from other ocular opportunistic infections. Retinal lesions are usually accompanied by a very mild anterior uveitis as well as a mild vitritis. If vitritis is severe, one should consider diagnoses other than CMV retinitis. Classic CMV lesions are hemorrhagic and necrotic and if untreated lead to loss of vision (Figs. 7–41 and 7–42). However, early lesions may have no hemorrhage and may have a granular appearance. Larger lesions in the periphery may have a white granular border surrounding an atrophic retinal scar (Figs. 7–43 and 7–44). Other unusual manifestations include a retinal periphlebitis, which can be present in areas of the retina unaffected by CMV and which resolves after CMV has been treated (Figs. 7–45 and 7–46). Patients may also present with a retinal detachment, examination of the retinal periphery revealing active retinitis with necrotic full-thickness retinal holes (Figs. 7–47 and 7–48).

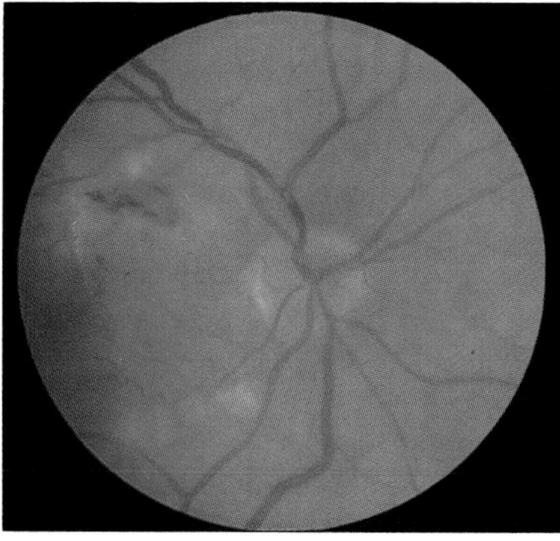

FIGURE 7–41. Cytomegalovirus retinitis
Cytomegalovirus retinitis, showing a fulminant hemorrhagic, necrotic lesion along the superotemporal arcade.

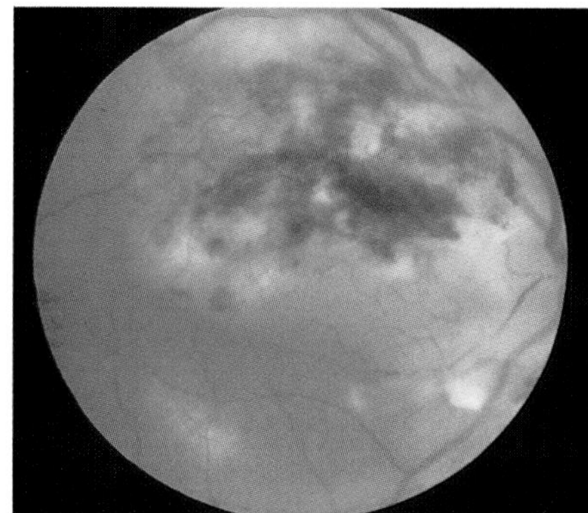

FIGURE 7–42. Cytomegalovirus retinitis
Enlargement of the lesion seen in Figure 7–41. Vision has decreased to 20/400 because of macular involvement.

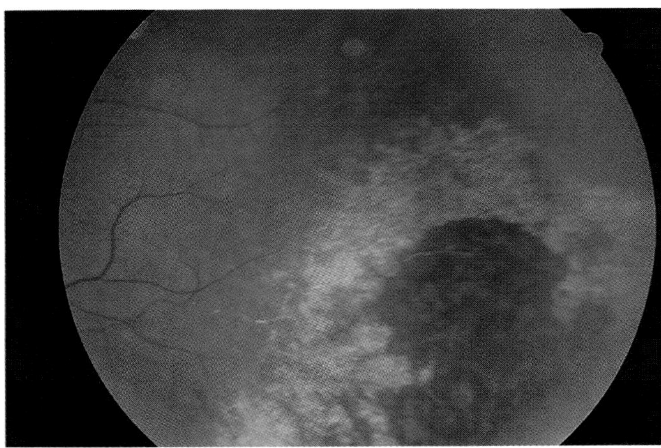

FIGURE 7–43. Cytomegalovirus retinitis

Cytomegalovirus retinitis, showing a granular lesion in the retinal periphery with a white border and atrophic center before treatment.

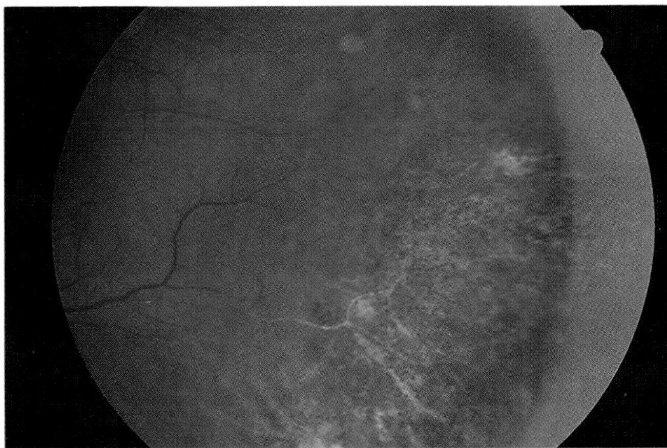

FIGURE 7–44. Cytomegalovirus retinitis

The lesion shown in Figure 7–43 after treatment. The borders are now atrophic.

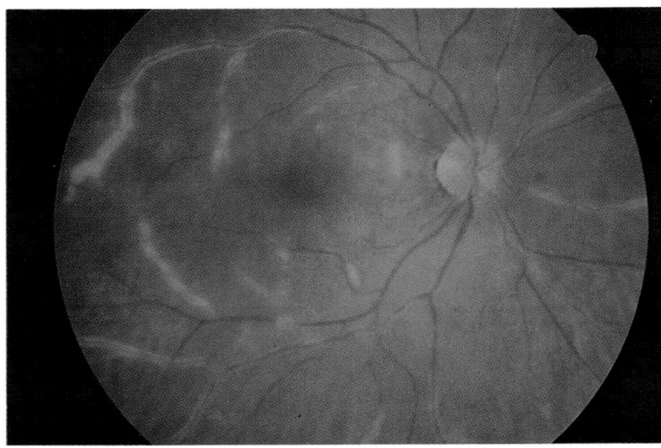

FIGURE 7–45. Retinal periphlebitis

Retinal periphlebitis in an area not affected with cytomegalovirus retinitis.

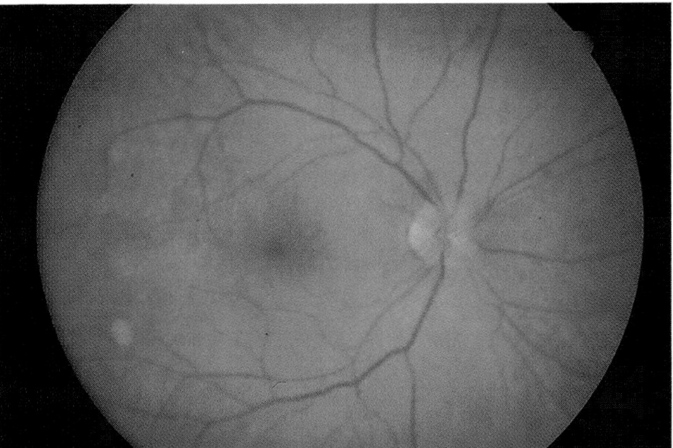

FIGURE 7–46. Retinal periphlebitis

Retinal periphlebitis has resolved after treatment for cytomegalovirus of the patient shown in Figure 7–45.

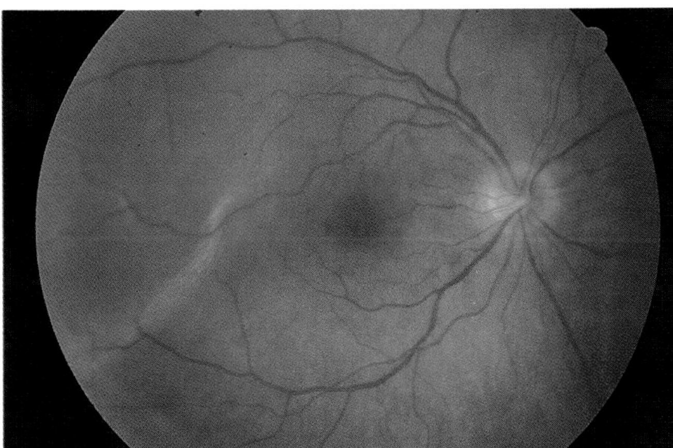

FIGURE 7–47. Retinal detachment

Retinal detachment in patient with cytomegalovirus retinitis. Note the elevated retina temporal to the macula.

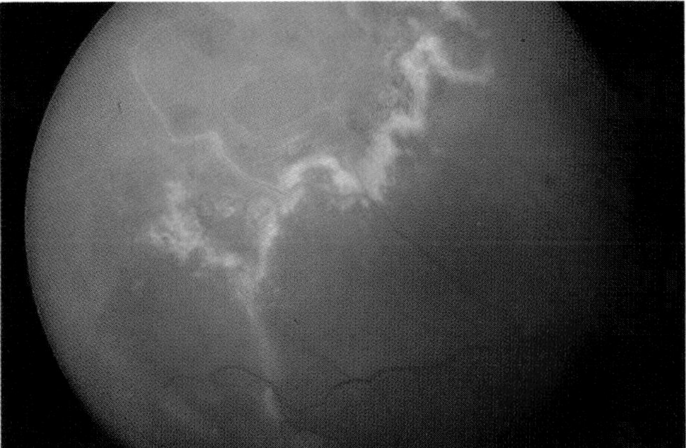

FIGURE 7–48. Retinal detachment

Retinal periphery of patient in Figure 7–47. Note the granular retinitis and full-thickness retinal holes.

The location of the infection influences the visual outcome; lesions involving the optic nerve or macula have the worst prognosis. In cases of CMV papillitis, an associated retinal edema can result in transient loss of vision. When the edema resolves after treatment, vision may return (Figs. 7–49 and 7–50). When the macula is destroyed, vision does not return (Fig. 7–51). Cytomegalovirus retinitis that appears in patients who are undergoing therapy for nonocular CMV manifests more subtly. Patients do not complain of flashes and floaters and may develop symptoms only when they have lost large areas of their visual field. Lesion borders may be minimally active with large areas of retinal atrophy. The silent manifestation of retinitis can be partially avoided by routine examination of patients being treated for extraocular CMV and by educating these patients to seek ophthalmic care if they notice even minor visual changes (Fig. 7–52).

Treatment of Cytomegalovirus Retinitis

Current therapy for CMV retinitis consists of lifelong treatment with either intravenous ganciclovir (Cytovene)[62–65] or intravenous foscarnet (Foscavir).[66–69] Treatment is divided into two phases: an induction phase, in which the drug is given two or three times daily for 2 or 3 weeks, and a maintenance phase, in which the drug is given once daily. Patients are monitored for the clinical improvement of retinitis and for the development of side effects of therapy. As with the treatment of other opportunistic ocular infections, the treatment for CMV retinitis requires a team approach. The goal of treatment is to convert an active infection into an atrophic scar (Figs. 7–53 and 7–54).

The most common side effect of ganciclovir is neutropenia, and patients must have complete blood counts with determination of absolute neutrophil count while on therapy. The use of colony-stimulating factors may reverse the drug-induced neutropenia; however, medication must be interrupted if counts fall to dangerous levels. Extreme caution is required when other marrow-suppressing drugs must be given with ganciclovir. Thrombocytopenia, anemia, and gastrointestinal disturbances are also reported with ganciclovir use. The most common side effect of foscarnet is nephrotoxicity. This is reduced by careful hydration, but serum creatinine must be monitored during treatment, and dosages should be adjusted carefully depending on renal function. Hypocalcemia and hypomagnesemia may be avoided by using oral supplements. During infusion, patients may experience signs of hypocalcemia such as tingling or perioral numbness even with normal serum calcium levels. This is due to a decrease in serum ionized calcium and frequently responds to calcium supplementation. Infusion-related nausea can often be controlled by using antinausea medications, slowing the infusion rate, or dividing doses. Patients who have seizures while on foscarnet should have careful central nervous system evaluations to eliminate treatable disease before attributing the seizure to drug toxicity.

A study comparing the efficacy of ganciclovir and foscarnet showed they were equivalent in their ability to delay progression of retinitis, and patients had similar visual outcomes on either drug. However, patients who were assigned to foscarnet had a median survival of 12.6 months compared with 8.5 months for those assigned to ganciclovir; but patients on foscarnet switched to ganciclovir at a higher rate because of toxicity or drug intolerance.[61,70] There have been several encouraging reports of the use of the combination of ganciclovir and foscarnet in patients with retinitis that was progressing on monotherapy.[71–77]

Because both ganciclovir and foscarnet are given intravenously and usually require the placement of an indwelling catheter, there has been a great deal of interest in the development of other forms of administration. Studies of oral ganciclovir, both for maintenance therapy of patients with stable retinitis[78,79] and as prophylaxis against the development of CMV disease, have been encouraging. Oral ganciclovir has been approved by the U.S. Food and Drug Administration for the maintenance treatment of CMV retinitis that has stabilized after intravenous induction therapy.

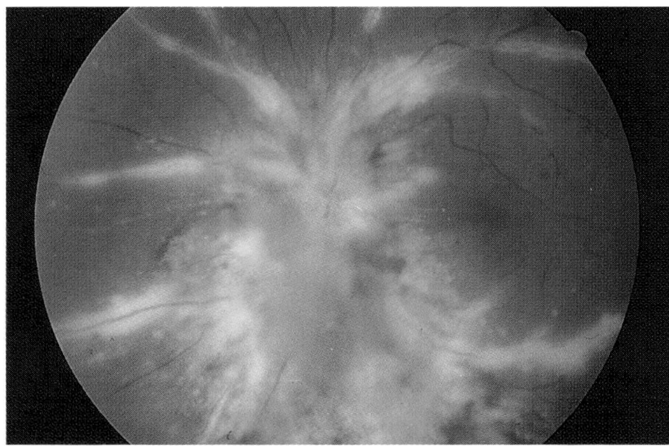

FIGURE 7–49. Cytomegalovirus papillitis
Cytomegalovirus papillitis with periphlebitis; visual acuity is 20/60.

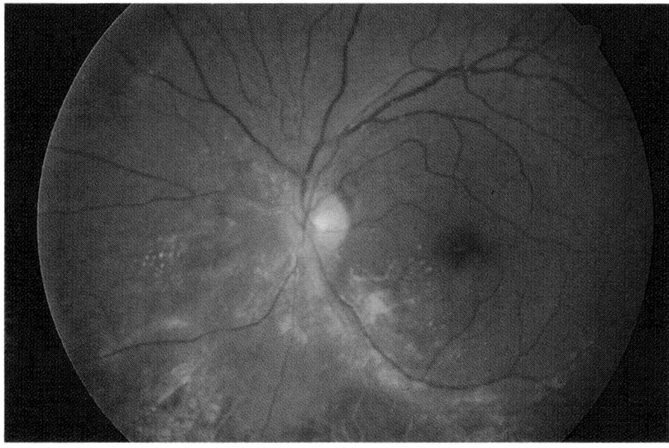

FIGURE 7–50. Cytomegalovirus papillitis
Cytomegalovirus papillitis after treatment (patient in Fig. 7–49). Visual acuity has improved to 20/25.

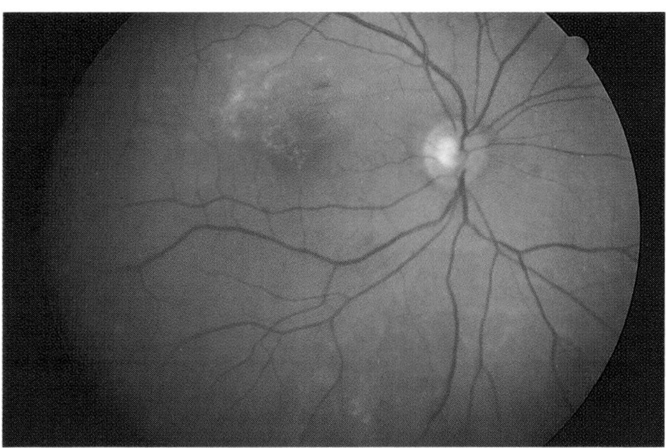

FIGURE 7–51. Cytomegalovirus retinitis
Cytomegalovirus retinitis involving the macula at presentation. Acuity is 20/200 and has not improved after therapy.

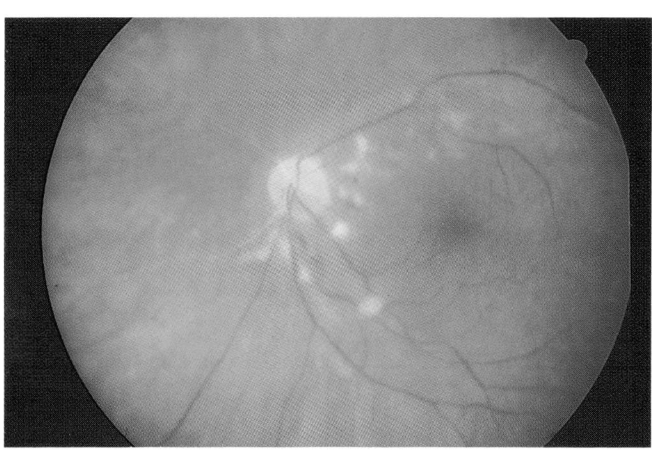

FIGURE 7–52. Cytomegalovirus retinitis
Cytomegalovirus retinitis manifesting in a patient who has been on therapy for cytomegalovirus colitis. He complained of loss of peripheral vision. Lesion borders are subtle.

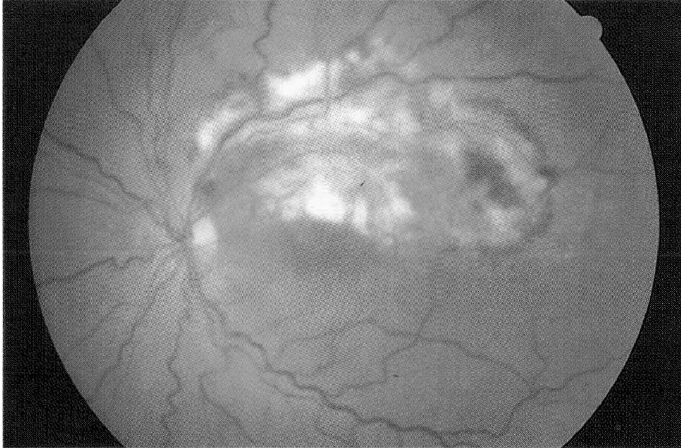

FIGURE 7–53. Cytomegalovirus retinitis
The active lesion of cytomegalovirus retinitis. Visual acuity is 20/200.

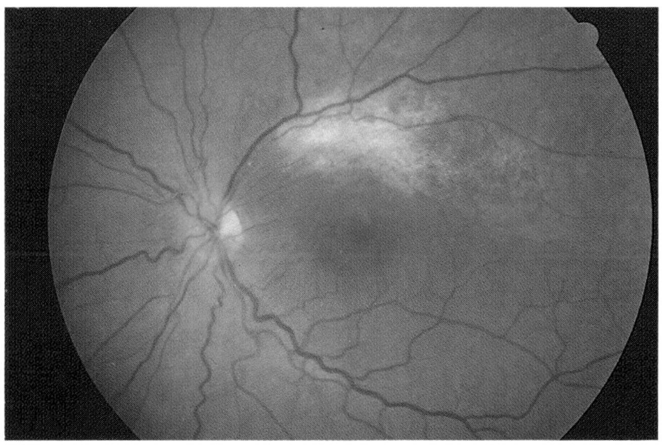

FIGURE 7–54. Cytomegalovirus retinitis
Atrophic scar after therapy in patient shown in Figure 7–53. Visual acuity is 20/30, and lesion has not changed for more than 18 months.

There has also been interest in the local administration of both ganciclovir and foscarnet directly into the vitreous.[80–87] This has been tried both in patients who were unable to receive systemic medication and in patients whose disease was progressing in spite of maximum doses of intravenous drug. A device has been developed that releases ganciclovir into the vitreous as a steady rate for about 8 months (Fig. 7–55).[88,89]

Other drugs for intravenous and intravitreal use are in development.[90,91]

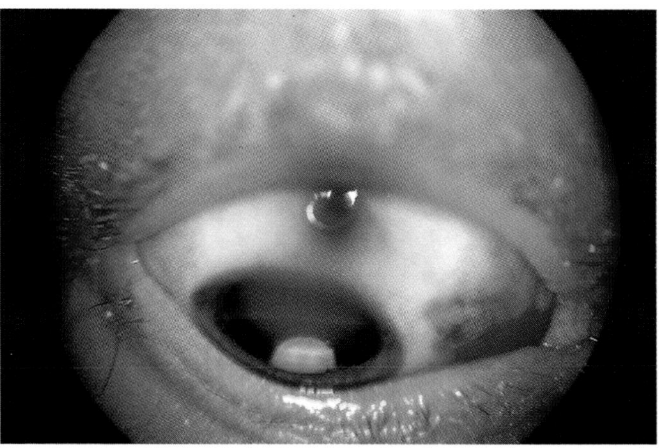

FIGURE 7–55. Intravitreal implant
Intravitreal implant in place. See the yellow half circle inferiorly.

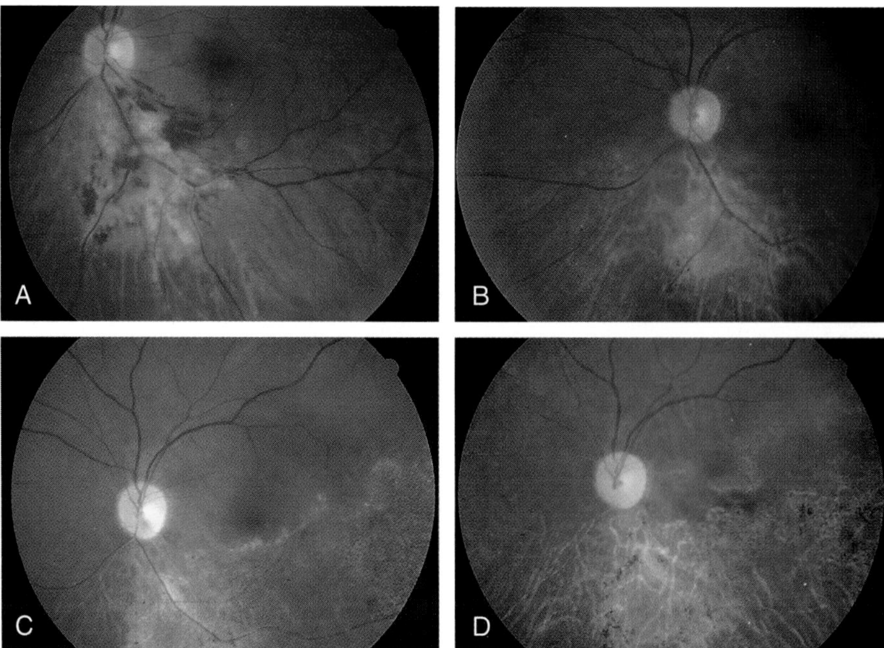

FIGURE 7–56. Cytomegalovirus retinitis
Cytomegalovirus retinitis smoldering in spite of aggressive therapy. *A,* Lesion at presentation (2/90). *B,* Reactivation nasal to atrophic scar; acuity is still 20/20 (6/90). *C,* Continued progression; acuity is 20/40 (11/90). *D,* Continued progression; acuity has dropped to 20/200 (6/91).

Long-Term Management of Cytomegalovirus Retinitis

In the ideal situation, treatment of CMV retinitis transforms an active lesion into an atrophic scar. However, most patients experience progression of their retinitis and require reinductions with the current drug that they are taking or change to another treatment with the other intravenous drug, as monotherapy or in combination, or addition of an intravitreal drug. Assessment of retinitis progression requires the careful study of serial retinal photographs.[73,74] Treated retinitis does not usually have the distinct borders that are seen in untreated disease, and retinal vascular and choroidal landmarks can be helpful in determining progression (Fig. 7–56*A–D*). Most patients with retinitis are evaluated monthly; if lesions are active or immediately sight threatening, more frequent evaluations should be scheduled. Patients should be advised to contact their ophthalmologist if they experience changes in vision.

Retinal detachments are also seen with increasing frequency in patients with treated retinitis. The larger the area of affected retina, particularly in the retinal periphery, the greater the incidence of retinal detachment. Patients with active lesions are more likely to develop retinal detachments than patients whose infection is quiescent.[92,93] Repair of these detachments using vitrectomy and silicone oil tamponade has resulted in more success than using conventional scleral buckling techniques[94,95] (Figs. 7–57 and 7–58). This technique is not without sequelae. Patients may develop cataracts, but these can be removed with standard cataract surgery techniques (Fig. 7–59).

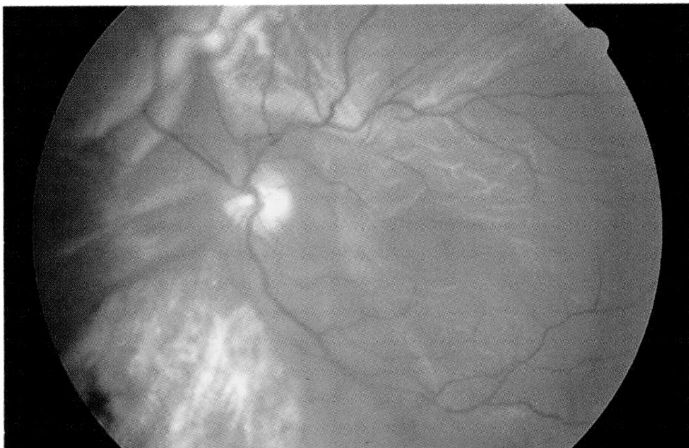

FIGURE 7–57. Retinal detachment

Retinal detachment in a patient with treated cytomegalovirus retinitis; note the atrophic scar of treated retinitis below the optic disk, preoperative.

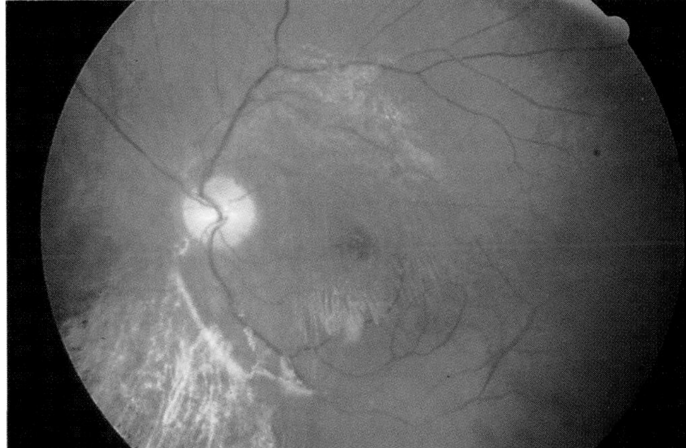

FIGURE 7–58. Repaired retinal detachment

Repaired retinal detachment of patient in Figure 7–57. Glinting reflexes above and below the macula are often seen after the use of silicone oil tamponade.

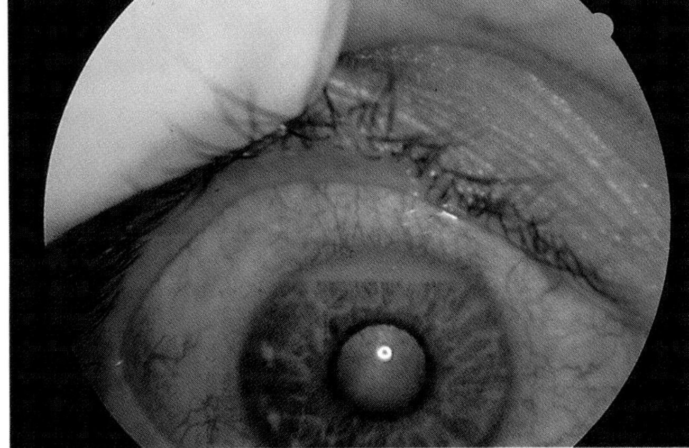

FIGURE 7–59. Mature cataract

Mature cataract and oil level at the superior limbus in a patient who had undergone retinal detachment repair with silicone oil.

Significant advances in the treatment of CMV retinitis have occurred in the last 10 years, and new therapies that hold promise are on the horizon. Prevention of CMV retinitis through successful prophylaxis regimen would reduce the incidence of infection. Aggressive therapy to limit the size of retinal lesions, perhaps with local administration of drug combined with systemic medication to prevent extraocular CMV using an oral drug or an intravenous preparation with a long half-life, would be a good starting point.

SUMMARY

Careful examination of the eye—externally for lesions of the lid skin, conjunctiva, and orbit and with the ophthalmoscope for the many retinal and choroidal ocular opportunistic diseases—often helps the physician treating a patients with AIDS to arrive at a nonophthalmic diagnosis. A close relationship between the patient's ophthalmologist and primary physician is paramount in managing the many ocular complications of HIV infection.

References

1. Shuler J, Holland G, Miles S, Miller B, Grossman I. Kaposi's sarcoma of the conjunctiva and eyelids associated with the acquired immunodeficiency syndrome. Arch Ophthalmol 1989; 107:858–862.
2. Shields J, De Potter P, Shields C, Komarnicky L. Kaposi's sarcoma of the eyelids: Response to radiotherapy. Arch Ophthalmol 1992;110:1689.
3. Itescu S, Brancato L, Buxbaum J, et al. A diffuse infiltrative CD8 lymphocytosis syndrome in human immunodeficiency virus (HIV) infection: A host immune response associated with HLA-DR5. Ann Intern Med 1990; 112:3–10.
4. Lucca J, Farris R, Bielory L, Caputo A. Keratoconjunctivitis sicca in male patients infected with human immunodeficiency virus type 1. Ophthalmol 1990;97:1008–1010.
5. Cole E, Meisler D, Calabrese L, Holland G, Mondino B, Conant M. Herpes zoster ophthalmicus and acquired immunodeficiency syndrome. Arch Ophthalmol 1984;102:1027–1029.
6. Melbye M, Grossman R, Goedert J, Eyster E, Biggar R. Risk of AIDS after herpes zoster. Lancet 1987;1:728–730.
7. Sandor E, Millman A, Croxson T, Mildvan D. Herpes zoster ophthalmicus in patients at risk for the acquired immune deficiency syndrome (AIDS). Am J Ophthalmol 1986;101:153–155.
8. Sellitti T, Huang A, Schiffman J, Davis J. Association of herpes zoster ophthalmicus with acquired immunodeficiency syndrome with acute retinal necrosis. Am J Ophthalmol 1993;116: 297–301.
9. Robinson M, Udell I, Garber P, Perry H, Streeton B. Molluscum contagiosum of the eyelids in patients with acquired immune deficiency syndrome. Ophthalmology 1992;99:1745–1747.
10. Charles N, Friedberg D. Epibulbar molluscum contagiosum in acquired immune deficiency syndrome. Ophthalmology 1992;99:1123–1126.
11. Dugel P, Gill P, Frangieh G, Rao N. Ocular adnexal Kaposi's sarcoma in acquired immunodeficiency syndrome. Am J Ophthalmol 1990;110:500–503.
12. Dugel P, Gill P, Frangieh G, Rao N. Treatment of ocular adnexal Kaposi's sarcoma in acquired immune deficiency syndrome. Ophthalmology 1992;99:1127–1132.
13. Hummer J, Gass J, Huang A. Conjunctival Kaposi's sarcoma treated with interferon alpha-2a. Am J Ophthalmol 1993;116:502–503.
14. Friedberg D, Stenson S, Orenstein J, Tierno P, Charles N. Microsporidial keratoconjunctivitis in acquired immunodeficiency syndrome. Arch Ophthalmol 1990;108:504–508.
15. Lowder C, Meisler D, McMahon J, Longworth D, Rutherford I. Microsporidia infection of the cornea in a man seropositive for human immunodeficiency virus. Am J Ophthalmol 1990; 109:242–244.
16. Ashton N, Wirasinha P. Encephalitozoonosis (nosematosis) of the cornea. Br J Ophthalmol 1973;57:669–674.
17. Pinnolis M, Egbert P, Font RL, Winter F. Nosematosis of the cornea. Arch Ophthalmol 1981;99:1044–1047.
18. Didier E, Didier P, Friedberg D, et al. Isolation and characterization of a new human microsporidian, *Encephalitozoon hellum* (n. sp.), from three AIDS patients with keratoconjunctivitis. J Infect Dis 1991;163:617–621.
19. Schwartz D, Bryan R, Hewan-Lowe K, et al. Disseminated microsporidiosis *(Encephalitozoon hellum)* and AIDS. Autopsy evidence for respiratory acquisition. Arch Pathol Lab Med 1992;116:660.
20. Schwartz D, Visvesvara G, Diesenhouse M, et al. Pathologic features and immunofluorescent antibody demonstration of ocular microsporidiosis *(Encephalitozoon hellum)* in seven patients with acquired immunodeficiency syndrome. Am J Ophthalmol 1993;115: 285–292.
21. Diesenhouse M, Wilson CGF, Visvesvara G, Grossniklaus H, Bryan R. Treatment of microsporidial keratoconjunctivitis with topical fumagillin. Am J Ophthalmol 1993;115:293–298.
22. Farrell P, Heinemann M-H, Roberts C, Polsky B, Gold J, Mamelok A. Response of human immunodeficiency virus–associated uveitis to zidovudine. Am J Ophthalmol 1988;106:7–10.
23. Saran B, Maguire A, Nicols C, et al. Hypopyon uveitis in patients with acquired immunodeficiency syndrome treated for systemic *Mycobacterium avium* complex infection with rifabutin. Arch Ophthalmol 1994;112:1159–1165.
24. Cohen JI, Saragas SJ. Endophthalmitis due to *Mycobacterium avium* in a patient with AIDS. Ann Ophthalmol 1990;22:47–51.
25. Charles N, Boxrud C, Small E. Cryptococcosis of the anterior segment in acquired immune deficiency syndrome. Ophthalmology 1992;99:813–816.
26. Berger J, Kaszovitz B, Post M, Dickinson G. Progressive multifocal leukoencephalopathy associated with human immunodeficiency virus infection. Ann Intern Med 1987;107:78–87.
27. Freidman D. Neuro-ophthalmic manifestations of human immunodeficiency virus infection Neurol Clin 1991;9:55–72.
28. Mansour A. Neuro-ophthalmic findings in acquired immunodeficiency syndrome. J Clin Neuro-ophthalmol 1990; 10:167–174.
29. Vitale A, Spaide R, Warren F, Moussouris H, D'Amico R. Orbital aspergillosis in an immunocompromised host. Am J Ophthalmol 1992;113:725–726.
30. Font R, Laucirica R, Patrinely J. Immunoblastic B-cell malignant lymphoma involving the orbit and maxillary sinus in a patient with acquired immune deficiency syndrome. Ophthalmology 1993;100:966–970.
31. Matzkin D, Slamovits T, Rosenbaum P. Simultaneous intraocular and orbital non-Hodgkin lymphoma in the acquired immune deficiency syndrome. Ophthalmology 1994;101:850–855.
32. Stanton C, Sloan DI, Slusher M, Greven C. Acquired immunodeficiency syndrome–related primary intraocular lymphoma. Am J Ophthalmol 1992; 110:1614–1617.
33. Mansour A, Jampol L, Logani S, Read J, Henderly D. Cotton-wool spots in acquired immunodeficiency syndrome compared with diabetes mellitus, systemic hypertension, and central retinal vein occlusion. Am J Ophthalmol 1988;106:1074–1077.
34. Freeman W, Chen A, Henderly D, et al. Prevalence and significance of acquired immunodeficiency syndrome–related retinal microvasculopathy. Am J Ophthalmol 1989;107:229–235.
35. Adan A, Goday A, Ferrer J, Cabot J. Diabetic retinopathy associated with acquired immunodeficiency syndrome. Am J Ophthalmol 1990;109:744–745.
36. Freeman W, Gross J, Labelle J, Oteken K, Katz B, Wiley C. *Pneumocystis carinii* choroidopathy. Am J Ophthalmol 1989;107:863–867.

37. Rao N, Zimmerman P, Boyer D, et al. A clinical, histopathologic, and electron microscopic study of *Pneumocystis carinii* choroiditis. Am J Ophthalmol 1989;107:218–228.
38. Friedberg D, Greene J, Brook D. Asymptomatic disseminated *Pneumocystis carinii* infection detected by ophthalmoscopy. Lancet 1990;336: 1256–1257.
39. Shami M, Freeman W, Friedberg D, Siderides E, Listhaus A, Ai E. A multicenter study of *Pneumocystis* choroidopathy. Am J Ophthalmol 1991; 112:15–22.
40. Holland G, Engstrom RJ, Glasgow B, et al. Ocular toxoplasmosis in patients with the acquired immunodeficiency syndrome. Am J Ophthalmol 1988; 106:653–667.
41. Holland G, Executive Committee of the American Uveitis Society. Standard diagnostic criteria for the acute retinal necrosis syndrome. Am J Ophthalmol 1994;117:663–667.
42. Forster D, Dugel P, Frangieh G, Liggett P, Rao N. Rapidly progressive retinal necrosis in the acquired immunodeficiency syndrome. Am J Ophthalmol 1990;110:341–348.
43. Margolis T, Lowder C, Holland G, et al. Varicella-zoster virus retinitis in patients with the acquired immunodeficiency syndrome. Am J Ophthalmol 1991;112:119–131.
44. Morley M, Duker J, Zacks C. Successful treatment of rapidly progressive outer retinal necrosis in the acquired immunodeficiency syndrome. Am J Ophthalmol 1994;117:264–265.
45. Johnston W, Holland G, Engstrom R, Rimmer S. Recurrence of presumed varicella-zoster virus retinopathy in patients with acquired immunodeficiency syndrome. Am J Ophthalmol 1993;116:42–50.
46. Gass J, Braunstein R, Chenoweth R. Acute syphilitic posterior placoid chorioretinitis. Ophthalmology 1990;97: 1288–1297.
47. Becerra L, Ksiazek S, Savino P, et al. Syphilitic uveitis in human immunodeficiency virus-infected and noninfected patients. Ophthalmology 1989; 96:1727–1730.
48. McLeish W, Pulido J, Holland S, Culbertson W, Winward K. The ocular manifestations of syphilis in the human immunodeficiency virus type 1-infected host. Ophthalmology 1990;97:196–203.
49. Passo M, Rosenbaum J. Ocular syphilis in patients with human immunodeficiency syndrome. Am J Ophthalmol 1988;106:1–6.
50. Blodi B, Johnson M, McLeish W, Gass D. Presumed choroidal tuberculosis in a human immunodeficiency virus infected host. Am J Ophthalmol 1989; 108:605–607.
51. Morinelli E, Dugel P, Riffenburgh R, Rao N. Infectious multifocal choroiditis in patients with acquired immune deficiency syndrome. Ophthalmology 1993;100:1014–1021.
52. Barondes M, Sponsel W, Stevens T. Plotnik R. Tuberculous choroiditis diagnosed by chorioretinal biopsy. Am J Ophthalmol 1991;112:460–461.
53. Helm C, Holland G. Ocular tuberculosis. Surv Ophthalmol 1993;38:229–256.
54. Schanzer M, Font R, O'Malley R. Primary ocular malignant lymphoma associated with the acquired immune deficiency syndrome. Ophthalmology 1990;98:88–91.
55. Davis J, Nussenblatt R, Bachman D, Chan C-C, Palestine A. Endogenous bacterial retinitis in AIDS. Am J Ophthalmol 1989;107:613–623.
56. Macher A, Rodrigues M, Kaplan W, et al. Disseminated bilateral chorioretinitis due to *Histoplasma capsulatum* in a patient with acquired immunodeficiency syndrome. Ophthalmology 1985;92:1159–1164.
57. Jabs DA, Enger C, Bartlett JG. Cytomegalovirus retinitis and acquired immunodeficiency syndrome. Arch Ophthalmol 1989;107:75–80.
58. Holland GN, Pepose JS, Pettit TH, Gottlieb MS, Yee RD, Foos RY. Acquired immune deficiency syndrome: Ocular manifestations. Ophthalmology 1983;90:859–873.
59. Palestine AG, Rodrigues MM, Macher AM, et al. Ophthalmic involvement in acquired immune deficiency syndrome. Ophthalmology 1984;91:1092–1099.
60. Kuppermann BD, Petty JG, Richman DD, et al. Correlation between $CD4^+$ counts and prevalence of cytomegalovirus retinitis and human immunodeficiency virus–related noninfectious retinal vasculopathy in patients with acquired immunodeficiency syndrome. Am J Ophthalmol 1993;115:575–582.
61. Studies of Ocular Complications of AIDS Research Group, in Collaboration with the AIDS Clinical Trials Group. Mortality in patients with the acquired immunodeficiency syndrome treated with either foscarnet or ganciclovir for cytomegalovirus retinitis. N Engl J Med 1992;326:213–220.
62. Holland GN, Sidikaro Y, Kreiger AE, et al. Treatment of cytomegalovirus retinopathy with ganciclovir. Ophthalmology 1987;94:815–823.
63. Jabs DA, Newman C, de Bustros S, Polk BF. Treatment of cytomegalovirus retinitis with ganciclovir. Ophthalmology 1987;94:824–830.
64. Orellana J, Teich SA, Friedman AH, Lerebours F, Winterkorn J, Mildvan D. Combined short- and long-term therapy for the treatment of cytomegalovirus retinitis using ganciclovir (BW B759U). Ophthalmology 1987;94:831–838.
65. Jacobson MA, O'Donnell JJ, Brodie HR, Wolsy C, Mills J. Randomized prospective trial of ganciclovir maintenance therapy for cytomegalovirus retinitis. J Med Virol 1988;25:339–349.
66. Jacobson MA, Causey D, Polsky B, et al. A dose-ranging study of daily maintenance intravenous foscarnet therapy for cytomegalovirus retinitis in AIDS. J Infect Dis 1993;168:444–448.
67. Jacobson MA, O'Donnell JJ, Mills J. Foscarnet treatment of cytomegalovirus retinitis patients with acquired immunodeficiency syndrome. Antimicrob Agents Chemother 1989;33:736–741.
68. Lehoang P, Girard B, Robinet M, et al. Foscarnet in the treatment of cytomegalovirus retinitis in acquired immune deficiency syndrome. Ophthalmology 1989;96:865–874.
69. Walmsley SL, Chew E, Read SE, et al. Treatment of cytomegalovirus retinitis with trisodium phosphonformate hexahydrate (foscarnet). J Infect Dis 1988; 157:569–572.
70. Studies of Ocular Complications of AIDS Research Group, in Collaboration with the AIDS Clinical Trials Group. Foscarnet-ganciclovir cytomegalovirus retinitis trial 4: Visual outcomes. Ophthalmology 1994;101:1250–1261.
71. Bachman DM, Bruni LM, DiGioia RA, et al. Visual field testing in the management of cytomegalovirus retinitis. Ophthalmology 1992;99:1393–1399.
72. Holland GN, Buhles WC, Mastre B, Kaplan HJ, Group UCRS. A controlled retrospective study of ganciclovir treatment for cytomegalovirus retinitis Arch Ophthalmol 1989;107:1759–1766.
73. Holland GN, Shuler JD. Progression rates of cytomegalovirus retinopathy in ganciclovir-treated and untreated patients. Arch Ophthalmol 1992;110: 1435–1442.
74. Keefe KS, Freeman WR, Peterson TJ, et al. Atypical healing of cytomegalovirus. Ophthalmology 1991;99:1377–1384.
75. Kuppermann BD, Flores-Aguilar M, Quiceno JI, Rickman LS, Freeman WR. Combination ganciclovir and foscarnet in the treatment of clinically resistant cytomegalovirus retinitis in patients with acquired immunodeficiency syndrome. Arch Ophthalmol 1993;111:1359–1366.
76. Weinberg DV, Murphy R, Naughton K. Combined daily therapy with intravenous ganciclovir and foscarnet for patients with recurrent cytomegalovirus. Am J Ophthalmol 1994;117: 776–782.
77. Dieterich DT, Poles MA, Lew EA, et al. Concurrent use of ganciclovir and foscarnet to treat cytomegalovirus infection in AIDS patients. J Infect Dis 1992;167:1184–1188.
78. Crumpacker C, Group SCOGS. Oral vs. intravenous ganciclovir as maintenance treatment of newly diagnosed cytomegalovirus retinitis in AIDS (abstract 538). First National Conference on Human Retroviruses and Related Infections, Washington, DC, 1993, p 154.
79. Spector S, Busch D, Follansbee S, et al. Pharmacokinetic, safety and antiviral profile of oral ganciclovir in HIV-infected persons (abstract 539). First National Conference on Human Retroviruses and Related Infections, Washington, DC, 1993, p 154.

80. Lieberman RM, Orellana J, Melton RC. Efficacy of intravitreal foscarnet in a patient with AIDS. N Engl J Med 1994;330:868–869.
81. Ussery FM, Gibson SR, Conklin RH, Piot DF, Stool EW, Conklin AJ. Intravitreal ganciclovir in the treatment of AIDS-associated cytomegalovirus retinitis. Ophthalmology 1988;95:640–648.
82. Cantrill HL, Henry K, Melroe H, Knobloch WH, Ramsay RC, Balfour HH. Treatment of cytomegalovirus retinitis with intravitreal ganciclovir. Ophthalmology 1988;96:367–374.
83. Cribbin K, Orellana J, Lieberman R. Intravitreal ganciclovir in patients resistant to ganciclovir and/or foscarnet (abstract no. PoB 3159). International Conference on AIDS. Amsterdam, July 19–24, 1992.
84. Diaz-Llopis M, Chipont E, Sanchez S, España E, Navea A, Menezo JL. Intravitreal foscarnet for cytomegalovirus retinitis in a patient with acquired immunodeficiency syndrome. Am J Ophthalmol 1992;114:742–747.
85. Heinemann M. Long-term intravitreal ganciclovir therapy for cytomegalovirus retinopathy. Arch Ophthalmol 1989;107:1767–1772.
86. Heinemann M. *Staphylococcus epidermidis* endophthalmitis complicating intravitreal antiviral therapy of cytomegalovirus retinitis. Arch Ophthalmol 1989;107:643–644.
87. Henry K, Cantrill H, Fletcher C, Chunnock BJ, Balfour HH. Use of intravitreal ganciclovir (dihydroxy propoxymethyl guanine) for cytomegalovirus retinitis in a patient with AIDS. Am J Ophthalmol 1987;103:17–23.
88. Smith TJ, Pearson A, Blandford DL, et al. Intravitreal sustained-release ganciclovir. Arch Ophthalmol 1992; 110:255–258.
89. Sanbourn GE, Anand R, Torti RE, et al. Sustained-release ganciclovir therapy for treatment of cytomegalovirus retinitis. Arch Ophthalmol 1992; 110:188–195.
90. Azad RF, Driver VB, Tanaka K, Crooke RM, Anderson KP. Antiviral activity of a phosphorothioate oligonucleotide complementary to RNA of the human cytomegalovirus major immediate-early region. Antimicrob Agents Chemother 1993;37:1945–1954.
91. Polis MA, Baird B, Jaffe HS, Fisher PE, Walker RE, Masur H. A phase I/II dose escalation trial of (s)-1-[3-hydroxy-2-(phosphonylmethoxy)propyl]-cytosine (HPMPC) in HIV infected persons with CMV viruria (abstract WS-B11-5). IXth International Conference on AIDS, Berlin, 1993, p 54.
92. Jabs DA, Engler C, Haller J, de Bustros S. Retinal detachments in patients with cytomegalovirus retinitis. Arch Ophthalmol 1991;109:794–799.
93. Freeman WR, Friedberg DN, Berry C, et al. Risk factors for development of rhegmatogenous retinal detachment in patients with cytomegalovirus. Am J Ophthalmol 1993;116:713–720.
94. Freeman WR, Henderly DE, Wan WL, et al. Prevalence, pathophysiology, and treatment of rhegmatogenous retinal detachment in treated cytomegalovirus retinitis. Am J Ophthalmol 1987;103: 527–536.
95. Orellana J, Teich SA, Lieberman RM, Restrepo S, Peairs R. Treatment of retinal detachments in patients with the acquired immunodeficiency syndrome. Ophthalmology 1991;98:939–943.

HIV INFECTION IN AFRICA

Elly T. Katabira
Robert Colebunders

8

EPIDEMIOLOGY

Infection with the human immunodeficiency virus (HIV) is becoming a major public health problem in nearly all sub-Saharan African countries. In 1994 the World Health Organization (WHO) estimated that 10 million Africans were infected with HIV.[1]

HIV-1 INFECTION

In large cities, HIV-1 seroprevalence rates among the general population range between 4 and 15% and among prostitutes between 20 and 80%. Initially, the HIV epidemic was recognized in central and eastern Africa, but now it is spreading rapidly to western and southern Africa as well. In West Africa, the situation is probably most serious in the Ivory Coast, particularly in Abidjan where 8% of pregnant women are infected with HIV-1. Infection with HIV-1 is now spreading from cities to rural areas.[2]

Acquired immunodeficiency syndrome (AIDS) has become the leading cause of hospital admissions in many large cities in sub-Saharan Africa. A study in Abidjan, a city in which the first AIDS cases were recognized as late as 1985, noted that AIDS had become the leading cause of death in men and the second leading cause of death in women, after deaths related to pregnancy and abortion.[3] Because of HIV infection, mortality in children remains the same or is increasing, which is in contrast with the 40% reduction predicted in 1970.

In Africa, HIV is essentially a heterosexually transmitted viral infection. Eighty percent of all infections are acquired by heterosexual intercourse. Several studies have suggested that genital ulcerations and nonulcerative sexually transmitted diseases such as gonorrhea, chlamydial infection, and trichomoniasis may enhance the risk of sexual transmission of HIV-1 by increasing both the infectiousness of an HIV-infected individual and the susceptibility to HIV of a noninfected sexual partner.[4]

The second most common route of HIV-1 transmission in Africa is mother to child transmission. Transmission rates observed in African studies vary from 30 to 40%.[5] These rates are higher than those observed in American and European studies. This discrepancy is only partially explainable by the differences in methodology between African and American or European investigators. Recent studies have estimated that breast-feeding may be responsible for increasing the transmission rate from mother to child by 14%.[6]

Blood transfusion is the third most important mode of transmission of HIV-1 in Africa. Despite the fact that HIV testing is becoming more widely available, a large proportion of the transfusions administered in Africa still are not screened for HIV.

The contribution of injections with contaminated needles and syringes to the spread of HIV in Africa is still unclear, although epidemiologic studies and age-specific HIV prevalence rates suggest that this is not a major route of transmission.

HIV-2 INFECTION

Infection with HIV-2 is prevalent in West Africa and mainly in Guinea Bissau. It is spreading much less rapidly than HIV-1 infection. In several countries of West Africa, HIV-1 infection is already more prevalent than HIV-2 infection. The explanation of this phenomenon is that HIV-2 is less pathogenic and is transmitted less easily (sexually and from mother to child) than HIV-1 infection.[7]

DIAGNOSING THE INFECTION IN AFRICA

In the past few years, the ability to diagnose HIV infection and to determine the related degree of immune deficiency has improved considerably, especially in the de-

TABLE 8–1. CLINICAL CASE DEFINITION OF AIDS

The following AIDS surveillance case definition could be used in countries in which serologic testing for HIV infection is not widely available. For epidemiologic surveillance, an adult (>12 years) is considered to have AIDS if at least two major signs are associated with at least one minor sign that are not known to be due to a condition unrelated to HIV infection.

Major Signs*

- Weight loss >10% body weight, or cachexia
- Chronic diarrhea >1 month
- Prolonged fever >1 month (intermittent or constant)

Minor Signs

- Persistent cough for >1 month†
- Generalized pruritic dermatitis
- History of herpes zoster
- Oropharyngeal candidiasis
- Chronic progressive and disseminated herpes simplex infection
- Generalized lymphadenopathy

* The presence of generalized Kaposi's sarcoma or cryptococcal meningitis is sufficient by itself for the diagnosis of AIDS.

† For patients with tuberculosis, persistent cough >1 month should not be considered a minor sign.

World Health Organization. Guidelines for HIV/AIDS Surveillance and AIDS Case Definitions in Adults. WHO/ERF/RES/SPA 1992.

veloped world. Unfortunately, these improvements have not been possible in Africa because of a lack of facilities to perform tests such as the enzyme-linked immunosorbent assay and CD4 lymphocyte counts on a regular basis. To overcome this handicap, the WHO arrived at a clinical AIDS case definition that was devised through a workshop in Bangui in 1985.[8] This definition, which was meant for epidemiologic purposes to help African countries count AIDS cases, has now been evaluated in many countries.[9,10] Based on these evaluations, a modified clinical AIDS case definition has been proposed by the WHO (Table 8–1).

For the diagnosis and management of patients with HIV infection and AIDS, this clinical WHO case definition of AIDS remains inadequate. Common conditions such as tuberculosis may be misdiagnosed as AIDS. For patient management purposes, the WHO has developed clinical guidelines to help health care workers at all levels recognize and offer appropriate treatment and counseling to those infected with HIV.[11] To add a prognostic indicator to the clinical diagnosis, in the absence of the CD4 lymphocyte counting facilities, the WHO has proposed a clinical staging system (Table 8–2).[12] This system uses simple parameters that can be applied easily by the ordinary health care worker. Evaluation of the system is under way.

TABLE 8–2. PROVISIONAL CLINICAL SYSTEM FOR HIV INFECTION AND DISEASE

Clinical Stage I

1. Asymptomatic
2. Persistent generalized lymphadenopathy
3. History of acute retroviral infection

And/or performance scale 1: asymptomatic, normal activity

Clinical Stage II

4. Weight loss <10% of body weight
5. Minor mucocutaneous manifestations (seborrheic dermatitis, prurigo, fungal nail infections, oropharyngeal ulcerations, angular cheilitis)
6. Herpes zoster within the last 5 years
7. Recurrent upper respiratory tract infections (e.g., bacterial sinusitis)

And/or performance scale 2: symptomatic, normal activity

Clinical Stage III

8. Weight loss >10% of body weight
9. Chronic diarrhea >1 month
10. Prolonged fever (intermittent or constant) >1 month
11. Oral candidiasis (erythematous or pseudomembranous)
12. Oral hairy leukoplakia
13. Pulmonary tuberculosis, within the past year
14. Severe bacterial infections (e.g., pneumonia, pyomyositis)

And/or performance scale 3: bedridden <50% of the day during the last month

Clinical Stage IV

15. HIV wasting syndrome,* as defined by the Centers for Disease Control and Prevention (CDC)
16. *Pneumocystis carinii* pneumonia
17. Toxoplasmosis of the brain
18. Cryptosporidiosis with diarrhea >1 month
19. Isosporiasis with diarrhea >1 month
20. Cryptococcosis, extrapulmonary
21. Cytomegalovirus disease of an organ other than the liver, spleen, or lymph nodes
22. Herpes simplex virus infection, mucocutaneous >1 month, or visceral any duration
23. Progressive multifocal leukoencephalopathy
24. Any disseminated endemic mycosis (e.g., histoplasmosis, coccidioidomycosis)
25. Candidiasis of the esophagus, trachea, bronchi, or lungs
26. Atypical mycobacteriosis, disseminated
27. Nontyphoid *Salmonella* septicemia
28. Extrapulmonary tuberculosis
29. Lymphoma
30. Kaposi's sarcoma
31. HIV encephalopathy,† as defined by the CDC

And/or performance scale 4: bedridden >50% of the day during the last month

(*Note:* Both definitive and presumptive diagnoses are acceptable.)

* HIV wasting syndrome: weight loss of >10% of body weight, plus either unexplained chronic diarrhea (>1 month), or chronic weakness and unexplained prolonged fever (>1 month).

† HIV encephalopathy: clinical findings of disabling cognitive and/or motor dysfunction interfering with activities of daily living, progressing over weeks to months, in the absence of a concurrent illness or condition other than HIV infection that could explain the findings.

Adapted from World Health Organization. Acquired immunodeficiency syndrome (AIDS). Interim proposal for a WHO staging system for HIV infection and disease. Wkly Epidemiol Rec 1990;65:221–228.

NATURAL HISTORY OF AIDS IN AFRICA

Several studies on the natural history of HIV infection in adults suggest that there is a higher progression rate to AIDS and a shorter survival time of persons with AIDS in Africa compared with those recorded in the West.[13–15] However, these reports have many shortcomings. In most studies, the time of infection was unknown, and definitions of AIDS that were used were different from definitions used in the West.

The mean incubation period for perinatally acquired AIDS is close to 5 years. The infant mortality rate of children born to HIV-seropositive mothers is very high in Africa: 15 to 40% die during the first year of life.[16]

As clinicians gain experience in caring for persons infected with HIV in Africa, they have become aware that this infection can run a prolonged course of up to 10 or

Text continued on page 210

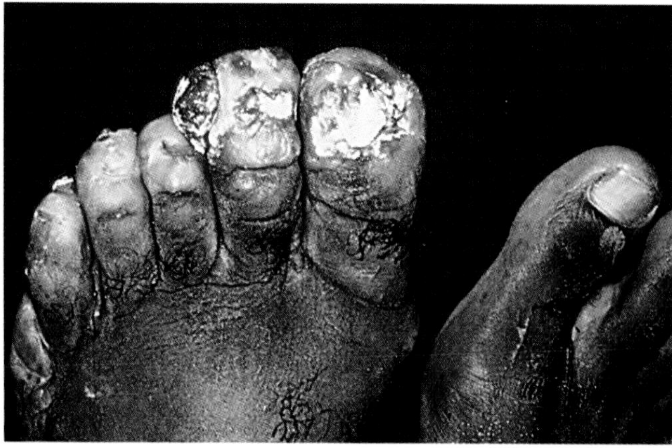

FIGURE 8–1. Kaposi's sarcoma
A 22-year-old Zairian HIV-seronegative male with Kaposi's sarcoma lesions localized at his left foot. He had no other symptoms.

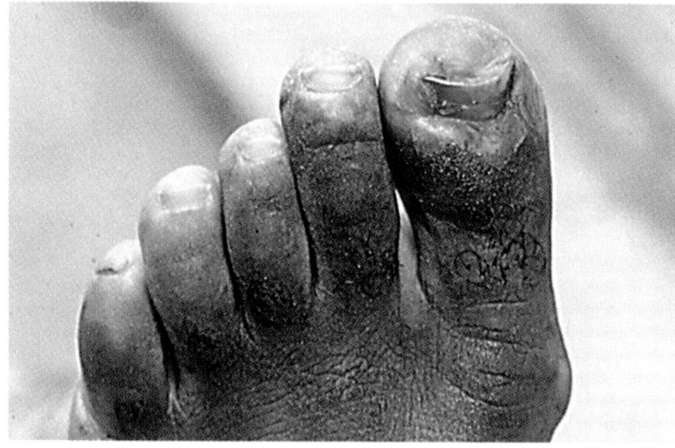

FIGURE 8–2. Kaposi's sarcoma
The same patient shown in Figure 8–1 after treatment with vincristine sulfate (Oncovin). A complete remission was obtained.

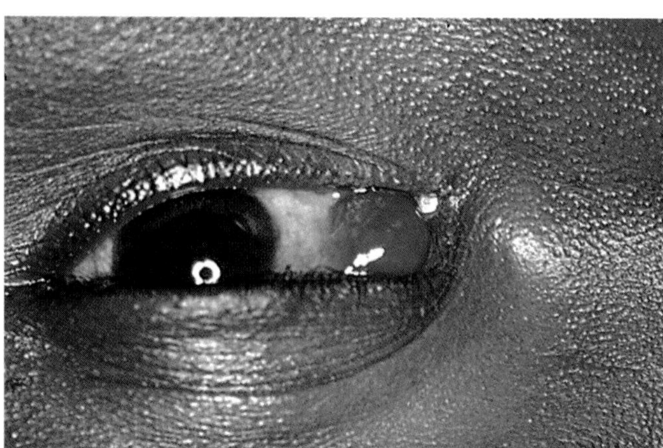

FIGURE 8–3. Kaposi's sarcoma
A 25-year-old Zairian woman with HIV infection and a Kaposi's sarcoma lesion localized at the conjunctiva.

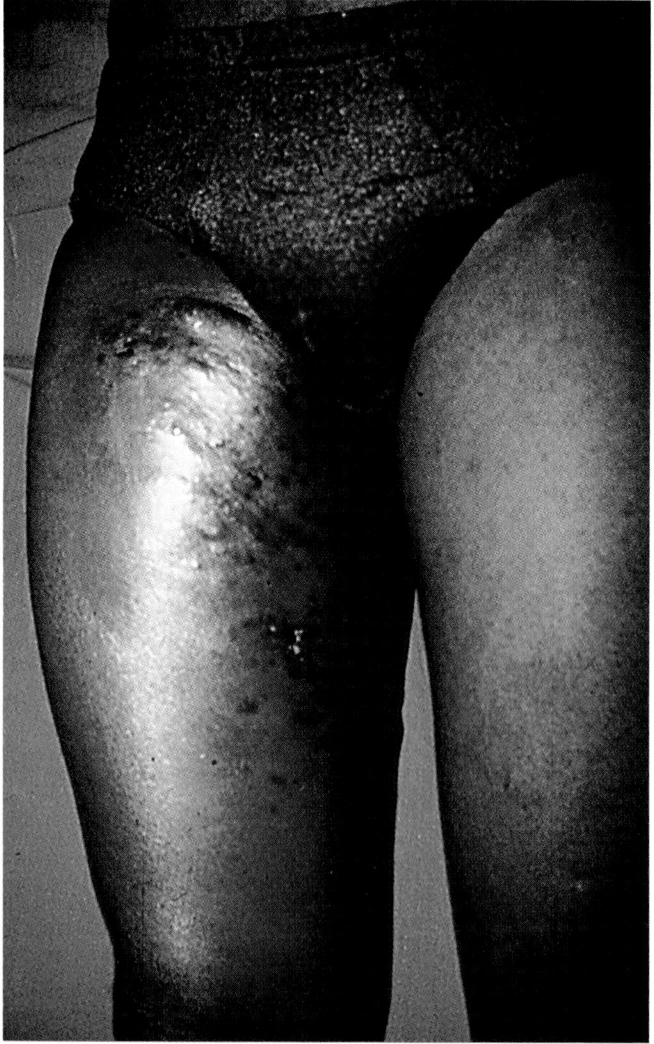

FIGURE 8–4. Kaposi's sarcoma
A 26-year-old Zairian man with HIV infection and Kaposi's sarcoma lesions localized at his right thigh. The lesions are associated with severe edema.

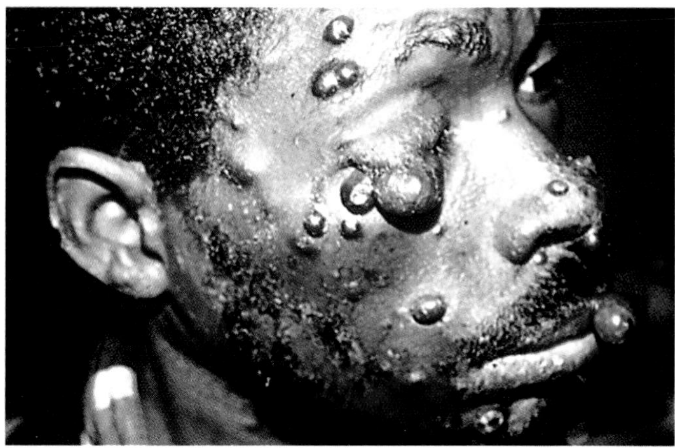

FIGURE 8–5. Kaposi's sarcoma
Nodular and tumoral Kaposi's sarcoma lesions in a Zairian male with HIV infection.

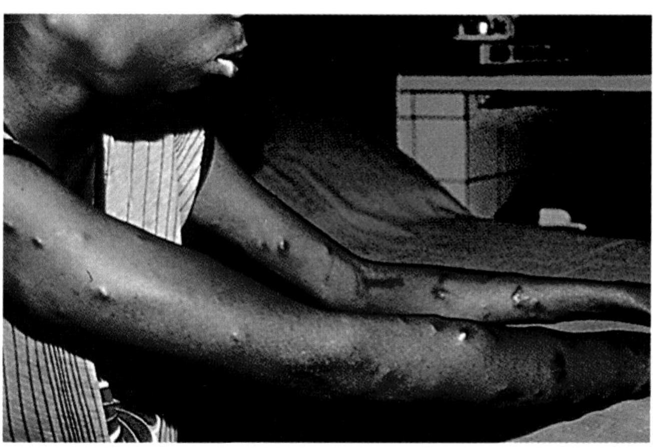

FIGURE 8–6. Kaposi's sarcoma
An HIV-infected Zairian woman with many Kaposi's sarcoma lesions on all parts of her body along with large polyadenopathies. A rapid increase of the Kaposi's sarcoma lesions had occurred during pregnancy.

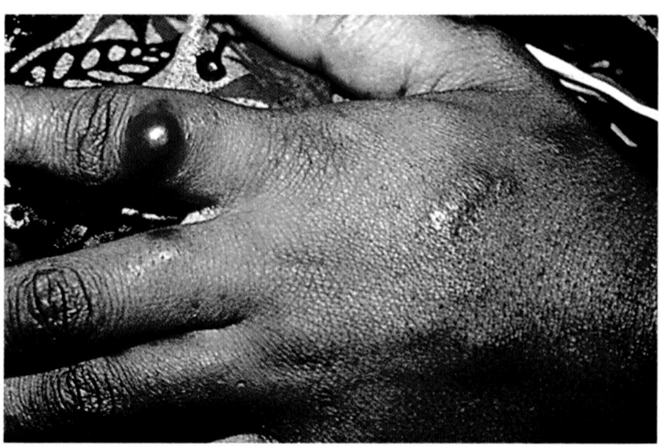

FIGURE 8–7. Kaposi's sarcoma
Same woman as shown in Figure 8–6. A nodular Kaposi's sarcoma lesion on her finger and a Kaposi's sarcoma plaque on the back of her hand are visible.

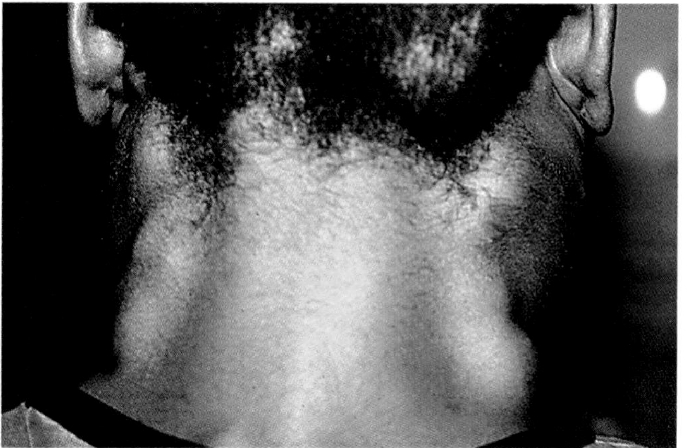

FIGURE 8–8. Kaposi's sarcoma
Same woman as shown in Figure 8–6. Important cervical adenopathies are evident.

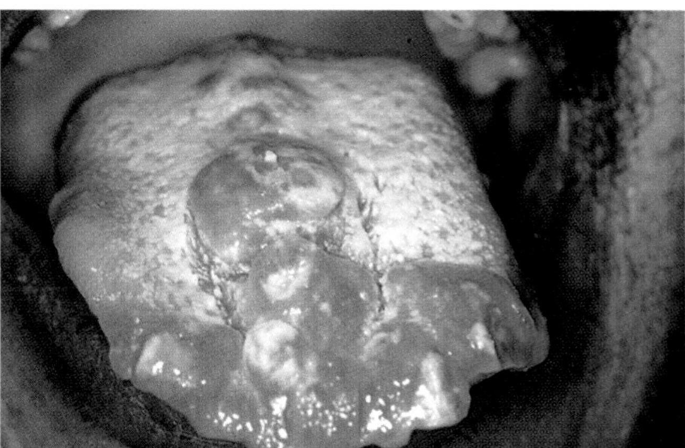

FIGURE 8–9. Kaposi's sarcoma
Zairian man with HIV infection and generalized Kaposi's sarcoma: Kaposi's sarcoma of the tongue and oral candidiasis can be seen.

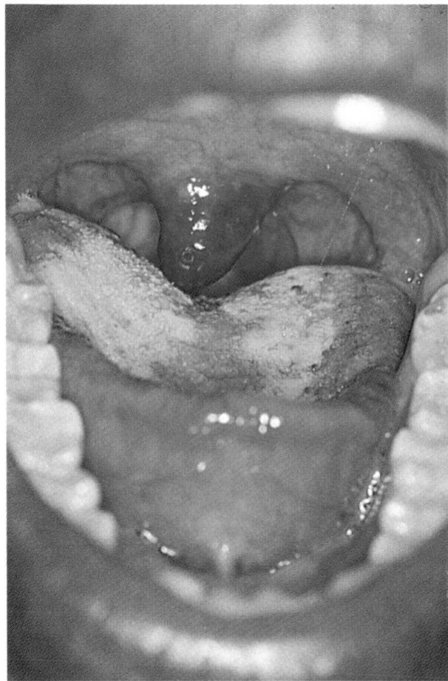

FIGURE 8–10. Kaposi's sarcoma
Kaposi's sarcoma affecting the uvula. Note the hyperpigmentation of the tongue.

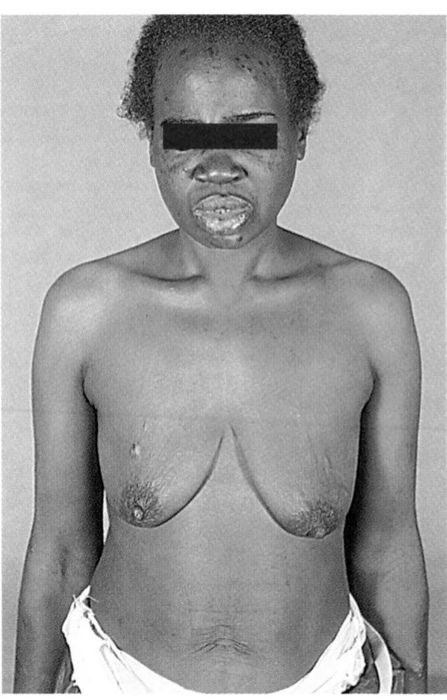

FIGURE 8–11. Kaposi's sarcoma
Disseminated Kaposi's sarcoma.

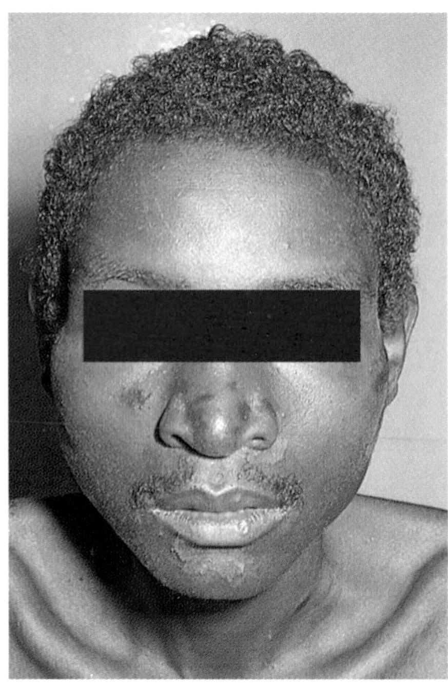

FIGURE 8–13. Kaposi's sarcoma
Silky hair changes and Kaposi's sarcoma lesions on the nose.

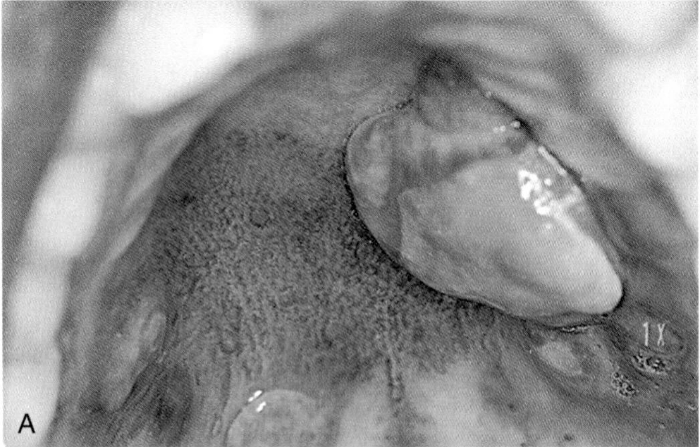

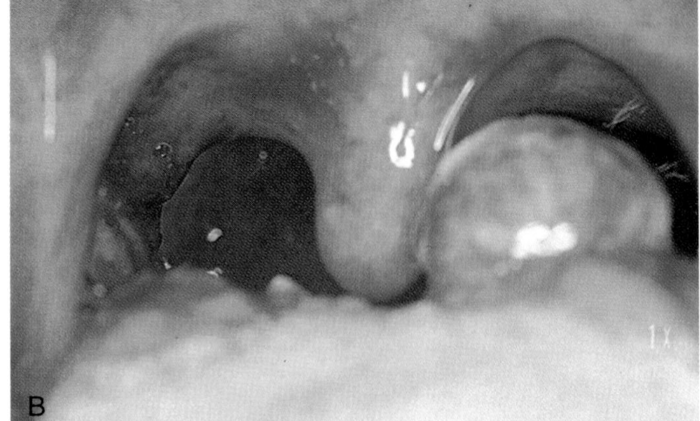

FIGURE 8–12. Kaposi's sarcoma
Oral Kaposi's sarcoma nodules. The hyperpigmented palate is not caused by the Kaposi's sarcoma lesions.

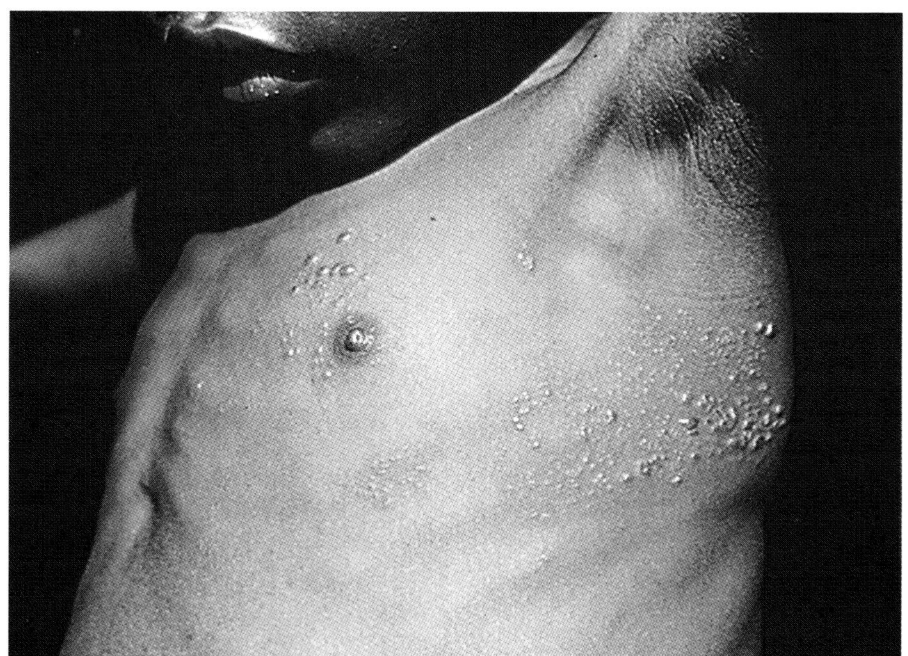

FIGURE 8–14. Herpes zoster
Thoracic herpes zoster infection in a Zairian child with HIV infection.

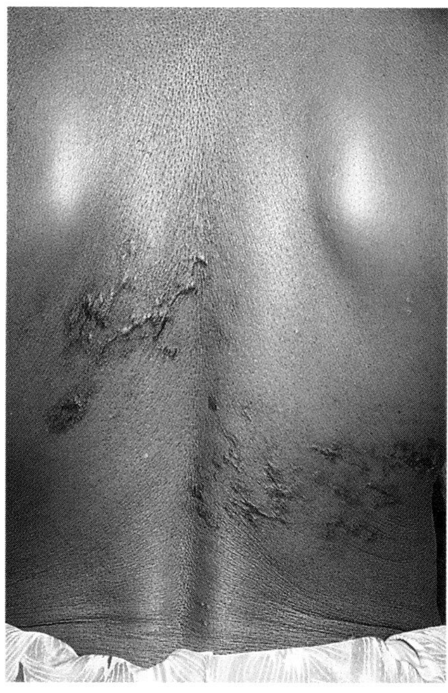

FIGURE 8–15. Herpes zoster
Recurrent herpes zoster with minimal keloid formation in a 50-year-old woman. Her first attack was in October 1989 and her second in April 1992.

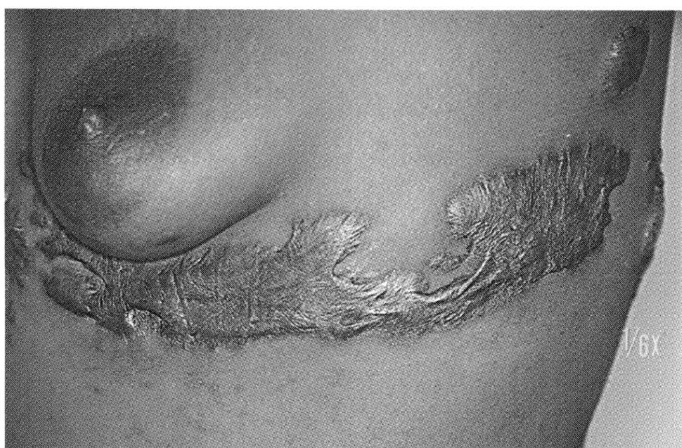

FIGURE 8–16. Herpes zoster
Herpes zoster scar with keloid formation. This is a common finding, reflecting the high tendency to keloid formation among African people.

more years. Access to good medical care is associated with prolonged survival. Unfortunately, most patients do not have access to any reasonable health care services. This means that even simple, easily treatable nonopportunistic infections such as pneumonia and salmonella sepsis may cause premature death in someone who still has a good immune status.[17] Other factors that may influence disease progression are the following:

1. The underlying immune status of the patient at the time of infection. Patients in the higher socioeconomic group who are healthy at the time of infection may have a better prognosis.

2. Coinfection with other sexually transmitted disease.[18]

As in the developed countries, some people in Africa can remain infected for a long time without developing symptoms. At the same time, some progress very fast to end-stage disease without any apparent reason.

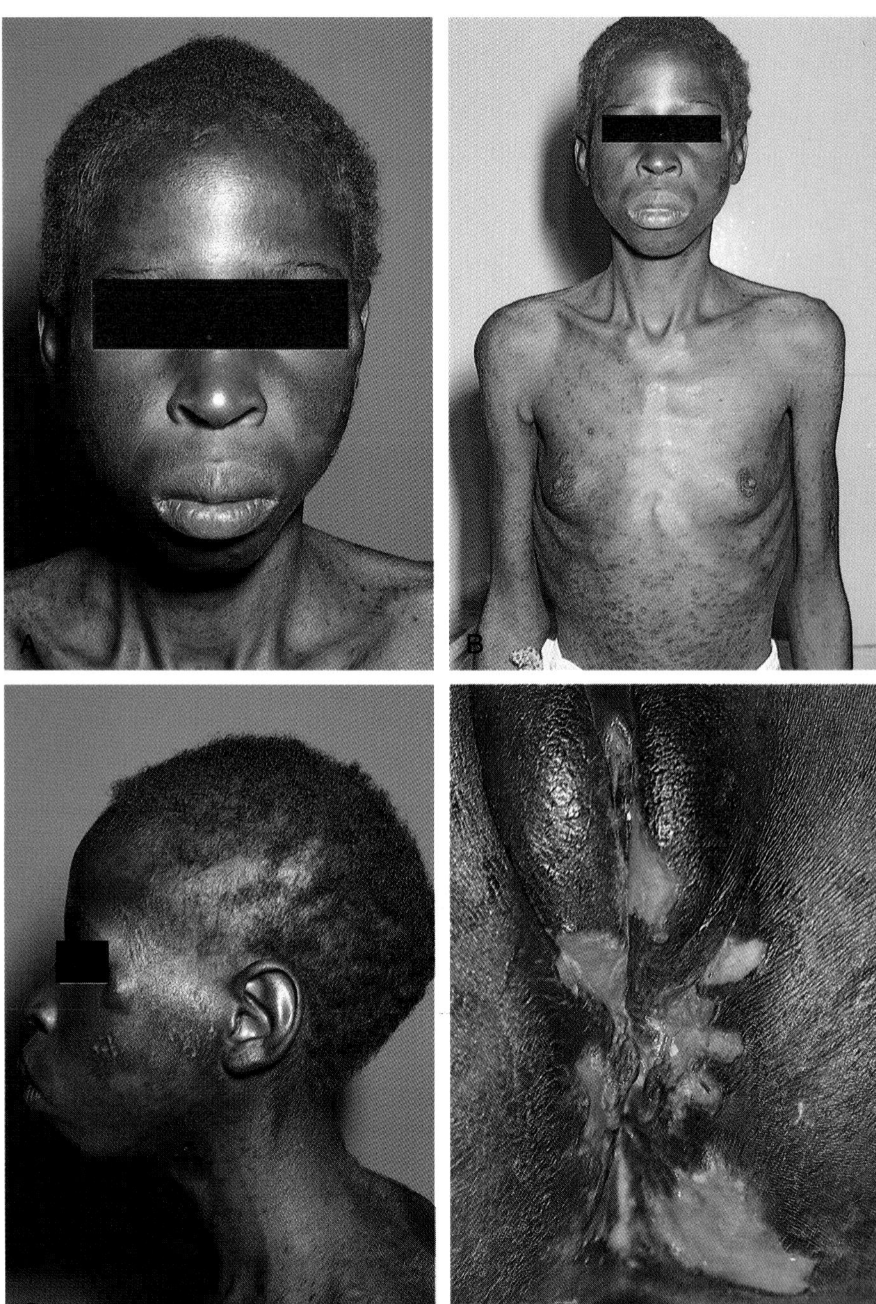

FIGURE 8–17. Cutaneous manifestations

A, Facial hyperpigmentation and silky hair changes, which often start at the frontal hairline. The changes can be disguised by hair treatment. *B,* Same patient, showing a severe weight loss and a chronic maculopruritic rash, especially over the abdomen. This rash is often very itchy and can be complicated by secondary infection, leading to recurrent and chronic skin sepsis. *C,* Close-up view, showing the hyperpigmentation and patchy hair loss. *D,* Extensive perineal ulceration caused by herpes simplex type 2 infection in the same patient. The ulcers are usually very painful. Initially, they may be recurrent, but as the patient's immune status worsens, they become persistent and can progress to affect the entire perineum.

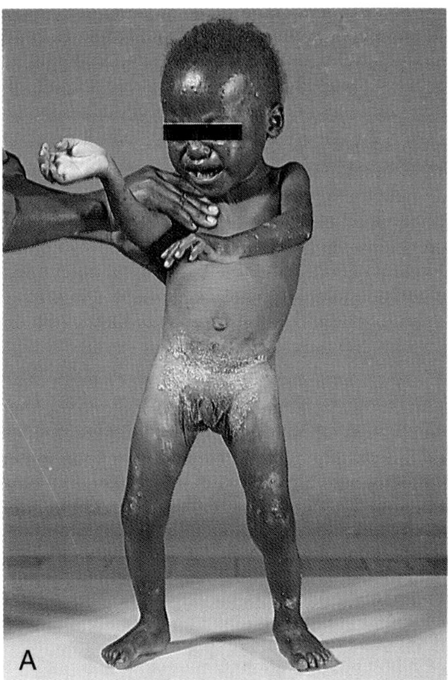

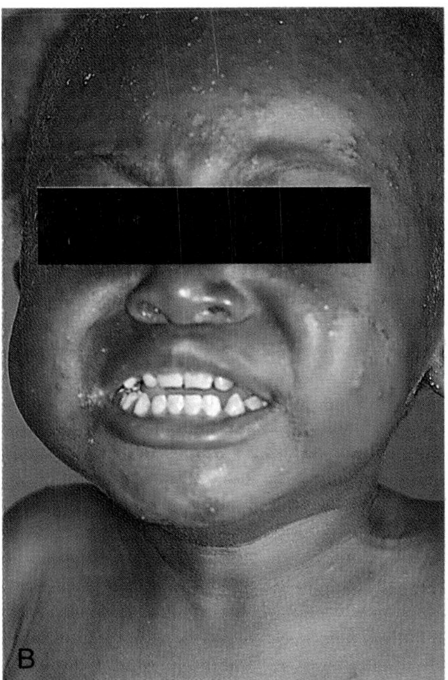

FIGURE 8–18. Skin rash
Growth retardation, weight loss, and facial rash in a child.

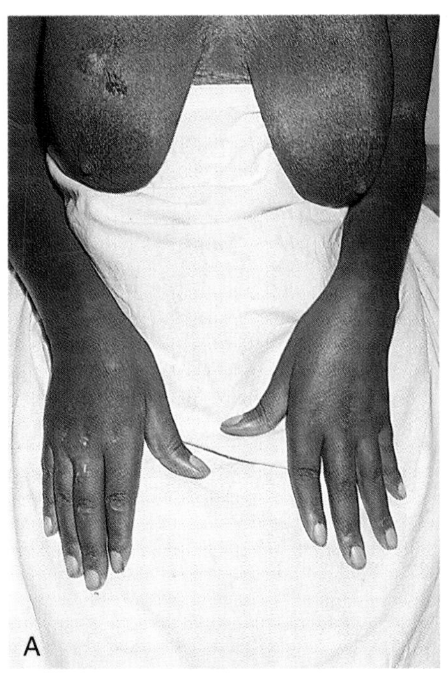

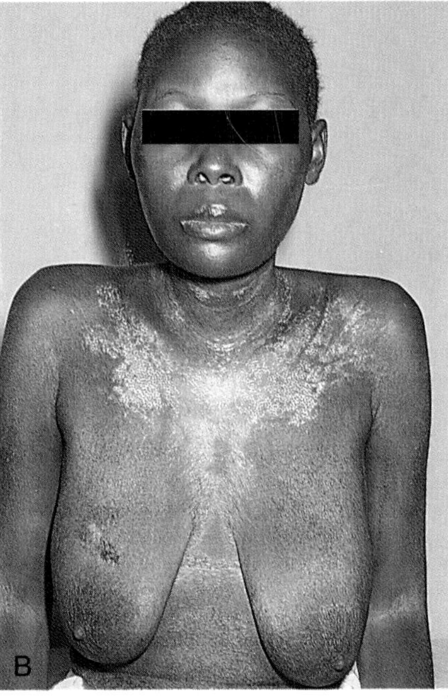

FIGURE 8–19. Scleroderma
Scleroderma in an HIV-infected woman. The features of scleroderma and alopecia developed in 1990 when the patient was probably already infected with HIV.

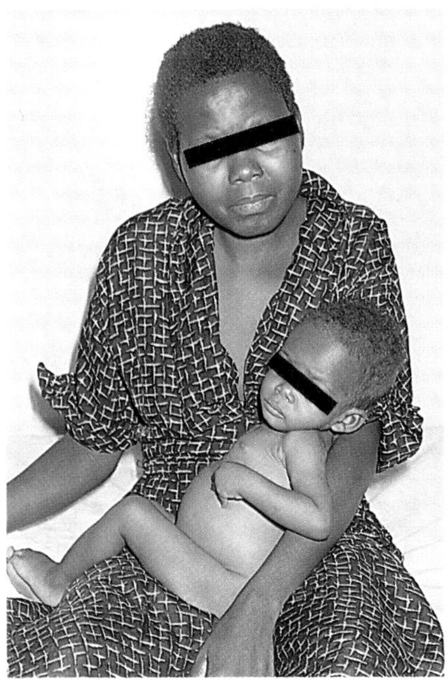

FIGURE 8–20. Symptomatic mother and child
Mother with her 10-month-old daughter, who has been sick since she was born. The mother herself has minimal signs and symptoms of HIV infection.

CLINICAL SPECTRUM OF HIV INFECTION

Clinical manifestations of HIV infection may vary from place to place in Africa depending on the common prevailing diseases in that region. Acute HIV infection, the so-called seroconversion syndrome, may be very difficult to recognize in many parts of Africa because of the many different types of febrile illnesses that can mimic acute HIV infection. In addition, many patients present to the health care worker so long after such an episode that they cannot remember it. To make things worse, quite often the results of the HIV test performed during the acute HIV infection may be negative, confusing the uninitiated health worker.

Neurologic manifestations may occur during an acute HIV infection.[19] These include confusional states and acute brain syndromes. Patients therefore may end up in psychiatric institutions, where they do recover only to present months or years later with a clinical picture of HIV infection. Some are managed as cerebral malaria patients because a positive finding on a blood slide for malarial parasites has been found. Yet in malaria-endemic areas, parasites are readily found in people without symptoms. Transverse myelitis, various types of encephalitis, and Guillain-Barré syndrome are also encountered in acute HIV infection.

After the acute HIV infection, many patients may remain asymptomatic for a long time. The average duration ranges from 1 to 8 years. However, during this period their immune status may be deteriorating. The onset of symptoms may be very insidious such that many patients may not easily recall when they first became ill. Recurrent fevers are very common, and these may be due to the HIV itself or to other intercurrent infections such as malaria, salmonella, and other bacterial or viral infections. In the early stages of HIV infection, many patients do recover from these attacks and may have long spells of well-being. In some, these attacks may trigger off a steady decline with gradual weight loss and development of other complications.

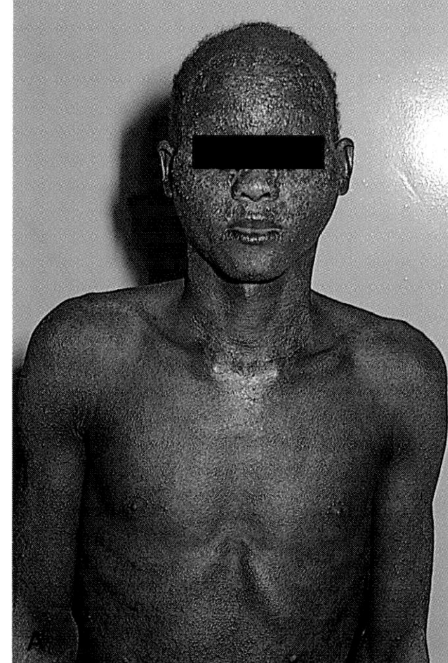

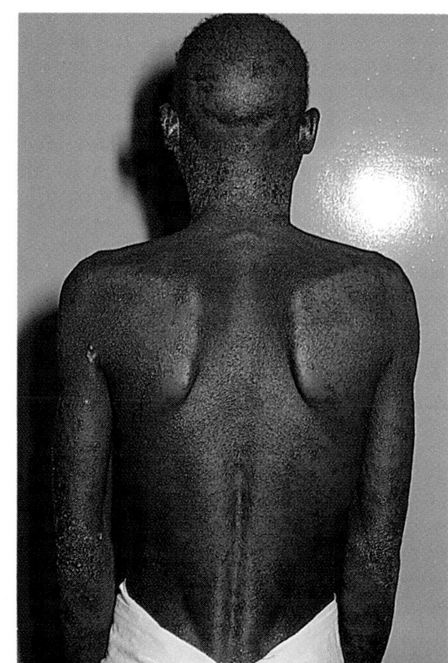

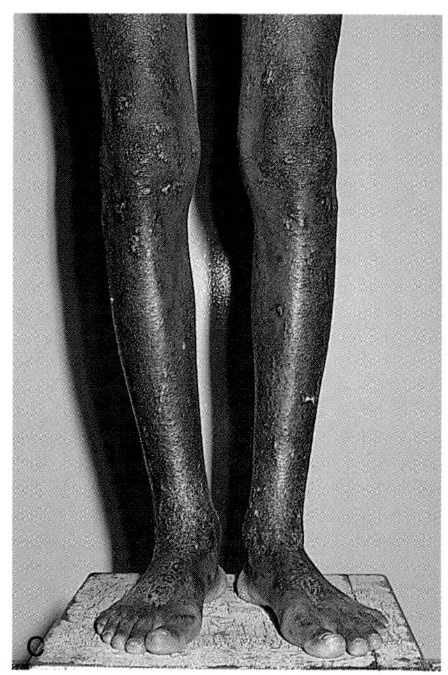

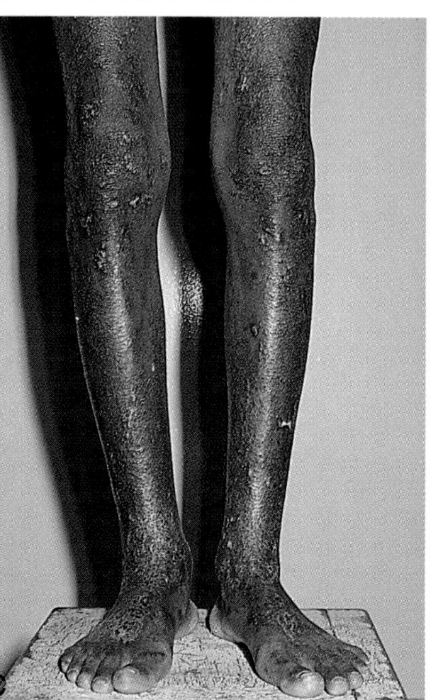

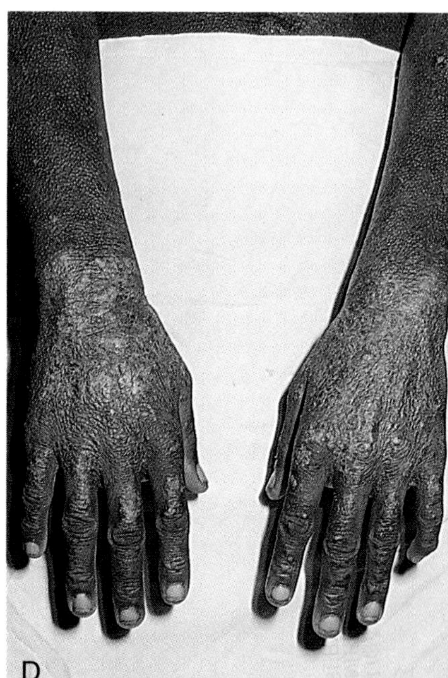

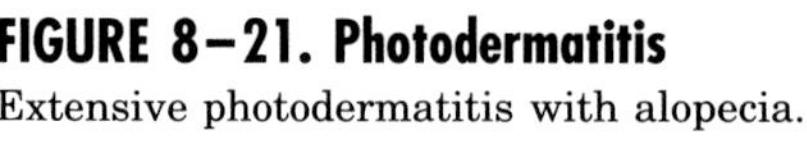

FIGURE 8–21. Photodermatitis
Extensive photodermatitis with alopecia.

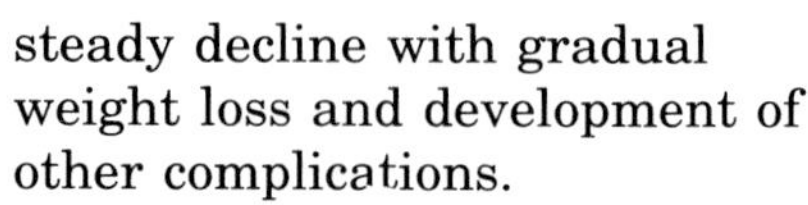

Chronic diarrhea, a recurrent or persistent papulopruritic eruption,[20] oral and esophageal candidiasis, and acute and chronic pulmonary infections including tuberculosis are among the com-

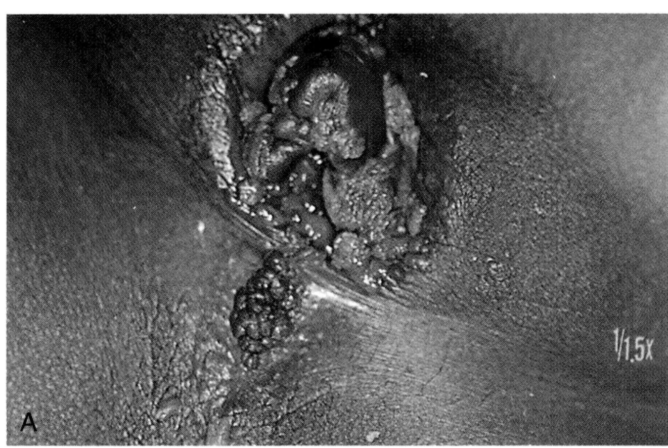

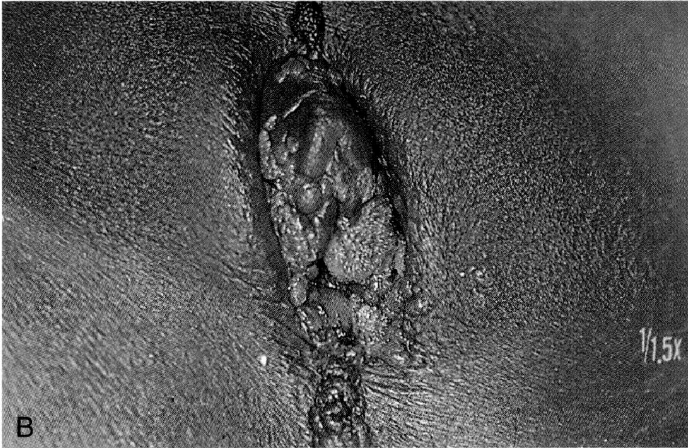

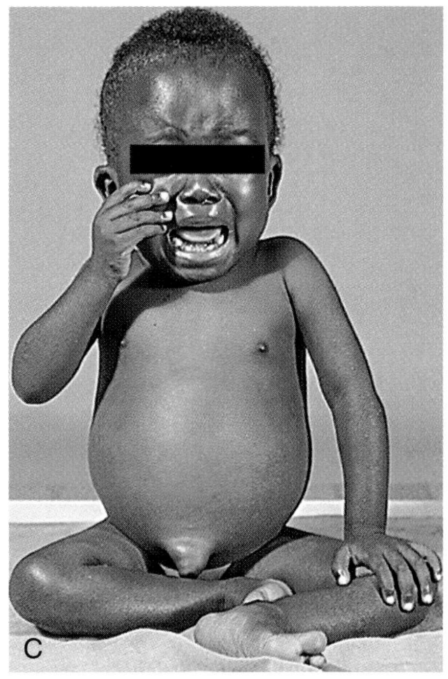

FIGURE 8–22. Vulvar warts

Vulvar warts in a seropositive symptomatic child.

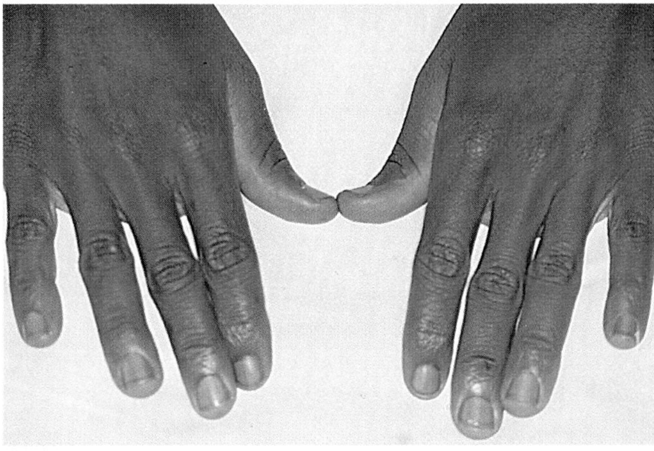

FIGURE 8–23. Nail changes

Nail changes often seen in persons infected with HIV. The presence of these changes usually signifies advanced immunosuppression, with $CD4^+$ cell counts of less than 200/mm^3. These changes are not due to fungal infection of the nail beds.

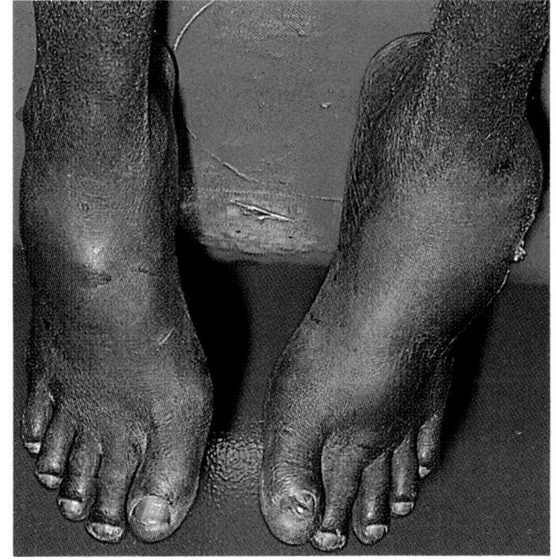

FIGURE 8–24. Abscess formation

Multiple abscess formation that affects both feet.

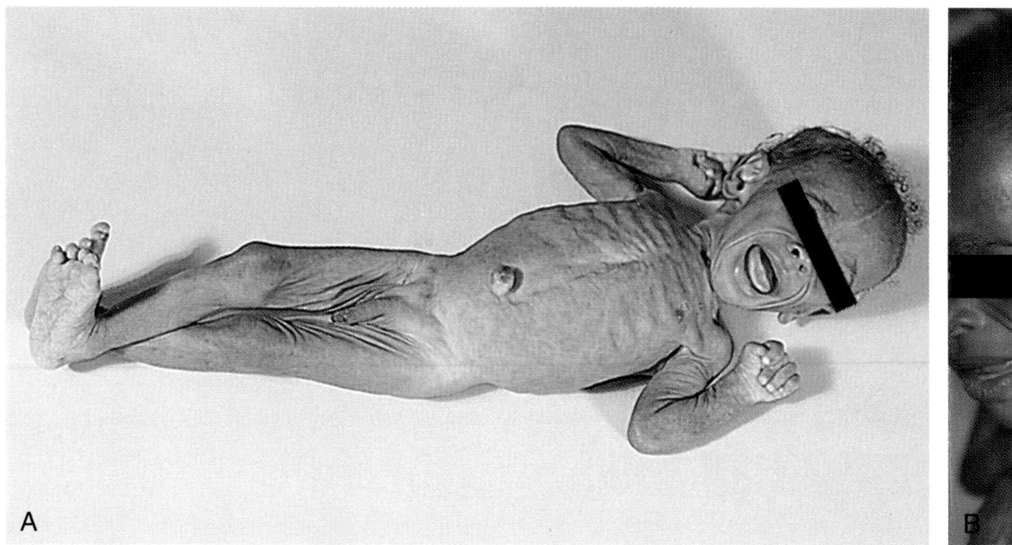

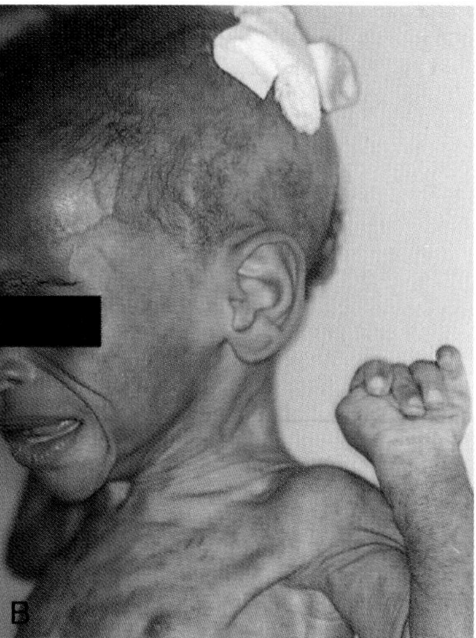

FIGURE 8–25. Growth retardation and maculopapular rash
A, Severe weight loss and growth retardation in a 7-month-old boy. *B,* This same child also has a maculopapular rash.

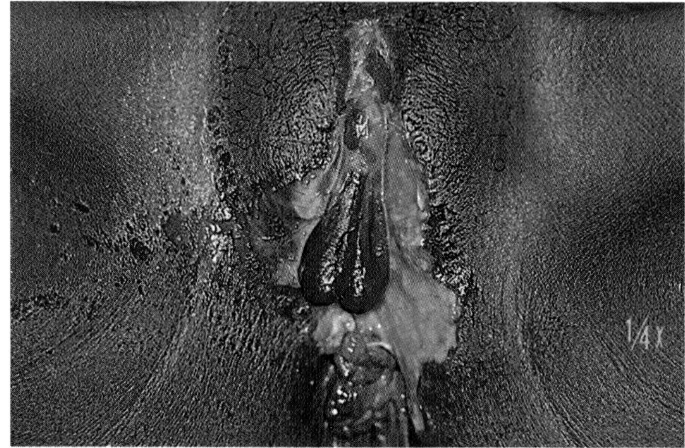

FIGURE 8–26. Herpes simplex type 2
Extensive genital sores due to herpes simplex type 2 infection.

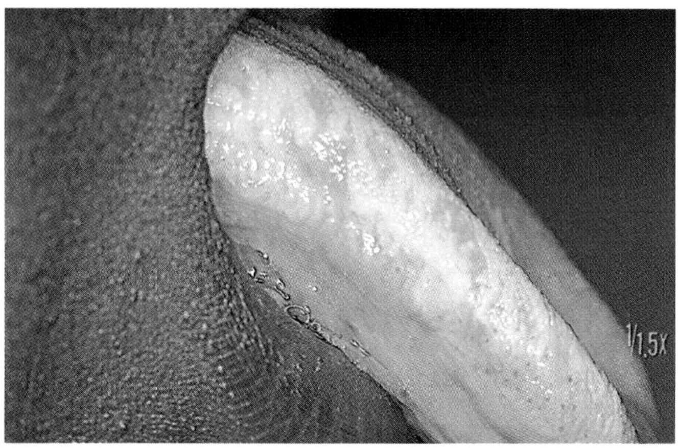

FIGURE 8–27. Oral hairy leukoplakia
Oral hairy leukoplakia in a female patient. These lesions are less common in African patients than in white patients in the West.

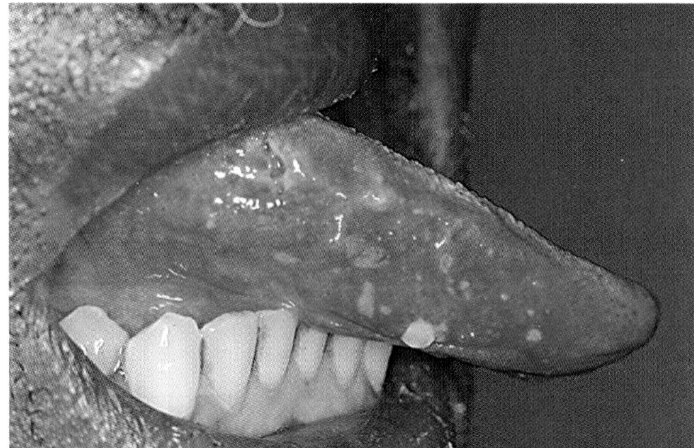

FIGURE 8–28. Aphthous ulcerations
Aphthous ulcerations that affect the tongue.

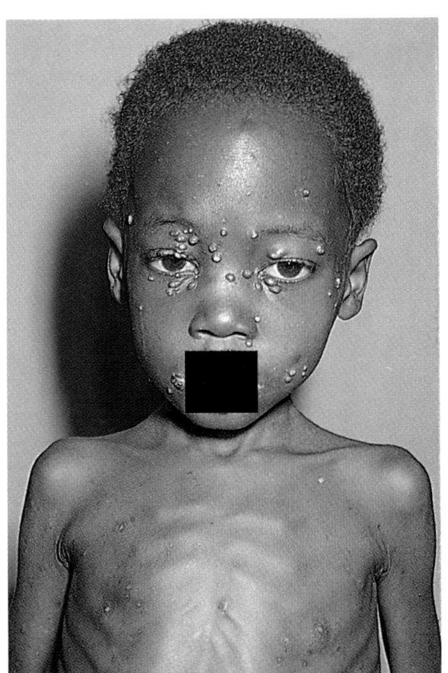

FIGURE 8–29. Molluscum contagiosum
Molluscum contagiosum in a 4½-year-old girl with Kaposi's sarcoma lesions on the forehead and the left cheek.

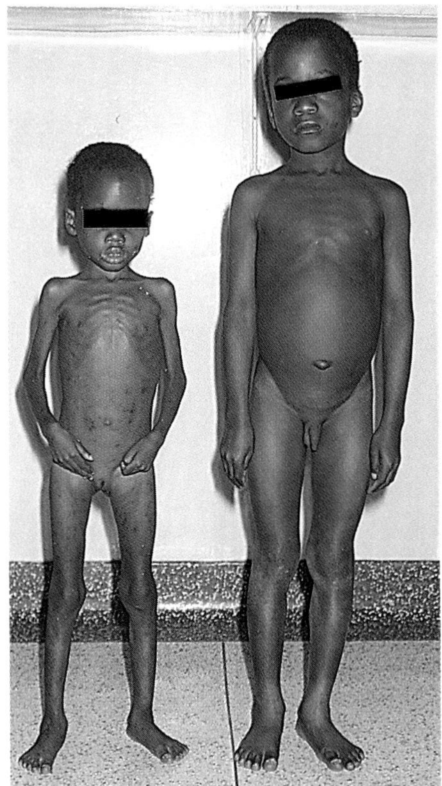

FIGURE 8–30. Discordant twins
An HIV-infected 4½-year-old girl with her uninfected twin brother. The girl has been sickly since shortly after birth. Both children were breast-fed by their mother, who is now mildly symptomatic.

mon clinical manifestations encountered in HIV-infected people in Africa. The diarrhea may be nonspecific initially, lasting for only a day or two, with long spells in between before the next attack. The patient (and sometimes the health care worker) may at first relate these early episodes to something eaten or drunk or to a change of diet. However, as time goes on, the duration of the bouts gets longer and the periods between the attacks get shorter. The diarrhea can be very profuse, often watery, in some cases blood stained or containing mucoid or frank pus. The associated emaciation was responsible for the term *slim disease* first described in Uganda in 1985.[21]

Recurrent attacks of upper respiratory infections are common, especially in the early stages of the HIV infection. With the progression of the immunosuppression, these attacks may become complicated in that patients go on to develop lower respiratory tract infections such as pneumonias due to bacterial, fungal, or viral organisms. Tuberculous infections of the lung or pleura are very common and are now one of the major health concerns in the Third World countries in which both HIV and tuberculosis are prevalent.[22,23] For unknown reasons, *Pneumocystis carinii* pneumonia, so common in the West, is infrequently reported in Africa.[24]

In severely immunosuppressed patients, infections such as cryptococcal meningitis are encountered.[25] Kaposi's sarcoma is the commonest cancer seen in HIV-infected persons in Africa.[26] This form of Kaposi's sarcoma is much more aggressive than the endemic type, which was well known in certain regions of Africa long before the HIV epidemic. Lymphomas do not seem to occur as commonly in Africa as in the United States.

THERAPY AND PREVENTION

So far, no drug has been developed that eliminates HIV from the human body. However, some antiviral agents, such as zidovudine, didanosine, and zalcitabine, have been shown to be beneficial for certain patients. Unfortunately, these drugs are too expensive for routine use by the average African HIV-infected patient. However, it has been demonstrated that by effectively managing the various intercurrent opportunistic and nonopportunistic infections commonly found in these patients and by counseling them, one can improve significantly their quality of life and their survival.[27]

The main mode of transmission of HIV in Africa is through heterosexual spread. Multiple sexual partners and high incidence of sexually transmitted diseases are cited as reasons why HIV is so prevalent in some parts of Africa. Preventing the further spread of the disease calls for a change in people's sexual behavior and practices. This is not easy and requires massive well-coordinated and well-organized health education campaigns. Vaccine development is still in its infancy, and it will take a long time before an effective vaccine is available and affordable for persons in Africa.

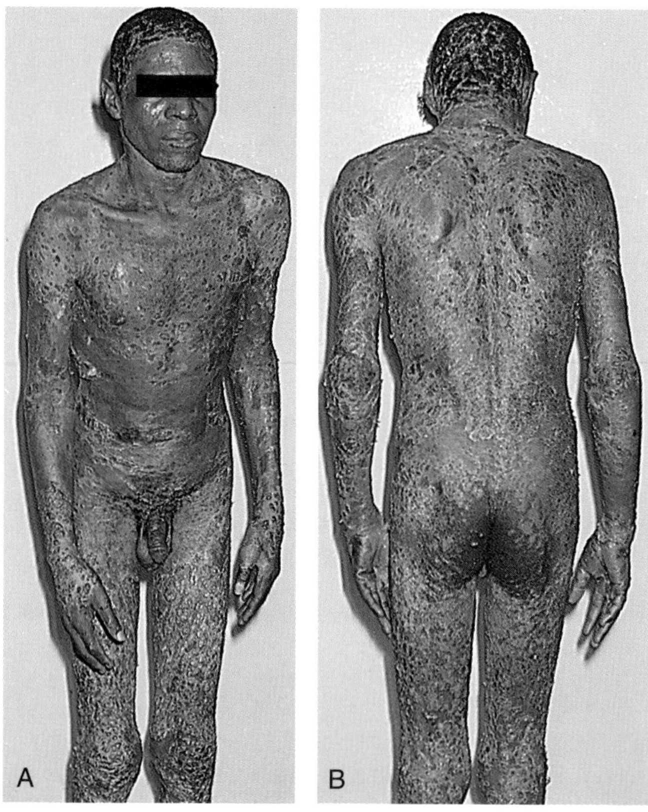

FIGURE 8–31. Seborrheic dermatitis
Extensive seborrheic dermatitis.

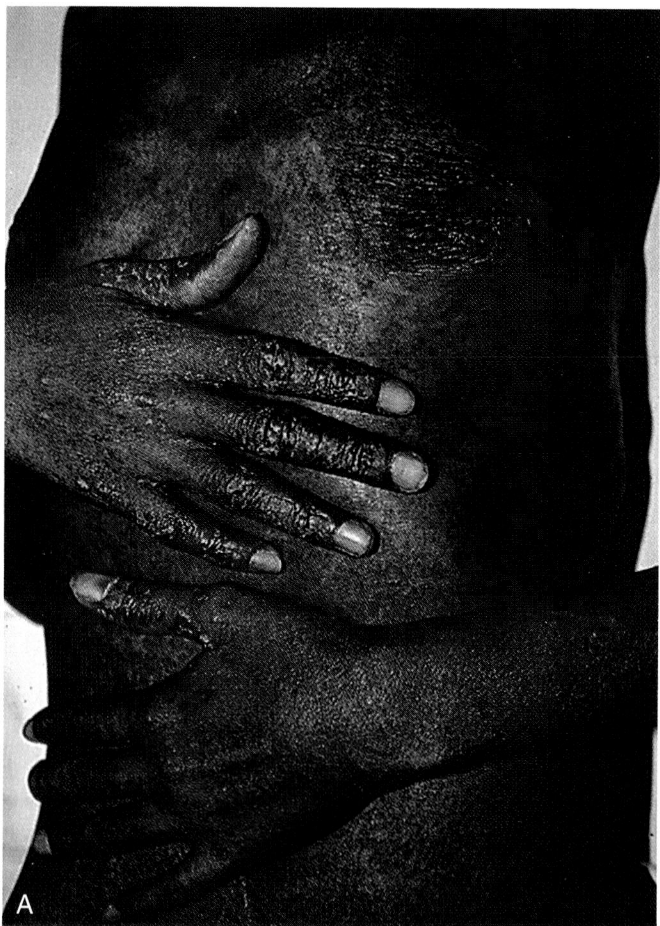

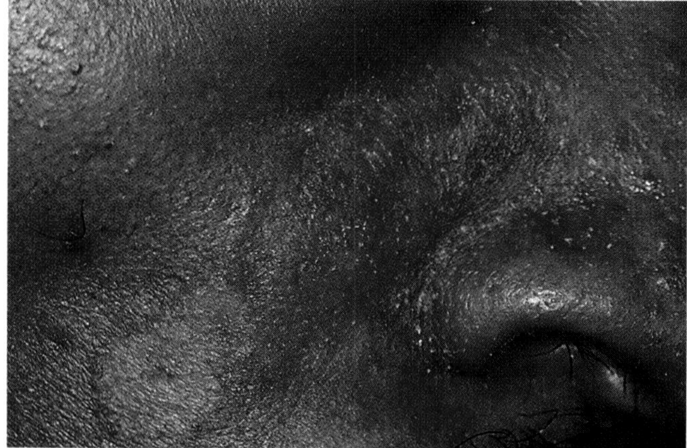

FIGURE 8–32. Seborrheic dermatitis
Seborrheic dermatitis in a Zairian man with HIV infection but without other complaints.

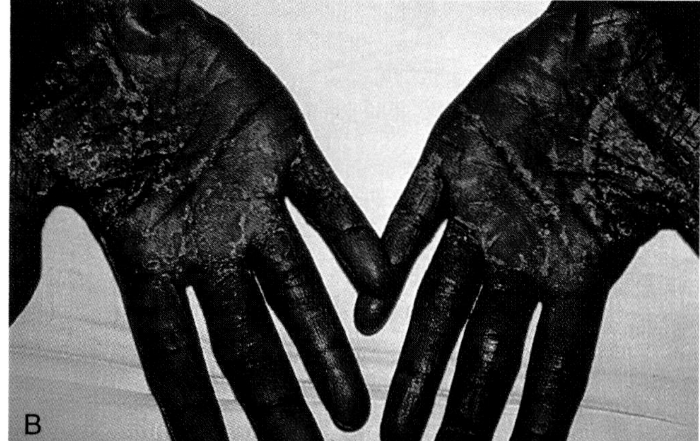

FIGURE 8–33. *Microsporum langeroni* infection
A 25-year-old HIV-infected Zairian woman with a generalized cutaneous fungal infection caused by *M. langeroni*. *A,* Lesions on the back of the hands and on the abdomen. *B,* Lesions on the palms of the hands. *M. langeroni* is a fungal infection observed only in central Africa.

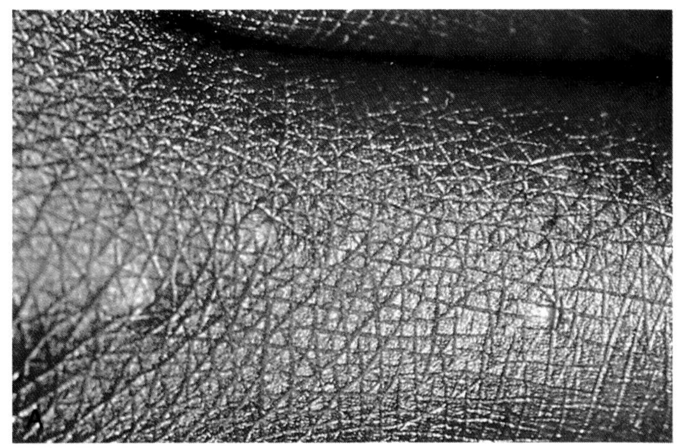

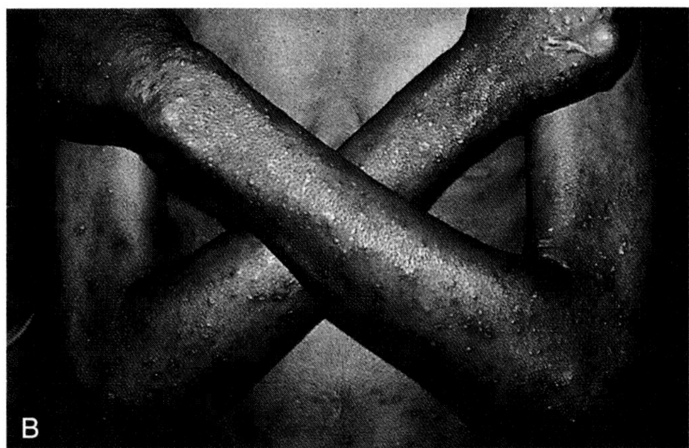

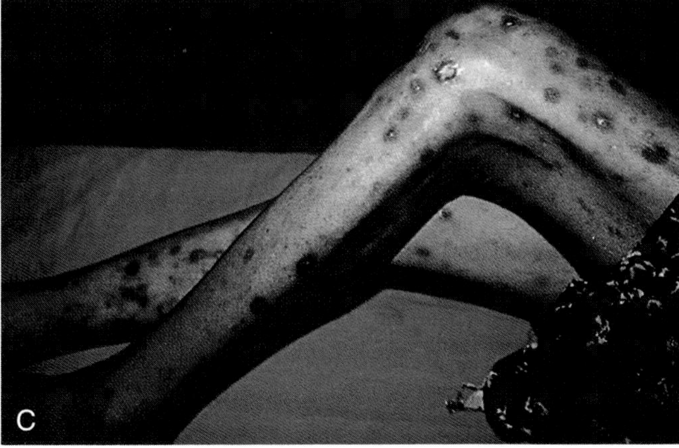

FIGURE 8–34. Papulopruritic eruption

A generalized papulopruritic eruption of unknown origin is observed in 10 to 20% of African patients with HIV infection. *A,* Initial lesions: small papules of 1 to 3 mm. *B,* A papulopruritic eruption in a 23-year-old Zairian male, mainly localized on the external surface of the arms. *C,* A cachectic 45-year-old HIV-infected woman in end-stage disease, with scars of a papulopruritic eruption on her legs (in end-stage disease, the pruritus often disappears spontaneously, and only scars remain).

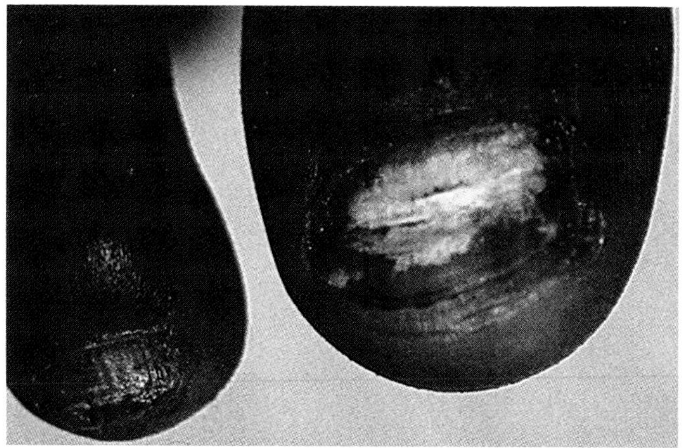

FIGURE 8–35. Onychomycosis
Onychomycosis affecting the toes.

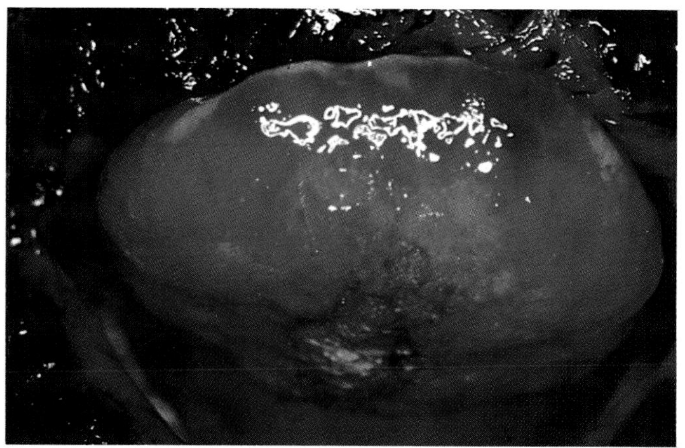

FIGURE 8–36. Stevens-Johnson syndrome
Stevens-Johnson syndrome that developed because of thiacetazone treatment for *Mycobacterium tuberculosis* infection in an HIV-seropositive person. Such reactions occur particularly frequently in persons with HIV infection.

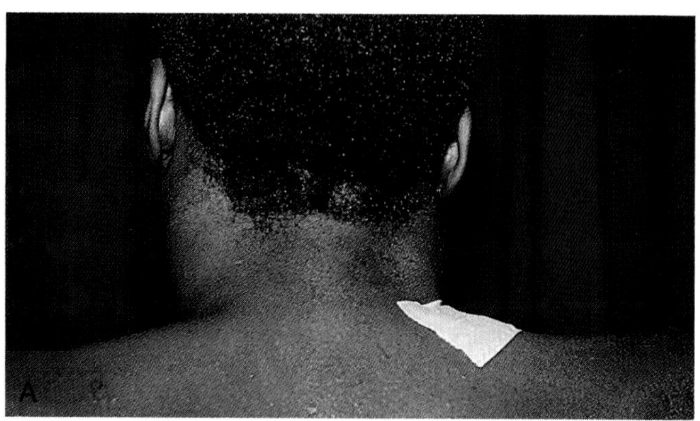

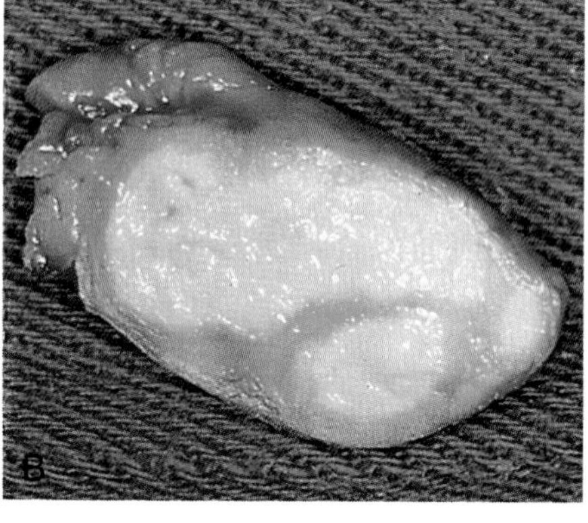

FIGURE 8–37. Tuberculous adenitis
A, A 26-year-old HIV-infected Zairian man with a large cervical polyadenopathy. *B,* A lymph node biopsy specimen from the patient shown in *A.* The lymph node is full of caseum because of *Mycobacterium tuberculosis* infection.

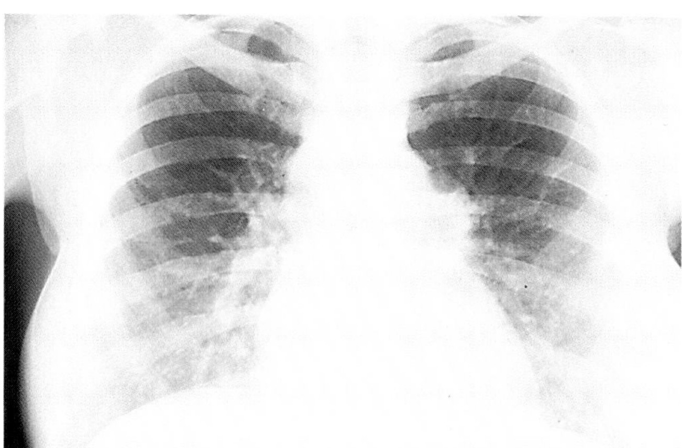

FIGURE 8–38. *Mycobacterium tuberculosis* infection
A chest radiograph of a 23-year-old Zairian woman with low-grade fever and fatigue. The hilar and mediastinal enlargement of lymph nodes is caused by *M. tuberculosis* infection. Such enlargement of lymph nodes is particularly frequent among HIV-seropositive persons with *M. tuberculosis* infection.

References

1. World Health Organization. The pandemic of HIV/AIDS: Current situation and future trends. WHO/GPA/RES/SFI/92.1:1–17.
2. Nkowane BM. Prevalence and incidence of HIV infection in Africa: A review of data published in 1990. AIDS 1991;5(suppl 1):S7–S15.
3. De Cock KM, Barreze B, Diaby L, Lafontaine MF, Gnaore E, Porter A, Pantobe D, Lafontant GC, Dago-Akribi A, Ette M, Odehouri K, Heyward WL. AIDS—The leading cause of death in the West African city of Abidjan, Ivory Coast. Science 1990;249:793–796.
4. Laga M, Nzila N, Goeman J. The interrelationship of sexually transmitted diseases and HIV infection: Implications for the control of both epidemics in Africa. AIDS 1991;5(suppl 1):S21–S28.
5. Ryder RW, Temmerman M. The effect of HIV-1 infection during pregnancy and the perinatal period on maternal and child health in Africa. AIDS 1991; 5(suppl 1):S75–S85.
6. Dunn DT, Newel ML, Ades AE, Peckham CS. Risk of human immunodeficiency virus type 1 transmission through breastfeeding. Lancet 1992;340:585–588.
7. De Cock KM, Brun-Vezinet F, Soro B. HIV-1 and HIV-2 infections and AIDS in West-Africa. AIDS 1991;5(suppl 1):S21–S28.
8. World Health Organization. Provisional WHO clinical case definition for AIDS. Wkly Epidemiol Rec 1986; 61:72–73.
9. Colebunders R, Mann JM, Francis H, Bila K, Lebughe I, Kakonde N, Kabasele K, Ifoto L, Nzilambi N, Quinn TC, van der Groen G, Curran JW, Vercauteren G, Piot P. Evaluation of the clinical case definition of acquired immunodeficiency syndrome in Africa. Lancet 1987;1:492–494.
10. Widy-Wirski R, Berkley S, Downing R, Okware S, Recine U, Mugerwa R, Lwegaba A, Sempala S. Evaluation of the WHO/CDC clinical case definition for AIDS in Uganda. JAMA 1988;260:3286–3289.
11. Wabitsch KR, Tarantola D, Mann J. Clinical management guidelines of HIV infection and AIDS, an algorithm approach (abstract 180). IV International Conference on AIDS and Associated Cancers in Africa. Marseille, France, October 1989.
12. World Health Organization. Acquired immunodeficiency syndrome (AIDS). Interim proposal for a WHO staging system for HIV infection and disease. Wkly Epidemiol Rec 1990;65:221–228.
13. Colebunders RL, Latif AS. Natural history and clinical presentation of HIV-1 infection in adults. AIDS 1991; 5(suppl 1):S103–S112.
14. Colebunders R, Ryder RW, Francis H, Nekwei W, Bahwe Y, Lebughe I, Ndilu M, Vercauteren G, Nseka K, Perriëns J, Van der Stuyft P, Quinn TC, Piot P. Seroconversion rate, mortality and clinical manifestations associated with the receipt of an human immunodeficiency virus infected blood transfusion. J Infect Dis 1991;164:450–456.
15. Mbaga JM, Pallangyo KJ, Bakari M, Aris EA. Survival time of patients with acquired immunodeficiency syndrome: Experience with 274 patients in Dar es Salaam. East Afr Med J 1990;67:95–99.
16. Lepage P, Hitimana DG. Natural history and clinical presentation of HIV-1 infection in children. AIDS 1991; 5(suppl 1):S117–S125.
17. Gilks CF, Brindle RJ, Otieno LS, et al. Life-threatening bacteraemia in HIV-1 seropositive adults admitted to hospital in Nairobi, Kenya. Lancet 1990;336:545–549.
18. Berkley SF, Widy-Wirski R, Okware SL, et al. Risk factors associated with HIV infection in Uganda. J Infect Dis 1990;160:22–30.
19. Howlett WP, Nkya WM, Nmuni KA, Missalek WR. Neurological disorders in AIDS and HIV disease in the northern zone of Tanzania. AIDS 1989;3:289–296.
20. Pallangyo KJ. Cutaneous findings associated with HIV disease including AIDS: Experience from sub-Saharan Africa. Trop Doct 1992;22:35–41.
21. Serwadda D, Mugerwa RD, Sewaknambo NK, et al. Slim disease: A new disease in Uganda and its association with HTLV-III infection. Lancet 1985;2:849.
22. Perriens JH, Mukadik Y, Nunn P. Tuberculosis and HIV infection: Implications for Africa. AIDS 1991;5(suppl 1):S127–S133.
23. Elliot AM, Luo M, Tembo G, et al. Impact of HIV on tuberculosis in Africa: A cross-sectional study. BMJ 1990;301:412–415.
24. Lucas S, Goodgame R, Kocjan G, Serwadda D. Absence of pneumocystosis in Uganda AIDS patients. AIDS 1989; 3:47–48.
25. Desmet P, Kayembe KD, De Vroey C. The value of cryptococcal serum antigen screening among HIV-positive/AIDS patients in Kinshasa, Zaire. AIDS 1989;3:77–78.
26. Desmon-Hellman SD, Katongole-Mbidde E. Kaposi's sarcoma: Recent developments. AIDS 1991;5(suppl 1):S135–S142.
27. Katabira ET, Wabitsch KR. Management issues for patients with HIV infection in Africa. AIDS 1991;5(suppl 1):S149–S155.

INDEX

Note: Page numbers in *italics* refer to illustrations; page numbers followed by (t) refer to tables.